PEDIATRIC PHYSICAL THERAPY

Second Edition

Jan Stephen Tecklin
M.S., P.T.

Associate Professor
Department of Physical Therapy
Beaver College
Glenside, Pennsylvania

With 14 Contributors

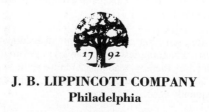

J. B. LIPPINCOTT COMPANY
Philadelphia

Acquisitions Editor: Andrew Allen
Coordinating Editor: Maureen Mohan
Production Editor: Virginia Barishek
Indexer: Maria Coughlin
Interior Designer: Susan Blaker
Cover Designer: William T. Donnelly
Production: P. M. Gordon Associates, Inc.
Compositor: Pine Tree Composition, Inc.
Printer/Binder: R. R. Donnelley & Sons Company/Crawfordsville

Second Edition

6 5 4 3 2 1

Library of Congress Cataloging-in-Publication Data

Pediatric physical therapy / [edited by] Jan Stephen Tecklin : with 14
    contributors. — 2nd ed.
        p.   cm.
    Includes bibliographical references and index.
    ISBN 0–397–54962–8
    1. Physical therapy for children.   I. Tecklin, Jan Stephen.
    [DNLM: 1. Physical Therapy—in infancy & childhood.   WB 460 P371
1994]
RJ53.P5P43   1994
615.8′2′083—dc20
DNLM/DLC
for Library of Congress   93–38932
                                                                  CIP

Any procedure or practice described in this book should be applied by the health-care practitioner
under appropriate supervision in accordance with professional standards of care used with regard to
the unique circumstances that apply in each practice situation. Care has been taken to confirm the
accuracy of information presented and to describe generally accepted practices. However, the authors, editors, and publisher cannot accept any responsibility for errors or omissions or for any consequences from application of the information in this book and make no warranty express or im-
plied, with respect to the contents of the book.

Every effort has been made to ensure drug selections and dosages are in accordance with current
recommendations and practice. Because of ongoing research, changes in government regulations
and the constant flow of information on drug therapy, reactions and interactions, the reader is cautioned to check the package insert for each drug for indications, dosages, warnings and precautions,
particularly if the drug is new or infrequently used.

In loving memory of my mother, Natalie Rosen Tecklin
August 20, 1925–February 28, 1992

Contributors

Dolores B. Bertoti, MS, PT
Assistant Professor and Academic Coordinator of
    Clinical Education
Alvernia College
Reading, Pennsylvania

Susan K. Brenneman, MS, PT
Education/Development Coordinator
Division of Physical Therapy
Department of Rehabilitation Medicine
University of Pennsylvania Medical Center
Philadelphia, Pennsylvania

Nancy Farmer Brockway, MA, OTR
Consultant to Prince William Parent-Infant Education
    Program and Fair Oaks Special Care Nursery
Burke, Virginia

Laurie Grigsby de Linde, OTR/L
Senior Staff Occupational Therapist
Burn Center and Plastic Surgery
St. Christopher's Hospital for Children
Philadelphia, Pennsylvania

Julaine M. Florence, MHS, PT
Research Assistant Professor
Department of Neurology
School of Medicine
Washington University
St. Louis, Missouri

Susan Kenville Lindeblad, MS, PT
Division of Physical Therapy
Department of Orthopedics and Rehabilitation
School of Medicine
University of Miami
Coral Gables, Florida

Christine R. Morgan, MPT
Staff Physical Therapist
St. Christopher's Hospital for Children
Philadelphia, Pennsylvania

Jodi Barkin Oren, MA, PT
Physical Therapist
University of Minnesota Medical Center
    formerly
Senior Physical Therapist
Children's Memorial Hospital
Chicago, Illinois

Shirley A. Scull, MS, PT
Director of Physical Therapy
Children's Seashore House
Philadelphia, Pennsylvania

Mary Soltesz Sheahan, MA, PT
Private Practice
Montgomery County, Maryland

Jane Styer-Acevedo, BS, PT
Self-employed
Neonatal/Early Intervention
Upper Darby, Pennsylvania

Elena Tappit-Emas, BS, PT
Physical Therapist
School District of Philadelphia
Philadelphia, Pennsylvania

Jan Stephen Tecklin, MS, PT
Associate Professor
Department of Physical Therapy
Beaver College
Glenside, Pennsylvania

Ann F. Van Sant, PhD, PT
Associate Professor and Chairperson
Department of Physical Therapy
College of Allied Health Professions
Temple University
Philadelphia, Pennsylvania

Preface

The acceptance within our profession of the first edition of *Pediatric Physical Therapy* is very gratifying, and I reiterate my thanks to the authors of that edition. Of course, the responsibility in preparing this second edition was great. I have tried to maintain the focus on the entry-level student and novice therapist, although there may be some portions that exceed that level. In an effort to broaden the scope of the text, chapters were added that discuss rehabilitation of the child with cancer and the child with a burn injury.

Chapter 1 is entirely rewritten, with numerous drawings. I am very grateful that Ann Van Sant was able to join the book and add a very thoughtful chapter on motor development. Chapter 2, by Susan Brenneman, is an update of her chapter in the first edition. Mary Sheahan and Nancy Brockway also updated their excellent chapter about high-risk infants. Jane Styer-Acevedo completely revised Chapter 4, about cerebral palsy. This was an enormous effort on her part, and she offers a very complete presentation. Chapter 5, Spina Bifida, was updated by Elena Emas with great emphasis on the role of and integration into overall care of the physical therapist. Chapter 6, written by Chris Morgan, is entirely new to this second edition and presents an overview of common childhood malignancies and their physical therapy management. Chapter 7, by Laurie de Linde, is also new and gives a very detailed description of acute care and rehabilitation for the child with a burn injury. Chapters 8 and 9 have both been updated, as have Chapters 10 and 11 by Shirley Scull and Dolores Bertoti, respectively. Julaine Florence, a new author in this edition, rewrote Chapter 12 on neuromuscular disorders. Jody Oren updated Chapter 13 on adaptive equipment, with an added section on wheelchairs. Finally, Susan Lindeblad rewrote Chapter 14 about physical therapy in the public schools. I offer my most sincere thanks and appreciation to each author.

I would like to acknowledge Dennis Kuronen, Associate Professor of Fine Arts at Beaver College, for the drawings in Chapter 1 and the drawing of the depth of burns in Chapter 7.

I would also like to thank the staff at J. B. Lippincott Company for their unflinching assistance. In particular, Andrew Allen, Miriam Benert, and Maureen Mohan have all been patient professionals.

Pediatric Physical Therapy, second edition, should provide a more complete and current version of the first edition so that entry-level students and novice practitioners will have the basic information necessary to gain a foothold in the practice of pediatric physical therapy.

Jan Stephen Tecklin, M.S., P.T.

Preface to the First Edition

Pediatric Physical Therapy is, first and foremost, a textbook directed towards the education of students in entry-level physical therapy curricula. The text is *not* intended to offer the knowledge nor present the skills needed for advanced or specialty practice in pediatric physical therapy. The material in the book is based on current practice in physical therapy and has been written by many of the recognized experts in clinical care in pediatric physical therapy.

Pediatric Physical Therapy is intended to fill a major void in current physical therapy literature. There exists virtually no textbook which offers as comprehensive a content area as this book. Other textbooks examine neurological disorders, developmental disabilities, orthopedic disorders, and other particular topics. Although they are generally excellent publications, they present a limited topic area at a level that is inappropriate for the entry-level student in physical therapy. *Pediatric Physical Therapy* examines a wide range of disabilities including neurological, musculoskeletal, developmental, neuromuscular, and cardiopulmonary prob-lems. Each chapter about a disability group provides current information about the disability and describes skills necessary for the student to evaluate and treat a child with the disability. In addition to the specific disabilities and diseases discussed, several chapters examine specific areas or types of practice. These special areas include developmental testing, the high-risk neonate, physical therapy in the schools, and sports-related injuries in adolescents. The choice for the specific topic areas and for the knowledge and skills presented comes from a document of the Section on Pediatric Physical Therapy of the American Physical Therapy Association. This document, adopted by the Section in the mid 1980s, is a position paper entitled "Entry Level Competencies in Pediatric Physical Therapy," and a suggested list of competencies and the major disability groups were therein identified. *Pediatric Physical Therapy* is an effort to examine those disability groups based upon the suggested entry-level competencies.

Jan Stephen Tecklin, M.S., P.T.

Contents

Pediatric Physical Therapy,
second edition, edited by Jan
Stephen Tecklin. J. B. Lippincott
Company, Philadelphia © 1994.

1

Ann F. Van Sant

Motor Development

What is motor development? Why is the study of motor development important to physical therapists? Why should I study motor development if I don't expect to work with children? Does any of this information relate to clinical practice outside the realm of pediatrics?

These questions are frequently asked by professional students in physical therapy as they begin to study motor development. They are very important questions and each is answered below.

What is motor development? *Motor development is the process of change in motor behavior that is related to the age of the individual.* The focus on the relationship between age and motor behavior makes the study of motor development unique from other viewpoints. Motor development includes age-related changes in both posture and movement, the two basic ingredients of motor be-

havior. Although this chapter concentrates on the motor development of infants and children, developmental processes occur throughout the human life span. Adolescents, young adults, and those in their thirties, forties, and fifties are also undergoing developmental changes in motor behavior.

What causes these changes? For many years, physical therapists attributed much of the change we see in motor behavior to changes occurring within the central nervous system (CNS). Developmental change in motor abilities was thought to reflect maturation of the CNS. Recently, however, we have started to realize that the nervous system is not the only structure that determines developmental change. Changes in other body systems, such as the musculoskeletal and cardiorespiratory system, also influence motor development. Of course, the environment in which we live also exerts a very strong and systematic influence on motor development. So the causes of motor development are many. Each system—whether a body system or a specific environmental system—interacts in complex and fascinating ways to effect change in motor behavior as one grows older.

Why is it important for a physical therapist to understand motor development? The changes that occur in the motor behavior of an infant are truly remarkable. At birth, the infant is almost helpless, but by the first birthday, the child has acquired an impressive degree of physical independence. The child has moved from helplessness to competence in sitting, creeping, and standing. Many children are walking by their first birthdays. The natural pattern of progression toward physical independence can be a very useful guide when designing a treatment plan to help individuals overcome their limitations and gain independence. *The planning of treatment is facilitated by an understanding of the natural process by which physical independence is acquired.*

Why should I study motor development if I don't expect to work with children? Does any of this information relate to clinical practice outside the realm of pediatrics? Physical impairments arising from disease or trauma may affect functional independence at any age. When independence is altered, the natural pattern by which individuals first gain self-sufficiency is a very useful guide as you help an individual regain physical independence. Knowing about motor development is just as important for those working with young adults or the elderly as it is for those who work with children or adolescents. To understand how one attains control over their posture and movements through acquisition of skills that are a part of our daily lives is useful information for therapists in every type of practice setting. What we know about developmental change in one period of the life span can be used to assist individuals of all ages.

This chapter reviews the motor behaviors characteristic of the prenatal period, infancy, and childhood. Beginning with the prenatal period, the discussion of the variety and clearly well-adapted movements of the fetus sets the stage for understanding the great change the individual undergoes as the force of gravity is experienced immediately upon birth. The remarkable progress of the infant in attaining a great degree of physical independence during the first postnatal year is outlined. The discussion will explore the range of factors known to influence motor behavior during the early periods of development. The motor accomplishments of childhood are reviewed and the important achievements are outlined. Finally, at the end of the chapter, a brief discussion of contemporary issues in motor development is included that will be helpful for all therapists trying to understand the factors that underlie motor behavior, regardless of the age of the individuals with whom they might work.

Prenatal Development of Motor Behavior

A distinct language has been developed to describe periods and characteristics of motor development before birth. The prenatal period of development is also known as the *gestational period.* The gestational period typically lasts between 38 and 40 weeks, which translates to approximately 9 months of pregnancy. The prenatal period is a time of rapid developmental change.

The age of the developing individual before birth is measured using a variety of different conventions. *Menstrual age* (MA) is the term used when the age of the individual is calculated from the first day of the mother's last menstrual period. Menstrual age is typically measured in weeks. The term *gestational age* (GA) is in more common use in recent years and is roughly equivalent to menstrual age. The prenatal stage of development can be divided into three distinct periods: the germinal period, the embryonic period, and the fetal period.

The *germinal period* begins at the time of fertilization and lasts 2 weeks. It is during this period that the fertilized egg, called the zygote, undergoes rapid cell division. The zygote travels through the fallopian tube to the uterus and, by the end of the germinal period, becomes attached to the uterine wall. The *embryonic period* begins 2 weeks after conception and lasts about 6 weeks. During this time the developing individual is known as an embryo. The embryonic period is characterized by rapid *morphologic changes.* This is the time when the cells are rapidly dividing, growing, and differentiating to take on specialized functions. At the end of the embryonic period, the developing individual is about 2 inches long and is recognizable as a human being. The *fetal period* begins at 7 weeks MA and ends at birth. It is during the fetal period that motor behavior first appears. During the fetal period the developing individual is referred to as a fetus.

Two Views of Motor Development During the Fetal Period

Before the 1970s, our knowledge of motor behavior during the fetal period was limited because we could not visualize the fetus. The methods used to record fetal activity included mothers' reports of fetal movements, listening through the uterine wall with a stethoscope, or, in some instances, electrocardiography or electromyography to detect movement through the mother's abdomen.

Without the ability to visualize the fetus in utero, physicians and researchers proposed that the motor behavior of aborted infants could be studied to understand fetal movement. Hooker (1944), an anatomist and researcher, studied aborted fetuses who were not able to sustain vital functions necessary for extrauterine life. His research served as a classic foundation for understanding how human motor behavior evolves before birth. Our early theorists in physical therapy, such as Margaret Rood and Dorothy Voss, studied Hooker's findings in order to understand more fully the earliest forms of human movement. They applied what they learned from Hooker to their assessments of motor behavior, as well as to sequence the motor skills they included in their treatment programs.

Development of Motor Responses to Stimulation

According to Hooker (1944), motor behavior can be evoked at the age of approximately 8 weeks MA. In his studies, the fetus was kept in an isotonic bath at body temperature. He used the tip of a hair to apply tactile stimulation to the skin of the fetus. He carefully filmed and recorded any motor response to the tactile stimulation. The earliest responses were obtained only when touch was applied around the mouth, the *perioral area.* The motor responses were characterized as withdrawal movements. The fetus laterally flexed and rotated the head so that the mouth was moved away from the site of the stimulus. Hooker termed these reflexes "avoiding" reactions. Applying stimuli to older fetuses, he found the area sensitive to tactile stimulation had spread from the mouth in all directions: up toward the nose, out to the sides of the face, down the chin and, in even older individuals, to the neck and upper chest. The spread of the area of cutaneous sensitivity was accompanied by an increasingly wider ranging withdrawal response. In older fetuses, not only was neck flexion and rotation seen, but the trunk and pelvis would also laterally flex and rotate away from the side of stimulation. These wide ranging responses were termed "total body responses." In 11-week-old fetuses, when the palms of the hands were touched, partial finger closure resulted. In fetuses of the same age or just slightly older, touch on the sole of the foot would bring about plantar flexion of the toes. As with the first responses seen in the perioral area, upper and lower limb responses were wider ranging in older fetuses, involving flexion and withdrawal from stimuli applied to the palm or sole. In older fetuses, areas of cutaneous sensitivity were found in more proximal areas of the limbs, eventually including the whole upper and lower limbs.

Responses of older fetuses encompassed an increasing number of body regions, and the character of the responses also changed. Rather than withdrawing from the site of stimulation, there was an increase in the frequency of responses that moved the face toward the source of stimulation. This gradual change in direction—from movements away from the stimulus at about 8 weeks to moving toward the stimulus by 12 weeks—has important consequences. The fetus that moves away from stimuli is demonstrating what might be interpreted as a very primitive survival function by protecting the area from harm. Yet after birth, the individual must not withdraw from all touch received in the perioral area or feeding would be impossible. In a relatively short time frame, by the age of 14 to 15 weeks MA, all the preliminary feeding movements, including mouth opening and closing, sustained lip closure, and tongue movements, were found to be present. In fetuses of 29 weeks MA, audible sucking was observed.

The character of trunk and limb responses was also different in older fetuses. Rather than continuing as widespread, total body responses, some actions were confined to local areas, and the responses were more variable in their form. In fetuses of 13 or 14 weeks MA, Hooker described the character of movement as being graceful and flowing. At this age, responses that involved action of the whole body could include complete sequences of action. For example, movements such as head and trunk extension were followed by rotation and flexion. The action sequences were described as "anticipatory" of postnatal life, as they seemed to include patterns of action typically seen after birth, such as rolling or reaching out.

Hooker's studies were long regarded by physical therapists as an important source of information regarding motor development during the prenatal period. Yet the assumption that the aborted fetus demonstrates behavior typical of intrauterine fetal behavior has been questioned. Some argue that the environment of the aborted fetus is drastically different from the intrauterine environment and that motor behavior observed outside the uterus is not representative of the normal motor development that occurs in the intrauterine environment. A second criticism of these studies is that the fetuses studied were in the process of dying during the study. Fetuses born as young as Hooker reported could not breathe to sustain life. Many of the reactions observed may have been a result of decreased oxygen in the blood. Further, the aborted fetus may have had serious abnormalities that triggered the early birth. If that was the case, the movements observed and described by Hooker may not be typical of the normal population of infants born at term or 37 to 42 weeks GA.

Development of Spontaneous Movements

Spontaneous movements represent a different class of movements than do reflexive responses. Rather than being evoked, spontaneous movements arise without an apparent stimulus. Reflexes are evoked responses, and depend on a stimulus to be initiated. Spontaneous movements arise without external stimuli, and can be considered to be self-initiated. Spontaneous movements are not necessarily "voluntary." In fact, the term "voluntary movement" can be problematic when discussing early development. Volition implies intent and purpose, and we have no reliable way of determining the intent of the very young individual.

Until recently researchers and physicians concentrated on describing reflexes or evoked responses of the fetus and young infants and ignored spontaneous actions. This tendency to focus on reflexes is likely a result of our scientific culture that values well-controlled experiments. The preference for the controlled experimental approach to documenting human behavior may have led to the general belief that infants were only capable of "reflexive movement." In an experimental approach to the study of movement, spontaneous movements were considered to be random events, nonpurposeful, and interfering with the study.

In the 1970s, the technologic advance of ultrasonographic monitoring of the fetus brought about a revolution in our understanding of the development of movement during the fetal period. Milani-Comparetti, an Italian pediatric neuropsychiatrist, was given the opportunity to observe and interpret the ultrasonographic records of more than 1000 pregnant women. These women went on to deliver normal healthy babies. Milani-Comparetti had, until the time of his ultrasound study, been a firm believer in reflexes as the fundamental unit of human motor behavior. Yet his observations of the ultrasonographic records of normally developing fetuses changed his most basic concepts of motor development. Milani-Comparetti was impressed with the spontaneous and frequent nature of early fetal movement. He could find no stimuli evoking the natural movements of the developing individual.

He described the sequential appearance of spontaneous action across the fetal period and contributed to a greater understanding of human movement by describing *"primary movement patterns (PMPs)."* According to Milani-Comparetti, PMPs are the fundamental units of action from which all human movements develop. These action patterns arise spontaneously and later become linked to sensory stimuli to form *primary automatisms.* A primary automatism is similar to a reflex. His concept that spontaneous movements arise *before* primary automatisms was revolutionary, particularly for those who felt the reflex was the basic unit of motor behavior from which all other movements originated.

Milani-Comparetti's colorful and rich descriptions of the well-adapted movements of the fetus while in utero is an excellent example of how modern technology can be applied to aid our understanding of human movement. He described earliest fetal movements as "jumping." Jumping appeared spontaneously in fetuses of about 10 weeks GA. A series of jumps continued in succession until the fetus had attained a new resting posture on the uterine floor. The earliest form of jumping involved extension of the lower limbs and flexion of the upper limbs. Later, apparently owing to fetal growth within confined intrauterine space, the upper limbs were brought forward and extended down in front of the body during jumping.

Locomotor movements, which enabled the fetus to climb up and over the placenta, were described as a part of the motor behavior at 17 weeks GA. Milani-Comparetti described a wide range of very well-adapted fetal movements, including exploring the face and body with the hands, reaching out to grasp and move the umbilical cord, and so forth. Spontaneous sucking of the thumb and swallowing movements were documented. Responses to auditory and visual stimuli appeared before birth. Sound or light were applied to the abdominal wall of the mother to examine responsiveness to stimuli. Initially, responses of alarm were observed, with both hands being raised to shield the face in a seemingly protective pattern.

Milani-Comparetti discussed how the earliest responses were used ultimately "to be born." Locomotion was used to move into position for birth with the head down, engaged in the pelvic outlet. The jumping movements were used to thrust against the uterine wall to initiate or cooperate in the birthing process. Breathing movements, sucking, and swallowing were preparatory for feeding following birth, and auditory and visual responsiveness prepared the infant for receiving information about the new postnatal environment. One cannot read his work without a general sense that the fetus is behaving in a manner that reflects progressive adaptation to the uterine environment, as well as anticipation of the birthing process that is to come at the end of the gestational period.

Summary

There are two distinctly different views of the fetal period and thus of the origins of human movement. One point of view is based on research conducted on fetuses outside the uterine environment, and one is based on research conducted on fetuses as they function within the uterus. The latter, more natural study of prenatal movements reveals a very active and spontaneously moving fetus. The research conducted in an extrauterine environment portrayed fetal movements as reflexes. These view points were influenced by the technology available to the researchers at the time they conducted their studies, but they were also influenced by the prevailing scientific perspectives of the times in which they were developed. Physical therapists have become interested recently in self-generated movement, after a long period of concentration on reflexes and reactions of our patients. We now realize how very important it is to foster self-initiated actions, for they are an integral part of human movement from the very beginning. As a result, the work of Milani-Comparetti in describing the very earliest of self-initiated movements is of great interest to therapists and revolutionary in nature. The unique perspective of Milani-Comparetti stands in direct contrast to the traditional view of the fetus as a passive, reflexive being.

Motor Development During Infancy

Infancy is considered to be the period from birth until the child is able to stand and walk. Typically, infancy lasts approximately 1 year. This period is very instructive for physical therapists. The neonate, essentially helpless in the face of gravity, develops gradually the ability to align body segments with respect to each other and with respect to the environment, achieving what is called the "normal posture" of upright stance. The gravity-filled environment in which the infant must function is almost completely conquered during that first year. The newborn infant, able to lift the head only momentarily, gains the ability to hold the head in an increasingly vertical posture. The flexed posture of the newborn gives way to the extended posture of upright stance. Along the way, infants acquire locomotor skills: first rolling, then crawling and creeping, then walking with support, until they finally achieve that important milestone of independent locomotion (Table 1-1).

In the following discussion, the motor accomplishments of the first year of life are discussed for each trimester during the first postnatal year. A trimester comprises a 3-month period. Therefore, there are 4 trimesters during the first year after birth. This division of the first year into four periods is a useful way of understanding the rapid motor accomplishments of the infant. In each trimester, the behavior of the infant will be discussed for each of four body positions: the supine position, the prone position, sitting, and standing. Rather than focusing on a sequence of motor milestones, the accomplishments of the infant in each trimester are outlined.

The First Trimester: Getting the Head Aligned

The newborn infant is termed a neonate. The neonatal period lasts 2 weeks. The posture of the neonate is characterized by flexion. This posture is thought to derive, to some degree, from the flexed posture imposed during the prenatal period, but it has also been attributed to the degree of nervous system development. Specifically, the regions of the brain responsible for the motor abilities in-

Table 1-1. *Milestones of Motor Development for the First Year of Life**

Functional Accomplishment	Average Age of Accomplishment (in Months)	Normal Age Range (in Months)
Holds head erect and steady	0.8	0.7–4
Turns from side to back	1.8	0.7–5
Sits with support	2.3	1–5
Turns from back to side	4.4	2–7
Sits alone (momentarily)	5.3	4–8
Rolls from back to stomach	6.4	4–10
Sits alone (steadily)	6.6	5–9
Early stepping movements (with support)	7.4	5–11
Pulls to standing position	8.1	5–12
Walks with help	9.6	7–12
Stands alone	11.0	9–16
Walks alone	11.7	9–17

*From Bayley N. Bayley Scales of Infant Development. New York: Psychological Corp.; 1969

volved in extending the body against the force of gravity are thought not to be fully developed at this time. During the first trimester following birth, antigravity activity begins, and the infant acquires the ability to lift the head against the force of gravity. This is a major accomplishment of the first trimester.

The Supine Position

When the infant is in the supine position, the head and upper trunk rest on the support surface with the head turned to one side (Fig. 1-1). The lower trunk is often flexed so that the buttocks do not fully contact the bed. Both upper and lower limbs are held in a relatively symmetric posture of acute flexion during the first few days following birth. The feet may be positioned close to the buttocks and the hands are often contacting the trunk. Typically the hips are held in flexion and kept up off the support surface by the action of the hip adductor muscles. The knees are flexed and the ankles are held in an acute degree of dorsiflexion. The arms are held in forward flexion close to the body. The elbows and hands are flexed.

Some resistance is encountered when the neonate's limbs are passively moved into extension. Elbows, knees, and hips rebound into flexion after being passively straightened. This tendency to hold a flexed posture and to rebound into flexion when released from an extended position is termed "flexor tone." The physiologic mechanisms responsible for this phenomenon are not clearly understood. The posture is thought to reflect both the elasticity of soft tissue that had been confined in a flexed posture during the late fetal period and CNS activity at this early point in postnatal development.

The acutely flexed posture of the newborn infant is normal, but gradually wanes. By the end of the first trimester, the degree of flexion in the limbs has lessened. The feet and arms are no longer held off the support surface. This change is thought to result from active extension movements on the part of the infant as well as the pull of gravity.

The posture of the infant's upper limbs changes during the first trimester. After a month or so, *when the head is in a relatively central or midline position,* the flexion of the upper limbs begins to give way to an abducted and extended arm posture. Initially, this posture is seen when the infant is sleeping or when the whole body moves in an expression of delight or happiness. If the infant cries, an acute flexion posture will reappear. *When the head is turned fully to the right or left,* an asymmetric posture of the upper and lower limbs may be seen. The upper limb toward which the face is turned is frequently abducted to the side with the elbow extended. The lower limb on the face side is extended. The other upper limb is abducted and laterally rotated so that it rests on the bed with the elbow flexed. This posture of the upper limbs is commonly called an asymmetric tonic neck reflex posture.

Movements in the first trimester involve bouts of stretching, kicking and thrusting of the extremities, and turning and twisting of the head and trunk. The frequency and degree of movement is related to the "state of the infant." Prior to feeding, infants tend to be most active. They are more quiet and sleepy after feedings.

Infants are capable of focusing on objects held a short distance from their face and will turn to track the object, bringing the head to a midline position but not beyond. The infant cannot track objects beyond the midline until the end of the first trimester.

It is not uncommon for an infant to roll from a supine to a side-lying position during the first trimester. This is usually the result of the coupling of

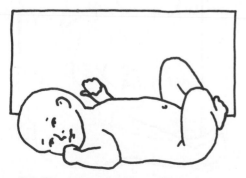

Figure 1-1. *First trimester, supine position.*

head turning with head and trunk extension. A roll from supine to prone is usually an accidental event early in the second trimester. Consistent rolling will not appear until late in the second trimester or during the third trimester.

The Prone Position

In the prone position, the newborn infant lies in flexion with the head turned to one side. The neonate has the capacity to lift and turn the head from one side to the other. A newborn infant placed prone will be able to keep the nose and mouth unobstructed and free for breathing. At the beginning of the first trimester, the upper limbs are held relatively close to the body in a flexed position. The lower limbs are flexed up under the infant, keeping the lower abdomen up off the bed. The hips and knees are acutely flexed and the feet are in dorsiflexion.

When awake and in the prone position, the infant spends much time actively extending the head and trunk against the force of gravity. The infant repeatedly lifts the head. It appears as if the infant is actively seeking a midline orientation, but the head is often off center and bobs up and down. Occasionally, the efforts are so great that the upper trunk is lifted as well so that the infant is supporting weight on the forearms, which are medially rotated and tucked under the trunk (Fig. 1-2). This so called *on-elbows posture* becomes increasingly frequent throughout the first trimester. With the increased frequency of active extension of the head and trunk comes attempts to straighten the elbows under the body and support the weight of the upper trunk on the hands. The infant frequently pushes up and then falls, rocking forward on the trunk with the arms flexed and pulled back in retraction. This sequence of pushing up and then falling into prone becomes increasingly common toward the end of the first trimester.

Sitting and Standing

During the first trimester, the infant cannot sit or stand alone. This is not a problem of strength, as the infant is able to develop sufficient tension in the

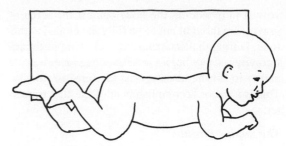

Figure 1-2. *First trimester, on-elbows position.*

muscles to fully support body weight in the standing position. Assistance is needed because the baby has no ability to balance. The sophisticated control and coordination of muscles that sustains the ability to balance is not developed at this time.

When held in a sitting position, the baby has a rounded back (Fig. 1-3). The head is typically held forward of the vertical in a flexed position. However, unless the infant is very sleepy, the chin does not droop; rather, it is held up off the chest by active contraction of the neck extensors. The head bobs, with intermittent loss of head position. Head bobbing seen during sitting is similar to the intermittent head lifting observed in the prone position.

During the course of the first trimester, the

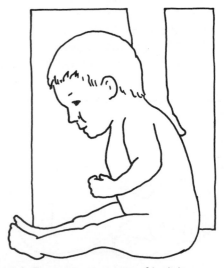

Figure 1-3. *First trimester, supported in sitting.*

steadiness of the head increases. By the end of the first trimester, most infants hold their heads steady in alignment with the trunk. The ability to keep the head aligned is termed "head control." Babies first straighten the head with respect to the trunk, but later they develop the ability to keep the head aligned with respect to gravity. That is, the baby can keep the head in what is called *a normal position.*

Although unable to stand alone, when provided support for balance, the newborn infant is able to maintain the standing position. This ability is referred to as primary standing (Fig. 1-4). Typically, this standing pattern is characterized by crossed feet and a bit of asymmetry in the lower limbs. The baby may stand on toes. Toward the end of the first trimester, this primary standing pattern begins to wane and is increasingly difficult to demonstrate. At that time, the baby is moving into a period of *astasia.* Quite literally, astasia means "without stance." When someone tries to stand the baby up, the legs give way and the infant sinks into flexion, not accepting or supporting weight through the lower limbs. Astasia may appear toward the end of

the first trimester and can last into the second trimester.

In summary, sitting and standing are not independent postures in the first trimester. But the infant shows promise of what is to come. By struggling against the force of gravity, the infant gains control of the head and has taken a large step toward conquering the force of gravity that rendered the baby helpless at the time of birth.

The Second Trimester: Pushing Up and Sitting Up

The second trimester is marked by great strides in combating the force of gravity. The infant begins this trimester with the competence to keep the head aligned with respect to the body and leaves with the ability to sit alone for brief periods and to push up onto hands and knees. These postures provide the foundation for later accomplishments, but in and of themselves, they permit a wider range of interaction with the surrounding world. Sitting and getting up on hands and knees are important milestones on the way to physical independence. Accomplishments in supine, prone, sitting, and standing positions are outlined in the following sections.

The Supine Position

When the infant is in the supine position, a great deal of activity can be observed. The baby frequently lifts the legs up off the support surface, bringing them toward the hands and face. The infant reaches out for the feet with the hands and struggles to bring the feet to the mouth for exploration (Fig. 1-5).

This struggle can lead to a loss of the supine position. The weight of the legs, if they are carried to the right or left, may turn the baby to a side-lying position. This apparent loss of control of the lower limbs during lifting may be one of the factors that leads to the ability to roll out of the supine position. Some infants accomplish this during the second trimester, but it is more often an achievement of the third trimester.

The infant also places the feet on the supporting

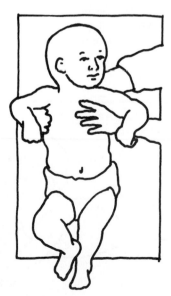

Figure 1-4. *First trimester, supported, primary standing.*

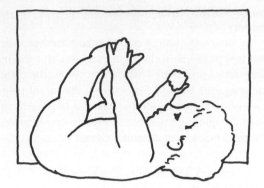

Figure 1-5. *Second trimester, supine position, reaching for feet.*

surface with the hips and knees flexed. This posture serves as a starting position for strong bursts of extension that lift the buttocks and spine off the surface. This is termed "bridging" (Fig. 1-6). Some babies push themselves to the far reaches of their cribs by a series of bridging movements. At other times, the infant will demonstrate strong rotation of the head and neck to one side, coupled with extension, as if to look up and over one shoulder. The action of turning and looking can also lead to rolling out of the supine position to a side-lying posture during the second trimester.

Although the infant does not consistently roll from the supine position, the extreme postures involving lifting of the lower limbs and extension with rotation of the head of the head and neck are precursors to the ability to roll.

The Prone Position

The intermittent lifting and bobbing of the head that is associated with the effort to gain an erect posture in the prone position during the first trimester gradually begins to involve the trunk musculature. The baby struggles in the prone position to elevate the trunk off the supporting surface, first getting up on elbows and then pushing up on hands. The baby spends a great deal of time pushing up (Fig. 1-7) and then dropping back into the prone position, pivoting on the stomach with arms and legs elevated off the support surface. This pivoting posture is termed "pivot prone" or the airplane position (Fig. 1-8).

It is not uncommon for the baby to push back while up on hands and thus to push across the support surface while in prone. This is termed *crawling,* defined as the locomotor pattern of moving forward or backward by pushing and pulling with the extremities while the abdomen is in contact with the support surface. Crawling begins during the second trimester. *Creeping* is a locomotor pattern characterized by elevation of the abdomen up off the support surface. Typically babies crawl before creeping. Crawling is a second trimester accomplishment, whereas creeping usually appears in the third or fourth trimester.

When crawling, babies tend to push backward first, later developing the capacity to move forward.

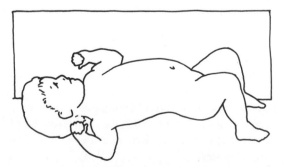

Figure 1-6. *Second trimester, bridging position.*

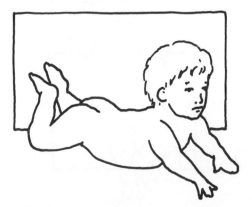

Figure 1-7. *Second trimester, pushing up to hands.*

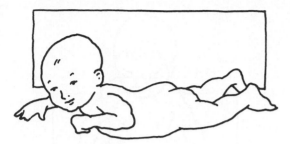

Figure 1-8. *Second trimester, pivot prone position.*

Initial attempts at crawling are characterized by a lack of coordination of the movements of the extremities. Soon a consistent pattern evolves that is very effective for moving about the floor.

American babies tend to spend more time in prone, particularly when compared to British children, who are more often placed in the supine position to play. Experience in a common or preferred position is an important determinant of the sequence of motor skill accomplishments. Often, children who spend a great deal of time in a preferred posture will demonstrate advances in the achievement of motor milestones accomplished from that posture, whereas skills in other postures might lag slightly. It is important to remember that some babies prefer the supine position, whereas others like sitting. In these instances, skills in the preferred posture often outdistance skills of the other postures. Differences in accomplishments among postures often reflect the child's preferences. These differences are to be expected as an expression of the infant's individuality and are a part of normal development.

The infant will also begin to push up on hands and knees during the second trimester. Usually this is accomplished by first pushing up on hands and then flexing the lumbar spine and hips, pulling the knees up under the chest. Initially, hands-and-knees is an unstable posture, but with time, the child becomes quite competent at pushing back into the hands-and-knees posture and will engage in bouts of rocking: repetitively shifting weight back and forth from the hands to the knees. Because the child does not have good control of the hips, if weight is

shifted to one side or the other, it is not uncommon for the child to fall out of the hands-and-knees posture. The rocking action seems to be a self-initiated balancing exercise and eventually leads to a very steady and stable hands-and-knees posture.

The Sitting Position

The second trimester is the time when the infant develops a steady and erect sitting posture. The infant's increasing ability to control the upper trunk is often manifested by the placement of the mother's hands while she supports the child in sitting. It is as though the mother knows intuitively how much freedom to allow the child to work against the force of gravity. The experience of struggling in a protected but challenging sitting posture helps the infant develop competence in sitting.

The baby first sits alone while propped forward on the hands (Fig. 1-9). The posture of the trunk and upper limbs is very similar to the posture attained when pushing up on hands in the prone position (compare Figs. 1-7 and 1-9). In both the prone push-up and the propped sitting position, the head is vertical with respect to gravity. The upper trunk is inclined forward of vertical, and weight is born on the hands. In propped sitting, the legs are commonly held in a ring position, with the hips ab-

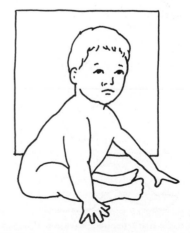

Figure 1-9. *Second trimester, sitting alone propped forward on hands.*

ducted and laterally rotated and with the feet in opposition to each other.

When given a supportive and protected environment, the infant will extend the trunk, retract the shoulder girdle, and flex the elbows to bring the arms into what is termed a "high guard" posture for brief instants of independent sitting (Fig. 1-10). During the second trimester, babies develop the capacity to sit with support for up to 15 to 20 minutes. Sustained periods of independent sitting will not be seen until the third trimester.

Developing at the same time as the ability to hold the trunk steadily in the vertical position is the capacity to extend the arms down to the support surface to catch and protect the body from falling. This is termed a "parachute" or "protective extension" reaction and is characterized by abducted arms with extension of the elbows, wrists, and hands. Protective reactions are fundamental for safe, independent sitting (Fig. 1-11).

The Standing Position

During the second trimester, the infant begins again to accept weight through the lower limbs and is able to stand with support. The standing posture that follows the period of astasia is termed "secondary

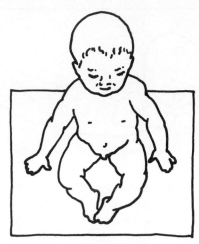

Figure 1-11. *Second trimester, "parachute" or "protective extension" position as viewed from above.*

standing." The secondary standing posture is characterized by abducted legs, extended knees, and a plantigrade posture of the feet (Fig. 1-12). In the plantigrade posture, the soles of the feet are in full contact with the support surface. The secondary standing posture differs from the primary standing seen during the first trimester. During primary standing, the feet are often crossed, and the infant will commonly stand on the toes, with the ankles plantar-flexed. In contrast, secondary standing is characterized by abducted lower limbs and a plantigrade posture of the feet.

Activity in standing increases across the second trimester. When supported under the arms, the child will first bounce up and down while standing; later in the trimester, the infant will begin to shift weight from side to side, picking up and stamping first one leg and then the other.

In summary, the accomplishments of the second trimester are impressive: moving across the support surface by bridging or crawling, sitting with support, getting up on hands and knees, and standing with support. The infant is gaining control of the body in fundamental postures that will lead to a greater range of mobility. A supportive environment allows the infant opportunities to explore the

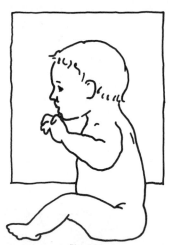

Figure 1-10. *Second trimester, "high guard" independent sitting for brief periods.*

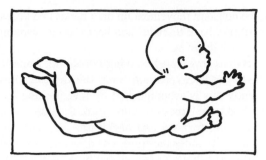

Figure 1-13. *Third trimester, rolling with head and upper trunk extension as viewed from directly above.*

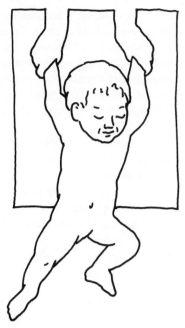

Figure 1-12. *Second trimester, standing with support.*

body and conquer the force of gravity evidenced by increasingly elevated and vertical postures.

The Third Trimester: Constant Motion

During the third trimester, the infant becomes mobile. With the ability to move about the environment, exploration is paramount. The drive to move up against the force of gravity seems to strengthen so that, by the end of the third trimester, babies are able to pull themselves up to standing. The world awaits discovery.

The Supine Position

Preference of the supine position is decreasing, particularly as the infant develops the capacity to roll out of supine into the prone position. The first roll may be accomplished either with a strong pattern of head and upper trunk extension and rotation, accompanied by the arm reaching up and over the shoulder (Fig. 1-13), or with a bilateral flexion pat-

tern of the lower limbs, carrying the legs up and over to one side (Fig. 1-14). Babies often stop in the side-lying position before completing the roll to prone. Some spend a great deal of time side lying, with the upper leg moving from behind the body to a position in front of the body. It is as though the baby is learning to balance in the side-lying position. Some infants will use rolling as a means of locomotion, but more commonly, creeping is seen.

The Prone Position

The third trimester begins with the child in a prone position, pivoting in circles on the stomach. The prone position soon becomes a transitional posture. Babies move through the prone position on their way to a hands-and-knees position, or to sitting or standing. As the trimester progresses, there seems

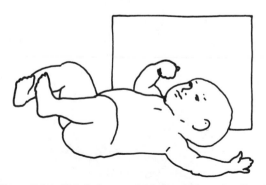

Figure 1-14. *Third trimester, initiating rolling using flexed legs.*

to be constant movement up onto hands and knees, to sitting, back to hands and knees, up to standing and back down again.

Babies accomplish moving into sitting from the hands-and-knees position during this trimester. Frequently this is accomplished by first pushing into the hands-and-knees posture; then, through a bout of rocking forward and backward, the knees are brought up under the trunk and the child sits back on the heels. Often while sitting back on the heels, the infant will drop down into a side-sitting posture with the legs flexed and rotated to one side. Initially, movement to the side-sitting position is unintended, but eventually the infant learns to control the movement and will move easily from hands and knees into side sitting without first sitting back on the heels. The hips are lowered to one side with control as the arms push the body weight back onto the buttocks. The arms are then lifted from the surface, and the baby may rotate the lower trunk and legs to achieve a symmetric sitting posture.

The Sitting Position

Maintaining an unsupported sitting position is now accomplished with ease. The child has developed balance abilities in sitting. The posture is steady and erect (Fig. 1-15). Sitting erect for as long as half an hour, the child will occasionally lean forward on the hands for support. The hands are more typically engaged in a variety of play activities: reaching out and grasping objects, banging them together, and bringing them to the mouth for exploration.

By the end of the third trimester, moving from sitting up into the hands-and-knees position is also accomplished with ease. By making use of the upper limb movement pattern that also serves as the protective extension or parachute reaction, the child reaches out to the side with the arms and transfers support from the buttocks to the hands. The lower trunk and buttocks are raised up off the support surface and rotated from the side into the symmetric hands-and-knees posture (Fig. 1-16).

Some children will hitch or scoot in sitting. While leaning on one hand and with one leg laterally rotated down onto the support surface and the other leg elevated with the foot in a plantigrade posture, the child steps out with the elevated leg, plants

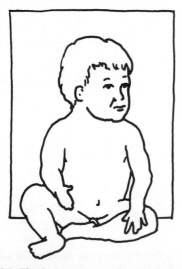

Figure 1-15. *Third trimester, unsupported sitting.*

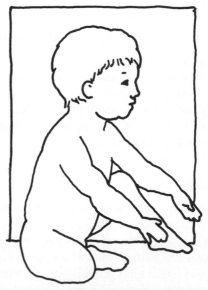

Figure 1-16. *Third trimester, transferring weight from buttocks to hands.*

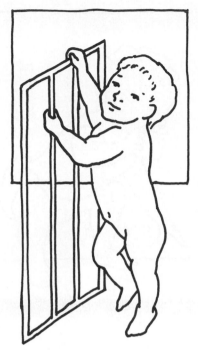

Figure 1-17. *Third trimester, pulling to stand.*

the foot and pushing with the other leg, slides the buttocks across the floor.

The Standing Position

The standing position is a favorite of babies during the third trimester. They are so captivated by this posture that they spend a great deal of time and effort pulling up to stand (Fig. 1-17). Initially the standing posture is characterized by a piked and unstable position of the hips. Later the hips are drawn forward under the shoulders and the standing posture is increasingly stable. Initially the child has no ability to get back down from standing. It is possible to find the child crying over the dilemma of how to get out of standing. The child will eventually discover how to fall by thrusting the buttocks backward and sitting down.

After pulling up the child spends great energy bouncing and actively disturbing balance. This up and down bouncing gradually gives way to shifting of the weight from side to side and taking steps beside the furniture. This is termed *cruising* and is the first form of independent walking (Figure 1-18).

The Fourth Trimester: Walking at Last

The Supine and Prone Positions

When the baby is awake, the prone and supine positions have become primarily transitional postures. The child spends such little time in them, they seem primarily to be passing points of stability on the way to more upright postures.

The hands-and-knees posture is the basis for creeping. This locomoter pattern comprises alternate action of the opposite arms and legs in forward mobility. Some infants become quite skillful as creepers and prefer this form of locomotion for months. Even the onset of walking will not preclude some children's preference for creeping.

Plantigrade creeping becomes a part of the

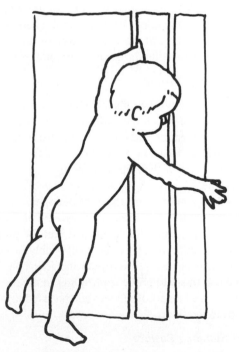

Figure 1-18. *Third trimester, "cruising" along a railing.*

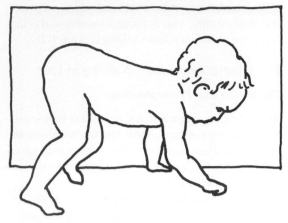

Figure 1-19. *Fourth trimester, "creeping" on extended arms and legs.*

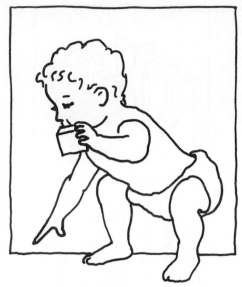

Figure 1-20. *Fourth trimester, moving from standing back down to sitting.*

child's repertoire. This form of locomotion involves creeping on extended arms and legs, with the feet in the plantigrade posture (Fig. 1-19). Plantigrade creeping is the next step in the gradual elevation of the trunk against the force of gravity. Full extension of the upper limbs led to the hands-and-knees posture, and now extension of the lower limbs leads to a plantigrade creeping position.

The Sitting Position

Sitting is a very functional position at this time, yet the ease with which the child moves in and out of the sitting posture—whether moving from sitting to the hands-and-knees posture, or pulling from sitting to kneeling and then up to standing—is quite remarkable.

Balance abilities are so well developed in sitting that the child will often pivot around in circles while sitting, using the hands and feet for propulsion. The child sits easily and comfortably in a high chair with the legs flexed onto the foot rest. The child can move to prone from sitting in the process of play or as a part of the movements used to stand up from the floor.

The Standing Posture

Standing is a preferred posture for most infants during the fourth trimester. Pulling to a standing position at furniture leads to cruising along the edge of furniture while holding on. The ability to move back down to sitting from standing is developed early in this trimester, and later in the trimester, the ability to move down to a squat-sitting posture from standing appears (Fig. 1-20). Children climb onto furniture from the standing position. They often can get up on chairs or low tables without difficulty by the end of the fourth trimester.

Stepping begins in a diagonally forward and sideward direction. This early stepping pattern can be seen in the first steps the child takes with the hands held (Fig. 1-21). Parents who walk children from behind with two hands held are in the best position to observe this diagonal stepping pattern, which leads the child first to one side and then to the other. Only with time do leg movements correct to a more forward direction.

The child progresses from walking with two hands held to walking with just one hand for support; with encouragement, the child lets go eventually and steps out alone. The first independent steps are also diagonal in nature, leading to a wide base of support. The feet land in a plantigrade position

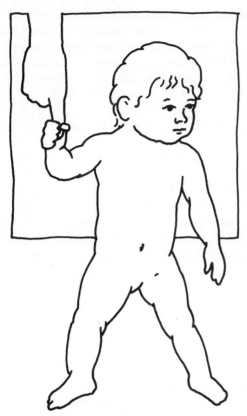

Figure 1-21. *Fourth trimester, forward and sideward stepping pattern.*

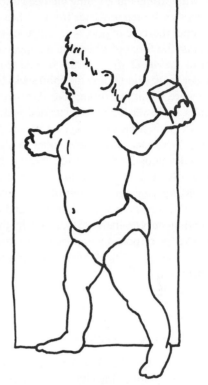

Figure 1-22. *Fourth trimester, independent steps with hands in high guard position.*

rather than in a heel-toe progression. The arms are held in "high guard" (Fig. 1-22).

While early attempts at walking are evidence of the precarious balance of the baby, the accomplishments of the first postnatal year are quite remarkable. In very short order the infant has moved from helplessness to independent mobility and active exploration of the world. With the onset of walking and climbing, even more of the world is within reach.

Within a few short months after the onset of walking the child will gain the ability to rise independently by rolling prone, getting onto hands and knees, and then assuming the plantigrade posture, and then pushing up with the arms to achieve independent standing. Climbing on and off objects, and

creeping up and down stairs become routine. Walking becomes smooth and coordinated. One can observe a progressively narrowing base of support, and forward-directed steps with a heel-toe pattern of foot contact. The arms move down from high, to middle, and finally to low guard, with a natural alternate-arm swing eventually appearing.

Summary

The transition from helplessness and physical dependence to independence during the first year after birth is of great importance to the child and family. As the infant gains control over the body and is able to resist the force of gravity, new worlds open up for exploration, and the baby is less dependent on parents to be held and carried. Antigravity control begins with lifting and aligning the head during the first trimester. It then proceeds from the head down to the upper thoracic region, with the arms extending against the force of gravity and supporting the weight of the upper trunk in the second trimester. The lower trunk extends and the child seeks the vertical posture of sitting during the third trimester. Gradually the lower limbs are extended as the child achieves a plantigrade creeping posture and pulls to standing. With increasing time spent in standing, the child develops the ability to balance in the posture and will let go of support to step out and walk. The cephalocaudal progression of antigravity extension to move into a vertical posture and the accompanying development of balance in the progressive series of postures represents an important pattern of accomplishment that leads to physical independence.

Motor Behavior During Early Childhood

Early childhood is the period from 2 years to 6 years. To this point in the chapter, most of the discussion has focused on the acquisition of new motor skills. Motor development during early childhood leads to the attainment of new skills but not necessarily new patterns of movement. It is as though the child has acquired all the fundamental movement patterns, but it is now learning to put them to use in meaningful activity.

Development of Locomotor Skills

In early childhood, the locomotor pattern of walking is refined and new locomotor skills are added: running, hopping, jumping, and skipping. These locomotor patterns require increasing amounts of balance and control of force for successful performance. The development of ability within each skill appears to depend on a combination of practice, growth of the body, and maturation of the CNS. The more refined the skill, the more practice must be devoted to develop the control needed.

Children require opportunities to exercise their developing abilities within fundamental motor skills.

Running is usually acquired between the ages of 2 and 4 years. Running differs from walking, specifically because of the "flight phase," during which there is no support of the body. The flight phase comes about by strong but careful application of propulsive force during the stance phase of the gait pattern. However, it is not until the age of 5 or 6 years that a degree of control in running is achieved: the ability to start, stop, and change direction with ease. Jumping first develops as the ability to jump down from heights. The child will first jump down off a box approximately 1 foot in height at about the age of $2\frac{1}{2}$ years. This skill is more characteristic of a stepping down pattern than an actual jump with two feet off the ground simultaneously. With time, the ability to jump to reach an object overhead emerges and later, the ability to jump for distance emerges. Across childhood, the height and distance jumped increases. In addition, the form of the movements used to jump change, becoming more efficient. Primitive jumpers demonstrate a very shallow preparatory crouch, while advanced jumpers demonstrate deep crouches. Initially, the arms appear to move to a high guard position in young jumpers, whereas in older and more experienced jumpers, the arms tend to be used to create momentum, being thrust up and overhead while jumping. Young and inexperienced jumpers demonstrate flexed heads and trunks during the jump. By contrast, older, more experienced jumpers utilize head and trunk extension during jumping actions.

Hopping seems to be an extension of the ability to balance while standing on one leg. Hopping is defined as elevation of the body off the ground and subsequent landing using a single foot. Hopping appears at about the age of $2\frac{1}{2}$ years, but is not well performed until the child is approximately 6 years of age, when a series of about 10 hops can be strung together. After a series of hops can be performed, children tend to incorporate them into games, such as hopscotch or dancing steps.

Skipping is a complex locomotor pattern that involves a step and a hop on one leg followed by a step and a hop on the other leg. Skipping is not achieved by most children until they are 6 years old. As with many of the locomotor skills, practice seems to be a significant factor in the acquisition of the skill. Older individuals who have not had the opportunity to practice the skill often are unable to demonstrate some of the more sophisticated loco-motor patterns.

Other Fundamental Skills of Childhood

Throwing and striking are two additional skills that undergo developmental change during early child-hood. Although throwing is a skill that is typically acquired during the first postnatal year, skillful throwing is still developing during early childhood. Sequences of change in movement patterns used to perform both throwing and striking tasks have been outlined for the trunk and lower limbs. Different steps in movement pattern development have been described for the action of the arms in throwing and striking. Across childhood, the distance of the throw becomes greater. The increase in distance is likely attributable to the emergence of movement patterns that more efficiently apply force to the ob-ject being thrown or struck. Catching and kicking are two additional skills that have been studied from a developmental perspective.

Catching begins to develop at about 3 years of age. The child initially holds the arms extended in front of the body and does not adjust the arms to account for the direction or speed of the object to be caught. Eventually the arms are used to scoop the object in toward the body, and gradually, the child can be seen to move and adjust the position of the body to intercept the object being thrown. With age and experience, the child anticipates the flight of the object, moves to arrive in time to intercept the object, and uses the hands to catch with a "give" that absorbs the force of the object.

Kicking requires balancing on one foot while transferring force to an object; such as a soccer ball. Early in the development of this skill, there is little preparatory backswing or follow-through in the kicking leg. With time, a backswing appears, first at the knee, and later involving the hip. Gradually, fol-low-through and a forward lean of the trunk be-come a part of the kicking action. These character-istics are typically seen in children at about the age of 6 years.

Performance Changes in Skills Acquired in Infancy

Age-related change in movement patterns used to perform skills first acquired during infancy contin-ues during early childhood and into later childhood and adolescence. A series of studies has docu-mented the movement patterns expected in tasks, such as rolling from supine to prone, moving from sitting on a chair to standing, and rising from supine to standing.

Rolling from Supine to Prone

During early childhood, the movement patterns used to roll from supine to prone are age-related. If the child were to roll from supine to prone moving over the left side, the roll would be characterized by a pushing pattern with the right lower limb, a trunk pattern in which the right side of the pelvis leads the movement, and the right upper limb would lift and reach up above the level of the left shoulder.

Rising from a Chair

When rising from a chair, the young child first lifts the legs up off the chair seat and then replaces them down on the floor. The trunk flexes forward until the buttocks are raised off the chair, at which time head and trunk extension begin to bring the child to the vertical standing posture. In children younger than 6 years of age, a push off of the chair seat would be expected. In children older than 6 years, the arms more commonly push on the legs during the rise.

Rising from a Supine Position

Young children rise to standing by coming forward from supine using a pattern of flexion with rotation of the head and trunk. One arm reaches forward while the other pushes against the support surface and the lower limbs assume a wide-based, medially rotated squat position. From squatting, the child extends to the vertical. This pattern of rising reaches a peak frequency at about the age of 7 years and then gradually declines in frequency during later childhood.

Motor Skill Development During Later Childhood and Adolescence

Later childhood is typically the period from 7 to 10 or 12 years of age. During later childhood, adolescence, and throughout the rest of the human life span, changes in the form of movements are related to age. It appears that the individual is constantly seeking the most efficient form of movement within skills that have already been attained, as growth and the individual's life-style changes.

Children have strong drives to develop self-esteem, to be accepted socially, to become skillful, and to explore the limits of their physical being. In school and in various recreational activities, the child moves into situations in which competition and cooperation are strong components of physical activity. Later childhood is a time of slow but steady physical growth that allows gradual mastery of motor skills. Skills are perfected and stabilized prior to adolescence. Preferences for various sports and athletic activities emerge.

Boys and girls tend to socialize to physical activity differently. Despite rapid change in schools that provide increasing opportunity for girls to participate in physical activities, boys still have greater opportunities available to them for pursuing an active life-style. But both boys and girls are more likely to be active if parents provide opportunities for them to engage in physical activity. Both boys and girls demonstrate improved performance within all fundamental skills of early childhood. However, boys typically demonstrate greater speed and strength at all ages when compared to girls.

Adolescence begins with the physical changes that hallmark puberty and ends when physical growth has ceased. The age of onset of adolescence is approximately 11 to 12 years in girls and 12 to 13 years in boys. Growth spurts occur that likely lead to the emergence of new patterns of movement within the skills already acquired. Even though the process of age-related change in motor behavior continues throughout adolescence and adulthood, the motor skills that permit physical independence are acquired primarily during the first year after birth. Later periods of development seem to provide opportunities for further refinement and development of control and coordination, leading to improved performance within skills.

Contemporary Issues in Motor Development

Physical therapists' concepts of development have undergone great change over the past 10 years. We view developmental sequences quite differently now, we no longer regard reflexes as the building blocks of motor behavior, and we look to patients to assume increasingly active roles in determining the goals and outcomes of physical therapy. New theories are emerging that offer different explanations of the process of development.

Developmental Sequences

For a number of years, physical therapists viewed the process of motor development as a simple reflection of maturation of the nervous system. The order of development of skills during the first year of life was believed to be inherently determined, and could not be changed. This affected the way in which therapists assessed and treated individuals with developmental disabilities. Through an examination, the individual's developmental level was determined and treatment was planned that would replicate the order of development of skills leading to the ability to walk independently. The sequence of development was used as a prescription for progressing patients to independence. It was believed that each skill in the sequence was a necessary precursor to the next skill, and that no step could be skipped if independence was to be achieved. This somewhat restrictive view of the developmental sequence is being replaced with a less strict interpretation of the developmental sequence. Currently, therapists view the developmental sequence as a guide for understanding the general process by which one attains the ability to control the body against the force of gravity. Age-appropriate skills are of greater concern than replication of the sequence of accomplishments during infancy. For example, creeping is a locomotor pattern that is most common during infancy and early childhood. In the past, creeping was viewed as a precursor to walking, and individuals of all ages who were unable to walk would be taught to creep as a natural step in the progression to walking. Currently, therapists are increasingly concerned with age-appropriate skills. Beyond the period of infancy and early childhood, in our culture, creeping is less commonly used as a form of locomotion. As a result, therapists today are less likely to require older individuals to creep as a prerequisite to walking than were therapists a generation ago.

Reflexes as Fundamental Building Blocks of Motor Behavior

The discussion of the emerging motor behavior of the fetus provides an excellent example of the change in thinking regarding reflexes. Until recently, reflexes were viewed as the fundamental units of motor behavior, from which volitional movements and skilled actions evolved. Milani-Comparetti's work interpreting the spontaneous movements of the fetus while in utero represents an increasing tendency to reject models of human development that do not recognize the primary and fundamental capacity of the individual to generate behavior. This recognition of the self-generation of movement is termed an *active organism* concept. It replaces the traditional view that the fetus and infant are incapable of generating movement and rejects the theory that the young individual is a reflexive being, dependent on external stimuli to activate the motor system—a *passive organism.*

The passive organism concept has permeated many treatment theories in physical therapy. The facilitation and inhibition of reflexes are outgrowths of this concept. For many years, facilitation procedures were the primary tools therapists used to remediate movement disorders. Recently, however, therapists have been attaching increased importance to movements that the patient generates. An emphasis on teaching and learning motor skills is replacing traditional facilitation approaches. Learning requires the individual to be an active participant, receiving and interpreting feedback and generating corrective action.

Coupled with the recognition of the patient's role in generating activity has been the increased recognition of the patient's role in determining the goals and outcomes of physical therapy. For young children, this translates to families assuming a greater role in determining the goals of treatment and carrying out treatment procedures for their child. Those receiving treatment are less passive and more active now than they were expected to be in years past.

New Theory of Motor Development

Contemporary theories do not rest as strongly on the CNS as the cause of motor development. Other body systems, such as the musculoskeletal system and the cardiorespiratory system, are also assumed to play a role in the process of motor development. Further, the environment represents a significant source of systematic change that influences motor development. Rather than simple singular causes of change, systems theories recognize the complex multiple causes of development. Although one factor might be found to be a catalyst for change, it is now recognized that no single agent is "the cause" of motor development. All systems are seen as undergoing constant change and are, therefore, dynamic. It is the interaction of these dynamic systems that promotes development of motor skills.

Therapists who formerly looked to the nervous system as the controller of motor skill development are now recognizing the influence of other factors, such as body size, motivation, and the environmental context in which skills occur, as important agents of developmental change. Systems theories are becoming increasingly well known and are beginning to guide research by physical therapists.

This switch to new theories promises to lead to a greater understanding of how motor skills evolve, not only during infancy but also during childhood and adolescence.

Bibliography

Albinson JG, Andrew GM, eds. *Child in Sport and Physical Activity.* Baltimore: University Park Press; 1976.

Asher C. *Postural Variations in Childhood.* Boston: Butterworths; 1975.

Bayley N. *Bayley Scales of Infant Development.* New York: Psychological Corp; 1969.

Bobath B. *Abnormal Postural Reflex Activity Caused by Brain Lesions.* London: Wm Heinemann Medical Books Ltd; 1965.

Caplan F. *The First Twelve Months of Life.* Princeton, NJ: Edcom Systems; 1973.

Casaer P. *Postural Behavior in Newborn Infants.* Philadelphia: JB Lippincott; 1979.

Corbin CB. *A Textbook of Motor Development.* Dubuque, IA: Little Brown & Co; 1973.

Espenschade AS, Eckert HM. *Motor Development.* 2nd Ed. Columbus, OH: Charles E. Merrill Publishing Company; 1980.

Falkner F. *Human Development.* Philadelphia: WB Saunders; 1966.

Gallahue DL. *Understanding Motor Development in Children.* New York: John Wiley & Sons; 1982.

Gesell A. The ontogenesis of infant behavior. In: Carmichael L, ed. *Manual of Child Psychology.* 2nd ed. New York: John Wiley & Sons; 1954.

Gesell A, Ames LB. The ontogenetic organization of prone behavior in human infancy. *J Genet Psychol.* 1940;56:247–263.

Haywood K. *Life Span Motor Development.* Urbanna, IL: Human Kinetics; 1987.

Holt KS, ed. *Movement and Child Development.* London: Wm Heinemann Medical Books Ltd; 1975.

Hooker D. *The Origin of Overt Behavior.* Ann Arbor: University of Michigan Press; 1944.

Humphrey T. Postnatal repetition of human prenatal activity sequences with some suggestions of their neuroanatomical basis. In: Robinson RJ, ed. *Brain and Early Behavior. Development in the Fetus and Infant.* New York: Academic Press; 1969.

Jacobs MJ. Development of normal motor behavior. *Am J Phys Med.* 1967;46:41–51.

Kugler PN, Kelso JAS, Turvey MT. On the control and coordination of naturally developing systems. In: Kelso JAS, Clark JE, eds. *The Development of Movement Control and Coordination.* New York: John Wiley & Sons; 1982.

Levine MD, Carey WB, Crocker AC, Gross RT, eds. *Developmental Behavioral Pediatrics.* Philadelphia: WB Saunders; 1983.

Lowry GH. *Growth and Development of Children.* 8th Ed. Chicago: Yearbook Medical Publishers; 1986.

MacDonald J. *Developmental Ordering of the Movement Patterns in Infants Rolling Supine to Prone.* Richmond: Virginia Commonwealth University, 1988. Thesis.

McGraw MB. *The Neuromuscular Maturation of the Human Infant.* New York: Hafner; 1963.

Milani-Comparetti A. Pattern analysis of normal and abnormal development: The fetus, the newborn, the child. In: Slaton DS, ed. *Development of Movement in Infancy.* Chapel Hill, NC: University of North Carolina, Division of Physical Therapy; 1981.

Payne VG, Issacs LD. *Human Motor Development: A Lifespan Approach.* 2nd Ed. Mountain View, CA: Mayfield Publishing Co; 1991.

Roberton MA, Halverson LE. *Developing Children—Their Changing Movement.* Philadelphia: Lea & Febiger; 1984.

Saint-Anne Dargassies S. *The Neuro-motor and Psychoaffective Development of the Infant.* New York: Elsevier; 1986.

Shirley MM. *The First Two Years: A Study of Twenty-five Babies.* Minneapolis: University of Minnesota Press; 1931.

Short-DeGraff MA. *Human Development for Occupational and Physical Therapists.* Baltimore, MD: Williams & Wilkins; 1988.

Smolak L. *Infancy.* Englewood Cliffs, NJ: Prentice Hall; 1986.

Stockmeyer S. An interpretation of the approach of Rood to the treatment of neuromuscular dysfunction. *Am J Phys Med.* 1967;46:900–956.

Tanner JM. *Fetus into Man: Physical Growth from Conception to Maturity.* Cambridge, MA: Harvard University Press; 1978.

Touwen B. *Neurological Development in Infancy.* London: Wm Heinemann Medical Books Ltd; 1976.

Van Sant AF. Life-span motor development. In: Lister M, ed. *Contemporary Management of Motor Control Problems.* Alexandria, VA: Foundation for Physical Therapy; 1991:77–84.

Voss, DE. Proprioceptive neuromuscular facilitation. *Am J Phys Med.* 1967;46:838–898.

Wickstrom R. *Fundamental Motor Patterns.* 3rd ed. Philadelphia: Lea & Febiger, 1983.

Wyke B. The neurological basis of movement: A developmental review. In: Holt K, ed. *Movement and Child Development.* Philadelphia: JB Lippincott; 1975.

Pediatric Physical Therapy, second edition, edited by Jan Stephen Tecklin. J. B. Lippincott Company, Philadelphia © 1994.

2

Susan K. Brenneman

Tests of Infant and Child Development

Physical therapists are important members of the professional team working with disabled children. They must have the skill and knowledge to contribute to the assessment of children, as the assessment process is a professional responsibility that serves the purpose of keeping the therapist's work current. *Assessment* is a continuing process of collecting and organizing relevant information in order to plan and implement effective treatment. It is important for therapists to base their treatment recommendations on appropriate tools of assessment.

A broad view of the child's difficulty and its functional significance is the most important aspect of the assessment. Children may present with a wide variety of behavioral difficulties, and the physical therapist must determine how best to help them function to their fullest potential. Although some aspects of the disability may be better dealt with by other disciplines, whereas other aspects are best handled by physical therapists, rigid division of labor among professionals is unwise. Depending on training and competence, the traditional roles of physical therapist, occupational therapist, and speech therapist may overlap. Most physical therapists, however, will be concerned mainly with the child's basic gross motor adaptation to the environment.[1]

The challenge for the physical therapist is to accurately assess and comprehend the significance of any delay that falls outside the limits of normal variability. Knowledge of the normal, orderly sequence of developmental achievement and patterns of integration is the basis upon which significant deviation in maturation is gauged.[2] The physical therapist, therefore, must be knowledgeable about normal development, as presented in Chapter 1. Understanding this broad developmental scope forms the basis for therapeutic intervention. Developmental milestones present the major clinical parameter of progressive growth and integration in the central nervous system (CNS). It is important to focus on those aspects of motor behavior that are of greatest concern. Because of the focus of their education, most physical therapists' emphasis is on muscles and joints, rather than on total patterns of motor behavior. However, it is not acceptable to deal with isolated parts, such as a foot, gait, or the spine.[1]

A battery of tests is required to assess a child adequately. Developmental assessment tests are only one type of test used. Another category of assessment that is addressed in this chapter is that of functional capabilities. Subsequent chapters will address assessment that are unique to a particular disability, completing the total assessment for the child with that disability.

Purposes of Developmental Testing

Use of developmental tests as screening tools promotes early intervention for deviations from normal growth and development in young children. Early identification of deviations facilitates the provision of anticipatory advice to parents, clinicians, and caregivers for future planning. Early recognition and a focused plan for intervention may prevent severe disability.

Developmental tests can assist in determining a diagnosis. Comprehensive scales, such as the Gesell scale,[3] specify problem areas and indicate whether a developmental problem is likely to include all areas of development or one focal area, such as gross motor development.

Developmental tests also facilitate the planning of a treatment program. Developmental scales provide valuable information about the level of operation of the child or the milestones reached. Developmental tests indicate where treatment should begin, and they provide information by which the progression of a therapeutic regimen can be guided. An explanation of developmental tests and their results may help parents understand the child's limitations—what can and cannot be expected—making it possible to establish common goals and to plan for the future. The results of developmental testing may reveal specific areas of deficit that require additional evaluation to discover the underlying cause of the delay.

Subsequent assessments will reveal the rate and trend of development of a child. After determining goals for the child, tests can be used to monitor progress and determine whether and when the child has achieved the goals. Therapists involved in research rely on developmental assessments to evaluate strategies for treatment and means of intervention. Research continues to evaluate the assessments themselves to ensure their reliability and validity. Developmental assessments. as well as being used as a clinical research tool, can also be used for evaluation of a program.

The ways in which test data are to be used should be determined before testing so that one can avoid the collection of superfluous data and so that all necessary information is obtained. It is a waste of time and effort to perform extensive tests just to be thorough, unless all the information gained will be used. As a therapist becomes skilled in the administration of developmental assessments, the ability to test what is appropriate will improve.

Basic Methods of Assessment

Decisions regarding intervention are usually based on information from various resources. Several basic methods are used to collect information about a child. A questioning mind is important in this process. Therapists must know what questions to ask both of themselves and of others. Guiding questions during clinical observation provides the foundation for all further screening or formal evaluation.

Among the most valuable skills a therapist can possess are the abilities to observe, to be flexible and spontaneous, and to be creative with play and other activities that foster intrinsic motivation in children.[4] Different methods and adaptations must be used for assessment because children are different from adults.

Orientation of the child and the parents to the environment is crucial. Both parent and child must feel comfortable with the therapist and the setting. This orientation is often best achieved by proceeding with the evaluation at a slow pace, and by adapting one's approach according to the reaction of the child.

During the assessment, the therapist needs to take a broad view of the child, whatever the disability. The child should not merely be labeled a "crutch walker," a "hemi," or "clumsy." Rather, the child is a person with a suspected disability, and the therapist's initial task is to be thorough and sensitive in discovering whether a disability or sensorimotor delay exists and what can be done to reduce the effects of the disability.[4]

Interview

An interview with the child and the parents provides important information about the development of the child. In many cases because of the young age of the child, the interview will be conducted exclusively with the parents. An interview should be friendly and informal rather than impersonal and inquisitive. The purpose of the interview should be clear, and the interviewer should know specifically what information is desired. A skillful and well-directed interview will help to fill in the gaps of an assessment. The therapist should be able to determine the area of greatest concern to the parents, and should note the age and circumstances in which the problem was first discovered.

History

A review of the child's developmental and medical history provides valuable information. A developmental history can be obtained through a questionnaire or an interview. The possible lack of reliability and bias of the parent should be considered in assessing the information gained in the history.

The medical records of a child may provide information regarding precautions, patient health status, previous medical history, suspected diagnosis, prognosis, medications, and other factors impacting on the child's health. The therapist should obtain information about the family and its genetic history; the pregnancy, labor, and delivery of the child; and the perinatal and neonatal events. This information will be useful in performing a comprehensive assessment.

Clinical Observation

Assessment begins by observation of the child at rest in various positions and during unstructured movement, as presented in Chapter 4. The therapist should also observe the child interacting with the environment, the child's social responses and communication, and the child's cognition. This observation can be done in a nonthreatening manner while the therapist is talking with the parents and establishing rapport with the child.

Tools for Assessment

After interviewing and observing the child, the administration of standardized and criterion- and norm-referenced assessments will yield an overall picture of the child's level of functioning. Tests of developmental assessment will help to identify which specific tests of functioning (e.g., goniometry, manual testing of muscles, or assessment of activities of daily living [ADL]) are needed. Those specific tests and methods used for various disabilities in childhood are reviewed in subsequent chapters.

Definitions

Terms for Understanding Standardized Assessments[5]

An *age-equivalent score* is the mean chronologic age represented by a certain test score. For example, a raw score of 52 on the Bayley Mental Scales represents an age equivalent of $4\frac{1}{2}$ months. Age-equivalent scores may be especially useful with developmentally delayed children for whom it may be impossible to derive a meaningful developmental index. Age-equivalent scores are easy for parents to understand, but they must be interpreted carefully because they can be misleading. Usually these children have qualitative differences in their behaviors, as well as a wide mixture of successes and failures on developmental tests.

The *criterion-referenced test* is one in which scores are interpreted on the basis of absolute criteria (e.g., the number of items answered correctly) rather than on relative criteria, such as how the rest of the normal group performed. Such tests are usually developed by the teacher or researcher and can be used for research involving a comparison of groups, just as norm-referenced tests are used. Criterion-referenced tests are used to measure a person's mastery of a set of behavioral objectives. The tests represents an attempt to maximize the validity or appropriateness of the content based on that set of objectives. The *developmental quotient* is the ratio between the child's actual score (developmental age) on a test and the child's chronologic age. An example is motor age/chronologic age equal to the motor quotient (MQ).

Norm-referenced or standardized tests use normative values as standards for interpreting individual test scores. The purpose of standardized tests is to make a comparison between a particular child and the "norm" or "average" of a group of children. Norms describe a person's test score relative to a large body of scores that have already been collected on a defined population. Examples of norm-referenced tests include the Bayley Scales of Infant Development,[6] the Denver II Screening Test,[7] and the Gesell Developmental Scales.[3]

The *percentile score* indicates the number of children of the same age or grade level (or whatever is used for a source of comparison) who would be expected to score lower than the child tested. For example, a child who scores in the 75th percentile on a norm-referenced test has done better than 75% of the children in the norm group.

A *raw score* is the total of individual items that are passed or correct on a particular test. On many tests, this will require establishing a basal and ceiling level of performance. The number of items required to achieve a basal or ceiling level varies from one test to another.

Reliability refers to consistency or repeatability between measurements in a series. Types of reliability include interobserver and test–retest. Interobserver reliability describes the relationship between items passed and failed, or the percentage of agreement, between two independent observers. Simply stated, interobserver reliability is an index of whether two different testers obtain the same score on a test. Test–retest reliability is the relationship of a person's score on the first administration of the test to the score on the second administration. Simply stated, this type of reliability determines whether the same or similar scores are achieved when the test is repeated under identical conditions.

Standard error of measurement (SEM) is a measure of reliability that indicates the precision of an individual test score. The SEM gives an estimate of the margin of error associated with a particular test score. For example, a Mental Development Index (MDI), from the Bayley Developmental Scales, at 12 months has an associated SEM of 6.7 points. This SEM means that one is 67% certain that the child's true MDI falls within 6.7 points of the obtained score.

Standard scores are expressed as deviations or variations from the mean score for a group. Standard scores are expressed in units of standard deviation. When using standard scores, information is needed concerning the mean and standard deviation of the standard score.

Validity is an indication of the extent to which a test measures what it purports to measure. *Construct validity* is an examination of the theory or hypothetical constructs underlying the test. *Content validity* assesses the appropriateness of the test or how well the content of the test samples the subject matter or behaviors about which conclusions must be drawn. The sample situations measured in the test must be representative of the set from which the sample is drawn. There are two types of *criterion-related validity*. *Concurrent validity* relates the performance on the test to performance on another well-known and accepted test that measures the same knowledge or behavior. *Predictive validity* means that the child's performance on the test predicts some actual behavior.

Sensitivity can be defined as the ability of a test to identify correctly those who actually have a disorder. High sensitivity results in few false-negative scores.

Specificity refers to the ability of the test to identify correctly those who do not have the disorder. High specificity results in few false-positive scores.

The positive predictive value of a test is defined as the proportion of true positives among all those who have positive results. *The negative predictive value* is the proportion of true negatives among all those who have negative screening results.

Guidelines for Selection of Tests

There is no lack of tests that purport to measure motor abilities of children. The problem is not quantity, but quality.[8] Careful and knowledgeable selection of tests is, therefore, important. If evaluators are unaware of the strengths, weaknesses, limitations, and restrictions of the tests being used, there is a high probability that an inappropriate test could be used, thus resulting in inaccurate or misinterpreted information.[9] Most published tests have some limitations or restrictions to their use, particularly regarding the ages and populations for whom they were developed and on whom they were standardized. The result of disregarding these restrictions could be the misuse of the test or misinterpretation of the outcomes.

In order to choose an appropriate test, some guidelines by which to evaluate a test are needed. Stangler and associates have proposed six criteria for evaluating a screening test that can be applied to any assessment test: (1) acceptability, (2) simplicity, (3) cost, (4) appropriateness, (5) reliability, and (6) validity. Every test may not fulfill each criterion; however, the test may be used knowledgeably if a therapist is aware of the limitations.

Acceptability is defined as acceptance to all who will be affected by the test, including the children and families screened, the professionals who receive resulting referrals, and the community. *Simplicity* is the ease by which a test can be taught, learned, and administered. *Appropriateness* of screening tests is based on the prevalence of the problem to be screened and on the applicability of the test to the particular population. *Cost* includes the actual cost of equipment, preparation and payment of personnel, the cost of inaccurate results, personal costs to the person being screened, and the total cost of the test in relation to the benefits of early detection.[10] In addition, tests must show both *reliability* and *validity*, as discussed previously.

Using Questions as Guidelines

A therapist can further ensure appropriate selection of the test by posing several questions regarding the test:

1. *For what purpose will the test be used?*
   - For diagnosis
   - For program planning
   - For research
2. *Who is the child?*
   - Age

- Suspected diagnosis
- Presenting disability

3. *What content areas need to be assessed?*
   - Gross motor
   - Fine motor
   - Speech
   - Muscle strength
   - Comprehensive assessment of functional capabilities

4. *What are the constraints for the examiner?*
   - Time
   - Training
   - Space and equipment
   - Money

Test Analysis Format

The Test Analysis Format developed by Clark and associates is another method for evaluating a test[4] (Display 2-1). An adapted version of this format is used to review the assessment tools in this chapter. After careful consideration of the aforementioned questions and criteria, the therapist should consult sources, including catalogs, books, and other therapists, to locate possible choices. The therapist should be sure to review several manuals thoroughly, to learn the tests and use them, and to evaluate the results.

Overview Test

Assessment may be considered in several broad categories. Screening tests are used to identify deficits in a child's performance that indicate the need for further services. Assessments of component functions address specific areas of functioning (e.g., gross motor ability or reflex status). Comprehensive developmental scales evaluate all areas of development. Functional assessments evaluate the essential skills that are required in the child's natural environments of home and school.

The rest of the chapter reviews selected tests that

Display 2-1
Test Analysis Format*

Title and authors:

What the test proposes to measure:

Population for whom the test was developed:

Test format

A. Type or instrument
B. Content of test
C. Administration
D. Scoring
E. Interpretation

Include information about the basic type of instrument that is being used—for example, interview, criterion-referenced or standardized test. Briefly discuss the basic guidelines for administration that pertain to the entire test. For example, is information obtained by a report from parents or by presenting tasks to children? How is the test set up? In general, are there time limits for items? Include basic information about procedures for scoring and interpretation.

Advantages of the test:

Disadvantages of the test:

Purchasing information:

References:

*Adapted by permission from Pratt PN, Allen AS: Occupational Therapy for Children. 2nd ed. St. Louis: CV Mosby; 1989.

---

are available. Some of the more widely known standardized evaluative procedures are presented, as are some tests which are not standardized, but which have proven useful in clinical practice. The categories just mentioned are used for organization.

Screening Tests

Screening tests are intended to differentiate between those persons who are normal and healthy in a particular respect from those who are not.[9] These tests typically raise more questions than answers, but the questions raised can be used to guide the selection of formal measures for evaluation.

Milani-Comparetti Motor Development Screening Test

The Milani-Comparetti Screening Test was developed by Italian neurologists Milani-Comparetti and Gidoni.[11] The original score form was modified by the staff at Meyer Children's Rehabilitation Institute, University of Nebraska Medical Center.[12] The current test manual, which is in its 3rd edition,[13] was written to provide additional clarification of the testing and scoring procedures, to document reliability data, and to revise the developmental milestones of the original score form to reflect a normative sample.

Test Measures and Target Population

Motor development is evaluated on the basis of a correlation between the functional motor achievement of the child and the underlying reflex structures.[11] The appropriate population for testing comprises children from birth to approximately 2 years of age.

Test Construction

The items included on the chart were not randomly selected or based on the statistical difference between normal and abnormal. Rather, Milani-Comparetti selected a parameter for study which involved items that were interrelated. This interrelatedness is described by a correlation between functional motor achievement and underlying reflex structures. The parameter chosen is called "standing," and is better translated from Italian to English to mean antigravity control of the body axis. This control includes head control and control while sitting, as well as control while standing. "Standing" was found to be a suitable parameter because it includes as essential and significant components a limited number of specific reactions, such as righting, parachute, and tilting reactions.[11] The original chart used in administering the test was developed after 5 years of experience in a child welfare clinic.

Test Format

TYPE. The test is criterion-referenced, and the 3rd Edition of the test provides manual normative data.[13] The examiner physically manipulates the child for a particular motor response. Parents can provide information if the child is uncooperative.

CONTENT. The illustrated manual developed by Meyer Rehabilitation Center provides instructions for test administration and scoring. The score chart can be reused at successive examinations (Fig. 2-1).

ADMINISTRATION. The original scoring chart developed by Milani-Comparetti has been revised to permit smoother, more rapid administration of the test. All of the original test procedures and scoring mechanisms are retained in the revision; they are simply placed in a different order for more efficient testing.[13] The chart integrates spontaneous behavior and evoked responses in a manner that is easy to follow and is based on the examination sequence. The child should be positioned for only the test items relevant to a particular age, expressed in months. Experienced observers can give the test in 4 to 8 minutes.

SCORING. The chart is a shaded graph indicating the time span during which a reflex or reaction is expected to be present. The child's age in months is used to score each item tested and is placed on the age line at which the child performs. Responses are judged as being either absent or present. Completion results in a graphic profile of the child's motor

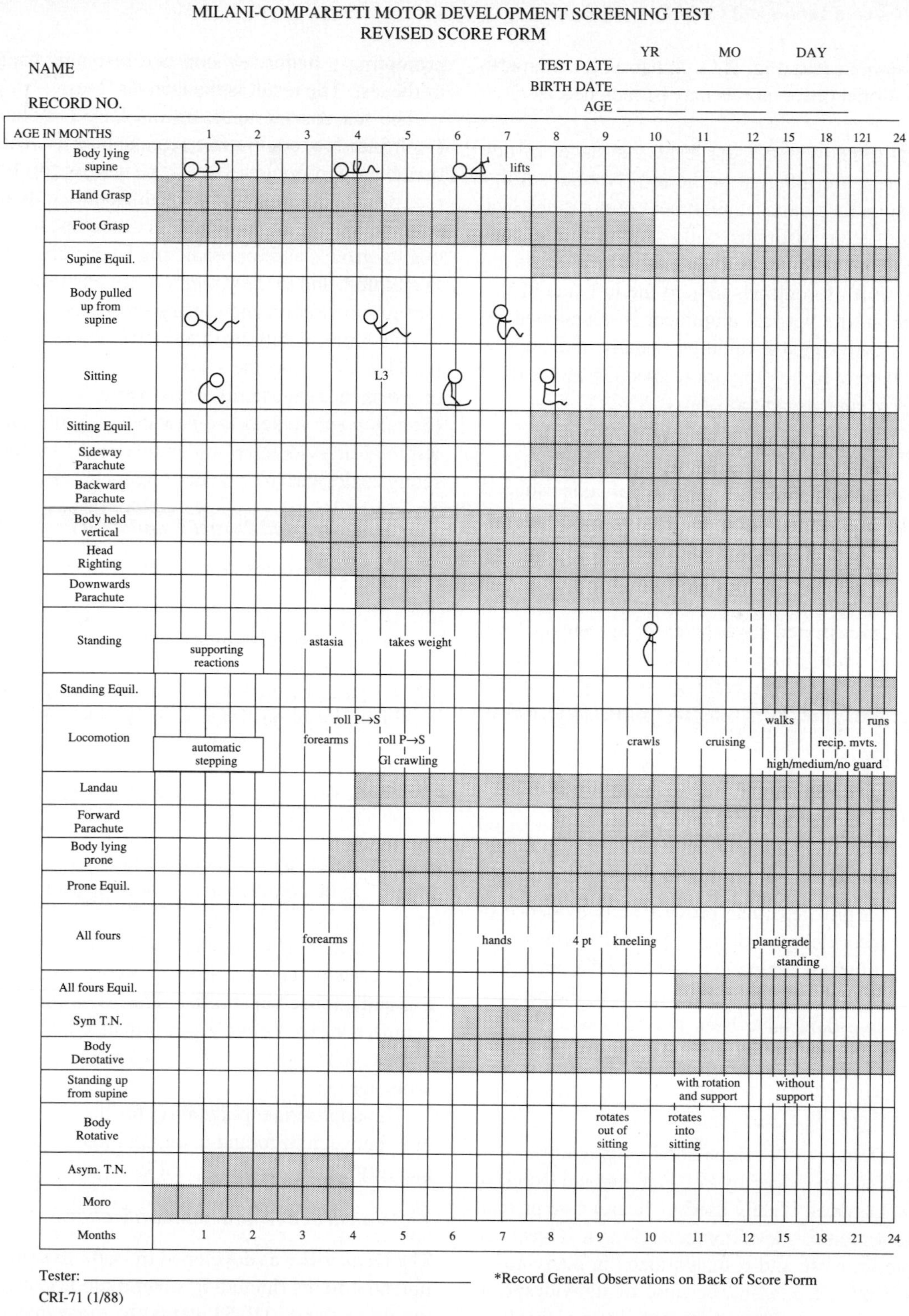

MILANI-COMPARETTI MOTOR DEVELOPMENT SCREENING TEST
REVISED SCORE FORM

NAME

RECORD NO.

	YR	MO	DAY
TEST DATE			
BIRTH DATE			
AGE			

AGE IN MONTHS	1	2	3	4	5	6	7	8	9	10	11	12	15	18	121	24
Body lying supine							lifts									
Hand Grasp																
Foot Grasp																
Supine Equil.																
Body pulled up from supine																
Sitting				L3												
Sitting Equil.																
Sideway Parachute																
Backward Parachute																
Body held vertical																
Head Righting																
Downwards Parachute																
Standing	supporting reactions		astasia	takes weight												
Standing Equil.																
Locomotion	automatic stepping		forearms / roll P→S	roll P→S / Gl crawling					crawls		cruising	walks / high/medium/no guard	recip. mvts.	runs		
Landau																
Forward Parachute																
Body lying prone																
Prone Equil.																
All fours	forearms		hands	4 pt	kneeling						plantigrade standing					
All fours Equil.																
Sym T.N.																
Body Derotative																
Standing up from supine									with rotation and support		without support					
Body Rotative							rotates out of sitting	rotates into sitting								
Asym. T.N.																
Moro																
Months	1	2	3	4	5	6	7	8	9	10	11	12	15	18	21	24

Tester: _____   *Record General Observations on Back of Score Form

CRI-71 (1/88)

Figure 2-1. *Revised scoring chart used for the Milani-Comparetti Motor Development Screening Test. (Stuberg W. The Milani-Comparetti Motor Development Screening Test. 3rd ed. Appendix B. Omaha: University of Nebraska Medical Center; 1992.)*

development (see Fig. 2-1). A narrative summary of additional observations may be included.

INTERPRETATION. Age levels for stages of development are inherent in the test. Normal results are shown by a vertical alignment of notations that are consistent with the child's chronologic age. Motor retardation usually appears as a homogeneous shift of notations toward the left side of the graph, but the vertical alignment is maintained. A wider scattering of findings usually indicates a more severe, or possibly more specific, motor dysfunction, such as cerebral palsy.

Reliability and Validity

Interobserver reliability results of one study[14] showed a high percentage of agreement, ranging from 79% to 98%. The most consistently high level of agreement was noted for active movement and postural control items. Overall, equilibrium reactions demonstrated lower levels of agreement, with standing equilibrium being the lowest scored item at 79%. Test–retest reliability results[14] showed percentages of agreement ranging from 82% to 100%.

Advantages

This screening test is practical and useful. It can be given quickly and does not require any special equipment or setting. The test can be learned quickly and is easily scored. By providing a developmental profile, it can provide early evidence of neuromotor delay or deficits, possibly indicating a need for further evaluation. The test relies on objective observations, rather than reports by the parents. Normative data have been provided with the 3rd Edition.

Denver II

The Denver Developmental Screening Test (DDST),[15] developed by Frankenburg and Dodds in 1967, has been widely used by health care providers to screen for developmental delays. It has been adapted for use and restandardized in many countries. Both despite and because of its widespread usage, there have been many criticisms of this tool,

prompting a major revision and restandardization of the test. The result is the Denver II test.[7,16]

The reasons for updating the DDST included: (1) the need for additional language items; (2) questionable appropriateness of 1967 norms for 1990; (3) changes in items that were difficult to administer or score; (4) appropriateness of the test for various subgroups and for predicting later performance in children, and (5) new methods for ensuring accurate administration and scoring of the test.[17]

The major additions to and differences between the Denver II and the DDST are: (1) an 86% increase in language items; (2) two articulation items; (3) a new age scale; (4) a new category of item interpretation to identify milder delays; (5) a behavior rating scale, and (6) new training materials.[17]

Test Measures and Target Population

The Denver II screens general development in four areas:

1. Personal-Social: Getting along with people and caring for personal needs
2. Fine Motor-Adaptive: Eye-hand coordination, manipulation of small objects, and problem-solving
3. Language: Hearing, understanding, and use of language
4. Gross Motor: Sitting, walking, jumping, and overall large muscle movement

Also included are five items documenting "test behavior" to be completed after administration of the test.

The Denver II is not an IQ test, nor is it designed to generate diagnostic labels or predict future adaptive and intellectual abilities. The test is best used to compare a given child's performance on a variety of tasks to the performance of other children of the same age.

The appropriate population for the test are children between birth and 6 years of age who are apparently well.

Test Construction and Standardization

The Denver II was developed by administering 326 potential items (including several modifications of the original 105 DDST items) to more than 2000 children who were considered to be representative of demographic variables within the Colorado population. Each item was administered an average of 540 times. Composite norms for the total sample and norms for subgroups (based on gender, ethnicity, maternal education, and place of residence) were used to determine new age norms. The *Denver II Technical Manual*[17] contains details of the standardization process.

Test Format

TYPE. The test is norm-referenced, with data presented as age norms, similar to physical growth curve.[16] Subnorms for various subgroups that differ in a clinically significant manner from norms depicted on the reference chart are presented in the Technical Manual.[17]

CONTENT. The Denver II has 125 items arranged on the test form in four sections: Personal-Social, Fine Motor-Adaptive, Language, and Gross Motor (Fig. 2-2). Age scales across the top and bottom of the test form depict ages, expressed in months and years, from birth to 6 years. Each test item is represented on the form by a bar that spans the ages at which 25%, 50%, 75%, and 90% of the standardization sample passed that item.[7] A standardized test kit, forms, and manuals are purchased to administer the Denver II.

ADMINISTRATION. This test generally depends on the examiner's observation of the child. Although certain items may be scored based on the verbal report of a parent (as indicated on the test form by an "R"), observation of the particular task is a more reliable method of scoring. Correct calculation of the child's age is important because correct interpretation of test results depends on accuracy of the age. Although the order of presenting the test items is flexible, the items must be given in the manner specified in the manual. The number of items given varies with the age and abilities of the child. The examiner should begin by administering every item intersected by the age line and at least three items nearest to and totally to the left of the

age line. Continued testing depends on whether the goal is to identify developmental delays or the relative strengths of the child.[7] "Test Behavior" ratings are scored after the completion of the test.

SCORING. Each item given should be scored on the bar at the 50% hatch mark. Items are scored as a pass (P), failure (F), no opportunity (N.O.), or refusal (R).

INTERPRETATION. The Denver II identifies the child whose development appears to be delayed in comparison to that of other children, and identifies changes in development within one child over time. Individual items should be interpreted first, with the entire test being interpreted last.

Individual items are interpreted as "advanced," "normal," "caution," "delayed," or "no opportunity." The entire Denver II test is interpreted as "normal," "suspect," or "untestable." A child whose scores are interpreted as suspect or untestable on the first test should be screened again before referral for further diagnostic evaluation.

The *Denver II Technical Manual* contains data regarding the results that might be expected so that, in cases when marked deviation is noted, the evaluator may compare with other experiences.

Reliability and Validity

Thirty-eight children from 10 age groups were tested twice on each of two occasions separated by an interval of 7 to 10 days. The mean examiner-observer reliability was found to be 0.99, with a range of 0.95 to 1.00 and a standard deviation of 0.016. The mean 7- to 10-day test–retest reliability for the same items was 0.90, with a range of 0.50 to 1.00 and a standard deviation of 0.12.[17]

The validity of the Denver II rests upon its standardization, not on its correlation with other tests, as all tests are constructed slightly differently.[17]

Advantages

Administration and scoring is done quickly and the test is acceptable to both children and parents. The *Denver II Training Manual*[7] gives detailed instruc-

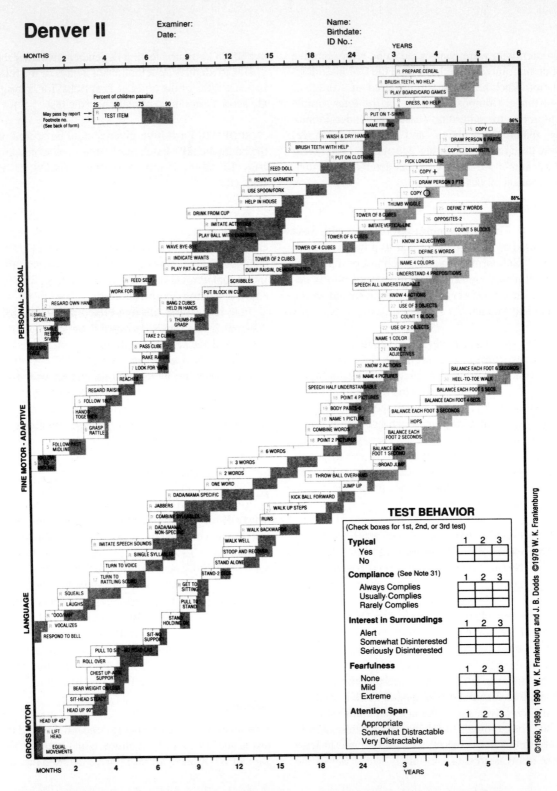

Figure 2-2. *Test form for the Denver II Screening test. (Frankenburg WK, Dodds J, Archer P, et al. Denver II Training Manual. Denver, CO: Denver Developmental Materials, Inc.; 1992.)*

tions for proper administration and interpretation of the tests. The *Denver II Technical Manual*[17] contains information on training personnel in the administration of the test and on the establishment of a community screening program. A videotaped instructional program and proficiency test have also been developed for the Denver II. This test is excellent for identifying children who are at risk for developmental problems and for monitoring a child longitudinally.

The authors of the Denver II stress that care should be taken not to use the test to generate diagnostic labels. Rather, it is more appropriately used as a "first step in tackling the problems of early detection, diagnosis, and treatment of developmental deviations in children."[17]

Tests of Motor Function

The physical therapist is concerned primarily with motor behavior. A large number of assessment tools are available that examine gross and fine motor function. The Movement Assessment of Infants, Peabody Developmental Motor Scales, and Bruininks-Oseretsky Test of Motor Proficiency are described.

Movement Assessment of Infants

The Movement Assessment of Infants (MAI) test was developed by Chandler and associates in response to the need for a systematic approach to the evaluation of motor function in infants who had been treated in a neonatal intensive care unit.[18]

Test Measures and Target Population

The test evaluates muscle tone, primitive reflexes, automatic reactions, and volitional movement in the first year of life. The MAI test, when given to infants at 4 months of age, provides an assessment of risk for motor dysfunction. According to the authors, the purposes of the test are (1) to identify motor dysfunction in infants up to 12 months of age, (2) to establish the basis for an early intervention program, (3) to monitor the effects of physical therapy on infants and children whose motor be-

havior is at, or below, 1 year of age, (4) to aid in research on motor development by using a standard system of assessment of movement, and (5) to teach skillful observation of movement and motor development through an evaluation of normal and handicapped children.[18] The test should not be used to identify the cause of any delay or to make a diagnosis.

The appropriate population for testing using the MAI are children birth through 12 months of age.

Test Construction and Standardization

The MAI test was created because of a need for a uniform approach to the evaluation of the high-risk infant. Over a period of 5 years of development and use, the MAI test was constantly modified and refined in order to improve its accuracy. When initially available, the test was still being developed and was distributed with a request by the authors for more research and revisions. Subsequent research studies[19–23] continue to refine and suggest revisions for the MAI.

Test Format

TYPE. The test is criterion-referenced. Results are obtained by direct handling and observation.

CONTENT. The test includes 65 items divided into four subtests: muscle tone, primitive reflexes, automatic reactions, and volitional movement. Muscle tone refers to the readiness of muscles to respond to gravity. Primitive reflexes are evaluated from fully integrated to reflex domination of movement. Automatic reactions include righting reaction, equilibrium reactions, and protective extension reactions. Volitional movement includes response to visual and auditory stimuli, production of sound, and typical motor milestones, such as hands to midline, fine grasp, rolling, and walking.

ADMINISTRATION. The MAI test is designed for use by physical and occupational therapists, physicians, nurses, psychologists, and others who have experience in the development of infants. Formal training is recommended for examiners using the

MAI test in research projects. A pleasant room with open space is needed, but little special equipment is required. The test manual describes the specific equipment needed. The MAI test requires 90 minutes for testing and scoring.

There is no particular order for giving items in the test. Items should be grouped by position in the test, by the amount of concentration required, and by the amount of distress. Observation of spontaneous activity and handling to assess postural tone and evoked behaviors are techniques used in testing.

SCORING. Numerical rating scales, which indicate the expected sequence of development, have been designed for each subtest. Each item has its own set of scoring criteria. Scoring should be done only by applying the criteria for the specific item. Scoring of all items must be based on the performance actually observed by the examiner.

INTERPRETATION. At this point in the development of the MAI test, no method is available for calculating a developmental score. A profile of a typical 4-month-old child is presented by the authors. This profile can be used for a comparison with the scores received by another child. An overall score indicating "degree of risk" of deviance from the norm is computed. At the four-month examination, the potential scores range from 0 to 48, with higher scores indicating greater deviance. The MAI authors suggest that children with total-risk scores of greater than 7 be identified as "at risk" in terms of motor development. Recent data on full term 4-month-old infants indicate a normal range of 0 to 13, with a mean of 6.0 and one standard deviation of 3.[21] An 8-month profile has also been developed by a group of researchers.[23]

Reliability and Validity

The test authors found an interobserver reliability of more than 90%.[18] Another study by Harris and associates showed an interobserver reliability of 0.72 and a test–retest reliability of 0.76.[24] Swanson and colleagues established interobserver reliability at a level of 0.90 agreement.[23]

Harris and associates studied the predictive validity of the MAI test by comparing test scores in infants at 4 months with specific diagnoses at 12 months of age.[25] They found an 11% rate of over-referrals and no under-referrals based on the MAI test scores at 4 months. Swanson and co-workers found strong correlations between MAI scores at 4 and 8 months and performance on the Bayley Scales at 18 months.[23] Sensitivity of the MAI was 83% at 4 months and 96% at 8 months. The specificity of the MAI at 4 months was 78%; this decreased to 65% at 8 months.

When working with at-risk infants, the most relevant information is afforded by the positive and negative predictive values of the test, which indicate the likelihood of normal or abnormal outcomes. The negative predictive value of the MAI is 85% and 91% at 4 and 8 months, respectively. The positive predictive value is 59% and 52% at 4 and 8 months, respectively, but is increased to 70% with sequential examinations.[23]

Advantages

The MAI test is a comprehensive and qualitative test of motor development. It is one of few assessment tools that consider the quality of movement. Recent studies show a high predictive validity for the MAI.

Disadvantages

The MAI test is lengthy to administer and requires extensive handling of the infant. Normative data are required to strengthen the ability to interpret and score the results. Studies have reported that numerous items have questionable reliability;[19,21,24] therefore, continued reliability and validity studies are needed to improve the usefulness of the MAI as a clinical tool.

Peabody Developmental Motor Scales

The Peabody Developmental Motor Scales (PDMS) and Activity Cards[26] represent a comprehensive program combining in-depth assessment with instructional programming. The test was developed by Folio and Fewell between 1969 and 1982.

Test Measures and Target Population

The PDMS provides a comprehensive sequence of gross and fine motor skills from which the therapist can determine the relative developmental skill level of a child, identify skills that are not completely developed or not in the child's repertoire, and plan an instructional program to develop those skills.[26]

Children from birth through 83 months of age are candidates for the text. The PDMS can be used with both able-bodied and disabled children.

Test Construction and Standardization

The PDMS was developed to improve on the existing instruments used for motor evaluation. Test items were obtained from validated motor scales, and new items were created based on studies of children's growth and development. The test was standardized on a sample of 617 children considered to be representative of the American population by geographical region, race, and sex.

Test Format

TYPE. The PDMS is an individually administered test. Instructions are provided that enable examiners to give the test to groups of children in a station-testing format. Although the PDMS is norm-referenced, it can be used as a criterion-referenced measure of motor patterns and skills.

CONTENT. The PDMS is divided into two components: the Gross Motor Scale and the Fine Motor Scale. The Gross Motor Scale contains 170 items divided into 17 age levels. The items are divided into five categories of skills, including reflexes, balance, nonlocomotor, locomotor, and receipt and propulsion of objects.

The Fine Motor Scale contains 112 items divided into 16 age levels. The items are classified into four skill categories that include grasping, use of hands, eye-hand coordination, and manual dexterity. Norms are provided for each skill category at each age level, as well as for total scores.

ADMINISTRATION. Both scales can be given to a child in approximately 45 to 60 minutes. Basal (item preceding earliest failure) and ceiling (item representing the most difficult success) rules are provided to eliminate unnecessary administration of items, thereby reducing the time taken for testing.

No specialized training is required to administer the scales and implement the activities, although the examiner should be thoroughly familiar with and have had practice in giving the test. In order to use the PDMS norms for valid interpretation of a child's performance, the scales must be given exactly as specified, including the presentation of materials, verbal instructions to the child, and adherence to basal and ceiling rules.[26] When instructional programming is the main purpose for testing, the directions can be adapted to fit the child's handicapped condition while retaining the intent of the item.

SCORING. The norms of the PDMS are based on scoring each item as 0, 1, or 2. Specific criteria are given for each item, as are the general criteria for the numerical scores. Scores are assigned as follows:

0—The child cannot or will not attempt the item.
1—The child's performance shows a clear resemblance to the item criterion, but does not fully meet the criterion. (This value allows for emerging skills.)
2—The child accomplishes the item according to the specified item criterion.

INTERPRETATION. Raw scores are determined and can be converted, by using the norms tables, to normative scores, which included percentile rank scores, standard scores, age-equivalent scores, and scaled scores. After the standard scores have been determined, they may be plotted on the Motor Development Profile. This profile provides a means of visually comparing performance on the Gross Motor Scale and Fine Motor Scale and on the skill categories in each scale.

Reliability and Validity

Test–retest reliability for the total score is 0.99 for both scales. The test–retest reliability is 0.95 for items given on the Gross Motor Scale and 0.8 for the Fine Motor Scale.[26] Interobserver reliability for total scores is 0.99 for both scales. When calculated on an item-by-item basis, the reliability coefficients are 0.97 for the Gross Motor and 0.94 for the Fine Motor Scale.[26] Subsequent research has shown similar results for interobserver reliability.[27] The strong reliability data indicate that PDMS is a highly stable assessment instrument.

According to the authors, the content validity of PDMS is based on established research into normal children's motor development and on other validated tests assessing motor development.[26] All of the data related to construct validity indicate that PDMS is a valid instrument for assessing motor development and that PDMS can discriminate motor problems from normal developmental variability.[26]

Advantages

The PDMS is a standardized, reliable, and valid assessment tool that is both norm-referenced and criterion-referenced and that allows the scales to meet the needs of various users. The three-point scoring system enables examiners to identify emerging skills and to measure progress in children who are slow in acquiring new skills. The scales are translated into a specific instructional program—the activity cards. Administration can be adapted for disabled children.

Disadvantages

Several drawbacks of the PDMS have been identified by its researchers and users.[27,28] The Peabody kit does not provide all of the items necessary for administration of the Fine Motor and Gross Motor scales, thus threatening standardization. The test manual does not provide clear criteria for each item for assigning a score of 1, thereby leaving the raters to decide whether there is a resemblance to the criteria needed for a successful performance.

Bruininks-Oseretsky Test of Motor Proficiency

The Bruininks-Oseretsky Test (BOT) of Motor Proficiency was developed by Dr. Robert H. Bruininks and is based partly on the American adaptation of the Oseretsky Tests of Motor Proficiency.[29] Although some similarity exists between the items in the two tests, the revised test reflects important advances in content, structure, and technical qualities.[29]

Test Measures and Target Population

The BOT is designed to assess gross and fine motor functioning in children so that a decision can be made about appropriate educational and therapeutic placement. The Complete Battery—eight subtests comprising 46 separate items—provides a comprehensive index of motor proficiency, as well as separate measures of both gross and fine motor skills.

This test is appropriate for children from $4\frac{1}{2}$ to $14\frac{1}{2}$ years of age. This test is designed for use with normal and developmentally disabled populations.

Test Construction and Standardization

Development and evaluation of the BOT has been extensive. The test has been standardized on a sample of 765 children who were carefully selected on the basis of age, sex, size of their community, and geographic location based on the 1970 census in the United States.

Test Format

TYPE. The BOT is norm-referenced and it involves individually administered tasks with direct observation and assessment of a child in a structured environment.

CONTENT. Each of the eight subtests is designed to assess an important aspect of motor development. The fine motor tests include coordination of the upper limbs, speed of response, visuomotor control, and speed and dexterity of the upper limbs. The subtests for gross motor skills assess speed and agility while turning, balance, bilateral coordination, and strength. The relationship of the eight sub-tests to the composites is shown in Figure 2-3.

ADMINISTRATION. The entire battery can be given in 45 to 60 minutes. Two short testing sessions are recommended for young children. A large area, relatively free from distraction, is required. Examiners do not need special training, but they must be familiar with the directions for giving the test. Procedures for administration and scoring of the test are well written and are shown in the manual. All of the materials needed to administer the BOT are provided in the standardized test kit.

SCORING. The person's raw scores are recorded during the administration of the test and are converted first to point scores, then to standard scores and approximate age equivalents (see Fig. 2-4 for a sample record form).

INTERPRETATION. Tables of norms are provided, and by comparing derived scores with the scores of subjects tested in the standardization pro-gram, users can interpret a person's performance in relation to a national reference group.

Reliability and Validity

Test–retest reliability scores average 0.87 for the complete battery. Interobserver reliability is excellent, with the results of two studies showing a reliability of 0.98 and 0.90.[29]

The validity of the BOT, according to Bruininks, "is based on its ability to assess the construct of motor development or proficiency."[29] In terms of motor proficiency, as measured by the performance of a particular child on a particular day, the BOT is a valid test.[8] The tests discriminate well between nonhandicapped populations and children learning who are disabled or mentally retarded.

Advantages and Disadvantages

The testing procedure is standardized and scores are normed. This is an excellent instrument for evaluating school-aged children who show motor problems but who do not have an obvious physical handicap. The test is valuable as a research tool be-

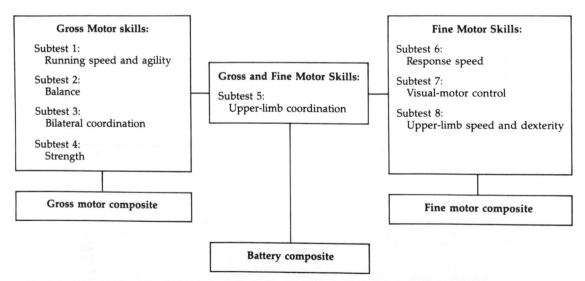

Figure 2-3. *Relationship of the eight subtests of the Bruininks-Oseretsky Test of Motor Proficiency to the composite test. (Adapted from Bruininks RH:* Examiner's Manual for Bruininks-Oseretsky Test of Motor Proficiency. *Circle Pines, MN: American Guidance Service; 1978:12.)*

SUBTEST 1: Running Speed and Agility

1. Running Speed and Agility[SF*]

TRIAL 1: __8.7__ seconds   TRIAL 2: __7.5__ seconds

Raw Score	Above 11.0	10.9-11.0	10.5-10.8	9.9-10.4	9.5-9.8	8.9-9.4	8.5-8.8	7.9-8.4	7.5-7.8	6.9-7.4	6.7-6.8	6.3-6.6	6.1-6.2	5.7-6.0	5.5-5.6	Below 5.5
Point Score	⓪	①	②	③	④	⑤	⑥	⑦	⑧	⑨	⑩	⑪	⑫	⑬	⑭	⑮

RECORD POINT SCORES FOR COMPLETE BATTERY ▼

⑧

POINT SCORE SUBTEST 1 (Max: 15)

RECORD POINT SCORES FOR SHORT FORM ▼

☐

SUBTEST 2: Balance

1. Standing on Preferred Leg on Floor *(10 seconds maximum per trial)*

TRIAL 1: __10__ seconds   TRIAL 2: _____ seconds

Raw Score	0	1-3	4-5	6-8	9-10
Point Score	⓪	①	②	③	④

④

2. Standing on Preferred Leg on Balance Beam[SF] *(10 seconds maximum per trial)*

TRIAL 1: __2__ seconds   TRIAL 2: __4__ seconds

Raw Score	0	1-2	3-4	5-6	7-8	9	10
Point Score	⓪	①	②	③	④	⑤	⑥

②

☐

3. Standing on Preferred Leg on Balance Beam—Eyes Closed *(10 seconds maximum per trial)*

TRIAL 1: __2__ seconds   TRIAL 2: __5__ seconds

Raw Score	0	1-3	4-5	6	7	8	9	10
Point Score	⓪	①	②	③	④	⑤	⑥	⑦

②

4. Walking Forward on Walking Line *(6 steps maximum per trial)*

TRIAL 1: __6__ steps   TRIAL 2: _____ steps

Raw Score	0	1-3	4-5	6
Point Score	⓪	①	②	③

③

5. Walking Forward on Balance Beam *(6 steps maximum per trial)*

TRIAL 1: __2__ steps   TRIAL 2: __4__ steps

Raw Score	0	1-3	4	5	6
Point Score	⓪	①	②	③	④

②

6. Walking Forward Heel-to-Toe on Walking Line *(6 steps maximum per trial)*

TRIAL 1: |I|0|0|0|I|0| = __2__ steps   TRIAL 2: |I|I|0|0|I|0| = __3__ steps

Raw Score	0	1-3	4-5	6
Point Score	⓪	①	②	③

①

7. Walking Forward Heel-to-Toe on Balance Beam[SF] *(6 steps maximum per trial)*

TRIAL 1: |I|0|0|0|0|0| = __1__ steps   TRIAL 2: |I|I|0|0|I|0| = __3__ steps

Raw Score	0	1-3	4	5	6
Point Score	⓪	①	②	③	④

①

☐

8. Stepping Over Response Speed Stick on Balance Beam

TRIAL 1: Fail (Pass)   TRIAL 2: Fail Pass

Raw Score	Fail	Pass
Point Score	⓪	①

①

⑯

POINT SCORE SUBTEST 2 (Max: 32)

*[SF] and the box in left-hand margin indicates short form.

Figure 2-4. *Recording form for the eight subtests of the Bruininks-Oseretsky Test of Motor Proficiency. (Adapted from Bruininks RH: Examiner's Manual for Bruininks-Oseretsky Test of Motor Proficiency. Circle Pines, MN: American Guidance Service; 1978:37.)*

cause of the ability to differentiate between populations.

One of the potential disadvantages of this test is that the space required to administer the BOT may limit its usefulness.

Comprehensive Developmental Scales

A basic component of any physical therapy assessment is a developmental evaluation. Developmental testing looks at the whole child, across all areas of development. These developmental areas include language, personal-social, fine motor, gross motor, self-help, and cognitive development. By using a comprehensive assessment, the therapist can develop strategies for treatment that address the whole child.

Gesell Developmental Schedules

The Gesell Developmental Schedules were developed by Arnold Gesell and his associates beginning in the 1920s. The original test items and procedures have been modified and updated through the years.[3] The Gesell schedules are the basis for future developmental scales.

Test Measures and Target Population

The test assesses behavior in the areas of adaptive, gross motor, fine motor, language, and personal-social development. It can be used to identify even minor deviations in children, and to determine the maturity and integrity of an individual's CNS.

The test is appropriate for children of ages 4 weeks to 36 months. Additional schedules are available to test children up to 60 months of age.

Test Construction and Standardization

During years of studying a large number of normal children, Gesell mapped the development of fetal, infant, and early behavior in children. The sched-

ules have been standardized by Gesell and associates.

Test Format

TYPE. The Gesell test is norm-referenced and involves direct assessment and observation by the examiner of the quality of and integration of behaviors.

CONTENT. Standardized materials can be obtained, or substitutes can be made according to the directions provided.[3] Developmental schedules show the behavioral characteristics of a key age and its two adjacent ages in three vertical columns. The key age occupies the central position (see Fig. 2-5 for an example of the key age of 16 weeks). Horizontally, the characteristics of behavior are grouped according to the five major behavioral fields.

ADMINISTRATION. As far as is possible, the standard sequences should be followed in the administration of the examination. The standard sequence differs depending on the maturity and age of the child. Examination procedures used in administering the individual items are well described and should be given in the prescribed, standardized manner[3] (Display 2-2).

SCORING. Two columns are provided on the developmental schedules for scoring: H for history, and O for observation. Some information is only available by report, particularly when it concerns language and personal-social behavior. A minus sign (−) indicates that the behavior does not occur, a plus sign (+) signifies the behavior occurs. And a plus-minus (±) notation is made if the behavior is just emerging but has not yet been fully integrated. A double plus sign (++) is recorded if a more mature pattern is observed.

INTERPRETATION. The final estimate of developmental maturity is based on the distribution of pluses and minuses. This estimate is not merely achieved by adding the pluses and minuses, but by

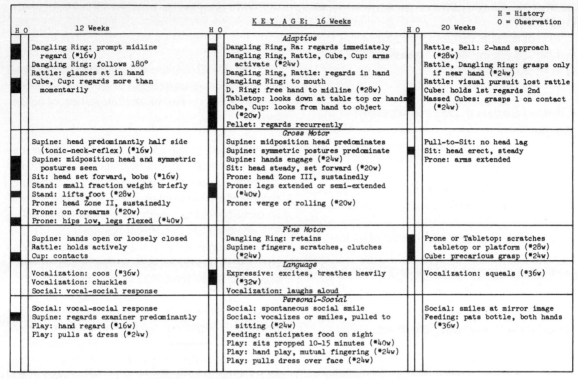

Figure 2-5. *Key Age chart from the Gesell Developmental Schedules for a 16-week-old child. (Knobloch H, Pasamanick B. Gesell and Armatruda's Developmental Diagnosis. 3rd ed. Philadelphia: JB Lippincott; 1974:42.)*

determining how well a child's behavior fits one age level rather than another. In any field of behavior, the child's maturity level is that point at which the aggregate of plus signs changes to an aggregate of minus signs.[3] The examiner assigns a representative age to each of the four areas, as well as an overall age. The ages can then be used to work out a developmental quotient (DQ), which is the age of maturity divided by the chronologic age.[30]

Reliability and Validity

Knobloch and Pasamanick reported that, on more than 100 clinical observations, a correlation of 0.98 was found between the DQs assigned by 18 pediatricians and those assigned by their instructor.[3] Test–retest reliability is reported to be 0.82 for 65 infants examined within 2 to 3 days of the initial date of testing.[3]

Correlations between infant and later examinations range from 0.5 to 0.85.[25]

Advantages and Disadvantages

The test's reliability and validity are generally excellent, and it is a good diagnostic tool. Testing procedures are standardized. This test is especially useful in research.

One disadvantage of the test is that the directions for testing are quite involved and require extensive practice and use in order to ensure valid results.

Bayley Scales of Infant Development

The Bayley Scales of Infant Development (BSID) were devised by Nancy Bayley and associates and are essentially a revision of Bayley's earlier work.[6]

Display 2-2.

Prescribed and Standardized Examination Sequence for the Administration of Test Items for the Gesell Developmental Schedules

Age: 12–16–20 Weeks	Situation No. (Appendix A-4)
Supine	1
Dangling ring	2
Rattle	3
Social stimulation	4
Bell ringing	5
Pull-to-sitting	6
Sitting supported	50
Chair—table top	
Cube 1, (2)	7,8
Massed cubes	11
(Cup)	16
Pellet	18
(Bell)	22
Mirror	24
Standing supported	51
Prone	52

Note: Italicized items appear for the first time in this sequence. Items in parentheses refer to situations sometimes omitted for special reasons.

(Normative behavior characteristic of the *key age: 16 weeks* and adjacent age levels is codified by the Developmental Schedule.)

*(Adapted from Knobloch H, Pasamanick B. Gesell and Armatruda's Developmental Diagnosis. 3rd ed. Philadelphia: JB Lippincott; 1974:43.

Test Measures and Target Population

The Bayley Scales are a comprehensive means of evaluating a child's current developmental status at a particular age. The scales are composed of three parts, each of which is designed to assess a separate component of the child's total development. The Mental Scale is designed to assess sensory-perceptual acuities, discriminations, and the ability to respond to these; the early acquisition of object constancy, as well as memory, learning, and problem-solving ability; vocalization and the beginnings of verbal communication; and early evidence of the ability to form generalizations and classifications, which is the basis for abstract thinking. The Motor Scale is designed to provide a measure of the degree of control of the body, and coordination of the large muscles and finer manipulatory skills of the hands and fingers. The Infant Behavior Record assesses the nature of the child's social and objective orientations toward the environment as expressed in attitudes, interests, emotions, energy, activity, and tendencies to approach or withdraw from stimulation.

The appropriate population for the BSID includes infants and toddlers between the ages of 1 and 30 months.

Test Construction and Standardization

The current scales represent the culmination of more than 40 years of research and clinical practice with small children.[6] The test has been standardized on a sample of 1262 children, distributed in approximately equal numbers among 14 age groups ranging from 2 to 30 months. The sample was selected to be representative of the population in the United States, as described in the 1960 United States Census of Population.

Test Format

TYPE. The test is norm-referenced. Information is obtained by direct observation and interaction with the child.

CONTENT. All materials needed for the test are included in the test kit except for stairs and a balance board. Materials have been selected carefully and casual substitutions are discouraged. A manual describes the procedures and progression of the test.

ADMINISTRATION. The time required for administration of the BSID varies with the number and complexity of items that must be presented. An average testing time for the Mental and Motor Scales is approximately 45 minutes, with some children occasionally requiring 75 minutes or more. After the child leaves, the researcher completes the Infant Behavior Record.

Changes may be made in the order of presentation, but no changes should be made in the specified manner of presenting test stimuli, as any such change would invalidate scoring. The Mental Scale is usually administered before the Motor Scale because the change in pace from sitting to moving about is the preferred sequence.

SCORING AND INTERPRETATION. Individual record forms are used to record a response on the test. For each item, the child is graded as follows: pass (P), fail (F), omit (O), refuse (R), or reported by mother (RPT). Only those items noted as passed are credited in scoring the test, but other results are useful in reviewing the adequacy of the test as an accurate measure of the child's performance. A basel level (item preceding earliest failure) and a ceiling level (item representing the most difficult success) are determined. The raw scores are changed to the Mental Development Index (MDI) and the Psychomotor Development Index (PDI) by consulting the norms for the child's particular age as derived by Bayley. An intelligence quotient should not be computed, because there is no evidence to support the interpretation of a figure of this kind derived from the BSID.[6]

Reliability and Validity

The reliability of the 1958 to 1960 version of the Mental and Motor Scales, the immediate predecessor of the current version of the BSID, was assessed by Werner and Bayley. Interobserver reliability rates for the Mental Scale and the Motor Scale were 89.4% and 93.4%, respectively. Test–retest reliability was 76.4% for the Mental Scale and 75.3% for the Motor Scale.

The correlation between results derived from the BSID and the Stanford-Binet Scale has ranged from minimal to moderate. Because the scales have limited value as predictors of future abilities, they are most useful in ascertaining the developmental status of a particular child at a particular age.

Advantages

Collectively, the BSID probably represent the best standardized techniques for behavioral assessment available for infants. These scales have been used extensively as an instrument for research, and are helpful in determining the developmental status of infants at a particular age.

Disadvantages

To administer the Bayley Scales, one must undergo training sessions and be validated as an examiner. The Bayley Motor Scale contains a small number of items for each level of development and omits stages that are generally accepted in the motor developmental sequence. For example, the Bayley Scales contain no items for running or kicking, and a single item incorporates all methods of the progression to walking. The Bayley Motor Scales, therefore, do not provide in-depth motor assessment nor do they delineate gross and fine motor development.[31]

Bayley II

After 24 years of use, the Bayley Scales of Infant Development have been revised. The changing nature of child care and the accumulation of information regarding children's abilities led to the revision. The *Bayley II* (not yet in wide clinical use) reflects current norms and allows diagnostic assessment at an earlier age.

The fundamentals of the test remain unchanged. It is a norm-referenced, standardized, three-part evaluation of the developmental status of children. The three parts are the Mental Scale, the Motor Scale, and the Behavior Rating Scale (formerly the Infant Behavior Record).

The revisions include: 1) revised norms, 2) age range extended downward to one month and upward to 42 months, 3) new items measuring a broader skill range, 4) updated stimulus materials that are more attractive and durable, 5) improved psychometric properties, and improved clinical utility, and 6) new scoring procedures.

Standardization

The *Bayley II* has been renormed on a stratified random sample of 1,700 children (850 boys and 850 girls) ages one month to 42 months, grouped at one-month intervals. The children came from all four geographic regions of the U.S. and closely parallel the 1988 U.S. Census statistics on the variables of age, gender, region, ethnicity, and parental education. These normative data enable the clinician to compare the infant's performance with same age peers and, if needed, help initiate intervention.

Clinical Validity

The Bayley Scales were originally designed to assess normal development in infants and young children. Because the primary use of developmental scales today is with children who are at risk or suspected of being at risk, an effort was made to gather more information about the use of the test with clinical samples.

The Bayley II Manual contains data for the following groups of children: children who were born prematurely, have the HIV antibody, were prenatally drug exposed, were asphyxiated at birth, are developmentally delayed, have frequent otitis media, are autistic, and/or have Down Syndrome.

Administration and Scoring

Although the fundamentals of the test remain unchanged, there have been some changes which facilitate the administration of the test. A second level of scoring was developed which is facet-based to match the content areas of cognition, language, person/social, and motor development. A developmental age for each facet can be obtained. This complements the traditional Mental/Motor Scale scoring. (From Bayley Scales of Infant Development, Second Edition: The *Bayley II*. The Psychological Corporation. San Antonio, TX. Harcourt Brace & Company, 1993.)

Neonatal Behavioral Assessment Scale

The Neonatal Behavioral Assessment Scale (NBAS), 2nd Edition,[32] was first developed by T. Berry Brazelton and published in 1973[33] with the help of many people who collaborated directly and indirectly. The second edition contains some additions and a few revisions designed to allay some of the criticisms of the first edition, as well as to restate some of the original purposes of the scale.

Test Measures and Target Population

The NBAS closely approximates a developmental evaluation of the neonate. It is intended to be a means of scoring interactive behavior rather than a formal neurologic evaluation, although the neurologic implications of such a scale make inclusion of some basic neurologic items necessary. The evaluation is primarily behavioral and is an attempt to score the infant's available responses to the environment, and, indirectly, the infant's effect on the environment.[32]

The NBAS is appropriate for the testing of children ages newborn to 1 month of age. It has been used to study both normal and premature infants, as well as infants from different national and ethnic groups.

Test Construction and Standardization

No formal standardization sample has been used in the development of the NBAS. As yet, the normative base for the NBAS is relatively limited.[32] Researchers using the scale have provided their own normative data with the population for which they were using the NBAS.

Test Format

CONTENT. The score sheet includes 28 behavioral items and 9 supplementary items (Display 2-3) that assess the neonate's capacity to organize states of consciousness, habituate reactions to dis-

Display 2-3.
Neonatal Behavioral Assessment Scale (NBAS)*

1. Response decrement to light (1,2)
2. Response decrement to rattle (1,2)
3. Response decrement to bell (1,2)
4. Response decrement to tactile stimulation of foot (1,2)
5. Orientation-inanimate visual (4,5)
6. Orientation-inanimate auditory (4,5)
7. Orientation-inanimate visual and auditory (4,5)
8. Orientation-animate visual (4,5)
9. Orientation-animate auditory (4,5)
10. Orientation-animate visual and auditory (4,5)
11. Alertness (4 only)
12. General tonus (4,5)
13. Motor maturity (4,5)
14. Pull-to-sit (4,5)
15. Cuddliness (4,5)
16. Defensive movements (3,4,5)
17. Consolability (6 to 5,4,3,2)
18. Peak of excitement (all states)
19. Rapidity of build-up (from 1,2 to 6)
20. Irritability (all awake states)

21. Activity (3,4,5)
22. Tremulousness (all states)
23. Startle (3,4,5,6)
24. Lability of skin color (from 1 to 6)
25. Lability of states (all states)
26. Self-quieting activity (6,5 to 4,3,2,1)
27. Hand-to-mouth facility (all states)
28. Smiles (all states)

Supplementary Items
29. Alert responsiveness (4 only)
30. Cost of attention (3,4,5)
31. Examiner persistence (all states)
32. General irritability (5,6)
33. Robustness and endurance (all states)
34. Regulatory capacity (all states)
35. State regulation (all states)
36. Balance of motor tone (all states)
37. Reinforcement value of infant's behavior (all states)

*The behavioral scale of the NBAS identifies the items examined and, in parentheses, the numbers of the appropriate states in which the assessment of each item on the scale can be made.

turbing events, attend to and process simple and complex events in the environment, control motor activity and postural tone while attending to these environmental events, and perform integrated motor acts.[32,34] The supplementary items have been developed for use with preterm, sick, fragile, and stressed infants, as well as to capture some of the more general characteristics of the infant's behavior in addition to the response of the examiner to the infant.[32] The test also includes 20 elicited (neurologic) responses (Display 2-4) that are based on Prechtl and Beintema's neurologic assessment of the infant.[35]

ADMINISTRATION. An important consideration throughout the tests is the state of consciousness or "state" of the infant,[32] classified according to six

stages: (1) deep sleep, (2) light sleep, (3) drowsy or semi-dozing, (4) alert, (5) active, (6) crying. The examiner attempts to bring the baby through an entire spectrum of states in each examination.

The examination usually takes 20 to 30 minutes and involves about 30 different tests and maneuvers. The examiner tries to elicit the best performance rather than an average performance from the infant; therefore, the examiner attempts to verify that the infant is incapable of a better response. The examiner must be flexible in the sequence of item administration to allow most of the items to be given at a time when the best performance will be achieved. Use of the NBAS requires direct training by experienced examiners. There are seven established reliability training centers.[32]

Display 2-4.
Elicited Responses of the Neonatal Behavioral Assessment Scale*

1. Plantar grasp
2. Hand grasp
3. Ankle clonus
4. Babinski response
5. Standing
6. Automatic walking
7. Placing
8. Incurvatum
9. Crawling
10. Glabella
11. Tonic deviation of head and eyes
12. Nystagmus
13. Tonic neck reflex
14. Moro reflex
15. Rooting (intensity)
16. Sucking (intensity)
17–20. Passive movements: right arm; left arm; right leg; left leg

*Items the examiner attempts to elicit during the examination.

SCORING. Most of the items are scored at the end of the examination. The elicited neurologic items are scored on a three-point scale designating low, medium, or high intensity of response. Asymmetry of response can also be noted. The behavioral items are each rated on a nine-point scale, with most of the items rated as optimal at the midpoint of the scale. A nine-point scale allows for a range of behavior that can bring out subtle differences among different groups of babies.

INTERPRETATION. The NBAS does not yield an overall score for an infant. Rather the results of the test are the scores for each of the items. The mean is related to the expected behavior of an "average" full-term, normal, white infant weighing 7 lb or more whose mother has not received more than 100

mg of barbiturates and 50 mg of other sedative drugs before delivery, whose Apgar scores were no less than seven at 1 minute, eight at 5 minutes, and eight at 15 minutes after delivery, who needed no special care after delivery, and who had an apparently normal intrauterine experience.[33]

Reliability and Validity

The reliability of independent testers trained at the same time is reported to range from 0.85 to 1.[20] Testers can be trained to a 0.9 criterion of reliability, and the level of reliability is still determined to be 0.9 or higher for a prolonged time.[32]

According to the author, test–retest reliability must be viewed in terms of the kinds of questions being posed when the NBAS is employed. It is clear that the standard psychometric criterion of a Pearson Product Moment Correlation Coefficient will yield low to moderate day-to-day stabilities. Conversely, an individually derived measure of day-to-day stability reveals quite a different and much more variable picture. Patterns of score changes over repeated examinations may well reveal important characteristics about individual infants and about groups of infants.[32]

In terms of validity, studies have shown that individual differences, as measured by the NBAS, are related to later individual differences.[32,33]

Advantages

The NBAS is an effective predictor of neurologic problems, as well as an effective teaching tool for parents. It is a valuable technique for differentiating the behavioral characteristics of normal neonates for research and clinical purposes.

Disadvantages

Among the disadvantages of the NBAS is that it is a difficult test to learn, and the tester must guard against overinterpretation when discussing test results with physicians and parents.[21] When the time required for scoring, interpretation of the test, and writing of the report is considered, the test becomes a lengthy process. The relationship between results on the NBAS and those derived from later functional testing has yet to be demonstrated.

Early Intervention Developmental Profile

The Early Intervention Developmental Profile (EIDP) was developed by an interdisciplinary team at the University of Michigan under the direction of Schafer and Moersch.[36]

Test Measures and Target Population

The EIDP is an infant assessment-based programming instrument made up of six scales that provide developmental norms and milestones in the following areas: perceptual or fine motor, cognition, language, social or emotional, self-care, and gross motor development. The profile should not be used to diagnose handicapping conditions, nor does it supply data that can predict future capabilities or handicaps. However, by examining a child's skills in six different areas, the profile helps to describe the child's comprehensive function, identifying relative strengths and weaknesses.[36]

Designed for children from birth to 36 months, the EIDP yields information that can be used to plan comprehensive developmental programs for children with all types of handicaps who function below the 36-month level.

Test Construction and Standardization

Test items were selected from well-known, standardized instruments for the evaluation of infants, including general developmental scales, motor scales, and language scales. Some original profile items were based on current developmental theories. The profile has not been standardized. Assignment of items to specific age ranges was based on standardizations or research from other instruments. The age-norm suggestions derived from the original source (i.e., Piaget) were used for original items.

Test Format

CONTENT. Each section of the profile is divided into age groupings, each of which covers 3 months within the first year of life and 4 months within the

second and third years. No consistent attempt was made to arrange items within age ranges in a developmental sequence.

The gross motor scale reflects a body of knowledge that constitutes the basis for the current treatment of cerebral palsy in infants and young children (e.g., Bobath and Fiorentino). There is an emphasis on neurodevelopmental theories of reflex development and integration of primitive reflexes into higher order righting reactions, protective responses, and equilibrium responses.[36]

The cognitive scale reflects the theories of Piaget, whereas the social-emotional scale reflects current theory on the emotional attachment between the mother and child and the child's gradual acquisition of ego functions during the first 36 months of life.[36]

ADMINISTRATION. The profile was designed to be given by a multidisciplinary team that includes a psychologist or special educator, physical or occupational therapist, and a speech and language therapist. Each member of the team can learn to give the entire profile, rather than being limited to only certain scales by one's chosen discipline. Administration of test items is thoroughly explained in the evaluation manual. References for each item are well documented. Test items are given until the child fails either six consecutive items or all items in two consecutive age ranges. The total time required for administration of the test may vary from 30 minutes to several hours. The materials needed for administration are described in the manual and should be available.

SCORING. Items are scored as a "pass" (P) when the criteria are met; however, when the child's behavior on an item does not meet scoring criteria, it is scored as a "fail" (F). A score of "pass-fail" (PF) indicates the emergence of a skill. An item is scored as "omitted" (O) when the evaluator must exclude an item.

INTERPRETATION. Ceiling levels (the age range containing the child's highest passed item) and basal levels (the age range preceding the child's earliest failure) are determined for each section. The ceiling and basal levels define a range of items on which the child's performance is inconsistent, which will provide the focus for programming efforts. Age levels for each area of performance are recorded on a composite table to yield a profile. Each testing booklet can be used for several subsequent evaluations, with the composite profile recorded with a different color or line notation each item to document progress.

Reliability and Validity

Interobserver and test–retest reliability values were assessed using small sample sizes; however, the results were generally excellent. Interobserver reliability ranged from a low of 80% to a high of 97%. Test–retest reliability ranged from 93% to 98%.[36]

Significant correlations were found between children's scores on the EIDP, the BSID, the Vineland Society Maturity Scale, and clinical motor evaluations. Thus, strong validity of content was found for the EIDP.

Advantages and Disadvantages

The combined results of the six scales provide a comprehensive record of the child's skills. Moreover, the completed profile lends itself well to the formulation of individualized objectives. The third volume of *Developmental Programming for Infants and Children: Stimulation Activities* is a comprehensive collection of sequenced activities designed to complement the Developmental Profile.[37] The EIDP reflects current developmental theory in the motor, cognitive, and social areas and is best used as a clinical instrument for interdisciplinary team planning.

The sample sizes for reliability and validity testing were small. Thus the EIDP cannot be used for diagnosis or for predicting future capabilities or handicaps.

Assessment of Functional Capabilities

Functional capabilities are views as skills that are essential within the child's natural environments of home and school. According to Haley,[38] the concept of disability and functional assessment incorporates the following key concepts:

1. A child may have serious motor impairments that are not always reflected by the level of functional limitation or disability.
2. Functional deficits may or may not lead to a restriction in social activities and important childhood roles.
3. Environmental factors, family expectations, and contextual elements of functional task requirements play an important role in the eventual level of disability and handicap of the child.

Comprehensive functional assessment instruments contain mobility, transfer, self-care, and social function items; they include measurement dimensions of assistance and adaptive equipment; and they incorporate developmental stages of functional skill attainment.[39] Pediatric physical therapists have long expressed the need for a functional approach to the assessment of children with movement disorders.

Pediatric Evaluation of Disability Inventory

The Pediatric Evaluation of Disability Inventory (PEDI)[40] was developed to meet the need for a reliable, valid, and norm-referenced instrument for assessing functional status in infants and young children by physical therapists and other rehabilitation personnel. The PEDI was designed to be a comprehensive yet clinically feasible instrument that can be used for clinical assessment, program monitoring, documentation of functional progress, and clinical decision making.[41]

Test Measures and Target Population

The PEDI measures both the capability and performance of functional activities in three content domains: (1) self-care, (2) mobility, and (3) social function. Capability is measured by the identification of functional skills for which the child has demonstrated mastery and competence (Display 2-5). Functional performance is measured by the level of caregiver assistance and environmental

---

Display 2-5.
Functional Skills Content of the Pediatric Evaluation of Disability Inventory*

Self-Care Domain	**Mobility Domain**	**Social Function Domain**
Types of food textures	Toilet transfers	Comprehension of word meanings
Use of utensils	Chair/wheelchair transfers	
Use of drinking containers	Car transfers	Comprehension of sentence complexity
Toothbrushing	Bed mobility/transfers	
Hairbrushing	Tub transfers	Functional use of expressive communication
Nose care	Method of indoor locomotion	
Handwashing	Distance/speed indoors	Complexity of expressive communication
Washing body and face	Pulls/carries objects	
Pullover/front-opening garments	Method of outdoor locomotion	Problem-resolution
	Distance/speed outdoors	Social interactive play
Fasteners	Outdoor surfaces	Peer interactions
Pants	Upstairs	Self-information
Shoes/socks	Downstairs	Time orientation
Toileting tasks		Household chores
Management of bladder		Self-protection
Management of bowel		Community function

*Used with permission from Haley SM, et al. Pediatric Evaluation of Disability Inventory (PEDI): Development, Standardization and Administration Manual. Boston; New England Medical Center Hospital and PEDI Research Group; 1992:13.

---

modifications needed to accomplish major functional activities (Display 2-6).

Children ranging in age from 6 months to 7.5 years may be tested. The PEDI is primarily designed for the evaluation of young children, but it can be used to evaluate older children whose functional abilities fall below those expected of 7.5-year-old children with no disabilities.

Test Construction and Standardization

The content and measurement scales of the PEDI underwent numerous revisions prior to the publication of the final version. Initially, content was identified based on the available literature, previous functional and adaptive tests, and the clinical experience of the authors and consultant involved. A Development Edition was field-tested on more than 60 handicapped children and their families. The scales' comprehensiveness and representativeness was evaluated by external content experts. Revisions based on the field testing and the content validity study were then incorporated into the final PEDI items to establish the Standardization Version.

Normative data for the PEDI were gathered from 412 children and families distributed throughout Massachusetts, Connecticut, and New York. The sample closely approximated most of the demographic characteristics of the U.S. population as defined by the 1980 U.S. census data. Additionally,

Display 2-6.
Complex Activities Assessed with Caregiver Assistance and Modifications Scales*

Self-Care Domain	Mobility Domain	Social Function Domain
Eating	Chair/toilet transfers	Functional comprehension
Grooming	Car transfers	Functional expression
Bathing	Bed mobility/transfers	Joint problem solving
Dressing upper body	Tub transfers	Peer play
Dressing lower body	Indoor locomotion	Safety
Toileting	Outdoor locomotion	
Bladder management	Stairs	
Bowel management		

*Used with permission from Haley SM, et al. Pediatric Evaluation of Disability Inventory (PEDI): Development, Standardization and Administration Manual. Boston; New England Medical Center Hospital and PEDI Research Group; 1992:13.

three groups of children (totaling 102) with disabilities composed clinical samples for validation purposes.

Test Format

TYPE. The test is norm-referenced, and it can also be used as a criterion-referenced measure of functional status.

CONTENT. The PEDI includes three sets of measurement scales: Functional Skills, Caregiver Assistance, and Modifications. These scales are used to assess the three content areas of self-care, mobility, and social function. The *Functional Skills Scales* were designed to reflect meaningful functional units within a given activity. The *Caregiver Assistance Scales* measure disability of children with respect to the amount of help they need to carry out functional activities. The *Modifications* section is not a true measurement scale, but rather a frequency count of the type and extent of environmental modifications the child depends on to support functional performance.

ADMINISTRATION. The PEDI can be administered by clinicians and educators who are familiar with the child, or by structured interview of the parent. The PEDI's focus on typical performance requires the respondent to have had the opportunity to observe the child on several different occasions in order to gain an accurate picture of the child's typical performance.[40] Administration guidelines, criteria for scoring each item, and examples are provided in the accompanying manual. Specific training is required to ensure that examiners are knowledgeable about the item criteria used in the instrument and the methods employed in determining the child's level of assistance.

SCORING. Scores are recorded in a booklet that also contains a summary score sheet that is used to construct a profile of the child's performance across the different domains and scales. A summary of rating criteria for the three sets of measurement scales is provided in Display 2-7.

INTERPRETATION. The PEDI provides two types of transformed summary scores: normative

Display 2–7.
Rating Criteria for the Three Types of Measurement Scales

Part I: Functional Skills	Part II: Caregiver Assistance	Part III: Modifications
(197 discrete items of functional skills)	(20 complex functional activities)	(20 complex functional activities)
Self-care, Mobility, Social Function	Self-care, Mobility, Social Function	Self-care, Mobility, Social Function
0 = unable, or limited in capability to perform item in most situations	5 = Independent	N = No Modifications
	4 = Supervise/Prompt/Monitor	C = Child-oriented (non-specialized)
1 = capable of performing item in most situations, or item has been previously mastered and functional skills have progressed beyond this level	3 = Minimal Assistance	R = Rehabilitation Equipment
	2 = Moderate Assistance	E = Extensive Modifications
	1 = Maximal Assistance	
	0 = Total Assistance	

Used with permission from Haley SM, et al. Pediatric Evaluation of Disability Inventory (PEDI): Development, Standardization and Administration Manual. Boston; New England Medical Center Hospital and PEDI Research Group; 1992:16.

standard scores and scaled scores. Separate summary scores are calculated for Functional Skills and for Caregiver Assistance in each of the three domains, thus yielding six normative standard scores and six scaled scores. Normative standard scores are transformed scores that take into account the child's chronological age, thereby providing an indication of the child's relative standing in relation to age expectations for functional skills and performance. Scaled scores, distributed along a scale from 0 to 100, provide an indication of the performance of the child along the continuum of relatively difficult items in a particular domain on the PEDI. Scaled scores are not adjusted for age and, therefore, can be used to describe the functional status of children of all ages. In addition, frequency totals of the four levels of modifications can be calculated. These totals provide descriptive informa-

tion on the frequency and the degree of modifications a child uses.

Reliability and Validity

The internal consistency reliability coefficients obtained from the normative sample range between 0.95 and 0.99. Inter-interviewer reliability in the normative sample was very high (ICCs = 0.96 to 0.99) for the Caregiver Assistance Scales. Agreement on Modifications was also quite high, except for Social Function, where it was still adequate (ICC = 0.79).[40] Further studies are planned to assess test-retest reliability and interobserver reliability between rehabilitation team members.

Content validity was examined using a panel of 31 experts[41] to validate and confirm the functional content of the PEDI. Data related to construct validity and concurrent validity[39] indicate that the PEDI is a valid measure of pediatric function. Preliminary data also support the discriminant and evaluative validity of the PEDI.[40]

Advantages and Disadvantages

The PEDI represents a standardized clinical instrument for pediatric functional assessment. Rigorous methodology during its development has resulted in an instrument that is both valid and reliable. The authors welcome input and feedback from users of the PEDI which will be useful to the authors as updated and revised versions are made available in the future.

Owing to the "newness" of the PEDI, further studies are needed to confirm its technical validity and to identify any needed changes or additions.

Integration of Information

Throughout the process of evaluation, physical therapists compile extensive information concerning their young clients. The final component of a thorough assessment is to organize, synthesize, and use the data to guide intervention. There are four possible uses for the information gained from evaluation:[42]

1. To plan a treatment program
2. To identify areas of progress or lack of progress
3. To identify or rule out the existence of a specific problem
4. To provide diagnostic information

Physical therapists are primarily involved with the first two areas. The way in which test data are to be used should help determine the data needed, thus assuring the collection of necessary data while avoiding superfluous information. As a result of the procedure for assessment, the physical therapist identifies specific areas of dysfunction in a particular child. Program goals and objectives can then be developed to address these areas of dysfunction. *Program goals* describe long-term expectations of treatment and relate to general areas of development. *Objectives* are short-term accomplishments,

written in behavioral terms, which enable the child to progress toward achievement of the long-term goals. A program for therapy is designed to meet the objectives identified by focusing on the activities required for the child to achieve the objectives.

The assessment process can be seen as an ongoing cycle. The information gathered from the formal assessment is used in the development of goals and objectives that guide the treatment program. Reassessments are periodically performed to review the appropriateness of the treatment program

---

Display 2–8.

Suggested Outline for a Narrative Report on the Results of Developmental Testing

1. Identification information: child's name, date of birth, current age, date of evaluation
2. Reason for evaluation and source of referral
3. History
   A. Perinatal history
   B. Significant medical history
   C. Developmental history as presented by parents or other historian
4. Clinical observations
   A. Neurologic development: reflex development, muscle tone, equilibrium, and protective responses
   B. Musculoskeletal status: range of motion, manual muscle test, anthropometric measurements
   C. Sensory status: results of sensory testing, visual ability, and auditory ability
   D. Functional abilities: daily activities (e.g., feeding, toileting, dressing), assistive devices
5. Results of developmental assessments: include developmental age.
6. Summary of findings
7. Recommendations

and to monitor the progress of the child. Reports of physical therapy assessments are usually presented in narrative form. The purposes of a report are to clarify what has been heard and observed, to give the data on which recommendations for treatment are based, and to transmit this information in a clear and understandable way to others. Certain information is included for all patients, but each child's report should provide a specific description of the distinctive abilities and disabilities of that child.[3] An outline of a narrative report is given in Display 2-8.

Summary

Several clinically useful and commonly used tools for assessment have been described, among them screening tests, tests of motor function, and comprehensive developmental assessments. The information gained from these assessments, when combined with the information obtained from an interview, medical and developmental history, and clinical observation, completes the comprehensive evaluation of a child. The guidelines presented for the selection of specific tests will aid the therapist in choosing the test most appropriate for the population to be assessed. The therapist should remember that a questioning attitude, based on and supported by knowledge of human growth and development, is necessary for a comprehensive evaluation.

References

1. Semans S. Specific tests and evaluation tools for the child with central nervous system deficit. *Phys Ther.* 1965;45:456–462.
2. Scherzer AL, Tscharnuter I. *Early Diagnosis and Therapy in Cerebral Palsy.* New York: Marcel Dekker; 1982.
3. Knobloch H, Pasamanick B, eds. *Gesell and Armatruda's Developmental Diagnosis: The Evaluation and Management of Normal and Abnormal Neuropsychologic Development in Infancy and Early Childhood.* Hagerstown, MD: Harper & Row; 1974.
4. Clark PN, Coley LI, Allen AS, Schanzenbacher KE. Basic methods of assessment and screening. In: Clark PN, Allen AS, eds. *Occupational Therapy for Children.* St. Louis: CV Mosby; 1985.
5. Connolly B, Harris S. Survey of assessment tools. *Totline.* 1983;9:8–9.
6. Bayley N. *Bayley Scales of Infant Development.* New York: The Psychological Corporation; 1969.
7. Frankenburg WK, Dodds J, Archer P, et al. *Denver II Training Manual.* Denver, CO: Denver Developmental Materials, Inc; 1992.
8. Gallahue D. Assessing children's motor behavior. In: *Understanding Motor Development in Children.* New York: John Wiley; 1982.
9. Lewko JH. Current practices in evaluating motor behavior of disabled children. *Am J Occup Ther.* 1976; 30:413–419.
10. Stangler SR, Huber CJ, Routh DK. *Screening Growth and Development of Preschool Children: A Guide for Test Selection.* New York: McGraw-Hill; 1980.
11. Milani-Comparetti A, Gidoni EA. Routine developmental examination in normal and retarded children. *Dev Med Child Neurol.* 1967;9:631–638.
12. Trembath J, Kliewer D, Bruce W. *The Milani-Comparetti Motor Development Screening Test.* Omaha, NE: University of Nebraska Medical Center; 1977.
13. Stuberg WA, et al. *The Milani-Comparetti Motor Development Screening Test.* 3rd ed rev. Omaha, NE: University of Nebraska Medical Center; 1992.
14. Stuberg WA, White PJ, Miedaner JA, Dehne PR. Item reliability of the Milani-Comparetti Motor Development Screening Test. *Phys Ther.* 1989;69:328–335.
15. Frankenburg WK, Dodds JB, Fandel AW. *Denver Developmental Screening Test Manual.* Denver, CO: LADOCA Project & Publishing Foundation; 1973.
16. Frankenburg WK, Dodds J, Archer P, et al. The Denver II: A major revision and restandardization of the

Denver Developmental Screening Test. *Pediatrics.* 1992; 89:1.

17. Frankenburg WK, Dodds J, Archer P. *Denver II Technical Manual.* Denver, CO: Denver Developmental Materials, Inc.; 1990.

18. Chandler LS, Andrews MS, Swanson MW. *Movement Assessment of Infants*—A Manual. Rolling Bay, WA: Chandler, Andrews, and Swanson; 1980.

19. Haley SM, Harris SR, Tada WL, et al. Item reliability of the movement assessment of infants. *Phys Occup Ther Pediatr.* 1986;6(1):21–38.

20. Harris SR. Early neuromotor predictors of cerebral palsy in low birthweight infants. *Dev Med Child Neurol.* 1987;29:508–519.

21. Schneider JW, Lee W, Chasnoff IJ. Field testing of the Movement Assessment of Infants. *Phys Ther.* 1988;68:321–327.

22. Piper MC, Pinnell LE, Darrah J, Byrne PJ, Watt MJ. Early developmental screening: Sensitivity and specificity of chronological and adjusted scores. *Dev Behav Pediatr.* 1992;13:95–101.

23. Swanson MW, Bennett FC, Shy KK, Whitfield MF. Identification of neurodevelopmental abnormality at four and eight months by the Movement Assessment of Infants. *Dev Med Child Neurol.* 1992;34:321–337.

24. Harris SR, Haley SM, Tada WL, Swanson MW. Reliability of observational measures of the Movement Assessment of Infants. *Phys Ther.* 1984;64:471–475.

25. Harris SR, Swanson MW, Andrews MS, et al. Predictive validity of the movement assessment of infants. *J Dev Behav Pediatr.* 1984;5:336–343.

26. Folio MR, Fewell PR. *Peabody Developmental Motor Scales and Activity Cards Manual.* Allen, TX: DLM Teaching Resources; 1983.

27. Stokes NA, Deitz JL, Crowe TK. The Peabody Developmental Fine Motor Scale: An interrater reliability study. *Am J Occup Ther.* 1990;44:334–340.

28. Harris SR, Heriza CB. Measuring infant movement: Clinical and technological assessment techniques. *Phys Ther.* 1987;67:1877–1880.

29. Bruininks RH. Bruininks-*Oseretsky Test of Motor Proficiency: Examiners' Manual.* Circle Pines, MI: American Guidance Services; 1978.

30. Self PA, Horowitz FD. The behavioral assessment of the neonate: An overview. In: Osofsky JD, ed. *Handbook of Infant Development.* New York: Wiley, 1979.

31. Palisano RJ. Concurrent and predictive validities of the Bayley Motor Scale and the Peabody Developmental Motor Scales. *Phys Ther.* 1986;66:1714–1719.

32. Brazelton TB. Neonatal Behavioral Assessment Scale. *Clin Dev Med.* 1984:88.

33. Brazelton TB. Neonatal Behavioral Assessment Scale. *Clin Dev Med.* 1973:50.

34. Stengel TJ. The Neonatal Behavioral Assessment Scale: Description, clinical uses, and research implications. *Phys Occup Ther Pediatr.* 1980;1:39–57.

35. Prechtl HFB, Beintema B. The neurological examination of the full-term infant. *Clin Dev Med.* 1964:12.

36. Rogers SJ, D'Eugenio DB. Assessment and application. In: Schafer DS. Moersch MS, ed: *Developmental Programming for Infants and Young Children.* Vol 1. Ann Arbor, MI: The University of Michigan Press; 1977.

37. Brown SL, Donovan CM. Stimulation activities. In: Schafer DS, Moersch MS, eds. *Developmental Programming for Infants and Young Children.* Vol 3. Ann Arbor, MI: The University of Michigan Press; 1977.

38. Haley SM: Motor assessment tools for infants and young children: A focus on disability assessment. In: Forssberg H, Hirschfeld H, eds. *Movement Disorders in Children.* Basel: S. Karger, AG; 1992;278–283.

39. Feldman AB, Haley SM, Coryell J. Concurrent and construct validity of the Pediatric Evaluation of Disability Inventory. *Phys Ther* 1990;70:602–610.

40. Haley SM, et al. *Pediatric Evaluation of Disability Inventory (PEDI): Development, Standardization and Administration Manual.* Boston: New England Medical Center Hospitals and PEDI Research Group; 1992.

41. Haley SM, Coster WJ, Faas RM. A content validity study of the Pediatric Evaluation of Disability Inventory. *Ped Phys Ther* 1991;3:177–184.

42. Stockmeyer S. A pattern for evaluation in the assessment of motor performance. *Phys Ther* 1965;45:453–455.

Pediatric Physical Therapy,
second edition, edited by Jan
Stephen Tecklin. J. B. Lippincott
Company, Philadelphia © 1994.

3

Mary Soltesz Sheahan and Nancy Farmer Brockway

The High-Risk Infant

- **The Environment of the Neonatal Intensive Care Unit**
- **Neonatal Development**
- **Synactive Model of Infant Behavior**
- **Risk Factors**
  Neurologic Conditions
  Respiratory Conditions
  Metabolic Conditions
  Cardiovascular Conditions
  Viral Infections of the Fetus and Neonate
  In Utero Substance Exposure
  Necrotizing Enterocolitis
  Retinopathy of Prematurity
  Neonatal Orthopedic Problems
- **Neonatal Assessment**
  Apgar Score
  Clinical Assessment of Gestational Age in the Newborn Infant

Neonatal Behavioral Assessment Scale
Assessment of Preterm Infant's Behavior
Neurologic Assessment of the Full-term and Preterm Newborn Infant
Morgan Neonatal Neurobehavioral Examination
Movement Assessment of Infants
Milani-Comparetti Motor Development Screening Test
- **Developmental Intervention**
  Therapeutic Handling
  Therapeutic Positioning
  Feeding
  Parent Education
- **The NICU Team**
- **Discharge Planning and Developmental Follow-up**

Recent advances in neonatology have reduced significantly the morbidity and mortality rates for high-risk infants. Premature infants, however, are at greater risk than infants born at term for developmental deficits and handicapping conditions. As a result of this risk, pediatric therapists have become increasingly involved in providing intervention in the neonatal intensive care unit (NICU). These therapists advocate early detection and remediation of neuromotor deficits to minimize or prevent further disabilities that emerge as compensations for initial movement disorders.[1]

The pediatric therapist's role in the NICU requires a good understanding of the medical needs of high-risk neonates. The ability to assess thoroughly the physiologic status of the neonate is crucial for successful implementation of developmental intervention. Therapists initially entering the NICU setting need close supervision from an experienced clinician. Advanced training in normal and abnormal development is also strongly recommended.

The chapter examines the role of the pediatric therapist working with high-risk infants in the NICU. A basic description of the high-risk infant is given and appropriate intervention techniques are presented. The term *high-risk infant*, as used in the context of this chapter, refers to those infants whose perinatal medical course might contribute to motor, cognitive, or social deficits. Some of the most common medical problems associated with the high-risk infant are described.

The Environment of the Neonatal Intensive Care Unit

A comparison between the intrauterine and NICU environment is necessary in order to appreciate the complexities of the problems faced by the neonate who is at high risk. The intrauterine environment is ideally suited for the development of the fetus for a variety of reasons. In utero, the fetus receives muted sounds generated by the mother, including rhythmical heart beats, respiratory sounds, and voice. Although sounds from the external environment are heard by the fetus, those sounds are dampened. Intrauterine visual input is limited to a dim red glow. The amniotic fluid provides an optimal environment for the elimination of gravity to provide for random movement, and the boundaries of the uterine wall provide deep proprioceptive input as the fetus moves. Maternal movement provides additional proprioceptive and vestibular input to the fetus. Fetal thermoregulation is controlled well in the intrauterine environment.

In stark contrast, the NICU environment is characterized by bright light and constant and offensive noise produced by medical equipment, voices, telephones, radios, alarms, and closing of incubator doors. The medically unstable infant experiences adverse tactile input from necessary invasive medical intervention. Gravity makes movement into flexed positions difficult for the often hypotonic neonate. The previous intrauterine boundaries are now absent and proprioceptive feedback changes. Postnatally, the infant is subjected to thermoregulation problems.

Neonatal Development

A basic understanding of the development of the premature and full-term infant is necessary in order to appreciate the rationale behind developmental intervention in the nursery. This section of the chapter provides a comparison of the development of a premature infant and that of a full-term infant. A complete discussion of normal development is found in Chapter 1.

The premature infant characteristically displays global hypotonia.[2] The level of hypotonia is related to the degree of prematurity.[3] For example, the infant of 28 weeks' gestation shows greater range of motion and flexibility in the shoulders, elbows, hips, and knees than infants born at later gestational ages. The extremities of the premature infant are typically postured in extension and abduction, with decreased flexor patterns and midline orientation. The reduced timespan spent in the tightly packed uterine environment contributes to the premature infant's lack of physiologic flexion. The force of gravity against weak muscle groups further reinforces the extended posture in premature infants. Primitive reflexes may be absent, reduced, or inconsistent, and spontaneous movement is minimal.[2] Infants maintained for long periods with mechanical ventilation may show increased hypertension of the neck, scapular elevation, retraction of the shoulders and upper extremities, arching of the trunk, and immobility of the pelvis.[4]

By contrast, the full-term infant displays strong physiologic flexion. The 40 weeks spent in utero allows for full development of flexor muscle tone. The tightly compacted uterine posture causes mild flexor contractures in the elbows and knees. These contractures are gradually reduced. Flexion of the wrist and dorsiflexion of the ankle increase in the full-term infant. At term, the infant's extremities are generally flexed and adducted. Spontaneous

Table 3-1. *Neurodevelopmental Profile of the Fetus and Premature Neonate**

1 Week

Implantation into the uterine wall

3 Weeks

Beginning of heart contractions

3–6 Weeks

Non-nervous (aneural) muscular activity
Spontaneous contractions of skeletal muscles are
more pronounced cephalad than caudal

4 Weeks

Heart pulsation and pumping of blood
Formation of backbone and spinal canal
Beginning of formation of digestive system
Length of ¾ inch

8–9 Weeks

Continuous trembling secondary to autonomous muscle
contraction without organization
Generalized avoidance reflexes resulting from stimulation
around lips and nose with a fine hair
Limbs that are beginning to show divisions (thigh, knee, calf,
foot)
Formation of umbilical cord
Disappearance of tail-like process
Length of 1 1/8 inches
Weight of 1/30 oz

9–12 Weeks

Primitive palmar grasp reflex
Mouth opening elicited by stimulation of lower lip area
Mouth opening, but not sucking, elicited by stimulation of both
lips
Global flexion and extension
Formation of nails on digits
External ears present
Almost full development of the eyes but persistent fusion of
eyelids
Length of 3 inches
Weight of 1 oz
Brain weight of 10 g

16 Weeks

Increased frequency of fetal propulsion—head rotation with
thrusting
Respiratory movements—mouth opening and head extension
with inspiration
Skin—bright pink and transparent; covered with a fine,
down-like hair
Length of 6 1/2 to 7 inches
Weight of 4 oz

17 Weeks

Initial appearance of sucking reflex

20 Weeks

Fully developed repertoire of movement patterns
Isolated, independent movements of the extremities and head
    Opens hands with extension of digits to explore surrounding
    surfaces
    Opens mouth; sucking and swallowing present
    Uses facial expressions—grimaces, wrinkles forehead
Protective or avoidance light reflex— turns away from light
even though eyes are closed
Length of 10 to 12 inches
Weight of 1/2 lb to 1 lb

22 Weeks

Initial myelination of the CNS and peripheral nervous system

24 Weeks

Lungs have matured to the degree that viability is possible
Length of 11 to 14 inches
Weight of 1 1/4 to 1 1/2 lb
Brain weight of 150 g

28 Weeks

Appearance of alert state— able to respond to stimuli
Remains dominated by sleep state
Movement
    Tremulous, random movements
    Slow, global movements with rapid, jerky, segmental
    movements
Muscle tone
    Moderate hypotonia segmentally and axially
    Extreme passivity, which is greater in the upper extremities
    than in the lower extremities
Excessive mobility—more pronounced in proximal segments
Length of 14 to 17 inches
Weight of 2 1/2 to 3 lb

32 Weeks

Spontaneous appearance of an alert state which may not
correlate with motor activity
More pronounced state differentiation
Movement
    Bursts of movement when in an awake state
    Movement dominated by trunk
    Creeping in isolette, especially to sides
    Marked decrease in tremulousness and clonic movements
    Attempted hand-to-mouth movements
Muscle tone
    Noted decrease in lower extremity hypotonia to hip joint
    Increased strength of weight bearing
    Ability to attempt to straighten head (life-saving reaction)

Table 3–1. *Neurodevelopmental Profile of the Fetus and Premature Neonate* (continued)*

36 Weeks

Vigorous, sustained cry

Continued improvement in behavioral state differentiation

Movement

    Spontaneous movement that is more limited and less varied in the upper and lower extremities

    Increased cocontraction of agonist/antagonist muscle groups causing a restraining quality

Muscle tone

    Hypotonia of the upper extremities and upper trunk in

comparison to the lower trunk and lower extremities (frog-like position)

40 Weeks

Sustained periods of a quiet-alert state

Improved state differentiation

Movement

    Less disorganizing and more uniform spontaneous movement

Muscle tone

    Diminished hypotonia in the upper extremities and upper trunk

Information has been compiled from the following sources: Comparetti AM. Prenatal and Postnatal Development of Movement: Implications for Developmental Diagnosis. Arlington, Va., 1982; Forslund M, Bjerre I. Neurological assessment of preterm infants at term conceptual age in comparison with normal full-term infants. Early Human Development 1983;8:195–208. Piper M, Byrne P, Pinnell L. Influence of gestational age in early neuromotor development in the preterm infant. Am J Perinatol 1989;6:405–411 and Saint-Anne Dargassies S. Neurological maturation of the premature infant of 28 to 41 weeks gestational age. In: Human Development. Philadelphia. WB Saunders, 1966.

movements can be limited by the strong physiologic flexion.[2]

As the premature infant develops, flexor muscle tone increases in a caudocephalic direction.[5] The premature infant usually does not achieve the full degree of flexor muscle tone seen in the full-term infant.[3] Therefore, the premature infant lacks the counterbalance of flexor tone to offset the normal progression of extensor muscle tone, thereby causing an imbalance between extensor and flexor groups. This imbalance may interfere with development of midrange control of the head, sitting balance, reaching skills, and bilateral coordination. Secondary to the decreased midline and reaching skills, body image and exploratory skills may be adversely affected (Table 3-1).[6]

Synactive Model of Infant Behavior

A synactive model of infant behavior has been postulated by Als et al. and is based upon a hierarchical interaction of four subsystems: (1) autonomic, (2) motor, (3) state, and (4) attentional/interactive, as described in Table 3-2.[7] Stability or equilibrium of the lower subsystems is required for the maturation and expression of the higher subsystems, but the expression of higher level subsystems can jeopardize the equilibrium or stability of the lower level

subsystems. For example, an infant struggling to maintain cardiorespiratory homeostasis will find it difficult or impossible to assume an alert state and to interact with the environment. Conversely, alertness and responses to environmental events may contribute to instability of the autonomic, motor, or state subsystems. As a result, the infant might have reactions, such as apnea, bradycardia, or loss of muscle tone. When interacting with the environ-

Table 3–2. *Synactive Theory of Neurobehavioral Organization: Four Subsystems*

Autonomic: Includes patterns of respiration, heart rate, thermoregulation, and digestion.

Motor: Includes posture, tone and activity of the trunk, extremities, and face. The infant's active movements can contribute to instability in the autonomic system.

State: This includes the range of states available to the infant, the transitions from one state to another, and the clearness and differentiation of states.

Attention/Interactive: This includes the infant's ability to assume and maintain an alert state, and take in and respond appropriately to environmental input, including social, cognitive, and emotional input.

From Als H, Leter BM, Tronick EZ, Brazelton TB. In: Fitzgerald H, et al. eds. Theory and Research in Behavioral Pediatrics. Vol 1. New York: Plenum; 1982 and 1985.

ment, the infant strives to regulate its responses to maintain a balance among the four subsystems.[7,8]

Als and associates have documented neonatal behavioral cues that act as indicators of either stress or stability (Table 3-3).[7,8] Physical therapists must be able to recognize these signals and modify treatment in response to these cues. Additionally, parents and all caregivers should be educated about appropriate responses to these infant cues.

Risk Factors

Neurologic Conditions

Asphyxia

Asphyxia is the result of an inadequate exchange of oxygen and carbon dioxide and can have many causes.[9,10] Events occurring during pregnancy and at the time of delivery can contribute to asphyxia. The impact of an episode of asphyxia on a neonate's brain is called *hypoxic-ischemic encephalopathy* (HIE). Hypoxia and ischemia usually occur concurrently or serially.[11,12] The major factors contributing to neonatal asphyxia are interference with umbilical blood flow and poor gas exchange from the mother's circulation through the placenta to the fetus. Failure of the infant's lungs to inflate, which can be caused by many factors, results in persistent fetal circulation (pulmonary hypertension), which may either contribute to, or be secondary to, neonatal asphyxia.[9] Hypoxic-ischemic injuries are the most common cause of severe, nonprogressive neurologic defects caused by perinatal events. Mental retardation, spasticity, choreoathetosis, ataxia, and seizure disorders are associated with asphyxia in the neonate.[12,13]

Cerebral ischemia refers to decreased blood flow to the brain and is typically related to systemic hypotension and decreased cardiac output.[3,5] *Hypoxemia*, or decreased arterial oxygen concentration, can result from perinatal asphyxia, recurrent apnea, or severe respiratory disease. Additionally, fetal hypoxemia depresses the myocardium, causing neonatal bradycardia and hypotension, which lead to further systemic ischemia. In particu-

Table 3–3. *Behavioral Indicators of Stress and Stability**

Signs of Stability or Approach Signals
  Smooth respiration
  Pink, stable color
  Animated facial expression
  Brightening of the eyes
  "Oh" face
  Cooing
  Smiling
  Hand-to-mouth activity
  Well-regulated muscle tone
  Smooth body movements, minimal movement
Signs of Stress
  Physiological indicators
    Color changes
    Circumoral cyanosis
    Skin mottling
    Change in respiratory rate or rhythm
    Change in heart rate
    Coughing
    Sneezing
    Yawning
    Vomiting
    Bowel movement
    Hiccups
  Motor indicators
    Sudden change in muscle tone
    Flaccidity (truncal, extremities, facial)
    Stiffness
      Leg bracing
      Opisthotonos
      Finger splaying
      Facial grimacing
      Tongue extension
      Hyperflexion
    Alterations in the quality of movement
      Disorganized movement
      Jitteriness
      Squirminess
  Behavioral Indicators
    Irritability (crying, inconsolability)
    Staring
    Gaze aversion
    Hyperalertness
    Roving eye movements
    Glassy-eyed appearance
    Sleeplessness and restlessness

*From ref 7 per Tecklin AlS, 1982.

lar, systemic ischemia affects the kidneys, liver, lungs, and gastrointestinal tract. Altered vascular autoregulation in the neonate increases the infant's vulnerability to ischemic injury.[14] When an asphyxial event occurs, the physiological systems offer the greatest protection to the brain. Systemic complications may occur even though the central nervous system (CNS) is spared. Asphyxia leads to metabolic disturbances, including hypoglycemia, hypocalcemia, and hyperkalemia.[9,10] Hypoglycemia generates lactic acid, which adds to the brain damage incurred by asphyxia. Lactic acid can then cross the blood–brain barrier, which can be beneficial for a short period, but which subsequently has serious deleterious effects, including brain damage.[13]

When the infant is traumatized by severe HIE at birth, immediate stupor or coma occurs after birth, often requiring mechanical ventilation. Seizures and severe apnea may occur within the first 12 to 24 hours after birth. Severe hypotonia and absence of spontaneous movement will be seen. Neonatal reflexes are absent or greatly reduced. Brain-stem–mediated ocular reactions may be disturbed. Mortality among these infants is high, and survivors have a high incidence of significant neurologic impairment.[11,12,15] Stupor or coma is associated with bilateral hemispheric disturbances. Recovery from the stupor may occur 12 to 24 hours after birth. At that time, seizures frequently increase in severity.[12] At 24 to 72 hours of age, the infant may reenter a stuporous or comatose state. Mortality of asphyxiated infants is highest at this stage. The most common causes of death after severe asphyxia are hypoxemia caused by pulmonary hypertension; intraventricular or intracerebral hemorrhage; disseminated intravascular coagulation (DIC) that causes uncontrolled hemorrhage, particularly in the lungs; arrhythmias or inadequate cardiac output caused by myocardial failure; and renal failure.

Infants who suffer moderate HIE at birth are usually lethargic and difficult to arouse during the first 12 hours of life. These infants have a history of acidosis and hypotension at delivery. They often require resuscitation at delivery and commonly need assistance to establish adequate respiration. Mechanical ventilation is usually short-term. Seizures and apnea are less likely to occur in those infants with moderate HIE than in those with the severe form. Infants with moderate HIE are often hypotonic with weak proximal musculature. Their muscle tone and level of arousal may improve within 2 to 3 days. They are at much less risk of mortality and long-term neurologic sequelae than are infants with severe HIE.[11,15] Necrotizing enterocolitis (NEC) and acute renal problems are among the significant risks for the moderately involved group.

Mild HIE is usually the result of asphyxia occurring immediately before delivery. Affected infants usually recover well and require minimal resuscitation. Acidosis and hypotension are less severe in this population. Reactions to mild HIE peak during the first 24 hours of life. Characteristically, these infants have a brief period of lethargy shortly after birth. Later, they may display jitteriness, hyperalertness, irritability, and exaggerated responses to stimulation. The Moro response may be hyperactive and easily elicited, or it may occur spontaneously, without an antecedent stimulus. Muscle tone and strength are likely to be normal, although deep tendon reflexes may be slightly hyperactive. Associated transitory hypoglycemia may be present and occasionally causes seizures. Infants with mild HIE do not incur long-term neurologic impairment.[9,16] Rapid recovery from a state of reduced consciousness and quick recovery of spontaneous respirations are associated with a more optimistic outcome.[9,12]

Lesions Associated with Hypoxic-Ischemic Encephalopathy

Lesions associated with HIE include selective neuronal necrosis, status marmoratus of the basal ganglia and thalamus, parasagittal cerebral injury, and periventricular leukomalacia (PVL).[17] Selective neuronal necrosis of the cerebral cortex, diencephalon, basal ganglia, cerebellum, and especially the brain stem in a characteristic but widespread distribution is a common result of a hypoxic-ischemic episode. As a result of neuronal necrosis, the gyri may decrease in size, and glial fibers may replace gray and white matter. Myelination of white matter may be sparse. Associated disorders include mental retardation, hypertonicity, and seizures. Ataxia associated with spasticity is related to cerebellar lesions.[17]

Status marmoratus is characterized by a marbled appearance of the thalamus and basal ganglia. Neuronal loss, gliosis, and hypermyelination typify the pathology found with this defect.[18] Hypoxemia contributes to the cause of status marmoratus. Extrapyramidal disturbances, including choreoathetosis and rigidity, accompany the condition. The abnormalities in tone tend to be symmetric, thus reflecting the symmetry and bilaterality of this lesion.[12]

Parasagittal cerebral injury (watershed infarcts) is mainly the result of decreased cerebral blood flow. The areas in which the lesions occur are associated with the peripheral branches of the major cerebral arteries. Although such lesions are bilateral, they may be asymmetric. Decreasing systemic blood pressure makes the parasagittal areas highly vulnerable to damage, and the posterior aspects of the cerebral hemispheres are even more susceptible to injury. The full-term infant is most likely to be affected by the watershed phenomenon. Clinical features related to parasagittal injury include spastic quadriplegia, delays in language, and visuospatial deficits.[13,15]

Unlike full-term infants, premature infants typically exhibit PVL as a result of decreased blood flow. PVL refers to necrosis of white matter in areas surrounding the lateral ventricles. Intraventricular hemorrhage and ventricular dilatation often accompany this defect. PVL may be transitory, although white matter lesions often reduce to cystic cavities and are highly correlated with cerebral palsy. Spastic diplegia is the most common form of cerebral palsy resulting from PVL owing to the proximity of the ventricular system of descending motor fibers that innervate the lower extremities.[12,19]

Intraventricular Hemorrhage

Intraventricular hemorrhage (IVH) is the most common brain lesion seen in infants less than 32 weeks of gestation and occurs in approximately 40% of all premature infants.[10] Infants with a low birth weight and those with a more complicated medical course are at greatest risk. Unstable respiratory status, especially when complicated by pneumothorax and hypoxemia, and difficult deliveries, especially breech presentation, are factors thought to contribute strongly to IVH. IVH also occurs as a result of frequent swings in blood pressure that cause alternating ischemia followed by reperfusion and hyperemia. The fragile cerebral vasculature of the premature infant is poorly supported in the gelatinous subependymal germinal matrix in the periventricular region. As a result, the swings in blood pressure and perfusion put stress on the fragile vasculature to the point of rupture. Hemorrhages usually originate in arterioles in the germinal matrix near the caudate nucleus. IVH may occur suddenly, or it may evolve and expand slowly for 1 to 3 days. Because blood has a higher acoustic impedance than cerebrospinal fluid and brain matter, IVH can be detected easily by a neurosonogram through the anterior fontanelle.[17,20] The extent of bleeding shown by the neurosonogram is graded as described in Table 3-4.

Neurologic outcome has been correlated with the severity of the hemorrhage. Infants with grades I and II IVH are considered to be at minimal risk for developing a long-term neurologic deficit. However, IVH of grades III and IV is associated with a significantly higher incidence of neurologic defi-

Table 3–4. *Grades of Intraventricular Hemorrhage**

Grade	Extent of Hemorrhage
I	Isolated germinal matrix hemorrhage
II	Intraventricular hemorrhage with normal ventricular size
III	Intraventricular hemorrhage with ventricular dilation
IV	Intraventricular dilation with parenchymal hemorrhage

Adapted from Papile L, Munsick-Bruro G, Shaefer A. Relationship of cerebral intraventricular hemorrhage and early childhood neurologic handicaps. J Pediatr. 1983;103:273–277.

cits, including hydrocephalus, cerebral palsy, and mental retardation.[21]

Respiratory Conditions

Respiratory Distress Syndrome

Respiratory distress syndrome (RDS), also called hyaline membrane disease (HMD) because of the appearance of the lungs at autopsy, is characterized by clinical signs that include chest wall retractions, cyanosis, expiratory grunting, flaring of the nares, and tachypnea. Apnea, hypotension, and pulmonary edema are also associated with RDS. Premature infants born at less than 37 weeks of gestation are most commonly affected.[22] RDS is a leading cause of death in premature neonates, but medical advances, especially the recent introduction of exogenous surfactant, have led to a significant reduction in morbidity and mortality.[23]

A decreased production of chemically mature levels of surfactant is associated with RDS. This lack of adequate levels of surfactant causes a reduced alveolar surface tension, which causes alveolar collapse on expiration. This atelectasis, which occurs repeatedly, requires a massive increase in work of breathing as the infant tries to reinflate the lungs. Eventually, the infant suffers from decreased oxygenation, asphyxia, metabolic acidosis, and acute respiratory failure, any one of which can be fatal.[22]

Bronchopulmonary Dysplasia

Bronchopulmonary dysplasia (BPD) is a chronic lung disease of infancy. The specific pathogenesis of BPD is controversial, but most neonatologists believe that iatrogenic factors, such as barotrauma associated with mechanical ventilation, elevated concentrations of administered oxygen, and endotracheal intubation, play a significant role in the development of BPD. Other factors, such as air leaks, patent ductus arteriosus, and fluid overload, are known to increase the likelihood of BPD.[24]

The process of BPD begins with the destruction of the respiratory tract cilia. Ciliary destruction is followed by necrosis of the cells of the respiratory epithelium as distal as the bronchioles. Capillary endothelial cells and cells lining the alveolar sacs may also be damaged. Pulmonary interstitial fibrosis may occur as early as 2 to 3 days in infants born between 25 to 26 weeks of gestation.[24] Recovery from the pulmonary damage of BPD is a slow process, with pulmonary impairment persisting for up to 1 year or longer.[25,26] The chronic lack of oxygenation in these babies often impairs neuromotor development.

Meconium Aspiration

In some cases, the fetus aspirates with its initial breath the thick meconium that it passed in utero. This meconium aspiration causes airway obstruction that can produce respiratory distress with chest wall retraction, grunting, tachypnea, and cyanosis. Infants born at term, or post-term, are at greatest risk. The incidence of meconium aspiration is approximately 5% to 15% of all live births.[27]

Metabolic Conditions

Metabolic Acidosis

Metabolic acidosis results from increased production or inadequate excretion of hydrogen ions which form acid, or from excessive loss of basic material, such as bicarbonate ions, in the urine or stools. The result of either is a reduction of pH in the body.[27]

Hyperbilirubinemia

Hyperbilirubinemia (jaundice) is the accumulation in the blood of excessive amounts of bilirubin. Causes include Rh factor or ABO factor incompatibility of blood, physiologic jaundice, reabsorption of blood, and infection. Physiologic jaundice is commonly seen in premature infants who have a limited ability to excrete bilirubin from their systems. Excessive hemolysis of red blood cells can lead to excessive amounts of bilirubin and occurs with maternal-fetal blood group incompatibility. This type of hyperbilirubinemia has been the leading contributor to neurologic sequelae of all the causes of jaundice. Recent prevention of Rh sensitization of mothers, as well as improved management of Rh incompatibility, has almost eliminated the disease and its neurologic consequences.[22]

Kernicterus, or yellow staining of the brain, is caused by the deposition in the brain of unconjugated bilirubin. Most frequently, damage caused by kernicterus occurs in the basal ganglia and hippocampus. The mortality rate of affected infants is high. Long-term neurologic sequelae include choreothetosis, rigidity, hypotonia, high-frequency deafness, and metal retardation.

Recent evidence indicates that decreased levels of bilirubin in the very preterm infant may have subtle effects on learning and development.[9,22,28] Psychomotor delays may occur even in the absence of overt kernicterus.[11,22]

Cardiovascular Conditions

Patent Ductus Arteriosus

In utero, the ductus arteriosus is a vascular connection that shunts blood from the pulmonary artery to the descending aorta, thereby bypassing the lungs which do not provide for gas exchange during fetal life. Typically, the ductus arteriosus closes shortly after birth. Its failure to close is the most frequent cause of congenital heart failure in neonates.[27]

Viral Infections of the Fetus and Neonate

The developing brain is highly susceptible to injury as a result of viral infection acquired in intrauterine or early neonatal life when cell structures are organizing and myelinating and the vascular system is proliferating. The result of these infections may be malformations or impeded growth of the brain. Viral infections may persist in the infant's system for an extended time and may cause further neurologic impairment. Common nonbacterial agents affecting the neonate have been reported to cause so-called TORCH infections. These include toxoplasmosis (T); other (O) infections, such as syphilis, rubella (R), cytomegalovirus (C), and herpes simplex (H). As additional microorganisms have been identified, the TORCH group actually represents only one subgroup of congenital infections.

Various neurologic sequelae are associated with congenital infections. Psychomotor retardation, microcephaly, learning disability, seizures, blindness, sensorineural hearing loss, and hydrocephalus are examples of these sequelae.[29]

Human immunodeficiency virus (HIV) has quickly become a major public health problem.[30] Of those children with acquired immunodeficiency syndrome (AIDS), 80% contracted the virus in utero via transplacental transfer.[31,32] Intravenous drug use is the major risk factor associated with mothers who give birth to HIV-infected infants. Maternal antibodies to the virus cross the placenta, and infants of infected mothers will have HIV antibodies whether or not the infants are infected.[32] Infants diagnosed with AIDS usually have specific clinical features, including opportunistic infections; interstitial pneumonitis with respiratory distress resulting from lymphocytic interstitial pneumonitis, microcephaly, and other neurologic abnormalities; and recurrent bacterial infections.[32] Infants with AIDS present a major challenge to the rehabilitation field, as more than 90% of these young patients show signs of static or progressive encephalopathy.[33,34] Therapists working in the NICU, as well as those in all areas of rehabilitation, must be informed of and adhere strictly to infectious disease control policies.

In Utero Substance Exposure

Fetal Alcohol Syndrome

Fetal alcohol syndrome (FAS) occurs in infants whose mothers consume more than 1 to 2 oz. of alcohol a day during their pregnancy.[17] The likelihood of the infant developing FAS increases if the mother smokes and drinks.[35]

The incidence of FAS is 1 in 750 live births.[36] FAS is the most common cause of birth defects that is completely preventable. Characteristics that babies with FAS demonstrate include poor motor control, tremulousness during the newborn period, mental retardation, facial dysmorphism, prenatal and postnatal growth deficiency, congenital hip dislocation, abnormalities of the joints, and attention deficit disorders.[4,13]

Cocaine Exposure; Maternal Cocaine Abuse

The recent epidemic of cocaine abuse, in all its various forms, including crack cocaine, has resulted in large numbers of infants being born after in utero exposure to cocaine. Serious effects of cocaine exposure have been reported in neonates. These effects include low birth weight, intrauterine growth retardation, reduced head circumference, preterm birth, hemorrhagic infarctions, cystic lesions, and congenital anomalies and malformations.[37–42] Additionally, increased obstetrical complications, especially placenta abruptio, have been reported.

Infants exposed to cocaine in utero may demonstrate withdrawal symptoms characterized by irritability, jitteriness, and vigorous sucking.[37,43] When the Neonatal Behavioral Assessment Scale (NABS) has been used to assess these neonates, they have shown deficits in the areas of orientation, motor ability, and regulation of state, including a low threshold for overstimulation.[38,44] In addition, abnormal reflex behavior and autonomic instability have been documented.[41] Diminished scores for orientation have been attributed to the infant's inability to attain an alert state.[38]

Neonatal Drug Withdrawal Syndrome

Infants born to mothers who abused narcotics during pregnancy may show symptoms of withdrawal when they are deprived of the drug after birth. Low birth weight has been reported in 50% of infants born to mothers addicted to heroin. Symptoms of withdrawal increase in infants if the maternal dosage is high, if the mother's last dose was within 24 hours of delivery, or if the maternal addiction is long-standing. Symptoms of withdrawal from heroin typically appear within the first 4 days of life, whereas withdrawal from methadone may appear slightly later.[17,45]

The classic symptom of withdrawal from heroin in a neonate is jitteriness, which is further delineated as being stimulus-sensitive, rhythmic, and easily stopped by passive flexion of the extremities.[17]

Other common signs and symptoms include hyperirritability, increased activity, hypertonicity, and reduced sleep. There is frequently a high-pitched cry and excessive sucking behavior. These infants are commonly poor feeders despite their tendency toward a strong sucking pattern. Gastrointestinal complications, including regurgitation and diarrhea, are common. Seizures are uncommon with withdrawal from heroin, but are more likely to occur with withdrawal from methadone.[33]

Necrotizing Enterocolitis

Necrotizing enterocolitis is a pathologic condition of the gastrointestinal tract that often occurs during the first 6 weeks of life in premature infants weighing less than 2000 g.[46,47] These infants have also suffered perinatal insults, such as asphyxia, sepsis, hypoxia, or respiratory distress. The disease process leads to intestinal mucosal ulceration and hemorrhage, necrosis, and epithelial sloughing. Intestinal perforation may occur.[48]

Retinopathy of Prematurity

Retinopathy of prematurity (ROP) is the main cause of childhood blindness and is a process by which abnormal growth of blood vessels occurs in the immature part of the retina in some premature infants. The cause of this abnormal vascular growth is not fully understood. High levels of administered oxygen are believed to have a detrimental effect on the infant's vulnerable intraocular vasculature. There is an increased incidence of ROP in low-birth-weight infants who have numerous medical complications during hospitalization in the NICU.

In most infants with ROP, the abnormal blood vessels heal by themselves during the first year of life and cause little or no visual impairment. Nearsightedness or strabismus will be the result in many of the patients in whom healing is incomplete. Scarring of the retina may also occur in patients who have only partial healing and who may have visual problems that cannot be corrected completely. In the most severe cases, retinal blood vessels continue their abnormal development and form scar tissue that may cause retinal detachment. Retinal detachment causes severe visual impairment and, occasionally, complete blindness. Only a small percentage of premature infants develop the severe form of the disease. ROP is graded according to its severity (see Table 3-5).

Prevention of prematurity is the only effective prophylaxis for ROP. Cryotherapy is effective in arresting many moderately severe cases (designated as Zone 1 or 2 and Stage 3 or 4+). Although cryotherapy does not always prevent retinal detachment, it decreases the incidence of poor outcome from 55.5% to 33.9% based upon visual acuity and from 47.4% to 25.7% based upon anatomical outcomes.[49]

Neonatal Orthopedic Problems

Brachial Plexus Injury

Brachial plexus injuries are classified as those injuries involving the upper plexus, Erb palsy, and those involving the lower plexus, Klumpke paralysis. Brachial plexus injuries occur in approximately 0.25% of all deliveries.[50]

Erb palsy involves the fifth and sixth cervical roots and accounts for most brachial plexus injuries.[50] Erb palsy occurs most frequently following difficult breech or forceps delivery. Spontaneous recovery is often seen within a few days or weeks.

Table 3–5. *Stages of Retinopathy of Prematurity*

Stage	Characteristics
I	Normal newborn eye demonstrating incomplete vascularization of the peripheral temporal retina
II	Active stage: early vascularization with engorged arterioles and venules
III	Advanced active phase: more advanced venules with vitreous proliferation and organization, as well as retinal traction
IV	Cicatricial phase: localized retinal detachment and severe retinal traction with "temporal dragging" of the macula vessels

From Eden R, et al. Assessment and care of the fetus. Norwalk: Appleton, Lange, 1990.

When recovery is delayed, contractures can occur at the shoulder or elbow, and atrophy is common in the affected muscle groups.[51] The infant will have weakness in external rotation, extension, and abduction at the shoulder; elbow flexion, forearm supination; and wrist extension.

A pediatric therapist usually instructs the parents to position the involved upper extremity in a neutral position by pinning the sleeve of the baby's tee shirt to the diaper. This position protects against further injury to the plexus and prevents overstretching of flaccid muscles, tendons, and ligaments. Although this pinned position may reinforce adduction and internal rotation of the shoulder, contractures can usually be prevented with gentle range of motion (ROM) exercises. A 2-week recovery period prior to rehabilitation is usually prudent.

Congenital Dislocation of the Hip

Congenital dislocation of the hip (CDH) is an abnormality in the relationship between the femoral head and the acetabulum. Subluxation occurs if the two structures are in partial contact, whereas dislocation occurs when there is complete loss of contact. The femoral head is usually displaced in a lateral, posterior, or superior direction owing to the pull of the major muscle groups. Seventy percent of cases occur in females. The incidence increases in breech deliveries. Dysplasia of the femoral head and acetabulum increases with growth.

Because successful correction of the deformity depends on treatment within the first 3 months of life, all neonates should be screened routinely for CDH. The Barlow maneuver, in which medial-to-lateral pressure on the proximal femur is used to test the stability of the hip joint, is the preferred method of screening. Treatment becomes more complicated and invasive if CDH is not detected until later in infancy or early childhood. If hip dysplasia or CDH is diagnosed within the first 3 months of life, it can be treated effectively with dynamic splinting that maintains the hip in a flexed, abducted position with the femoral head seated in the acetabulum. Some of the most commonly used splints were designed by Pavlic, Ilfeld, and Von

Rosen. Subluxation may be treated by using double or triple diapers on the infant or by using a Frejka pillow.[52-54]

Talipes Equinovarus (Clubfoot)

Talipes equinovarus, a foot deformity, has three components. Plantar flexion (equinus) occurs at the joint where the talus articulates with the distal tibia and fibula. Inversion (varus) occurs primarily at the subtalar, talocalcaneal, talonavicular, and calcaneocuboid joints. Supination occurs at the mid-tarsal joint. All three components must be present for the diagnosis of classic talipes equinovarus.[55]

The incidence of talipes equinovarus is approximately 1 in 800 to 1000 live births. Approximately 10% of cases are associated with a hereditary pattern. The deformity is often associated with a neuromuscular disorder (e.g., myelomeningocele). When clubfoot is detected, the infant should be examined carefully for other anomalies, particularly those involving the spine.

Talipes equinovarus can be corrected most rapidly if the treatment is begun shortly after birth, while the foot is still malleable. Treatment consists of manipulation with gentle stretching of the contracted muscle tissues of the medial and posterior aspects of the foot. Manipulation and exercise is often followed by splinting to maintain the desired position, or serial casting. If treatment is delayed, surgery may be necessary to lengthen the tightened soft tissue structures of the foot.[54]

Metatarsus Varus

Metatarsus varus consists of adduction of the forefoot, which occurs primarily at the midtarsal joint (the talonavicular and calcaneocuboid joints). The severity of this deformity depends on the relative flexibility or rigidity of the joint. A more rigid deformity, unable to be manually corrected past midline, may be treated with serial casting. Passive ROM exercise may be adequate for a more flexible deformity. The role of the pediatric therapist will often include instruction in proper exercise technique for the infant's caregiver.[55]

Tibial Torsion

Tibial torsion, often described as "toeing in," consists of excessive internal rotation of the tibia. The problem is more pronounced in premature infants who have low muscle tone. Prone positioning may exacerbate tibial torsion. This deformity is often corrected by using an external rotation splint that is worn at night. Laxity of the ligaments of the knee in young children may also cause tibial torsion.[55,56]

Neonatal Assessment

A thorough assessment of the infant's neurodevelopmental and behavioral status is the initial step in establishing an intervention program for the infant. Neurologic development of both the premature and full-term infant occurs in a predictable sequence. This sequence provides expectations of an infant's performance at various gestational and corrected ages.

The authors of the first neurologic assessments of the neonate, including Amiel-Tison, Prechtl, and Saint-Anne Dargassies, mainly examined muscle tone and reflex development as manifestations of neurologic function.[57-59] Assessment of behavior as a reflection of more complex neurologic function has now been included in evaluations of the newborn infant. The therapist can draw from various tools of assessment to conduct a comprehensive neurodevelopmental evaluation. Special emphasis is given to muscle tone, development of reflexes, the quality of motor responses, and state organization.

Some general guidelines should be remembered when initiating the assessment process. First, it is important to capture the infant's optimal performance during the assessment.[60] This necessitates flexibility in scheduling. Periods of assessment should be scheduled midway between the infant's feedings. The schedule for other medical procedures, such as heel sticks for blood samples, should be considered when planning a schedule for assessing the infant. A knowledge of the effects on the infant's performance of medications and the overall medical condition are essential for accurate interpretation of assessment procedures. For example, some recovery of asphyxiated infants is expected for up to 2 weeks after birth. Assessment before the end of this recovery period must take into account the neurologic delay associated with asphyxia in order not to underestimate the capabilities of these infants.

Age corrected for prematurity is appropriate when interpreting the results of a neurodevelopmental assessment. Full-term gestation is considered to be 40 weeks. Infants are considered to be premature if they are born before the completion of 37 weeks of gestation.[22] The corrected age is established by subtracting the estimated number of gestational weeks less than 40 from the chronologic age. For example, 4 weeks after birth, an infant born at an estimated 32 weeks of gestation, or 8 weeks earlier than 40, has a corrected age of 36 weeks (4 weeks chronologic age minus 8 weeks equals 36). The same infant, 24 weeks after birth, is corrected to 24 weeks minus 8 weeks, which equals 16 weeks, or 4 months.

Use of corrected age for interpreting assessment procedures in both the neonatal period and throughout infancy varies among institutions. Our policy is to correct ages until the chronologic age of 18 months; however, this interpretation can artificially inflate assessment scores, thus disguising developmental delays. The experienced therapist must be aware of the quality of movement patterns and must look for subtle signs of neurologic deviations.

A brief discussion of the most commonly used neonatal assessments follows. Several of these tools require additional training in their administration and interpretation. In all cases, supervised experience is suggested to improve reliability. A detailed discussion of assessment tools can be found in Chapter 2.

Apgar Score

The Apgar score is a quantitative assessment of the neonate's medical status that is usually performed at 1 and 5 minutes of age and, occasionally, at 10 and 15 minutes of age as well. A score of eight or more at 1 minute of age means that the baby will not require extensive resuscitation. A score of zero to two indicates severe asphyxia and may indicate the need for intubation and cardiac massage. Scores of five to seven may indicate a need for less intense resuscitation, such as vigorous stimulation and administration of supplemental oxygen (Table 3-6).[36,46,61,62]

Clinical Assessment of Gestational Age in the Newborn Infant

The Clinical Assessment of Gestational Age in the Newborn Infant, developed by Dubowitz, Dubowitz, and Goldberg, is the most widely used

Table 3–6. *Apgar Score for Condition of the Newborn Baby**

Sign	Score		
	0	*1*	*2*
Heart rate	Absent	Slow (<100 bpm)	>100 bpm
Respiratory effort	Absent	Sow, irregular	Good, crying
Muscle tone	Limp	Some flexion of extremities	Active motion
Reflex irritability			
Response to catheter in nostril	No response	Grimace	Cough or sneeze
Response when feet are stimulated	No response	Some motion	Cry
Color	Blue, pale	Body pink, extremities blue	Completely pink
			Total score

**From Apgar V. Proposal for new method of evaluation of newborn infant. Anesth Analg 1953;32:269; Avery G, ed: Neonatology, Pathophysiology and Management of the Newborn. Philadelphia: JB Lippincott; 1975:117.*

and accepted scale for determining gestational age.[63] The scale involves evaluating 11 external characteristics or 10 neurologic criteria. These characteristics appear predictably with gestational age. The results of this assessment are then compared to obstetric records and prenatal sonograms to establish the gestational age. The determined gestational age is then plotted against the infant's height and weight to determine whether intrauterine growth was adequate or retarded.

Neonatal Behavioral Assessment Scale

The Neonatal Behavioral Assessment Scale (NBAS),[60] designed by Brazelton, permits the examiner to measure an infant's ability to respond to environmental events. Intrinsic to this assessment is the concept that the neonate is a complex organism capable of protecting itself from negative environmental stimuli while still being able to respond to positive input. The neonate also has the capacity to elicit responses from people in the environment. Despite the inclusion of some neurologic items, Brazelton does not consider the tool to be a formal neurologic evaluation. Brazelton was a pioneer in establishing the need to elicit an infant's best performance, rather than relying on average performance. The examiner is responsible for altering the infant's environment to attain an optimal response to a stimulus. Ideally, the examiner brings the infant through various behavioral states beginning with the infant in light sleep, progressing to an alert state, then to an active and crying state, and then back to a quieter state. This tool was developed for use with infants between 36 and 44 weeks' gestational age. Reliability in administering and scoring the NBAS is achieved through specific training and supervised practice.

Assessment of Preterm Infant's Behavior

Adapted from the NBAS, the Assessment of Preterm Infant's Behavior (APIB) evaluates the developing behavioral organization of the premature infant.[7] The APIB is based upon the synactive model of newborn behavioral organization discussed ear-lier. This assessment uses graded maneuvers to assess the functioning and interplay of five subsystems, including physiologic, motor, state, attentional-interactive, and self-regulatory. Like the NBAS, reliability in administering and scoring the APIB depends upon the extensive training and supervised practice.[8]

Neurologic Assessment of the Full-term and Preterm Newborn Infant

The Neurologic Assessment of the Full-term and Preterm Newborn Infant[64] investigates the infant's capabilities for habituation, movement and muscle tone, reflexes, and neurobehavioral responses. It provides diagrams in chart format for recording, and is based on a five-point scale for categorizing results. The tool was designed to meet four specific requirements. First, minimal training in neonatal neurology is required to administer this test. Second, it assesses both premature and full-term infants. Third, there is high test-retest reliability. Finally, administration of the assessment takes no longer than 10 or 15 minutes. The authors of the test have correlated results of assessments with the development of IVHs. The ability of this assessment device to document progression or resolution of neurologic abnormalities raises the possibility that this tool may be used to predict prognosis.

Morgan Neonatal Neurobehavioral Examination

The Morgan Neonatal Neurobehavioral Examination is divided into three sections: tone and motor patterns, primitive reflexes, and behavioral responses. Similar to the Dubowitz Neurologic Assessment, the Morgan examination is provided in chart format to expedite recording. Each of the three sections has nine items that are scored based on the level of maturity of a normal response or on the abnormality of a response. This assessment is applicable for infants between the ages of 34 and 44 weeks' gestation or corrected age. A numerical quotient, which Morgan has correlated with developmental outcome, can be obtained from the assessment (Table 3-7).[65]

Movement Assessment of Infants

Movement Assessment of Infants (MAI) provides a uniform approach to the evaluation of high-risk infants. It is used for infants between the ages of birth and 12 months. This assessment requires extensive handling of the infant, which makes the MAI very time-consuming.[66]

Milani-Comparetti Motor Development Screening Test

The Milani-Comparetti motor assessment test is used to test reflexes and motor milestones of infants from birth to 2 years of age. This assessment is relatively easy to administer and has a high reliability.[67]

Developmental Intervention

Numerous theories of intervention have been proposed by various experts who work in NICUs. Neurodevelopmental and sensorimotor approaches are the bases for most interventional programs implemented by physical and occupational therapists. Both approaches take into account the fact that infant neuromotor development is a unique and individualized process. Treatment, therefore, is designed to meet the specific problems and needs of each infant.

Neurodevelopmental treatment, as designed by Bobath, uses handling to inhibit abnormal responses while facilitating automatic reactions.[68] Handling techniques are used with the neonate to provide normal sensory and motor experiences that will provide the basis for motor development. Movement experience is frequently limited or disturbed in the premature or medically unstable infant. Disruptions and abnormalities of the normal patterns of movement may interfere with the development of head control, trunk stability, oculomotor coordination, eye-hand coordination, and social interaction.

With sensorimotor approaches, specific sensory input is administered to elicit a desired motor or behavioral response. Sensory integration techniques, originally developed for treatment of learning disabled children, are sometimes incorporated into sensorimotor programs. Sensorimotor intervention can be applied to the high-risk infant in various ways (e.g., linear rocking on a small beach ball might be used to stimulate the vestibular system and promote an alert state). If an infant is tightly swaddled, deep tactile and proprioceptive input can promote calming and self-regulating behavior.

Common goals of developmental intervention in the NICU include the following:

1. To promote state organization
2. To promote appropriate parent-infant interaction
3. To enhance self-regulatory behavior through environmental modification
4. To promote postural alignment and more normal patterns of movement through therapeutic handling and positioning
5. To enhance oral-motor skills and assist with oral feedings
6. To improve visual and auditory reactions
7. To prevent iatrogenic musculoskeletal abnormalities
8. To provide appropriate remediation of orthopedic complications
9. To provide consultation to team members, including the nursing staff and parents, regarding developmental intervention
10. To participate in interagency collaboration in order to facilitate transition to the home environment.

Success of intervention depends on individualization of treatment techniques to meet the infant's specific needs. The suggestions that preceded and that follow are not a "cookbook" to be used for solutions to particular problems. No activity is appropriate for all infants, and all activities must be adapted to respond to the infant's unique reactions to handling. For best results, therapeutic handling must be incorporated into routine care activities, such as rolling the infant or lifting and carrying the infant.

As previously emphasized, the therapist must have a complete understanding of normal and ab-

Table 3–7. *Morgan Neonatal Neuro-Behavioral Examination**

Name _____

Date of Birth _____ Gestational Age _____

Date of Exam _____ Chronological Age _____

Timing of Exam _____ Corrected Age _____

STATES
1. Deep sleep, no movement, regular breathing
2. Light sleep, eyes shut, some movement
3. Dozing, eyes opening and closing
4. Awake, eyes open, minimal movement
5. Wide awake, vigorous movement
6. Crying

Tone and Motor Patterns	1 (< 32 Wks)	2 (32–36 Wks)	3 (>36 Wks)	A (Abnormal)
Posture (Predominant)	Total extension	LE flexed, UE extended	Total flexion	Opisthotonus / Tonic extension
Arm recoil Infant supine. Take arms and extend parallel to the body; hold several seconds and release.	No flexion within 5 sec	Partial flexion at elbow >100° within 4–5 sec	Arms flex at elbow to <100° within 2–3 sec	Difficult to extend / Jerky flexion
Scarf Infant supine, head in midline. Bring arm across chest until resistance is met.	No resistance	Limited resistance past midline	Resistance at or before midline	Tonic flexion / Shoulder retraction
Popliteal angle Infant supine. Approximate knee and thigh to abdomen; extend leg by gentle pressure with index finger behind ankle.	180°–135°	90°–135°	90°–60°	<60°
Ankle dorsiflexion Infant supine. Flex foot against shin until resistance is met.	Limited 60°–90°	Partial 30°–60°	Complete <30°	Equinus >90°

A. Tone and motor patterns _____
   Abnormal patterns _____
B. Primitive reflexes _____
   Abnormal patterns _____

C. Behavioral responses _____
   Responsiveness _____
   Temperament _____
   Equilibration _____

(continued)

Table 3–7. *Morgan Neonatal Neuro-Behavioral Examination* * *(Continued)*

Tone and Motor Patterns	1(<32 Wks)	2(32–36 Wks)	3(>36 Wks)	A (Abnormal)
Prone suspension Hold infant in ventral suspension, observe curvature of back and relation of head to trunk.	Complete	Partial	Near horizontal	Tonic extension
Slip-through Hold infant in vertical suspension under axillae. Observe the amount of support required to prevent infant from "slipping."	Complete	Partial	None	Shoulder retraction
Pull-to-sit Pull infant toward sitting posture by traction on both arms.	Complete head/leg	Partial flexion	Occasional alignment	Tonic extension Shoulder retraction
Head righting Place infant in sitting position, allow head to fall forward, then wait 30 seconds	No attempt to raise head	Unsuccessful attempt to raise head upright	Occasional alignment	Head cannot be flexed forward.
Primitive Reflexes				
Root	Absent	Mouth opening, partial head turning	Full head turning with mouth opening	Tongue thrust
Suck	Weak	Inconsistent, irregular	Strong regular sucking in bursts of 5 or more movements	Clenching-tonic bite
Grasp	Absent	Sustained flexion	Traction	Thumb adduction
Positive support	Astasis	Inconsistent, partial	Full extension	Equinus
Walking	No response	Some effort, but not continuous with both legs	At least two steps	Scissoring
Crossed extensor	No response	Withdrawal and flexion	Flexion and extension	Tonic extension
Moro	No response	Abduction only	Abduction and adduction	Tremor only
Tonic neck	No response	Legs only	Arms and legs respond	Obligate
Cry	Absent	Whimpering	Sustained cry	High pitched

SCORING
1. Total responses to the 9 items in each area; A scored as 1⁻
2. Behavioral subtest scored 3, if 2 of three items are scored 3
3. Behavioral subtest scored 1, if 2 of three items are scored 1
4. Behavioral subtest scored 2 if neither of the above criteria are met
5. Score number of abnormal patterns

Tone and Motor Patterns	1 (<32 Wks)	2 (32–36 Wks)	3 (>36 Wks)	A (Abnormal)
Behavioral Responses				
Responsiveness/alertness	**1 (<32 wks)** Inattentive or brief responsiveness (4 or less)		**2 (32–36 wks)** Moderately sustained alertness; may use stimulation to come to alert state (5,6)	**3 (>36 wks)** Sustained and continuous attentiveness (7–9)
Orientation to face and voice	Does not focus or follow stimulus, brief following (4 or less)		Inconsistent or jerky following horizontal 30° (5,6)	Sustained, smooth following 60° horizontally and occasionally vertically (7–9)
Defensive reaction to cloth over face	No response, nonspecific activity with long latency (1–3)		Rooting, head turning (5,6)	Swipes with arms (7–9)
Temperament	1-Flat	1-Labile		
Irritability	No cry (1)	Cries to 6 stimuli (7–9)	Cries to 4 or 5 stimuli (5,6)	Cries to 1–3 stimuli (2–4)
Peak of excitement	Low level of arousal never > state 3 (1,2)	Insulated crying in response to stimuli (8,9)	Predominantly state 4—may reach state 5 with stimulation (3,4)	Predominantly state 5; reaches state 6 with stimulation (5–7)
Cuddliness	No moulding (3)	Resists, arches (1,2)	Molds with movement and handling (4,5)	Molds and nestles spontaneously (6–9)
Equilibration				
Self-quieting	Cannot quiet self (1–3)		Occasional success (4–6); no sustained crying	Quiets self on two or more occasions (7–9)
Consolability	Inconsolable (1)		Consoles with holding and rocking (2–5), consoling not needed	Consoles with talking or handling in crib (6–9)
Tremors	Tremors in all states (8,9)		Tremors occasionally with aversive stimuli (6,7)	No tremors or tremors only with crying (1–5)

*After Morgan A: Neuro-Developmental Approach to the High-Risk Neonate (Notes from a seminar). Williamsburg, VA, Nov 3–4, 1984. **LE,** lower extremities; **UE,** upper extremities.

normal development before entering the NICU. When handling, positioning, or feeding an infant, the therapist must be aware of the signs of physiological stress (see Table 3-3). Therapy must be modified or deferred if signs of stress are noted. Periodic rest breaks during the treatment session may help the infant to maintain physiologic homeostasis.

Therapeutic Handling

The primary goals of therapeutic handling in premature infants are to decrease hyperextension of the neck and trunk, reduce elevation of the shoulders, decrease retraction of the scapula, and reduce extension of the lower extremities. Activation of the primary flexor muscle groups must occur simultaneously.

In the supine position, neck and trunk hyperextension can be reduced by gently flexing the hips and knees. Extreme care must be taken with this activity to avoid hyperflexion of the neck, which can cause airway obstruction and pulmonary compromise in premature infants. Elevation of the shoul-

ders can be reduced in the supine position by bringing the infant's hands toward the buttocks. With the lower extremities flexed and the hands on the buttocks, weight bearing through the shoulder girdle can be introduced, as can subtle weight shifts. Alignment of the head and trunk should be maintained, especially during weight shifts (Fig. 3-1).

The side-lying position is advantageous for accomplishing several therapeutic goals. Neck and trunk hyperextension can be reduced in sidelying, and deep proprioceptive input can be applied through the shoulders and hips to promote postural stability. Additionally, scapular protraction (abduction) and upper extremity midline activities can be enhanced in the side-lying position (Fig. 3-2A). Weight bearing through the shoulders, hips, and feet provides proprioceptive input that may promote the development of more normal muscle tone and increase proximal stability (Fig. 3-2B).

Several therapeutic goals can be achieved using a technique called hammock handling. This handling technique is used to activate flexor muscle groups, facilitate head righting, and facilitate alerting. A hammock-like sling is made with a doubled

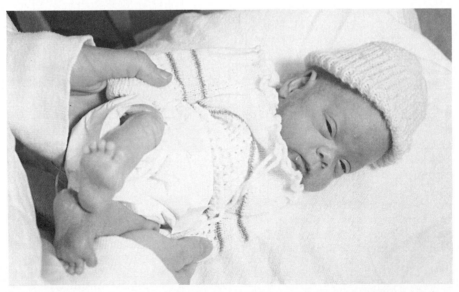

Figure 3-1. *Weight bearing through the shoulder girdle to promote proximal stability. Lateral weight shift provides a valuable sensorimotor experience.*

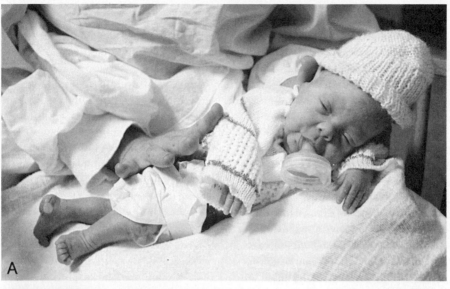

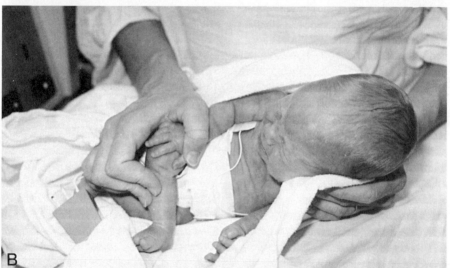

Figure 3-2. A. *In a side-lying position, disassociation not only between shoulder and pelvic girdles, but also between the lower extremities, can be achieved.* B. *Incorporation of weight bearing through the foot helps reduce tactile hypersensitivity of the foot.*

blanket whose sides have been rolled toward the infant for stability. The infant is placed in the hammock in a supine position and is elevated slowly to a semi-sitting position, after which the infant is lowered back to a supine position. This activity must be done slowly to fully elicit the desired head righting reactions. Promotion of an alert behavioral state through stimulation of the vestibular system is an additional benefit of the linear rocking that occurs with raising and lowering. A desired response to the hammock activity is activation of anterior neck and abnormal musculature to promote flexion.

In addition, scapular retraction and shoulder elevation can be reduced, and upper extremity midline skills can be increased with this activity (Fig. 3-3).

By placing the infant in a prone position, weight bearing and weight shifting can be introduced. The upper extremities of the infant should be held near the body in a flexed posture. The lower extremities should be flexed and adducted at the hip in order for the knees to be placed in position under the abdomen. By using this position, the infant's center of gravity is placed forward at a point near the cheek, similar to that of a full-term infant. The therapist's hands are placed along the infant's trunk to provide important tactile and proprioceptive cues that reinforce symmetry and facilitate graded extension of the neck and trunk. Subtle shifts in weight in lateral and anterior or posterior directions can be facilitated by the therapist, who should hold the infant on his or her lap while gently raising and lowering his or her own legs. Downward pressure through the infant's shoulders serves to elongate the cervical musculature. Stroking of the cervical extensor mus-

cle groups promotes head-turning reactions. If hyperextension of the neck or trunk or increased elevation of the shoulder is elicited in this position, handling must be altered to incorporate a greater degree of flexion into the infant's posture.

Supported sitting offers an opportunity to increase the infant's ability to assume and maintain an alert state. The upright or semi-upright position, because of vestibular input, encourages arousal and alert behaviors. This allows the infant to begin to interact with the environment, and may improve visual and auditory responses. Again, it must be stressed that coming to an alert state may contribute to loss of stability in the motor and autonomic subsystems. Therefore, the infant must be monitored closely. Adequate support of the trunk during supported sitting is essential to help prevent the elevation or retraction of the scapula, which is often seen in infants in an attempt to compensate for poor control of the head.

Head righting may become a realistic goal for more long-term hospitalized infants and can be fa-

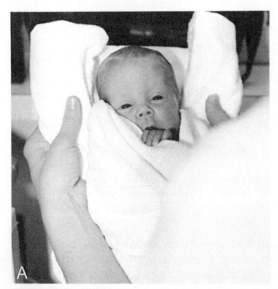 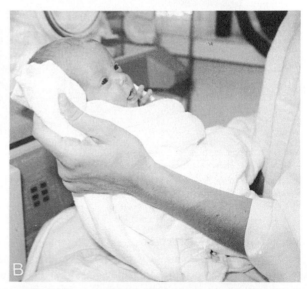

Figure 3-3. A. *and* B. *Hammock handling to improve head-righting reactions and to increase flexor responses. Vestibular input facilitates alert behavior state (origination of this technique is unknown to these authors).*

cilitated with work in prone and supported sitting. In a supported sit, extension of the trunk may be facilitated through subtle lateral shifting of weight over the ischial tuberosities. The trunk must be erect and aligned with the head before attempts are made to facilitate trunk extension. Anterior flexion of the neck can be stimulated by slowly shifting the infant's weight in a posterior direction, whereas extension of the neck can be achieved by anteriorly shifting the infant's weight.

Premature infants often show hypersensitivity to tactile input. The oral motor area, the palms of the hands, and the soles of the feet are especially prone to tactile hypersensitivity. Essential but aversive medical intervention, such as prolonged intubation, repetitive gavage feedings, and frequent heel sticks, may contribute to the infant's hypersensitivity. Various methods can be used to decrease the neonate's hypersensitivity. Deep rhythmical tactile and proprioceptive input, rather than light touch when handling the infant, will effectively reduce defensive behaviors. Light touch tends to be disorganizing, and may elicit a sympathetic nervous system response ("fight or flight"). Conversely, deep and rhythmical tactile sensation provides the discriminative tactile input and tends to be more organizing.[69]

Early deep stroking of the perioral area may be appropriate even if the infant is being mechanically ventilated. Stroking, for example, can be done from the temporomandibular joint toward the mouth, and deep pressure can be applied to the upper lip. Infants have a variable tolerance to this technique and should be monitored closely. Weight bearing and other forms of deep proprioceptive input also may help to normalize the neonate's tactile system. Deep pressure to the soles of the feet assists in reducing hypersensitivity in that area. Lotions and oils are usually contraindicated during tactile activities because they may irritate the skin.

In some instances, an infant's stay in the NICU may extend well past the neonatal stage. It may then become necessary to address higher level motor, cognitive, and social skills. For example, in the 4- to 6-month-old infant (adjusted age), the therapist might introduce counterrotation of the shoulder girdle and pelvic girdle in sidelying, as this improves coordination between flexor and extensor muscle groups. Similarly, the counterrotation provides the infant with early sensorimotor experience in dissociation between the shoulder and pelvic girdles and dissociation between the lower extremities. These experiences provide the infant with a foundation for higher level, more complex motor skills (see Fig. 3-2A).[70]

Infants who have deficits in state and behavioral organization are frequently referred for therapy. Infants included in this group of referrals may be lethargic or hyperirritable, such as those infants suffering from drug withdrawal syndrome. Calming techniques, such as tight swaddling and slow, rhythmical rocking, have been effective in soothing hyperirritable infants. Deep proprioceptive input may also promote calming. A pacifier can be soothing for infants and its use is recommended, particularly for infants addicted to drugs. Techniques to increase the alertness of lethargic infants may include carefully graded, but arrhythmic vestibular input, such as bouncing, light tactile input to the face and body, and upright positioning. Modulated stimulation may be indicated for all sensory systems. The infant's response must always be monitored carefully to avoid overstimulation.

Therapists rarely need to be concerned about the development of contractures in infants in the NICU. Ligamentous laxity in newborn infants typically protects them from permanent loss of joint mobility. Sloughing of skin and soft tissue that is the result of an infiltrated intravenous site, however, may cause contractures if located directly over a joint. Gentle ROM exercise can be provided to minimize contractures. The integrity of the area of sloughing must be respected during exercise. Infants who receive medications to cause paralysis (e.g., those receiving mechanical ventilation) will require ROM exercises if the medication is used for a long time. In order to minimize the number of different people handling the critically ill infant, the physical therapist may instruct the nursing staff in proper exercise techniques.

Therapeutic Positioning

Proper positioning of the high-risk and premature infant reinforces the therapist's goals to enhance flexor patterns, increase midline orientation, and promote state organization. Positions are changed frequently to offer the infant various sensorimotor experiences. The infant's medical status determines both the readiness for certain positions and the tolerance for a change of position. Careful attention must be given to protect the respiratory capacity of the infant. Hyperflexion of the neck and trunk, for example, can compromise both upper airway patency and diaphragmatic descent. Depending on the specific needs of the infant, individualized instructions in positioning should be made easily accessible to the infant's primary caregivers (Fig. 3-4).

The side-lying position has been strongly recommended for the infant in the NICU. In side-lying, the effects of gravity are reduced, thus promoting midline and flexor responses. Blanket rolls, bags of intravenous fluid, and sandbags can help provide stability for the infant. Symmetric development can be enhanced by using alternate right and left side-lying. The infant should be placed on the right side to facilitate gastric emptying after feeding (Figs. 3-5 and 3-6).

The desired flexor response can also be reinforced with the infant in a prone position. A small washcloth or diaper roll placed under the pelvis and below the abdomen increases flexion of the hip and knee to approximate the posture of a full-term infant. This position also minimizes excessive abduction and external rotation of the hip. Iatrogenic changes in the lower extremity, arising from extended abduction and external rotation of the hip, are also reduced. Rolls placed along the infant's sides help to reinforce symmetry (Figs. 3-7 and 3-8). The premature infant tends to be more organized, shows improved regulation of sleep and wake

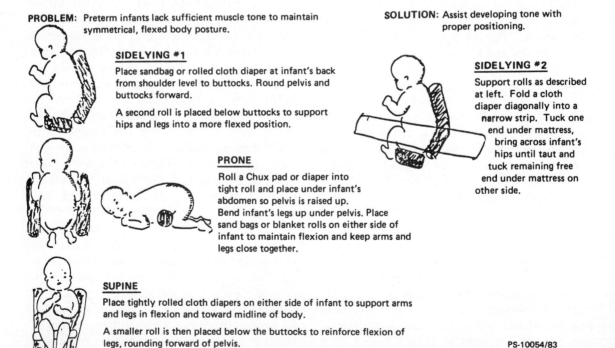

PROBLEM: Preterm infants lack sufficient muscle tone to maintain symmetrical, flexed body posture.

SOLUTION: Assist developing tone with proper positioning.

SIDELYING #1

Place sandbag or rolled cloth diaper at infant's back from shoulder level to buttocks. Round pelvis and buttocks forward.

A second roll is placed below buttocks to support hips and legs into a more flexed position.

SIDELYING #2

Support rolls as described at left. Fold a cloth diaper diagonally into a narrow strip. Tuck one end under mattress, bring across infant's hips until taut and tuck remaining free end under mattress on other side.

PRONE

Roll a Chux pad or diaper into tight roll and place under infant's abdomen so pelvis is raised up. Bend infant's legs up under pelvis. Place sand bags or blanket rolls on either side of infant to maintain flexion and keep arms and legs close together.

SUPINE

Place tightly rolled cloth diapers on either side of infant to support arms and legs in flexion and toward midline of body.

A smaller roll is then placed below the buttocks to reinforce flexion of legs, rounding forward of pelvis.

PS-10054/83

Figure 3-4. *Primary caregivers should receive individualized instructions for positioning an infant.*

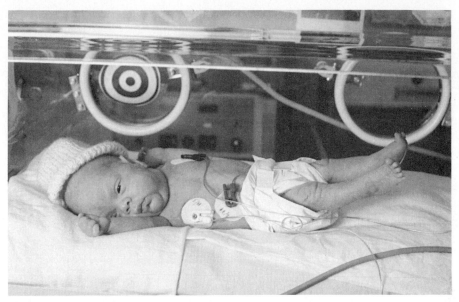

Figure 3-5. *Infant shows the excessive extensor posturing that is commonly seen in premature infants. The influence of the asymmetric tonic neck reflex is apparent in the upper extremities.*

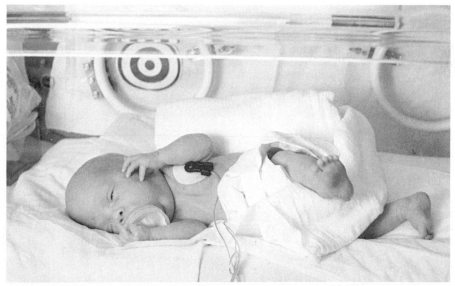

Figure 3-6. *Positioning the infant in a side-lying position using diaper and blanket rolls for support reduces extensor posturing and encourages flexion and midline orientation.*

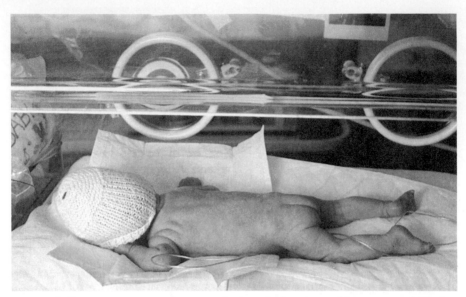

Figure 3-7. *Extensor patterns continue to predominate in the posture of the premature infant in the prone position.*

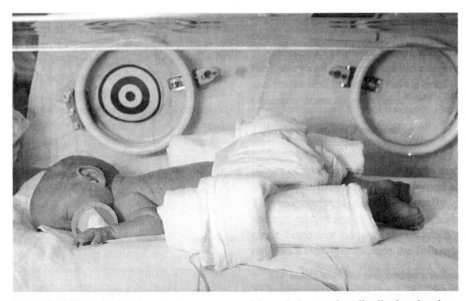

Figure 3-8. *Flexor tone and symmetry are promoted through the use of small rolls placed under the pelvis and along the infant's sides.*

patterns, and demonstrates better self-calming skills in the prone position.[71]

The medically unstable infant is often placed in a supine position for better accessibility for medical procedures. With the infant in a supine position, the force of gravity strongly enhances extensor postures and impedes random flexor movements. By placing blanket rolls along the infant's sides and under the shoulder girdles for support, antigravity flexor patterns are fostered in the upper extremities. Another roll under the knees helps to increase flexion of the hip and knee. Care must be taken to ensure that the airway stays open (Figs. 3-5 and 3-9).

Infant seats provide experience in the upright position, which helps promote an alert state. Adaptations of the seat are usually necessary to accommodate the low-birth-weight infant and to increase flexor positioning. Infant seats made for dolls can

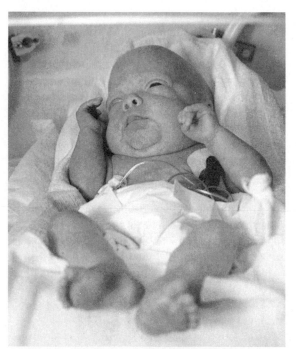

Figure 3-9. *Rolls placed along the infant's sides, below the scapulae, and under the knees encourage flexion, symmetry, and an alert state of behavior.*

be effective for low-birth-weight babies, and they often fit into the isolette. Various commercial positioning devices are also available.

Feeding

The pediatric therapist plays a crucial role in evaluating oral-motor skills, neurobehavioral readiness to feed, and establishment of successful feeding programs. The suck-swallow reflex emerges by 28 to 30 weeks of gestation. At this early stage, the reflex is weak, poorly coordinated, and lacks rhythmicity. Nippling at this time is unsafe.[2] Usually not until 33 to 35 weeks estimated gestational age has there occurred sufficient coordination of suck, swallow, and breathing to initiate oral feedings.

The therapist should do a comprehensive assessment of the infant's readiness to feed before oral feedings begin. An assessment of oral-motor reflex development is crucial. The presence of an effective gag reflex, which is a primary defense against aspiration, must be ascertained. The gag reflex is often either hyperactive or hypoactive as a result of prolonged endotracheal intubation and repetitive gavage feedings. The infant may not accept the nipple if a hyperactive gag reflex is present.[72]

Additional reflexes that should be assessed before feeding include rooting and suckling. Depending on the infant's gestational age, these reflexes may be absent, depressed, or incomplete. A feeding assessment also includes an evaluation of oral-motor muscle tone; tongue configuration; coordination of suck, swallow, and breathing; and excursion of the jaw. Because a quiet, alert state is optimal for effective feeding, the infant's state should also be considered in the assessment of feeding.

Feeding skills of premature infants are adversely affected by decreased flexor and proximal muscle tone, decreased buccal fat pads, limited endurance, and a low state of arousal. Infants who are mechanically ventilated tend to display high arched palates that further impede their ability to express liquid from the nipple. Tactile hypersensitivity in the oral motor area is commonly observed.

Preparation for oral feeding can begin soon after

birth through graded tactile stimulation. This procedure can be begun even with the infant who is mechanically ventilated. Nonnutritive sucking, when encouraged during gavage feeding, has been shown to facilitate earlier oral feeding and weight gain.[73]

Therapeutic positioning and handling are used to enhance development of normal oral-motor skills. Placing the infant in an upright position with the neck elongated is encouraged. Hyperflexion of the neck must be avoided because occlusion of the infant's airway will be the result. Positioning and handling during feeding should provide for depression of the shoulder and should encourage midline orientation. Specific oral-motor techniques can be used to facilitate closure of the lips, stability of the jaw, suckling, and swallowing (Fig. 3-10). The infant's respiration, heart rate, color, and other physiologic signs should be monitored constantly

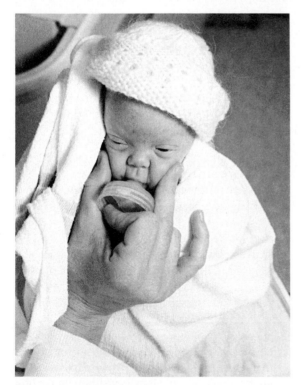

Figure 3-10. *External support to the infant's cheeks increases the strength of the infant's ability to suck and encourages greater approximation of the lips. Pressure is applied downward and forward toward the mouth.*

during feeding. When first attempting oral feeding, the infant's nurse and suctioning equipment must be nearby.

Various nipples are available for use with premature infants and infants with structural problems of the mouth, such as cleft palate. Some of these nipples are shown in Figure 3-11. Selection of the proper nipple depends on the infant's ability to suck, strength of sucking, endurance, and preference. Nipples vary in firmness, size, and the rate of flow. Occupational therapists and/or speech pathologists may be consulted for oral-motor and feeding intervention.

Parent Education

Parent education is an essential component of developmental intervention in NICU. Enactment of the amendments of the Education of the Handicapped Act (P.L. 99-457) has changed the focus of infant intervention from infant-centered to family-centered care.[74] The therapists now view parents as team members, and encourage participation to the extent the family wishes to participate in their infant's care. The therapist needs to be sensitive to variations in a family's ability or willingness to share in their infant's care, and must maintain a nonjudgmental attitude. Additionally, diversities in culture, values, and background must be respected. The major goals of parent education are to strengthen the parents' feelings of competency and to improve parent-infant interactions.

Open communication with the family is essential and can be facilitated using verbal and written means. Some therapists have found it useful to attach a communication booklet to the isolette in order to share information with parents who may visit after usual treatment hours. This may also serve to maintain an updated Individualized Family Service Plan (IFSP) as required by P.L. 99-457. Personal contact and telephone calls will keep parents informed of the infant's progress or developmental changes. The therapist involved in the NICU may need to consider flexible work schedules to guarantee family contact.

To improve parent-infant interaction, it is essen-

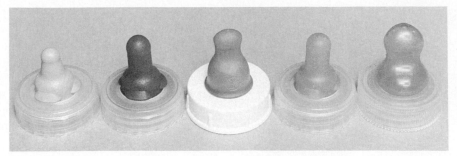

Figure 3-11. *Available nipples vary in size, shape, firmness, and rate of flow.*

tial that the family be informed of the infant's behavioral cues and signs of stress. Showing the family techniques to foster alertness as the infant's medical and behavioral stability increases is recommended. The parents may be shown positions that enhance social interaction, such as holding the infant in a semi-reclined, face-to-face position. Parent education can be enhanced with the use of commercially available literature designed for family use.

Emphasis is placed on instruction in therapeutic positioning and handling techniques, rather than on specific exercise regimens. The positioning and handling techniques can be incorporated into daily caregiving activities. By alerting the parents to the differences between desired and unwanted postures, the therapist can facilitate the parents' implementation of the various therapeutic techniques; furthermore, parents can become creative and inventive in analyzing and responding to the infant's motor needs. The parents, for example, must understand the objectives of each of the various recommended positions; thus, if an infant is arching into trunk extension in the side-lying posture, the parent will realize that extension is an unwanted position and will modify the position to better facilitate flexion. If parents do not understand the objectives, the fact that side-lying is a recommended position may be considered more important than the infant's arching into extension, and the position may be maintained, thereby reinforcing extension.

Parents spend many hours holding and carrying their infants. Therapeutic goals can be reinforced through proper carrying techniques. A parent will foster flexion and midline orientation by cradling the infant in the crook of the arm (Fig. 3-12). One of the infant's arms is often allowed to wrap around the body of the parent. This position of the upper extremity reinforces scapular retraction and should be discouraged. The infant should be carried on alternating sides of the parent's body to foster symmetric development. Parents commonly hold infants against their chest in a posture of total extension. This position should be modified to incorporate some components of flexion.

If specific exercises are recommended, they should be done only by persons who have been instructed by the therapist. Parents and others instructed in exercises must also be instructed in the recognition of signs of infant distress and signs of good tolerance. Discretion must be used by therapists because not all parents can successfully interpret and replicate th exercise regimen suggested. The skilled and sensitive therapist should be aware of the parent's level of understanding and responses and proceed accordingly. Instruction may be limited in some instances to rolling the infant from a prone to a supine position, or to picking up the infant. Written instructions with diagrams should facilitate both understanding and follow-through with the program.

The therapist should explain to the parents the difference between chronologic age and corrected age. This knowledge may help the parent establish realistic expectations about the infant. For example, knowing that their 8-week-old premature infant will perform, at 6 months of age, more like a 4-month-old baby, may help relieve the anxiety of a parent.

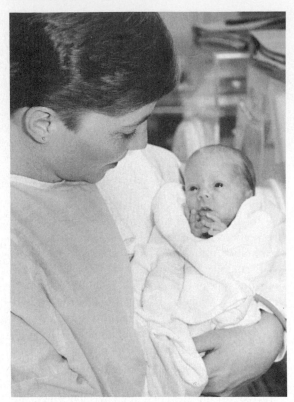

Figure 3-12. *Parents are encouraged to cradle infants in a flexed and upright position. Swaddling promotes an organized and alert state of behavior. Infants are swaddled with the hands toward midline and the lower extremities flexed.*

The NICU Team

Optimal care is facilitated by a coordinated team approach. Team members may include the parents, physicians, nurse practitioners, nurses, physical therapists, occupational therapists, speech pathologists, respiratory therapists, social workers, infant educators, and child life specialists. Communication among team members is essential for successful team interactions.

Staff education and training is an integral part of the role of the physical therapist in the NICU. Education can be achieved through formal in-service programs, direct and indirect consultation, and informal communication. In order for the therapist's program to be effective, staff support is essential to assist in carrying out the program. Frequently, owing to the fragility of the infant, specific handling performed by the therapist may be limited to 10- or 15-minute sessions. This minimal time is inadequate to achieve most therapeutic goals. The therapist must rely on the nursing staff to incorporate therapeutic positioning and handling into their routine care activities. General recommendations regarding development can benefit all infants in the NICU, even those who are not receiving direct physical therapy and occupational therapy services.

In-service training for the nursing staff regarding infant development and the goals of therapeutic intervention better enables the nurses to incorporate

---

Table 3–8. *Criteria for Referral for Physical Therapy Intervention in the Neonatal Intensive Care Unit*

Birthweight ≤ 1500 g

Gestational age ≤ 32 weeks

Severe perinatal asphyxia with Apgar scores of 5 or less at 5 minutes of age

Evidence of intraventricular hemorrhage, intracranial hemorrhage, or periventricular leukomalacia

Hydrocephalus or microcephalus

Dystonia (hypertonia, hypotonia, asymmetry)

Recurrent neonatal seizures (5 or more)

Intrauterine growth retardation or small for gestational age (two standard deviations below the mean in growth charts corrected for gestational age)

Peripheral nerve injury (injuries to the brachial plexus)

Musculoskeletal abnormalities (arthrogryposis, congenital hip dislocation, congenital torticollis, talipes equinovarus)

Myelodysplasia (spina bifida)

Neuromuscular diseases (Werdnig-Hoffmann disease, myotonic dystrophy)

Symptomatic neonatal drug withdrawal

Persistently poor nipple feeders

Chromosomal abnormalities affecting development (trisomy 21)

Abnormal behavior persisting for longer than 48 hours and suggestive of disturbances in the central nervous system (irritability, tremor, lethargy)

Failure to thrive

therapeutic goals into their care of all premature and high-risk infants. The nursing staff must be informed about the benefits of proper positioning. Members of the nursing staff must also be aware of the impact that their interventions may have on the infant's behavioral organization, as well as the effects of the infant's behavioral organization on his or her physiological system.

A system of primary care nursing has been established in many NICU settings. An infant's primary care nurse not only provides most of the care, but is responsible for facilitating communication between staff and family members. Maintaining good, open communication with the primary care nurse is effective in integrating the therapeutic program into the nursery setting.

Another major role for the therapist is increasing the awareness of neonatologists, pediatricians, resident physicians, and nursing staff to the role of physical therapists in the NICU. This process should include educating the nurse and physicians as to the criteria and procedure for referring infants for physical therapy. Some criteria for referral are suggested in Table 3-8.

Discharge Planning and Developmental Follow-up

To facilitate a smooth transition to home, it is essential that all members of the team coordinate discharge plans. Some nurseries provide rooming-in arrangements for parents prior to hospital discharge to allow them to begin to assume care of their infant. A home visit by a discharge planning nurse may be helpful prior to discharge.

Close developmental follow-up may be warranted depending on a variety of risk factors, including neurologic and social risk factors. An infant's neurodevelopmental status at discharge may necessitate continuation of ongoing direct therapeutic intervention. Both public and private resources for payment for therapy should be researched and taken into account when referrals are made.

Developmental follow-up programs are often available through the discharging NICU. Additionally, comprehensive developmental programs may be available through local counties and university-affiliated programs. Developmental programs are designed to supplement, but not supplant, the medical care provided by the infant's primary physician.

Summary

This chapter has discussed major disorders affecting infants in the NICU. Guidelines and specific tests of assessment have been described. Goals for developmental intervention have been presented and numerous therapeutic techniques have been discussed. Therapeutic handling, positioning, and feeding are reviewed as they relate to the goals for developmental intervention. The importance of parent and staff education and training, as well as team collaboration, has been emphasized. The need for well-coordinated discharge planning and developmental follow-up has also been emphasized. The NICU offers a major challenge to the physical therapist. The morbidity and mortality rates of these fragile infants are constantly being improved through advances in medical technology.

References

1. Salek B. Sensorimotor pathology in infancy and early childhood. In: Braun MA, Meyer-Palmer M, eds: *Detection and Treatment of the Infant and Young Child with Neuromuscular Disorders.* New York: Therapeutic Media; 1983.

2. Saint-Anne Dargassies, S. *Neurological Develop-*

ment in the Full-Term and Premature Neonate. Amsterdam: Excerpta Medica; 1977.

3. Carter RE, Campbell S. Early neuromuscular development in the premature infant. *Phys Ther.* 1975; 55:1339.

4. Anderson J, Auster-Liebhaber J. Developmental therapy in the neonatal intensive care unit. *Phys Occup Ther Pediatr.* 1984;4:100.

5. Amiel-Tison C, Grenier A. Neurological assessment during the first year of life. New York: Oxford University Press; 1986.

6. Scherzer AL, Tscharnuter I. *Early Diagnosis and Therapy in Cerebral Palsy: A Primer on Infant Developmental Problems.* New York: Marcel Dekker; 1982.

7. Als H, Lester BM, Tronick EZ, Brazelton TB. Manual for the Assessment of Preterm Infants' Theory and Behavior (APIB). In: Fitzgerald H, et al., eds. *Theory and Research in Behavioral Pediatrics,* Vol 1. New York: Plenum; 1982:65–132.

8. Als H, Lester BM, Tronick EZ, Brazelton TB. Toward a research instrument for the assessment of preterm infants' behavior (APIB). In: Fitzgerald H, et al., eds. *Theory and Research in Behavioral Pediatrics.* Vol 1. New York: Plenum; 1982:35–61.

9. Fenichel G. *Neonatal Neurology.* New York: Churchill Livingstone; 1985.

10. Phibbs R. Delivery room management of the newborn. In: Avery G, ed. *Neonatology: Pathophysiology and Management of the Newborn.* Philadelphia: JB Lippincott; 1981:182–201.

11. Volpe J. In: Avery E, ed. *Neonatology: Pathophysiology and Management of the Newborn.* Philadelphia: JB Lippincott; 1981.

12. Fitzhardinge P, Pape K. Follow-up studies of the high-risk newborn. In: Avery E, ed. *Neonatology: Pathophysiology and Management of the Newborn.* Philadelphia: JB Lippincott; 1981.

13. Menkes J. *Textbook of Child Neurology.* Philadelphia: Lea & Febiger; 1985.

14. Lou HC. Perinatal hypoxic-ischemic brain damage and periventricular hemorrhage. In: Harel S, et al., eds. *The At-Risk Infants.* Baltimore: Paul H. Brookes; 1985:153–157.

15. Volpe JJ. *Neurology of the Newborn.* Philadelphia: WB Saunders; 1987.

16. Robertson C, Finer N. Term infants with hypoxic-ischemic encephalopathy: Outcome at 3–5 years. *Dev Med Child Neurol.* 1985;27:473–484.

17. Malamud N. Status marmoratus: A form of cerebral palsy following either birth injury or inflammation of the central nervous system. *J Pediatr.* 1950; 37:610.

18. Bozynski ME, Nelson MN, Matalon TAS, et al. Cavitary periventricular leukomalacia: Incidence and short-term outcome in infants weighing less than 1200 grams at birth. *Dev Med Child Neurol* 1985; 27:572–577.

19. McMenamin JB, Shackelford GD, Volpe JJ. Outcome of neonatal intraventricular hemorrhage with periventricular echodense lesions. *Ann Neurol.* 1984; 15:285–290.

20. Bjar R, Coln R. *Brain Insults in Infants and Children.* Orlando, FL: Grune & Stratton; 1985.

21. Papile L, Munsick-Bruno G, Schaefer A. Relationship of cerebral intraventricular hemorrhage and early childhood neurologic handicaps. *J Pediatr.* 1983;103:273–277.

22. Evans HE, Glass L. *Perinatal Medicine.* Hagerstown, MD: Harper & Row; 1976.

23. Corbet AJ, Bucciarelli R, Goldman S, Mammel M, Wold D, Long W. Decreased mortality rate among small premature infants treated at birth with a single dose of synthetic surfactant: A multicenter controlled trial. *J Pediatr.* 1991;118:277–284.

24. Singer D. Morphology of hyaline membrane disease and its pulmonary sequelae. In: Stern L, ed. *Hyaline Membrane Disease.* Orlando, FL: Grune & Stratton; 1984:81–83.

25. Reid L. Bronchopulmonary dysplasia—Pathology. *J Pediatr.* 1979;95:836–841.

26. Vohi BR, Bell EF, Vih W. Infants with bronchopulmonary dysplasia: Growth patterns and neurologic and development outcome. *Am J Dis Child.* 1982;136:443–447.

27. Behrman RE, Vaughan VN. *Textbook of Pediatrics.* 13th ed. Philadelphia: WB Saunders; 1987.

28. Scheidt PC, Mellits ED, Hardy JB, et al. Toxicity to bilirubin in neonates: Infant development during the first year in relation to maximal neonatal serum bilirubin concentration. *J Pediatr.* 1977;91:292.

29. Griffith JF. Nonbacterial infections of the fetus and newborn. *Clin Perinatol.* 1977;4:117–130.

30. Prose NS. HIV infection in children. *J Am Acad Dermatol.* 1990;22:1223.

31. Grossman M. Children with AIDS. *Infect Dis Clin North Am.* 1988;2:533.

32. Pahwa S. Human immunodeficiency virus infection in children: Nature of immunodeficiency, clinical spectrum, and management. *Pediatr Infect Dis J.* 1988;7:S61.

33. Curless RG. Congenital AIDS: Review of neurologic problems. *Children's Nervous Syst.* 1989;5:9.

34. Diamond GW. Developmental problems in children with HIV infection. *Ment Retard.* 1989;27:213.

35. Wright JT, et al. Alcohol consumption, pregnancy, and low birth weight. *Lancet.* 1983;1:663.

36. Silk A (Fair Oaks Hosp, VA). Personal communication, July 1992.

37. Bingol N, Fuchs M, Diaz V. Teratogenicity of cocaine in humans. *J Pediatr.* 1987;110:93.

38. Chasnoff IJ, Griffith DR, MacGregor S, Dirkes K, Burns KA. Temporal patterns of cocaine use in pregnancy. Perinatal outcome. *Am Med Assoc.* 1989; 261:1741.

39. Chouteau M, Namerow PB, Leppert P. The effect of cocaine abuse on birth weight and gestational age. *Obstet Gynecol.* 1988;72:351.

40. Dixon S, Bejar R. Echoencephalographic findings in neonates associated with maternal cocaine and methamphetamine use: Incidence and clinical correlates. *J Pediatr.* 1989;115:770.

41. Eisen L, Field T, Bandstra E. Perinatal cocaine effects on neonatal stress behavior and performance on the Brazelton Scale. *Pediatrics.* 1991;88:427.

42. Little BB, Snell LM, Klein VR, Gilstrap LC III. Cocaine abuse during pregnancy: Maternal and fetal implications. *Obstet Gynecol.* 1989;73:157.

43. Van der Bor M, Walther FJ, Sims M. Increased cerebral blood flow velocity in infants of mothers who abuse cocaine. *Pediatrics.* 1990;85:733.

44. Lane SJ. Prenatal cocaine exposure: A role for occupational therapy. *Devel Disabil Special Interest Section Newslett* June 1992;15:1–2.

45. Zelson C, Rubio E, Wasserman E. Neonatal narcotic addiction: 10-year observation. *Pediatrics.* 1971; 48:178.

46. Lake AM, Walker WA. Neonatal necrotizing enterocolitis: A disease of altered host defense. *Clin Gastroenterol.* 1977;6:463–480.

47. Touloukian RJ. Neonatal necrotizing enterocolitis: An update on etiology, diagnosis, and treatment. *Surg Clin North Am.* 1976;56:281–298.

48. Neu J. Gastrointestinal problems and nutrition in neonatal and pediatric intensive care. In: Vidyasagar D, ed. *Neonatal and Pediatric Intensive Care.* Boston: PSG Publishing; 1985;299–300.

49. Fanaroff A, Martin R. *Neonatal-Perinatal Medicine.* St. Louis: Mosby-Yearbook; 1992.

50. Eng GD. Brachial plexus palsy in newborn infants. *Pediatrics.* 1971;48:18.

51. Nellhaus D, et al. Neurologic and muscular disorders. In: Kempe CH, ed. *Current Pediatric Diagnosis and Treatment.* Los Altos: Appleton and Lange; 1982:615.

52. Coleman SS. *Congenital Dysplasia and Dislocation of the Hip.* St Louis: CV Mosby; 1978.

53. Weiner D, et al. Congenital dislocation of the hip: The relationships of premanipulation, traction, and age to avascular necrosis of the femoral head. *J Bone Joint Surg.* 1977;59A:306.

54. Gartland J. *Fundamentals of Orthopedics.* Philadelphia: WB Saunders; 1974.

55. Hoppenfeld S. *Physical Examination of the Spine and Extremities.* New York: Appleton-Century-Crofts; 1976.

56. Kempe CH, et al. *Current Pediatric Diagnosis and Treatment.* Los Altos, CA: Lange Medical Publications; 1982.

57. Amiel-Tison C. Neurological evaluation of the maturity of newborn infants. *Arch Dis Child.* 1968; 43:89–93.

58. Prechtl H. *The Neurological Examination of the Full-term Newborn Infant.* 2nd ed. Philadelphia: JB Lippincott; 1977. Clinics in Developmental Medicine, No. 63.

59. Andre-Thomas CY, Saint-Anne Dargassies S. *The Neurological Examination of the Infant.* London; National Spastics Society; 1960. Little Club Clinics in Developmental Medicine, No.1.

60. Brazelton TB. *Neonatal Behavioral Assessment Scale.* 2nd ed. Philadelphia: JB Lippincott; 1984.

61. Apgar, V. Proposal for a new method of evaluation of newborn infant. *Anesth Analg.* 1953;32:260.

62. Drage JS, Berendes H. Apgar scores and outcome of the newborn. *Pediatr Clin North Am.* 1966;13:635.

63. Dubowitz LMS, Dubowitz V, Goldberg C. Clinical assessment of gestational age in the newborn infant. *J Pediatr.* 1970;77.

64. Dubowitz L. Neurological assessment of the full-term and preterm newborn infant. In: Harel S, Anastasiow N, eds. *The At-risk Infant.* Baltimore: Paul H. Brookes; 1985:185–196.

65. Morgan A. *Neuro-Developmental Approach to the High-Risk Neonate.* (Notes from a seminar presented in Williamsburg, VA; Nov 3–4, 1984.

66. Chandler LS, et al. *Movement Assessment of Infants: A Manual.* Rolling Bay, WA: Chandler LS et al.; 1980.

67. Milani-Comparetti A, Gidoni EA. Routine developmental examination in normal and retarded children. *Dev Med Child Neurol.* 1967;9:631.

68. Bobath K. *A Neurophysiological Basis for the Treatment of Cerebral Palsy*. Philadelphia: J B Lippincott; 1980.

69. Ayres AJ. *Sensory Integration and Learning Disorders*. Los Angeles: Western Psychological Services; 1972.

70. Gilfoyle EM, Grady AP, Moore JC. *Children Adapt*. Thorofare, NJ: Charles B. Slack; 1981.

71. Als H. Lecture notes. George Washington University, Washington, DC: Feb 21, 1985.

72. Evans MS, Stockdale WS. Problems of cerebral palsy and oral-motor function. In Wilson JM, ed. *Oral-Motor Function and Dysfunction in Children*. Chapel Hill: University of North Carolina at Chapel Hill Division of Physical Therapy; 1977: 163–166.

73. Field T, et al. Nonnutritive sucking during tube feedings: Effects on preterm neonates in an intensive care unit. *Pediatrics*. 1982;70:381–384.

74. The Education of the Handicapped Act Amendments of 1986. Public Law No. 99–457 (1986).

Pediatric Physical Therapy,
second edition, edited by Jan
Stephen Tecklin. J. B. Lippincott
Company, Philadelphia © 1994.

4

Jane Styer-Acevedo

Physical Therapy for the Child with Cerebral Palsy

- Definition
- Incidence
- Etiology
- Classification
- Associated Problems
- Assessment of the Child with Cerebral Palsy
    Assessment of Movement
    Assessment of Reflexes
    Assessment of Postural Tone
    Musculoskeletal Assessment
    Evaluation of Gait
    Assessment of Fine Motor and Adaptive Skills
    Considerations of Speech and Language
- Establishing Goals of Treatment
- Therapeutic Intervention
    Therapeutic Exercise
- Equipment Uses and Considerations
    Mats
    Benches
    Balls and Bolsters
    Tilt Boards and Equilibrium Boards

    Adaptive Equipment
- Lower Extremity Orthoses
    Bivalved Short-Leg Cast (Inhibitive Cast)
    Knee-Ankle-Foot Orthosis
    Molded Ankle-Foot Orthosis
    Articulating Ankle-Foot Orthosis
    Anterior Shell Ankle-Foot Orthosis
    Supramalleolar Molded Orthosis
    Shoe Inserts
    High-top Orthopedic Shoe/Phelps Short-Leg Brace
- Neurosurgical Intervention for Children with Cerebral Palsy
- Orthopedic Surgery for Children with Cerebral Palsy
    The Hip
    The Knee
    The Ankle and Foot
- Home Management
- Consultation with the School
- Other Disciplines Involved in the Care of Children with Cerebral Palsy

Definition

"Cerebral palsy is not a disease, but is, rather, a category of disability including patients with one kind of problem: chronic nonprogressive disorders of movement or posture of early onset. The anatomic sites of involvement, degree of motor disability, associated dysfunctions, and cause are heterogeneous."[1] "Cerebral palsy is often associated with other neurologic difficulties, including mental retardation."[2]

Incidence

The United States Collaborative Perinatal Project conducted by the National Institute of Neurologic and Communicative Disorders and Stroke included a study of 54,000 pregnant women from 12 urban teaching hospitals in the United States between 1959 and 1966.[3] Of the women in the study, 46% were white, 46% were black, and most of the rest were Puerto Rican. The socioeconomic status of the sample was lower than that of the general population. The children born to these women had a regular schedule of examinations, including a general physical examination and a neurologic examination at both 1 and 7 years of age. Among the 38,533 children whose outcome was known at 7 years of age, 202 met criteria for cerebral palsy (CP). Of the 202 children, 24 (12%) children had an acquired motor deficit secondary to a variety of factors in the early developing years, rather than congenital motor deficits occurring as a result of in utero factors or events at the time of labor and delivery. Infectious meningitis and trauma were the most common causes of acquired CP. In addition to the 202 children with CP who were alive at 7 years of age, 24 children with CP, most commonly with spastic quadriplegia, had died before 7 years of age. The following figures indicate the prevalence of CP based on the National Collaborative Perinatal Project:

5.2:1000—diagnosed as having CP
4.6:1000—when acquired cases of CP are excluded
2.6:1000—excluding mildly afflicted children. (This figure more closely represents the prevalence of handicapping congenital CP.)

Further study of the population in the United States Collaborative Perinatal Project indicated that there are "relatively low risks for cerebral palsy (1.3–2.9 per 1000) among children who had no abnormal signs, whether or not they had low 5-minute Apgar scores or whether or not they had seizures in the nursery period."[4] Other authors have found the incidence of CP to be 2 per 1000 infants in the United States.[5]

Etiology

Despite a marked increase in perinatal intervention aimed at reducing intrapartum asphyxia in recent years, CP rates have not shown a consistent decrease either in the United States or in Australia.[1] There has been a reduction in the perinatal mortality rate over the past decade owing to improvements in obstetric management, but this reduction has not been accompanied by a decrease in the prevalence of CP. In an effort to confirm the study regarding perinatal asphyxia by Ellenberg and Nelson,[4] the California Child Health and Development Studies group monitored 19,044 pregnancies to evaluate their long-term outcome. The children underwent follow-up for 5 years. Forty-one (0.2 percent) were found to have CP that was not the result of a progressive disease or a neural tube defect. Thirty-two (78 percent) of the children with CP did *not* have birth asphyxia, and the 22 percent who had asphyxia had other perinatal risk factors that may have compromised their recovery. Of the control infants 2.9% had birth asphyxia but recovered without neurologic damage. The authors believed that the strongest predictors of CP were the presence of a congenital anomaly, low birth weight, low placental weight, and an abnormal fetal position. All of these conditions are antecedents to the birth process and strong indicators of a fetus who is compromised prior to labor or delivery.[6] Melone and associates, in another study, confirmed that the intrapartum period is an infrequent source of CP.[5]

Others have investigated several areas in both

full-term and premature infants in an attempt to identify the risk factors and sources for CP. Their findings include, but are not limited to, abnormal neonatal signs;[7] hypoxia or ischemia;[1,6,8,9] chronic lung disease requiring 28 days or more of supplemental oxygen;[10] low Apgar scores;[2,11] neurosonographic abnormalities, such as severe intracranial hemorrhage,[10,11] increased periventricular leukomalacia,[12] increased periventricular echogenicity,[13,14] and periventricular cysts;[12–14] the need for mechanical ventilation,[13,14] and prematurity/gestational age.[13,15]

Predicting the long-term outcome of infants in the neonatal period continues to be difficult based upon the available data. In general, the higher the risk associated with a characteristic, or constellation of characteristics, the lower the prevalence of that characteristic or constellation.[4]

Classification

Scherzer and Tscharnuter describe how the motor pattern type of CP may take several forms.[15]

The spastic variety is most common and indicates a fixed lesion in the motor portion of the cerebral cortex. Athetosis or dystonia reflects involvement in the basal ganglia. Athetosis frequently involves intermittent tension of the trunk or extremities and a variety of uninhibited movement patterns—sometimes a basis for confusion in classification. Ataxia refers to a cerebellar lesion. Mixed types are also common. These may include combinations of spasticity with athetosis or ataxia. Rigidity suggests a severe decerebrate lesion.[15]

Scherzer and Tscharnuter have included in their work the definitions that are in common use for various clinical neurologic lesions:[14]

Monoplegia—involvement of one extremity
Hemiplegia—upper and lower extremity involvement on one side
Paraplegia—involvement of both lower extremities
Quadriplegia—equal involvement of upper and lower extremities
Diplegia—quadriplegia with mild involvement of the upper extremities

These authors further state that "Type, distribution, and severity are essential aspects of the cerebral palsy diagnosis. They give meaning and direction to treatment and management of the patient."[15]

The Bobaths'[16] description of the distribution of the various types of CP is similar to that of Scherzer and Tscharnuter,[15] but includes the trunk in the description of motor involvement. Molnar[17] identifies several major groups of children with CP based upon clinical signs. **Spastic CP** includes hemiparesis, diplegia, and quadriparesis. **Dyskinetic forms** include *athetosis* (slow, writhing movements of the face and extremities, particularly affecting the distal musculature), *dystonia* (rhythmic, twisting distortions and changes in tone involving primarily the trunk and proximal extremities and causing slow, uncontrolled movements with a tendency toward fixed postures), *choreiform movements* (rapid, irregular, jerky motions most commonly seen in the face and extremities), *ballismus* (coarse flailing or flinging motion of the extremities characterized by a wide amplitude of motion), and *tremor* (fine shaking motion of the head and extremities). Rarer types of cerebral palsy include **ataxia, rigidity, and atonia.** Clinical types of CP with mixed neurologic signs typically involve spastic athetosis, spastic ataxia, or spastic rigidity.[17]

Associated Problems

Strabismus is present in 20% to 60% of children with CP; the highest incidence is in the diplegic and quadriplegic populations. *Esotropia,* deviation of the eyes toward the midline, is more prevalent than exotropia. Homonymous hemianopsia occurs in 25% of children with hemiplegia.[17,18] Nystagmus is most common in children with ataxia. Mental retardation is more common in children with CP than in normal children. Of children with CP, 40% to 60% have some degree of retardation, with the highest proportion of severe deficits seen in children with quadriplegia, rigidity, and atonia.[17] Seizure disorders occur in as many as 50% of children with CP, with the severity and incidence varying across the different types of CP.[17] Significant communication disorders may be present in children with CP. These disorders may be secondary to poor oral-motor control of speech, central language dysfunction, hearing impairment, or cognitive deficits. Growth disturbances in both longitudinal and cross-sectional directions, and accompanying sensory deficits, have been shown in the involved limbs of children with hemiplegia. Disturbances in longitudinal growth were greatest in the radius, followed by the humerus and tibia. Cross-sectional area of the involved limb segments was decreased by 16% to 19%. Limb muscle atrophy increased with age. Although these findings are well documented, the causes, which may include neurotrophic and vascular changes, are obscure.[19–21]

Assessment of the Child with Cerebral Palsy

In this era of high technologic intervention, it is essential that therapists become very sensitive to the possible neurologic deficits in any infant or child with developmental delay or behavioral difficulties. According to Kitchen, 10% of very low birth weight (VLBW) infants weighing between 500 and 1500 g can be expected to develop CP. Kitchen further states that there may be a high rate of fetal aberration associated with the abnormal event of premature birth.[22] Several authors suggest that infants who are at increased risk for the development of CP can be predicted through the use of ultrasonography of the head.[12–14,23–26] Cystic lesions found in the occipital region confer a very high risk of severe CP.[25] Periventricular cystic lesions probably reflect damage to the white matter fibers of the cerebral corticospinal tracts and may appear clinically as spasticity. (Fig. 4-1).[23,25] When findings cited earlier are noted in an infant in the nursery, they should be used to guide the discharge plan for the infant and family. The goal of this early diagnosis is to provide early therapeutic intervention for the child with CP. This intervention should be in the form of developmentally based therapy, including physical, occupational, and speech therapies. Many practitioners recommend that graduates from neonatal intensive care units (NICUs) who have the neurologic signs just mentioned should be closely monitored

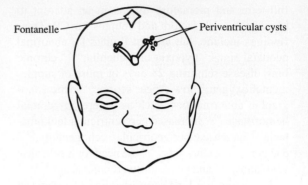

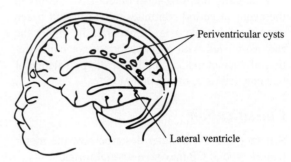

Figure 4-1. *Location of periventrical cysts which are thought to affect the corticospinal tracts and cause spasticity. (Compliments of Leonard Graziani, MD)*

after discharge. Of course, normal findings in an evaluation can be very reassuring for parents and caregivers alike. However, abnormal neonatal examination results cannot be used to diagnose CP definitively in the neonatal period. Rather, the results should be used to identify infants who are at increased risk for later developmental disability and who will require closer monitoring and possibly, early intervention programs.[27]

There is disagreement in the literature and in practice regarding how early an infant can be diagnosed with CP. Burns et al. believe that a diagnosis of very mild CP should be possible at 8 months of age.[28] Identification depends upon a combination of suspicious and abnormal signs revealed during comprehensive assessment of motor attainments, neurologic signs, primitive reflexes, and postural reactions. Children with persistent subtle or mild signs should be monitored closely until the possible outcome is clear.[28] Harris, using the Movement Assessment in Infants (MAI), found that certain items can help to distinguish the infant with CP from the nonhandicapped infant at 4 months of age.[29] Items of diagnostic value include neck hyperextension and shoulder retraction, ability to bear weight on the forearms while prone, ability to maintain a stable head position in supported or independent sitting, and the infant's ability to flex the hips actively against gravity.[29,30] Seven of the 17 MAI items that Harris found to be highly significant predictors are observational items. Both Harris and Milani-Comparetti found that watching the infant move against gravity is of greater diagnostic value than intrusive handling or attempts to stimulate a response.[29,30] Harris compared the diagnostic value of the MAI to the Bayley Scales in infants at 4 months of age and found that the MAI was more sensitive than the Bayley Scales.[29] However, the Bayley Motor Scale was extremely sensitive at 1 year of age. Nelson and Ellenberg[31] studied children who were diagnosed with CP at 1 year of age who subsequently "outgrew the cerebral palsy." They found that children with mild motor impairment at 1 year of age and those thought to have CP were all free of CP by the age of 7 years. However, all who were diagnosed with severe CP, and many with moderate CP, still carried the same diagnosis at the age of 7 years. Those who "outgrew" the CP were likely to have neurologic problems, such as mental retardation, nonfebrile seizures, or difficulty with speech articulation.[31] These findings substantiate the fact that any infant or child who demonstrates neurologic or behavioral abnormalities should undergo follow-up until early school age.

In order to understand the abnormal movement and motor control that occurs in children with CP, the therapist must understand the acquisition of motor control against gravity; the development of righting, equilibrium, and protective reactions; and musculoskeletal development in normal children. This information is presented in Chapter 1. Abnormal development has been described by many authors, including numerous sources cited within this chapter.[15,17,32–46] Bly has described in great detail the kinesiology and progression of abnormal development.[32]

The purpose of the assessment is to provide information so that the therapist can formulate goals for treatment and a treatment plan. Goals should be written in behavioral terms, be functional in nature, and be measurable. The physical therapist must develop an organized method of observation in order to determine the baseline function of the child, as well as the quality of movement. The therapist uses an accurate, organized set of observations to plan a treatment session that will address the problem areas and assist the child to achieve the stated goals. These observations should assist the therapist in differentiating between primary problems and secondary problems, and should help organize the treatment session.

Assessment of Movement

Much of the information about a child's movement and posture can be gathered by an observant therapist who watches the child entering the treatment area. The child can also be observed while the therapist is taking a history and discussing with the parents the various concerns that have brought them to a habilitation program.

Observation of the young baby being held in the mother's arms or lap can reveal information related to several questions that can begin to provide the basis for setting goals and planning of treatment. These questions might include the following:

1. How does the mother hold the baby? Does she support the head and trunk, or does she hold the baby at the pelvis?
2. Are the baby's head and trunk rotated or collapsed consistently to one side?
3. Do the baby's arms come forward to hold the mother or play with a toy in midline? Are the arms held behind the body with the scapulae adducted or are the arms flexed and adducted against the trunk?
4. While being held, does the baby thrust backward into trunk extension or collapse forward into trunk flexion?
5. How are the lower extremities held: are they ad-

ducted tightly in extension or are they floppy in flexion and abduction?
6. Is there isolated movement at the toes or ankles, or are the ankles held in plantar flexion or dorsiflexion? Is the foot everted or inverted and are the toes held loosely or tightly curled?

This type of observational analysis is not limited to the child held in the mother's arms. When the child arrives at the physical therapy department in a wheelchair, there are additional questions that may add to the baseline information.

1. Did the child independently propel the wheelchair or did someone help him or her?
2. In addition to mobility, does the wheelchair provide total postural support for major segments of the body? If the segments are free of support from the wheelchair, do those segments of the body seem in good postural alignment and do they move freely?
3. Does the child tend to thrust backward in the chair into trunk extension? Is the pelvis positioned in a posterior tilt? If the child does behave in this manner, is there similar thrusting and tightness in the extremities?
4. Is the child seated in a reasonably symmetric position or are there significant asymmetries in the posture?
5. Does the child seem comfortable in the chair?

Children with less severe movement disorders may ambulate into the department. Another group of questions will be helpful in assessing the movement of the ambulatory child.

1. Did the child ambulate with or without an assistive device, such as a walker, cane, or crutches?
2. Did the child need physical assistance from another person while ambulating?
3. Does the child's gait pattern appear stable and is the child safe?
4. When assessing temporal parameters, such as length of step, stance time, swing time, or base of support, does the gait pattern appear grossly symmetric or asymmetric?
5. Does the child's trunk collapse into lateral flexion on weight bearing on one or both legs, or is the trunk maintained in a proper antigravity extension?
6. Does the child have a heel-toe gait pattern? Does the child stand on the balls of the feet?

7. Are the hips and knees extended during stance phase, or are they flexed with the child in a crouched position?

These questions will provide the basis for the gross movement assessment portion of the total assessment. In addition to the gross observational assessment described, the therapist should examine individual aspects of motor function as part of the overall evaluation of the child. The therapist should begin with the aspect of function appropriate to the child's age and level of ability. The following list of positions provides a guideline by which to assess functional antigravity control:

Prone
Supine
Side-lying
Sitting—short sit, long sit, side sit
Quadruped
Kneeling
Half-kneeling
Standing
Walking

If the child possesses higher level skills the evaluation should be extended to include the following:

Climbing stairs
Navigating ramps or curbs
One-foot stance
Tandem gait
Running
Jumping
Hopping
Skipping

The child who functions from a wheelchair should be evaluated in terms of the following parameters:

Alignment and mobility of body
Shifting of weight
Propulsion of wheelchair
Management of wheelchair and its parts
Transfer to and from wheelchair

The qualitative aspects of movement evaluation commonly include, but need not be limited to, the following items:

Antigravity movement of head, trunk, and extremities
Base of support related to lateral dimensions of the trunk

Ability to elongate trunk on the weight-bearing side

Direction of weight shifts and resultant righting, equilibrium, or protective reactions

Effort required and endurance in movement

Speed and fluidity of movement, particularly during transitions between postures

Consistent compensations used for lack of proximal stability

Associated reactions

Various postures assumed and maintained

Degree of assistance required and reasons for the assistance

Assessment of Reflexes

Reflex behavior provides a major assessment of brainstem function and may provide the earliest indication of fixed motor deficit consistent with cerebral palsy long before any discrete motor signs are present. Two major categories function dynamically as the central nervous system develops toward maturation of higher centers. The first is a group of primitive reflexes present at birth and without which the infant would not be viable. These normally disappear within four to six months with maturation as the postural reflexes become manifest. The latter are closely associated with and underlie rolling, sitting, crawling, and walking.[15]

Primitive Reflexes

There is disagreement in the literature about which primitive reflexes have the greatest diagnostic value when evaluating infants. Scherzer and Tscharnuter give major consideration to the startle reflex, Moro reflex, palmar grasp, rooting, sucking, and asymmetric tonic neck reflex (ATNR).[15] Any of those reflexes persisting beyond 4 to 6 months of age should elicit a strong index of suspicion. (Formal testing for these reflexes is presented in other sources, and so will not be discussed here.)

Postural Reflexes

RIGHTING REFLEXES. Magnus described *righting reflexes* in the 1920s after his work with animals. These reflexes bring the head and trunk into a normal position in space and in relation to the ground.[41] Labyrinthine righting reflexes provide for normal orientation of the head in space (i.e., face vertical and mouth horizontal, with gravity being the controlling factor). Body-righting reflexes acting on the head also orient the head in space in relation to the ground. Asymmetric tactile stimulation throughout the body is the stimulus for this reflex. Neck-righting reflexes orient the body (trunk) in relation to the head. Dorsiflexion (extension) of the head causes extension of the vertebral column, whereas ventroflexion (flexion) of the head causes flexion or rounding of the vertebral column. Lateral inclination of the head toward one shoulder causes lateral curvature of the spine with the concavity directed toward the same shoulder. Rotation of the neck causes a reflex whereby the thorax is brought into symmetry with the head. Optical righting reflexes allow the head to be brought into a normal position by using visual cues in the environment as a stimulus.

The result of displacement of the center of gravity in a person with an intact nervous system, normal postural tone, and normal muscular coordination is that the person is able to use the righting reflexes. Righting reflexes are expressed through muscular control. The child with CP has abnormal muscle tone, spinal immobility, and poor coordination, and is usually unable to use righting reflexes effectively. In attempting to attain good righting reflexes in the child with CP, a therapist must first work to normalize postural tone and balance the flexors against the extensors. This can be achieved by increasing tone that is too low, decreasing tone that is too high, and stabilizing tone that fluctuates. The usual case is that axial (trunk) tone is too low to support posture or movement. Postural tone can be improved with approximation and movement against gravity while maintaining good postural alignment. The movement against gravity will facilitate the righting reflex. Anterior displacement of the body's center of gravity requires bilateral, symmetric activation of axial extensors with elongation of axial flexors in the effort to overcome the pull of gravity and right the head and trunk. The normal position of the body in response to an anterior displacement is shown in Figure 4-2. Bilateral, symmetric activation of axial flexors with elongation of axial extensors is necessary to correct the head and trunk when there is a posterior displacement of the

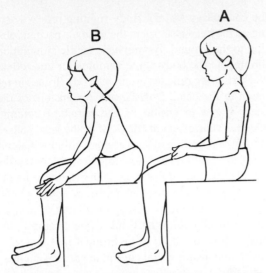

Figure 4–2. A. *Child in upright, midline sitting position.* B. *A posterior righting reaction in an attempt to return to position A after anterior displacement of the body.*

center of gravity. The normal position of the body in response to a posterior displacement is shown in Figure 4-3. In order to right the head and trunk when a lateral displacement of the center of gravity occurs, the child must produce a symmetric and balanced activation of the flexors and extensors on one side of the body to produce lateral flexion of the trunk with pelvic elevation. The normal position of the body in response to a lateral displacement of the body is shown in Figure 4-4. It is most important to remember that both activation, a shortening contraction, and elongation, a lengthening contraction, are active and dynamic and help to maintain alignment. Compare Figures 4-5 and 4-6 with Figures 4-3 and 4-4, respectively. Figures 4-5 and 4-6 each show a collapse into gravity on the "shortened" side and poor holding producing excessive length on the "elongated" side. These abnormal responses are the result of inadequate mobility of the spine, inadequate postural control or poor activation of muscles. These symptoms of movement indicate a need for greater external control by the therapist in order to help maintain align-

ment and achieve a better contraction to achieve more complete muscle shortening.

Note the position of the lower extremities during righting responses for anterior, posterior, and lateral displacements. For anterior and posterior displacements, the lower extremities are symmetric, as are the trunk reactions. With lateral displacement, lower extremity responses are asymmetric in hip rotation. External rotation occurs in the weight-bearing side and internal rotation on the non–weight-bearing hip.

EQUILIBRIUM REACTIONS. An *equilibrium reaction* is an automatic response requiring an adaptation by the entire body to restore balance after displacement of the center of gravity of the body.[42] The restoration of the center of gravity causes the body's return to a midline position. Movements of the trunk needed during an equilibrium reaction require rotation and activation of both the flexor and extensor muscle groups. In the continuum of automatic movement, equilibrium reactions require the greatest coordination and efficiency of muscular ef-

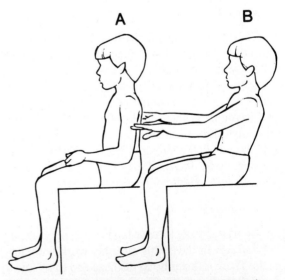

Figure 4–3. A. *Child in an upright, midline sitting position.* B. *An anterior righting reaction in an attempt to return to position A after posterior displacement of the body.*

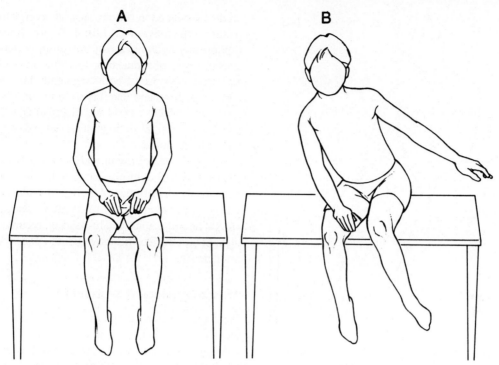

Figure 4-4. A. *Child in an upright, midline sitting position.* B. *A lateral righting reaction in an attempt to return to position A after lateral displacement of the body.*

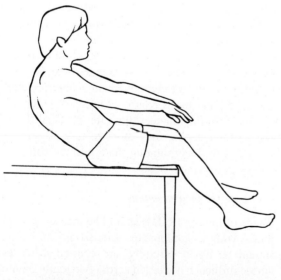

Figure 4-5. *Excessive lumbar and thoracic flexion with neck extension during a forward righting reaction.*

fort. By 12 months of age, equilibrium reactions are present in all positions except standing.[43]

Assessment of Postural Tone

Postural tone should be assessed with the child at rest and during movement and in both recumbent and upright positions. Tone should be assessed through the neck and trunk and throughout the extremities. Tone is often described as the resistance to passive movement and can be evaluated by moving the child's body segments. One specific method of assessment of tone requires that the therapist move body segments through their various planes of movement while the child is supine, prone, or seated. For example, with the child supine, a therapist might feel resistance to the following movements:

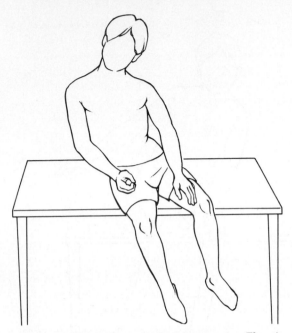

Figure 4-6. *Poor-quality lateral righting reaction. There is excessive lateral flexion of the neck and trunk in response to gravity. Note the external rotation of the hip on the left in an attempt to prevent a complete weight shift to the right side.*

Cervical flexion as the child's head is lifted from the supporting surface

Shoulder flexion and adduction with the shoulders depressed

Extension of the elbow, wrist, and fingers

Supination of the forearm

Movements required to engage the hands in midline activity and to bring hands to the mouth

Flexion, abduction, and external rotation of the hip

Flexion of the knee

Dorsiflexion of the ankle

Movements required to touch hands to either knees or feet

Lumbar flexion: movements used to elevate the pelvis from a supporting surface

The therapist can use a similar approach using functional postures and transitions through prone, sitting, side-lying, kneeling, and standing. Signs of increased postural tone in the moving child may include associated reactions, use of compensatory patterns of movement, distal fixing (increased flexion in fingers or toes), thrusting, or having a spasm. Signs of reduced or low tone may include excessive collapse of body segments, loss of postural alignment, and inability to move or to sustain a posture. When a child has fluctuating levels of postural tone, signs of both increased and decreased tone may be noted.

The presence of involuntary movement, athetosis, or ataxia should also be noted. It is useful to describe the distribution of these involuntary movements and responses and to identify conditions—weight bearing, non–weight-bearing, recumbent, or upright—in which the movements either increase or decrease.

Musculoskeletal Assessment

Persistent shortening of a muscle or group of muscles without adequate activation of antagonists—resulting from spasticity, abnormal reflex activity, weakness, or static positioning—places the child at risk for soft tissue contractures and, over time, bony deformity. With an awareness of the sequence usually seen in abnormal motor development and with knowledge of the postural and movement consequences, the physical therapist must be alert for areas of the body that are at risk for contracture and deformity. It is helpful, too, if older children or adolescents with CP who have acquired any form of mobility are taught the movement sequences typically used and those groups of muscles which are overused. In this manner, both the physical therapist and the patient may more readily note those areas at risk, incorporating them into the patient's goals and treatment plan.

Goniometric Measurements

Range of motion (ROM) should be measured at all joints with a goniometer. Limitations in range should be noted carefully and charted. Muscles whose influence is exerted across two joints should be examined and elongated over both joints when measurements are taken. When moving the child's limb through the range, the movement should be slow and steady to avoid eliciting a strong stretch reflex response and increased spasticity, thus adding to the limitation in motion.

Evaluation of the Spine

Mobility of the spine is necessary in all planes for correct alignment and movement of the spine, for good quality of righting and equilibrium reactions, and for full ROM of the extremities. Evaluation of the child's passive and active movement of the trunk is an essential part of the evaluation.

Passive spinal lateral flexion and spinal extension can be assessed in sitting or in standing dependent on the child's functional level.

Active spinal motion is assessed by having the child move through or maintain various functional positions. The therapist should notice which areas of the spine appear to be limited in mobility or are immobile and interfere with correct alignment and smoothly coordinated weight shifting. Children with CP often have tightness and limitation in cervical and capital flexion, thoracic extension, and lumbar flexion, lateral flexion, and rotation.[37]

The therapist must also document decreased or exaggerated curvatures of the spine—both laterally and in the anterior or posterior directions. When abnormal curvature is found, the treatment program should include appropriate measures to reduce or maintain the curves, depending on whether they are functional or structural.

Thoracic Movement

An area of special concern for the child with CP concerns the coordinated motion of the thorax that occurs during the breathing cycle. In normal babies younger than 6 months of age, there is an approximate 90-degree angle between the ribs and the spine. As control of the head and trunk develops in the normal baby, and as the baby begins to develop a more upright posture, there is a change in this 90-degree relationship. Owing to both gravity and the forces of the axial musculature in resisting gravity, there is a posterior to anterior downward slant to the ribs. As a result of this slant, there is an increased ability to expand the diameter of the thorax in both an anterior-posterior (pump-handle motion) and lateral direction (bucket-handle motion). In addition to this ability to change the inspired volume, the thoracic (external intercostal) and abdominal (obliques) muscles act to fix the rib cage. This fixation facilitates more complete contraction of the diaphragm, thus increasing lung volume. Children with CP typically have low postural muscle tone in the axial muscles. They also tend to have decreased active control of trunk flexors or extensors when in an upright position. As a result of this lack of thoracic muscle tone, there are differences in motion of the chest wall during inspiration. First, the downward slant of the ribs never fully develops, thus minimizing the mechanical advantage of the pump-handle and bucket-handle motions of inspiration. Second, without the muscle tone necessary to fix the rib cage, the diaphragmatic fibers, particularly the sternal fibers, serve an almost paradoxical function—that is, they cause depression of the xiphoid process and the sternum during inspiration. The lack of thoracic expansion, in conjunction with the sternal depression, causes shallow respiratory efforts. Vocalizations will be of short duration and will be low in intensity because of poor breath support. Examination of the respiratory excursion of the thorax is a critical portion of the motor assessment for the child with CP. As with other movements, thoracic and respiratory function should be assessed with the child in various functional positions. It may be useful to assess thoracic excursion in a young child while the child is crying. The "crying vital capacity" is a reasonable index of lung expansion in the infant.[44] The therapist should develop interventions aimed at increasing postural tone throughout the trunk. The therapist must specifically facilitate antigravity control of both axial extensor and flexor muscles, particularly the oblique abdominal muscles that aid in the forceful expiration needed for coughing and sneezing.

Evaluation of the Shoulder Girdle and Upper Extremity

The child with CP with excessive axial extension and poor activation of cervical and capital flexors, upper chest flexors, and abdominal muscles will likely demonstrate tightness and limitation of the shoulder girdle. Tightness of the pectoralis major, especially the sternal portion, seems to occur once the child assumes or maintains a sitting position. Poor extension of the trunk in a sitting position causes the child to collapse into gravity, with resultant rounding of the thoracic spine and tightness of the pectoralis major and rectus abdominus muscles. Dynamic scapular stability fails to develop and the scapulae become fixed in downward rotation and a forward-tipped position. These fixed positions will restrict motion at the sternoclavicular and acromioclavicular joints.[37] Full shoulder motion cannot be achieved with these limitations. The child with CP is likely to be limited in passive flexion, abduction, and external rotation of the shoulder. Elevation of the shoulder, which is used to stabilize the head, may produce limitations in scapulothoracic movement needed for depression of the shoulder. Moving distally, the therapist often finds limitations in extension of the elbow, supination of the forearm, and extension of the wrist and fingers.

Examination of the Hip

The child with CP commonly has tightness in the hip flexors, adductors, and internal rotators, with resultant limitation in extension, abduction, and external rotation of the hip. The Thomas test is used to identify a flexion contracture of the hip, which is common in children with CP. Abduction and adduction of the hip should be assessed with the hip and knee extended. Internal and external rotation should be assessed with the hip extended and the knee flexed while the child is in a prone position.

Femoral Anteversion

Femoral anteversion is a torsion or internal rotation of the femoral shaft on the femoral neck. Other terms that may be synonymous with femoral anteversion include fetal femoral torsion and persistent fetal alignment of the hip.

At birth, an infant has approximately 40 degrees of femoral anteversion, as measured by the angle between the transcondylar axis of the femur and the femoral axis of the neck. The neonate also has 25 degrees of flexion contracture of the hip owing to intrauterine positioning and physiologic flexor tone. In the progression of normal development, hip flexors lengthen as the result of gravitational pull while the child is lying in either a prone or supine position. Active extension and external rotation of the hip tighten the anterior capsule of the hip joint, thus producing a torque or torsional stress that decreases the anteversion that is present from birth.[45] In addition to the effects of the tightened hip capsule, the hip extensors and external rotators insert near the proximal femoral growth plate. When activated, the extensors and external rotators pull on the plate and help to decrease the torsion on the femur. The result of the various forces is that the adult value of 15 degrees of femoral anteversion is reached by 16 years of age.[46,47] Femoral anteversion is determined by biplane roentgenograms. Anteversion may be suspected on the basis of a simple clinical test. Internal and external rotation of the hip are tested with the hip in a position of extension (i.e., with the child in a prone position with knees flexed). Femoral anteversion may be suspected when external rotation at the hip is substantially less than internal rotation.

The child with CP often has overactivity and shortening of the flexors of the hip and poor control of extensors and of external rotators of the hip. Beals, in 1969, studied 40 children with CP and found that the degree of femoral anteversion was normal at birth.[48] However, this study also revealed that the amount of anteversion did not decrease over the first few years of life, as occurs with normal children. After 3 years of age, there was no significant change in anteversion with either age or ambulation status. The sample of children with CP had a mean of 14 degrees greater anteversion than the children without CP.[48]

Staheli and associates found greater angles of anteversion of the femur in the involved lower extremity of a group of children with CP than was found in their uninvolved limb.[20] Children with hemiparesis also commonly show poor activation of extensors and external rotators of the hip, with or without flexion contractures of the hip.

Examination of the Knee

The child with CP may have limited knee flexion or extension as a result of inadequate length of the quadriceps or hamstrings. Length of the medial and lateral hamstrings and the rectus femoris, all of which cross two joints, should be assessed by elongating the muscle over the knee and the hip. Passive straight leg raising or measurement of the popliteal angle will indicate the degree of hamstring tightness. If hamstring tightness is excessive, the child may be unable to sit on the ischium with 90 degrees of flexion of the hip, and stride length may be limited during ambulation.

Tightness of the quadriceps, which limits flexion of the knee, can be identified by looking for a patella that is located more superiorly than normal and by assessing the degree of flexion of the knee with the child in a prone position.

Tibial Torsion

Tibial torsion (tibial version) describes a twist of the tibia along its long axis so that the leg is rotated internally or externally. The specific angle of torsion is determined by the intersection of a line drawn vertically from the tibial tubercle and a line drawn through the malleoli.

Like the femur, the tibia undergoes developmental torsional changes. The malleoli are parallel in the frontal plane at birth. During infancy and early childhood, the tibia rotates externally, which places the lateral malleolus in a posterior position relative to the medial malleolus. Normal values for this gradual rotation, as suggested by Staheli and Engel, are presented in Table 4-1.[48]

The "unwinding" of the tibia, or the progression from relative internal to external tibial torsion, is attributable to changes in force on the tibia arising

Table 4-1. *Normal Values for External Rotation of the Tibia*

Age	Degree of External Rotation
0–3 months	4
3–6 months	6
6–12 months	7
2 years	11
9 years	13
10 years–adult	14

from the decrease in femoral anteversion that occurs as the child grows.

Examination of the Foot

Dorsiflexion of the ankle is often limited in the child with CP because of spasticity affecting the plantar flexors, mainly the gastrocnemius. Dorsiflexion of the ankle should be assessed with the subtalar joint maintained in a neutral position. Neutral alignment will prevent hypermobility of the forefoot while ensuring excursion of the hindfoot.[49]

Midtarsal movement can be assessed by stabilizing the hindfoot with one hand while passively supinating and pronating the forefoot with the other. Toes should be straight and mobile with approximately 90 degrees of extension available at the first metatarsophalangeal joint.

With the child standing, the calcaneous should be vertical or slightly inverted in relation to the lower one third of the leg. Children should begin to show a longitudinal arch at $3\frac{1}{2}$ to 4 years of age. Depression of the medial longitudinal arch is caused by adduction and plantar flexion of the talus with relative eversion of the calcaneous. These deformities are also associated with internal rotation of the lower extremity. Another mechanism for malalignment during standing occurs in children with extensor spasticity who have tightness of the plantar flexors. Their calcaneous is often maintained in some degree of plantar flexion and does not truly participate in weight bearing. The talus stays plantar-flexed with "apparent full weight bearing" with pronation achieved through hypermobility into extension through the midtarsal joint.[49,50] These two mechanisms must be examined carefully when considering an orthosis for standing or ambulation.

Discrepancy in Leg Length

Measurement of leg length should be done with the pelvis level in all planes, the hips in neutral rotation and abduction or adduction, and the knees fully extended. Measurements are taken from the anterosuperior iliac spine to the distal aspect of the medial malleolus.

Staheli and associates studied the inequality in the leg lengths in 50 children with spastic hemiparesis.[20] Of the 16 children who were older than 11 years of age, 70% had a significant discrepancy in leg length. Ten children had a discrepancy of 1 cm or more, and two children had discrepancies of greater than 2 cm between the involved and uninvolved limbs.

Correction of a discrepancy in the leg length by using a shoe lift is not advocated by some sources.[45] However, children with CP who have asymmetry in tone, muscle activation, posture, and movement are placed at even greater risk for muscle shortening and scoliosis when a discrepancy in leg length exists. Such a child will try to equalize the length by ambulating with the shortened limb in plantar flexion with the heel off of the floor, thus maintaining muscles with increased tone—the plantar flexors—in a continually shortened position. When a full-length shoe lift is used to correct the discrepancy in length, the child should be assessed in a standing posture for symmetry of the posterior iliac spines and the iliac crests. When the child wears an orthosis, the shoe-lift thickness must take this added measurement into account. Shoe lifts can be applied to shoes and sneakers in an attractive way at a minimal cost.

Evaluation of Gait

A baby prepares for ambulation by acquiring antigravity movement components of the neck, trunk, and extremities while in prone, supine, and side-lying positions. These movement components are also practiced by the baby in higher level positions against gravity (i.e., sitting, quadruped, kneeling, and standing). Stability of the joints increases as strength is gained in the surrounding musculature. Weight shifting has been practiced by the baby and is mastered in all directions along with appropriate righting and equilibrium responses.

From the onset of independent ambulation until approximately 3 years of age, the young child's gait pattern will continue to change with the acquisition of mature components in gait. An early, immature gait pattern is characterized by the following:

Uneven length of step
Excessive flexion of the hip and knee during swing phase
Immobility of the pelvis without pelvic tilting or rotation
Abduction and external rotation of the hips throughout swing phase
Base of support that is wider than the lateral dimensions of the trunk
Pronation of the foot as a consequence of the wide base
Contact with the floor that is made with the foot flat
Hyperextension of the knee throughout stance phase
Upper extremities in a high-, medium-, or low-guard position[51]

Sutherland[51a] and colleagues described five kinematic gait characteristics that change in normal childhood development during the ages of 1 to 7 years:

1. The duration of single-limb stance increases with age (especially up to the age of 2.5 years).
2. Walking velocity increases steadily (especially up to the age of 3.5 years).
3. Cadence (and its variability) decreases with age.
4. Step length increases (especially until the age of 2.5 years).
5. The ratio of body width to stride width (computed from the "pelvic span," which is measured from the level of the anterosuperior iliac spines, and the "ankle spread," which is the distance between left and right ankle centers during double-limb support) increases rapidly until the age of 2.5 years. It then increases more slowly until the age of 3.5 years, and then plateaus.

Furthermore, the *step factor* (step length divided by limb length) increases during the first 4 years of life and is suggested as a measure of neuromuscular maturation.[52]

Thelen and Cooke maintain that there is "a gradual evolution from the simple pattern generation of the newborn period," and that "an essential process is the individuation of joint action from the obligatory synergy of the newborn period."[53] In an earlier publication, Thelen also states that "Learning to walk is a complex, gradual process of maturation of motivation, the integration of subcortical pattern-generating centers with neural substrate for control of posture and balance, and important changes in body proportions and tone and muscle strength."[52]

To gain the stability not yet available at the trunk and pelvis, an early ambulator maintains a certain degree of scapular adduction, either bilaterally or unilaterally. The high-guard position (Fig. 4-7) consists of adduction of the scapula; extension, abduction, and external rotation of the shoulder; and flexion of the elbow. This position affords the greatest stability by maintaining maximal scapular adduction leading to strong extension of the trunk

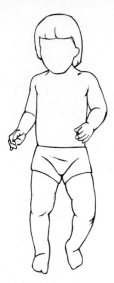

Figure 4-8. *Child ambulating with the upper extremities in a medium-guard position.*

with an anterior, immobile pelvis. A medium-guard position (Fig. 4-8) reduces the degree of scapular adduction. Shoulders continue to be held in extension, abduction, and external rotation, and elbows are flexed with forearms pronated. The low-guard position (Fig. 4-9) consists of scapular adduction with the arms at the sides.

The mature components of gait provide a useful framework for evaluating the gait of a child with CP.[54]

1. *Pelvic tilt.* A downward tilt of the pelvis from the horizontal plane occurs on the non–weight-bearing side. This tilt allows the center of gravity to be lowered as the body passes over the stance limb, thus reducing vertical oscillations of the body.
2. *Pelvic rotation.* Transverse rotation of the pelvis in an anterior direction occurs with internal rotation of the lower extremity at the end of the swing phase. This rotation contributes to a narrowing of the base of support and changes the distribution of weight during stance phase to the lateral border of the foot.
3. *Knee flexion at midstance.* This position permits a more fluid, smoother gait pattern.
4. *Heel strike.* Ankle dorsiflexion near the end of the

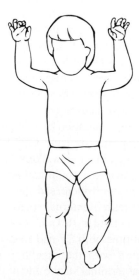

Figure 4-7. *Child ambulating with the upper extremities in a high-guard position.*

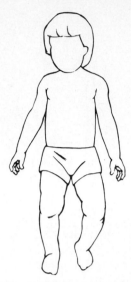

Figure 4-9. *Child ambulating with the upper extremities in a low-guard position.*

swing phase readies the foot for contact with the floor made at the heel.

5. *Mature mechanism of the foot and knee.* These mechanisms consist of an extension of the knee just before or at heel strike, flexion of the knee in a midstance position, and extension of the knee at heel-off.

6. *Mature base of support.* The base of support narrows to within the lateral dimensions of the trunk.

7. *Synchronous movement of the upper extremities.* Arm swing achieves a reciprocating movement with the lower extremities. Movements of the upper extremities balance out the leg advance and pelvic rotation that produce angular momentum to the lower body.[58]

Gait in Cerebral Palsy

One of the most frequently asked questions from parents and caregivers upon being told their child has CP is, "When will my child walk?" This prediction can be very difficult and should be approached with caution. Watt and co-workers attempted to determine the usefulness of early prognosis.[55] They discovered that predictions made at 1 year of age were the least useful, and that predictions made at 3.5 years of age did not significantly increase in ac-

curacy over the information which was available at 2 years of age. They found that the age at which the child sat, the type of CP, certain reflexes (tonic labyrinthine, ATNR, symmetrical tonic neck, and Moro), and two postural reactions (foot placement and parachute) all had a statistically significant correlation with ambulation at 8 years of age. However, no absolute value could be placed on the items.[55]

There are several classic gait patterns that are characteristic of the different types of CP. Variations do exist within each type, however. The classic gait patterns are described in the following section.

Many children with spastic diplegia have limited mobility in their lumbar spine, pelvis, and hip joints and show limited asymmetric pelvic tilt or pelvic rotation during gait.[36] In an effort to compensate for the lack of mobility of the lower body, these children shift their weight and maintain balance by using excessive mobility through the head, neck, upper trunk, and upper extremities. Their hips stay flexed during stance, and full extension of the hip is never achieved. Excessive adduction and internal rotation of the hip are frequently found; in severe cases, the medial aspect of the knees may approximate. Depending on the function of the pelvic, lumbar, and ankle musculature, the knees may be either flexed or hyperextended during stance. The feet may be in valgus outside the lateral dimensions of the trunk, or they may be close together in a narrow base of support in plantar flexion with the heels off of the floor. There can be concern and confusion regarding the differentiation between idiopathic toe walking and spastic diplegic CP. Hicks et al.[56] found that idiopathic toe walkers typically have heel cord contracture but minimal or no hamstring tightness, along with increased knee extension in stance and increased external rotation of the foot with increased plantar flexion. Conversely, they found that children with CP had an essentially normal gait pattern with the exception of sustained knee flexion at terminal stance and initial contact.[56] Although children with more severe involvement may require an assistive device for ambulation, most children ambulate without any devices, or with only a shoe insert or orthosis. Generally, children with spastic diplegic CP ambulate at about half the speed of children without CP, and the self-selected velocity is usually the most efficient rate of ambulation.[57]

Asymmetry is the most obvious feature of the gait of a child with hemiplegia, with most of the body weight borne on the uninvolved lower extremity. Shifting of weight to the involved side is brief and incomplete. Limbs on the involved side are retracted or rotated posteriorly, when compared to the shoulder and pelvis on the contralateral side. Arm swing occurs only on the uninvolved side, with the involved upper extremity held in shoulder hyperextension and elbow flexion as part of an associated reaction. The lower extremity can vary between stiffness in extension to greater mobility with flexion. Almost all children with spastic hemiplegia ambulate without assistive devices, but many use a shoe insert or an orthosis.

Children with milder cases of athetosis without significant spasms have underlying low postural tone that fluctuates to high tone. The gait pattern in the lower extremity is poorly graded and in total patterns of movement. The lower extremity is usually lifted high into flexion and placed down in stance into extension with adduction, internal rotation, and plantar flexion. The hips stay slightly flexed, the lumbar spine is hyperextended, the thoracic spine is excessively rounded, and the cervical spine is hyperextended with the chin jutting forward.[36]

Assessment of Fine Motor and Adaptive Skills

Assessment of the fine motor and adaptive skills of the child with CP is traditionally one of the main areas of concern for the occupational therapist, as well as for the physical therapist. If a treatment center or a school does not have an occupational therapist as a member of the staff, the physical therapist should have the basic skills to assess this area of movement and development. Questions to the parents or other caretakers that may alert the therapist to the need for intervention relate to the level of the child's self-sufficiency during feeding, dressing, toileting, and bathing. Additional firsthand information may be obtained by having the child undress and dress (including shoes, socks, and shirt) independently before and after the assessment session. As the child moves to attempt these tasks, the therapist can evaluate sitting balance, pelvic weight shifting, and righting actions of the head and trunk. Other parameters that can be evaluated as the child removes clothes include the ability to reach as well as various modes of grasp—depending on the object, the ability to release an object, and bimanual skills, such as buttoning and unbuttoning. During the evaluation process, the therapist should ascertain the following:

1. Whether the particular skill can be accomplished
2. The degree of assistance required
3. At what point in the movement assistance was necessary
4. *Why* the assistance was necessary

Consideration of Speech and Language Abilities

A comprehensive assessment of speech and language is not within the scope of practice of the physical therapist. However, the physical therapist can offer important information to the speech and language pathologist regarding the speech and language abilities and quality of respiration of the child based on observations made during physical therapy assessment and treatment. In obtaining this information, the physical therapist should consider the following questions:

- Did the child appear to hear your voice or other environmental sounds by becoming quiet or looking in the direction of the stimulus?
- Did the child understand questions asked during the evaluation, and did he or she follow step-by-step directional commands?
- Did the child vocalize or verbalize during the assessment? What types of sounds were made? Did the child repeat or appear to stutter speech sounds?
- If the child was verbal, were the words intelligible? Was breath support adequate for speech, or was the child able to speak in only one- or two-word utter-

ances owing to poor control of respiration? Do the expressive language skills appear to be delayed for the child's chronological age?

- If the child was nonvocal, was there another means of communication used (i.e., gestures, manual language board, electronic communication system)? Did the child use eye localization, pointing, or another means within this alternate system?
- Was the child's communication at a functional level?

The therapist should also ask if the parents have noted any problems with the child's speech or related functional areas, such as difficulty sucking, swallowing, chewing, feeding, or drinking.

These observations and questions can assist in making an informed referral to a speech and language pathologist who will perform a more detailed assessment. If appropriate, the speech and language pathologist can institute a therapeutic program that can be augmented during physical therapy sessions.

A comprehensive assessment of the thorax can be very beneficial to the child and can assist the speech and language pathologist in attaining the goals established for the child. The mobility of the vertebral column and the rib cage has a great impact on the effectiveness of respiration and breath support for vocalization. It also has an impact on pulmonary hygiene, as improved rib cage mobility and deeper respirations help air to flow in the lungs and can prevent or help cure pneumonia. Rib cage mobility and abdominal support provide a good basis for speech control and voice quality. Co-treatment with the speech and language pathologist can be very beneficial to the child, often resulting in more rapid progress. Addressing the child's musculoskeletal problems can assist the speech and language pathologist in planning therapy for communication and respiration issues.

Establishing Goals of Treatment

A thorough assessment leads to the establishment of specific long- and short-term goals for the child. Goals should be functional, objective, and expressed in behavioral terms. The goal should also address the qualitative aspects of movement. The time span considered as "long-term" may differ significantly, depending on the setting in which the child is seen. For a hospitalized child, a long-term goal might be the functional goal for the entire period of hospitalization. For the child in a school setting, a long-term goal might be a semester's expectation. Short-term goals would be written to identify goals of an intermediate nature that fall within the time span covered by the long-term goals. The short-term goals should relate functionally and qualitatively to the long-term goal. A therapist may find it helpful to perform a task analysis of the functional long-term goal, with the individual movement components, or tasks, serving as the short-term goals. Included in the statements of the goals should be the degree of assistance and the amount of support that is expected to be needed with the functional skill. The following examples illustrate the types of goals that might be appropriate. Notice that each short-term goal (STG) is a component that leads to the accomplishment of the long-term goal (LTG).

LTG
(child's name) will make the transition from short-sitting on a chair to standing at a table, given minimal assistance, with shoulders moving anteriorly over the knees and single upper extremity support.

STG 1.
(child's name) will right the head, trunk, and pelvis in response to imposed slow, moderate-range displacement in the anterior, posterior, and lateral directions while in a short-sitting position.

STG 2.
(child's name) will maintain the scapulae on the thoracic wall with an imposed weight shift in all directions when lying prone over a ball with upper extremities extended to bear weight on the floor.

STG 3.
(child's name) will shift the pelvis in an anteroposterior direction while in a short-sitting position, given minimal assistance, with righting of the head and trunk and with feet kept flat on the floor at hip width.

STG 4.
(child's name) will demonstrate righting of the head and trunk while standing with minimal imposed weight shift in all directions, with feet at shoulder-width

and heels on floor, and with single upper extremity support.

STG 5.

(child's name) will make the transition from short-sitting on a chair to standing at a table, given minimal assistance, with shoulders moving anteriorly over the knees and with bilateral upper extremity support.

Therapeutic Intervention

The therapeutic team should consist of the family, various allied health professionals (depending on the child's functional abilities), and school staff (according to the child's age). The family is of paramount importance to the success of the child. The physical therapist must take advantage of the child's functional assets, promote compensatory adaptations, and try to prevent secondary consequences of disabilities.[62] Physical therapy can minimize the need for or postpone orthopedic surgery, thereby reducing the number of surgeries a child may need.[63] The age of the child or adolescent becomes a factor when providing physical therapy services. Some authors believe that the physical therapy services provided should be most intensive in the early childhood and early school years, with gradual tapering. The rationale for this is that most children reach their expected functional capacity in terms of ambulation and daily activity skills by the time they reach school age. A burst of physical therapy is required after orthopedic interventions. Formal physical therapy should be supplemented, if not replaced, in early adolescence and adulthood in those with mild to moderate impairment by alternative activities, such as recreational pursuits.[62,63]

Therapists must be very clear about what services are indicated and how these services are changing the child's function. According to Fetters, we need a new way to look at treatment, and we need ecologically valid movement goals to guide treatment of motor dysfunction, as well as research in motor control.[64] The parameters that therapists have been using to guide their treatment sequences may need to be altered to achieve documented quality improvement in terms of functional goals. Kluzik and colleagues looked at the kinematic

properties of reaching in spastic quadriplegic children with CP and were able to show that, in using the neurodevelopmental treatment approach, the children experienced an immediate improvement in reaching at the end of the session.[65]

Kamm and colleagues address treatment from a dynamic systems approach, considering the goal of treatment to be working on the system when it is in transition.[66] According to their approach, the therapist would complete an assessment, after which he or she would attempt to predict under what conditions and how patients will change. The physical therapist would also anticipate system-wide responses to small changes in a control parameter. For example, placing an orthotic device in a shoe may alter the pattern of weight bearing, thus influencing the posture of the knee, hip, pelvis, and trunk. "When patients are able to explore and use the limits of postures to actively engage in tasks, they are adaptive and independent."[66]

General suggestions are made in this chapter as to various methods of treatment intervention, including therapeutic exercise and handling, equipment, ambulation aids, orthoses, orthopedic surgery, and home management. No specific treatment program for a particular type of CP is presented in this chapter, as each child has a unique set of functional skills and deficits. Tables 4-2 through 4-5 present major physical problems and general goals of treatment for four major types of CP. The focus of treatment presented in these tables is not intended for use as specific goals for any one patient, but should be used as general guidelines when writing goals for a treatment program. The information included in these tables is derived from numerous sources.[16,32,33,40,59-61]

Therapeutic Exercise

Neurodevelopmental therapy is one form of treatment that is frequently used in pediatrics. The theory was initially developed in the 1950s by the Bobaths in England. It has continued to develop over time to keep pace with our increased understanding of the central nervous system (CNS) and

Table 4-2. *Physical Problems of the Child with Spasticity*

Problems

Low tone in trunk musculature

Spasticity in extremity musculature

Incomplete righting reflexes, equilibrium reactions, and protective responses

Extremities maintained in midrange

Stereotypical (patterned) movement

Slow, laborious movement

Associated reactions present

At risk for orthopedic deformities secondary to muscle and joint tightness

Fearful of movement

Focus of Treatment

Increased tone in trunk musculature

Reduced tone throughout the extremities

Full range of motion in extremities

Increased spinal mobility

More varied and differentiated movement patterns

Provision of weight-bearing experience with movement

Inhibition of associated reactions

Avoidance of static postures

Child to initiate movement

Provision of different movement experiences—varying positions, speed and direction, and equipment while ensuring safety

Anticipate sites of muscle shortening and joint immobility. Work for muscle elongation, joint mobility, proximal stabilization, and active function of muscles around the joint.

motor control. The following is a list of current theoretical assumptions based on current scientific concepts as agreed upon by the Neurodevelopmental Treatment Association Instructor Group in 1992:

1. The CNS controls movements, not muscles. Changes in muscle properties will limit the capability for movement.
   Clinical Assumption:
   A. Patterns of movement are most easily learned and retained in a self-initiated, functional context.

2. The sensory system affects motor function. (Includes all sensory modalities: proprioceptive, visual, tactile, vestibular)
   - Sensory experience and correct interpretation of sensory information are necessary for motor learning.
   - Attention and interpretation are necessary for voluntary motor control.
   - Automatic motor control relies on motor programs and is relatively independent of sensory feedback.
   Clinical Assumptions:
   A. Training of movement control may require teaching the patient to interpret sensory information correctly.
   B. Patients with CNS dysfunction may have an abnormal ability to receive and interpret sensory information.

Table 4-3. *Physical Problems of the Child with Athetosis*

Problems

Fluctuating level of muscle tone (hypotonia → normal)

Involuntary movement

Lack of co-contraction of muscles

Lack of grading of movement

Inability to hold segment at various points within the range of motion

Asymmetry in both posture and movement

Greater involvement of head, trunk, and upper extremities than lower extremities

Movement of head affecting trunk and limbs

Incomplete righting reflexes, equilibrium reactions, and protective responses

Focus of Treatment

Balance postural muscle tone.

Develop midline and symmetric muscle action.

Develop increased muscle control in ranges away from midline position.

Hold posture or motion at various points within the range during movement transitions.

Smooth grading of movement.

Aim for independent movements of the head on a stable trunk.

Develop smoothly coordinated automatic reactions.

Table 4-4. *Physical Problems of the Child with Ataxia*

Problems

Usually hypotonic, but some have increased tone

Poor co-contraction and sustained holding of postures

Dysmetria

Poorly coordinated righting reflexes, equilibrium reactions, and protective responses

Goals of Treatment

Balanced postural tone

Midline and sustained holding throughout range of movement

Smoothly coordinated automatic reactions

Table 4-5. *Physical Problems of the Child with Hypotonia*

Problems

Poor head control

Very poor trunk stability and control

Shallow breathing

Absent or slow righting reflexes, equilibrium reactions, and protective responses

Joint hypermobility

Focus of Treatment

Increased postural tone

Improved head and trunk control against gravity

Improve automatic reactions

Smooth coordinated movement of the extremities in gravity-eliminated positions and in positions against gravity with trunk stabilized

Permit child to react to imposed movement

Stabilization of joints in neutral alignment

3. Functional movement requires complex CNS processes. Self-initiated functional movement incorporates an idea, decision, program, plan, and execution.
   Clinical Assumptions:
   A. Initiation of movement is self-directed.
   B. The interplay between "handling" and self-directed movement depends on the patient's specific impairment and capabilities.
4. Abnormal tone, resulting from CNS dysfunction, affects movement performance. Abnormal tone occurs with changes in the intrinsic properties of muscles, with reflexive alterations of muscle tension, and with voluntary alterations of muscle tension.
   Clinical Assumption:
   A. Modification of tone through handling techniques is a component of functional treatment.
5. Acquisition of functional skills in normal infants and children provides a system for analysis of abnormal movement in patients with CNS dysfunction.
   Clinical Assumptions:
   A. The developmental sequence is not used as a method of treatment, but as a guide to understanding the relationships of normal movement components.
   B. Treatment is aimed at reaching functional, age-appropriate goals, not at following or mimicking the developmental sequence.
6. Damage to the CNS leads to predictable neurologic impairments. Neurologic impairments can lead to further secondary impairments in the musculoskele-

tal, cardiopulmonary, and integumentary systems.
   Clinical Assumptions:
   A. Effective treatment must address both the motor deficit and the secondary impairments.
   B. Treatment may be limited by the lesion.
7. Automatic postural control is necessary for normal movement.

Based on these assumptions, a therapeutic exercise program plays a vital role in the habilitation/rehabilitation of a child with CP. The exercise program should be developed in relation to the assessment of the child and the subsequently identified long- and short-term goals. It is similar to other forms of exercise in that the therapist must upgrade the difficulty of the program to progress the child to greater achievement in strength, endurance, and coordination. In order to increase the child's strength, the therapist has two available options: (1) to progress the movement from a gravity-eliminated movement to one that is working against gravity, and (2) to alter the amount of assistance given by the therapist so that the child has to use greater force and control. Increasing the number of repetitions of a movement or lengthening the time of exercise will help to improve endurance. Coordination should improve with an increase in strength and endurance, depending on the lesion.

Gravity

The therapist can use the effects of gravity as a force against which the child must move and function. The therapist places the child in a position so that any movement of the head and trunk, or the limbs, must be done against gravity. Of course, this technique requires that the child have postural tone that is strong enough to function against gravity, yet not too strong to prevent active movement. The motion can be made in a position with no gravity if the child's "strength" is inadequate, if the movement is poorly coordinated, or if the movement is performed with associated reactions. An example of progression against gravity is shown when the child attempts to progress from a sitting position to kneeling, then to standing. Each progression requires greater strength to stabilize the trunk owing to the increasing height of the center of gravity from the floor.

Weight Shift

A *weight shift,* or a displacement of the center of gravity of the body, can be used to offer increased difficulty of movement for the child with CP. The child has several options to respond to this displacement of the body mass. The options are selected based on the speed, range, and direction of displacement, the child's strength and coordination, and the cognitive desire to respond. The movement options in response to a weight shift include:[59]

1. A righting response
2. An equilibrium reaction
3. A protective extension response
4. A fall

Variables that can be manipulated in shifting weight include:

1. Range of displacement
2. Speed of displacement
3. Direction of displacement

These variables can be used individually or in combination to increase or decrease the difficulty of a movement. The therapist must continually reevaluate the child's response based on the variables presented. For example, a righting reaction is the expected response to a slow, small range displacement in sitting. If a protective extension response was seen, the therapist would need to reevaluate the possible reasons for the response and modify the position and support of the child. The displacement would be repeated to determine if modifications produced the more appropriate righting reaction.

Dissociation or Differentiation

Therapeutic exercise should be directed toward dissociation of one extremity from the opposite limb and the limbs from the body to achieve greater muscular coordination. Emphasis should be placed on achieving greater differentiation of the joints within the dissociated limb, as well.

External Support

The therapist's hands or a piece of equipment may be used to provide initial support to inhibit excessive tone, maintain alignment, initiate a weight shift, support a movement, or aid smooth transitions of movement. This external support should be altered intermittently at first to provide the child with an opportunity to practice the movement independently.

Support of the child's body to inhibit tone and to facilitate movement can be moved from a proximal point such as the trunk, shoulder, or pelvis, which provides a greater amount of support, to a more distal point along the limb. By moving the point of support more distally, the therapist expects that the child will assume a greater degree of control over muscle tone and movement at the unsupported joints.

Sensory Systems

It is necessary to address the child's sensory system (proprioceptive, visual, tactile, and vestibular) specifically as it affects motor function. The child with CP may have difficulty in receiving and interpreting sensory feedback and is, therefore, at a disadvantage for motor output. The therapist should provide the child with movement experiences and sensory input that will help to teach the child correct interpretation of sensory stimuli. The experience should begin as exact stimulation for the child who has great difficulty interpreting or receiving sensory stimuli. The kinds of sensory stimuli can be broadened with improvement.

Secondary Musculoskeletal Changes

A child's difficulty in performing functional tasks may be attributable to an inability to work against gravity or to control self- or therapist-imposed weight shifts. However, this difficulty may also be the result of changes within the musculoskeletal system. An assessment should identify which muscles are shortened, which joint capsules are tight, and where the fascia has thickened over time owing to injury or stress of movement. These areas should be addressed so that smoothly coordinated motor tasks can be accomplished. It is beyond the scope of this chapter to address joint mobilization techniques or myofascial release. Joint mobilization techniques are highly specialized for the pediatric client and should not be attempted without specific instruction. Myofascial release, once learned, can be more easily adapted to the pediatric client.

Other Considerations

The therapist should avoid prolonged holding in static positions during treatment. Smoothly graded transitions in movement with brief holding of midline or neutral alignment is more desirable than extended periods in static postures. Imposed weight shifts and transitions in movement should be varied, both in speed and range, so that the child cannot anticipate rhythmical displacements. Weight shifts and transitions in movement must be practiced in different positions for improved function. Initiation of weight shifts and transitions in movement are important parts of treatment, particularly for the child with spasticity. Active movement and much repetition are needed for a child to "learn" a movement.

Equipment Uses and Considerations

Equipment may be used as an aid to therapeutic exercise and handling. The therapist may use equipment to place the child in a position to enhance movement, inhibit undesirable responses, introduce instability into the context of movement, assist in controlling the amount of instability and the degree of freedom,[66] or assist in the handling and movement of larger patients. The positions and movements available to the therapist are limited only by the therapist's creativity and handling skills.

Mats

A firm mat provides a good working surface on the floor against which the child can push or work in attempting to attain specific postures or movements against gravity. The mat provides proprioceptive and tactile feedback so that the child has better sensory information regarding movement.

Benches

Benches of various heights can be used for short-sitting, table-top activities, stepping, climbing, cruising, and so on. One bench can be adjustable in height, or the therapist may wish to have several benches of graduated height to accommodate the table-top and climbing activities.

Balls and Bolsters

Firm balls and bolsters provide mobile surfaces that can aid the therapist in facilitating automatic reactions of the child. The direction in which the ball is moved and the position of the child on the ball can be varied to facilitate movement of the head and truck into flexion, extension, lateral flexion, and/or rotation. It is essential to remember that the ball has a curved weight-bearing surface so that lateral displacement of the ball will result in weight bearing through the ischium that is on top of the ball. The weight-bearing side of the trunk should be elongated. Varied use of the ball and its infinite possibilities for movement allows the therapist to control the degree to which the movement is assisted by or performed against gravity. Figures 4-10 through 4-14 give visual examples of ways in which such a ball can be utilized.

Tilt Boards and Equilibrium Boards

A tilt board offers a surface on which the child may lie recumbent, sit, kneel, stand, or maintain a quadruped position while being rocked in an anteroposterior or mediolateral direction. A slowly rocking tilt board may be used to elicit a righting reaction, whereas a more rapid tilt will elicit an equilibrium reaction.

Adaptive Equipment

Adaptive equipment is often a necessary and useful adjunct to treatment of the child with CP. Equipment may be provided to offer postural support to the child, or it may aid functional skills and mobility. Any equipment used should be comfortable, safe, easy to use, and attractive. Adaptive equip-

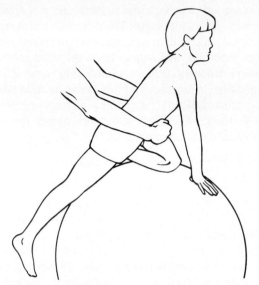

Figure 4-11. *Child in the prone position being supported on a ball with lower extremities dissociated, extension throughout the spine, shoulders flexed, and elbows extended.*

ment and its use should coincide with and reinforce therapeutic goals for the child. The equipment should be reassessed frequently with the aim of reducing support systems as the child gains active control.

Chapter 13 provides a comprehensive review of the theory and concepts behind adaptive equipment and resources; therefore, only a brief description of common items appears here.[40,61,67]

Equipment to Aid Positioning

SIDE-LYING. Side-lyers are usually made of two pieces of wood or tri-wall, a triple-thickness corrugated paper material, that are joined at 90 degrees. This supporting corner is usually padded with sponge rubber and is covered with vinyl or heavy cloth. Important considerations when positioning a child in a side-lyer include the following:

- The head should be elevated on a pillow to maintain its alignment with the trunk. This elevation will also reduce excessive pressure, which may compromise circulation in the underside arm.

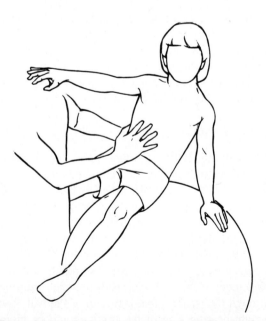

Figure 4-10. *A child who is supported on a ball responds to a lateral displacement by using a lateral righting reaction. Weight is centered over the left ischium.*

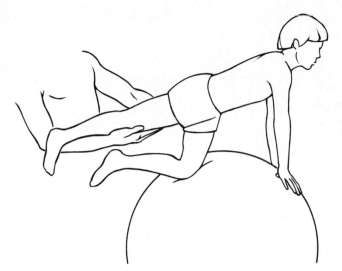

Figure 4-12. *Forward weight shift onto extended upper extremities with lower extremities maintained in dissociated position. This is designed to facilitate trunk extension with abdominal holding and shoulder flexion with elbow extension without excessive extension through the lower extremities.*

- Support of the anterior trunk will help maintain alignment in a frontal plane and will provide tactile input to the abdominal muscles.
- Support between the thighs will help dissociate the lower extremities while supporting the uppermost flexed leg in neutral alignment. The support in neutral alignment will prevent a position of adduction and internal rotation at the hip. These two positions often lead to subluxation of the hip joint.
- Toys should be placed at chest level or lower to avoid hyperextension of the neck and to promote eye-hand regard.

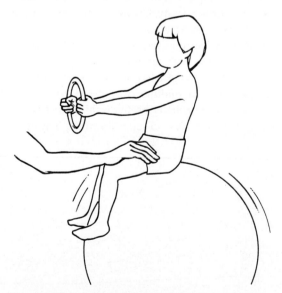

Figure 4-13. *A forward righting reaction in response to backward displacement. The position of the upper extremities facilitates activation of the abdominal muscles.*

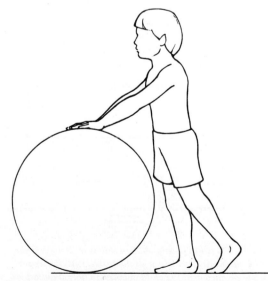

Figure 4-14. *Older child assuming a forward stance position while weight bearing on a mobile surface.*

- Arms should be in a forward position for play and exploration. A child positioned in a side-lyer is depicted in Figure 4-15.

PRONE POSITION. Use of the prone position must be monitored carefully. Wedges and bolsters commonly used to elevate and support the upper body may cause undesirable postures, such as hyperextension of the neck, forward jutting of the jaw, excessive thoracic rounding, hyperextension of the lumbar spine, and anterior tilt of the pelvis with flexion of the hip. These postures may occur when the equipment used is placed too far cephalad, thus producing a high center of gravity; they also occur when the child has inadequate axial flexors—neck flexors, pectorals, abdominals—to counter the axial extension. A child is shown in proper alignment in Figure 4-16, whereas in Figure 4-17, poor positioning is shown on a prone support.

SITTING. There have been great technologic advances in the past 5 to 10 years concerning the materials and equipment available for appropriate seating. It is beyond the scope of this chapter to address current wheelchair designs and seating. However, the basic concepts that must be considered when adapting a seat for a child will be presented. There is currently disagreement within the field about the most functional seated position for a child. Myhr and von Wendt have found that, when

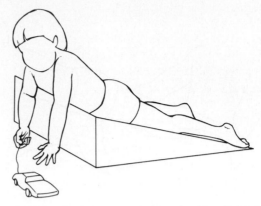

Figure 4-16. *Proper prone positioning is achieved with the assistance of a wedge.*

the head, trunk, and upper extremities are anterior to the ischial tuberosities, pathologic movements (e.g., ATNR) are minimized, postural control is increased, and arm and hand function are best.[68] This positioning was achieved through the use of a forward-tipped seat, firm backrest, arms supported against a table, and the feet permitted to move backward. The study included 23 children in six different sitting positions. This positioning concept warrants further study. However, the more traditional approach will be presented here.

Functional sitting occurs when the pelvis is in a neutral position with the hips and knees at 90 degrees of flexion, the head aligned over the trunk, and the trunk at midline over the pelvis so that weight is borne equally on the ischial tuberosities, with the feet resting on a support surface. The upper

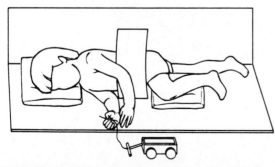

Figure 4-15. *Child positioned in a side-lyer. Note that the head is maintained in line with the trunk, with the upper extremities forward, the child engaged in activity in a position in which gravity is eliminated, and with the lower extremities dissociated.*

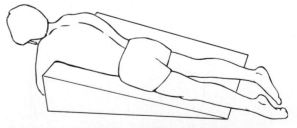

Figure 4-17. *A child that is poorly positioned prone over a wedge. Note the thoracic kyphosis, internal rotation of the shoulders, and flexion of the cervical spine.*

extremities should be allowed to move freely for functions, such as wheelchair propulsion or table-top activities. The aim of adaptive seating is to approximate this positioning as much as possible to allow the child the greatest degree of function. Possible additions/adaptations to the chair may include the following:

- Solid seat to promote neutral alignment of hips
- Solid back for adequate support of the trunk and scapulae. Contoured styles are available to facilitate forward arm placement, lumbar extension, and ease of wheelchair propulsion. The height of the seatback should be no higher than the top of the shoulders in a wheelchair that is upright (not reclined).
- Head support as required by the child's ability to maintain the head in midline
- Tilt-in-space feature whereby 90-degree hip flexion is maintained, but the entire body is tipped posteriorly. This is indicated when the child is unable to hold the trunk upright against gravity. This can also be accomplished by adding a wedge under the thighs in a reclining wheelchair (Fig. 4-18).
- Lateral supports for the hips that can be extended to-ward the knee to control excessive abduction. These supports should keep the hips in a midline position.
- Lateral trunk supports to aid the child in maintaining the trunk erect and in good alignment against gravity. The trunk supports should not be used without hip supports so as to keep the pelvis in proper alignment.
- A seatbelt should be used at the level of the pelvis where it can assist in maintaining weight bearing on the ischial seats. This belt may be at a 45-degree angle to the hips or over the proximal thighs. Figure 4-19 illustrates a child using lateral trunk and hip supports with a pelvic seatbelt.
- Chest support may be required for a child who does not have the endurance to maintain an upright position against gravity for extended periods of time. A variety of straps and supports are available. The therapist must choose one that does not interfere with upper extremity function, but rather gives proximal stability to allow for distal mobility. The H strap is one possibility (Fig. 4-20). It must be fastened to the solid back and provides a posterior and inferior pull to the shoulders.
- Removable trays, when placed on adjustable-height armrests, allow for the child to perform table-top ac-

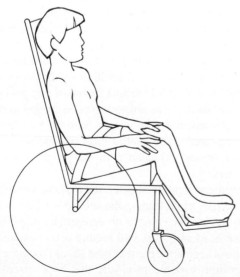

Figure 4-18. *Child is reclining in a wheelchair with a seat wedge to maintain 90 degrees of flexion of the hips.*

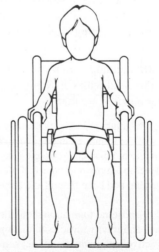

Figure 4-19. *Child is sitting in a wheelchair with hip blocks and lateral trunk supports that are placed asymmetrically to maintain the trunk in neutral alignment against gravity.*

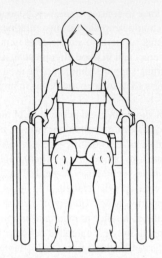

Figure 4-20. *Child is positioned securely in wheelchair with an H strap.*

tivities at a comfortable height. The level of the tray should be ascertained by having the child bend the elbow to 90 degrees of flexion to allow for comfortable forearm placement.

This section is not intended to be a comprehensive list of all possible adaptations for seating. Rather, it should be used as a general guideline when developing a seating system for a child.

STANDING. Standing is a useful and therapeutic activity for the child with CP. Some of the benefits of a standing position are that it:

1. Increases the angle of inclination between the shaft and neck of the femur, changing the position of the hip from one of coxa valga to coxa vara
2. Helps develop a more normal acetabulum
3. Elongates hip and knee flexors and ankle plantar flexors
4. Normalizes postural tone throughout the body and stimulates antigravity muscles of the hip and knee
5. Allows active antigravity use of neck, trunk, and upper extremities
6. Provides a new visual perspective of the environment for the child

Children with CP often have abnormal methods of standing and bearing weight. The following are some typical standing postures:

1. Asymmetric weight bearing
2. Hips flexed, adducted, and internally rotated; knees flexed and in valgus; ankles excessively dorsiflexed; feet pronated and abducted ("crouched gait")
3. Stiff extension in lower extremities; hips adducted and internally rotated; ankles in a position of equinovarus
4. Ankles plantar-flexed (heels on the floor); feet pronated; knees hyperextended; hips flexed
5. May not accept weight on their lower extremities

Symmetric standing is a goal for many children with CP. The desired positions include neutral alignment of the feet; extension of the knees and hips; neutral alignment of the pelvis, trunk, and head; upper extremities forward of the body; and a base of support either within or just slightly outside the lateral dimensions of the trunk. For many children with CP, achieving this position is impossible without some means of external support. For many, the prone-stander or supine-stander supports the well-aligned position described. With each type of stander, there is a means of controlling the degree of incline away from vertical, thus providing for optimal alignment. Both standers include straps to secure the trunk and pelvis, and lateral supports to control the trunk. A tray or table should be used to encourage a forward position of the upper extremities. If the child cannot maintain a neutral position of the foot, an orthosis may be needed to provide alignment during weight bearing. Standing is not indicated if the neutral positions cannot be attained or approximated with the prone or supine standers.

While in a prone-stander, the child bears weight on the feet while leaning the anterior surface of the body against the equipment. Antigravity movement of the head and trunk will require active extension of those segments. the therapist should monitor the extension response to ensure that hyperextension throughout the spine does not occur. This response can lead to anterior pelvic tilt, which is commonly associated with flexion of the lower extremities in children with CP. Figure 4-21 shows a child in good alignment in a prone-stander, whereas Figure 4-22 shows a child in improper alignment.

When placed in a supine-stander, the child bears weight on the feet, but the posterior surface of the body leans against the equipment. A major benefit of the supine-stander is that its use involves the activation of the abdominal muscles, particularly when the child works with the upper extremities above the waist. Children with limited head control are better placed in a supine-stander that provides posterior support for the head.

Assistive Devices to Aid Ambulation

Several devices are available to assist a child in ambulation and to make ambulation as functional, energy-efficient, and least cumbersome as possible. A study by Rose et al. documented a linear relationship between oxygen uptake and heart rate throughout a wide range of walking speeds for children

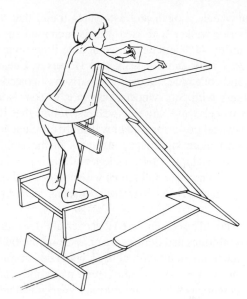

Figure 4-22. *Poor alignment in a prone stander. Note the excessive anterior pelvic tilt and flexion of the lower extremities.*

with and children without CP.[69] They suggested that heart rate be used to evaluate the child's fitness and to measure energy expenditure. This may be a good method to aid in the decision about which assistive device should be used for the child.

WALKERS. Traditional walkers are forward walkers, sometimes known as rollator walkers. They have two wheels in front and the child pushes it in front of him or her. A recurrent problem with this type of walker is anterior trunk lean, so that the body's line of gravity is anterior to the feet and the hips are held in flexion.[70,71] Sometimes, vertical handles are added to facilitate more forearm supination, shoulder depression, and thoracic extension. However, posterior walkers have proven to be more energy-efficient, and have resulted in improved upright posture. The shoulders are held in greater depression with extension, the scapulae tend to be more adducted, and greater thoracic extension is noted. The posterior walker may have either two or

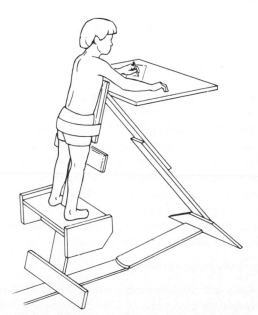

Figure 4-21. *Child is properly aligned in a prone stander.*

four wheels. Logan and associates found that the posterior walker with two wheels increased stride length by 41% and decreased double limb support by 39% over anterior walkers.[70] However, Levangie and colleagues, in their comparison of posterior walkers with four wheels, posterior walkers with two wheels, and anterior walkers, found that the four-wheel posterior walker was more efficient and allowed more significant increases in the child's velocity, right and left stride length, and left step length.[71] The results obtained with anterior walkers and posterior walkers with two wheels were similar.[71]

It should be remembered that each child's ambulation abilities and deficits are unique and should be evaluated on an individual basis when determining which walker affords the greatest stability and safety while providing for the most energy-efficient gait pattern.

CRUTCHES AND CANES. Axillary and forearm crutches are rarely used for the child with CP because the child's balance must be significantly better than when a walker is used. The child with improved balance often prefers using no assistive device and having the upper extremities free to assist in maintaining balance. Forearm crutches tend to facilitate rounding of the shoulders and forearm pronation with a forward leaning trunk. When excessive effort is needed to maintain balance, the lower extremities will tend to adduct and the hips will internally rotate. When combined with hip flexion, the child is at risk for hip subluxation and dislocation.

Canes are typically not indicated as assistive devices for the child with CP. When balance reactions are adequate for safe ambulation without a walker, the child will typically choose to shift weight with the trunk and upper extremities, keeping the upper extremities free for functional use. When the child has adequate balance reactions for safe ambulation most of the time, but inconsistently loses his balance (e.g., when on rough terrain), a cane may be useful. It may also be indicated for hemiplegic children who have functional use of one upper extrem-

ity and impaired or slow balance reactions through the trunk.

INFANT WALKERS. There is great controversy over the use of infant walkers for any infant owing to the accidents associated with their use. The Canadian Medical Association has requested that their government ban the sale of walkers. They believe that their use is too risky, recognizing that 2 of 5 children (30% to 45%) who use walkers have mishaps ranging from finger entrapment to falls down stairs.[72] Kauffman and Ridenour have shown that use of a walker enables an infant to commit substantial mechanical errors, yet succeed in bipedal locomotion.[73] Some physicians believe that walkers adversely affect muscle development, cognitive development, and coordination, which can lead to a delay in walking alone, along with other developmental problems.[74]

Infant walkers should not be used for infants with CP. Despite the fact that manufacturers are altering walkers, making them adjustable in height, and providing a more supportive seat, walkers still promote abnormal movement patterns. Walking on the toes is common for any infant while in a walker, but a child with CP is more likely to have lower extremity extension with ankle plantar-flexion. This pattern typically includes arching of the back and adduction of the scapulae with humeral extension for counterbalance. Propulsion in the walker is achieved by pushing with the feet when the body is supported by the tray or sides of the walker.[75] The infant has not acquired the motor control and balance necessary for walking and has not mastered any skill that is transferable to independent ambulation. The infant with CP may actually be reinforcing abnormal patterns of movement, which can cause further developmental delays or even lead to deformity, such as hip subluxation.

Equipment for Mobility

Infants and children have a strong desire to move through the environment. This movement allows the child to explore the surroundings, to retrieve a toy lost during play, and to interact with others for comfort and play. The child with CP may lack a means of independent mobility, may have poor endurance in whatever means of mobility may exist, or may exert such effort as to produce an increase in tone that may limit other body functions, such as upper extremity function or vocalization. Adaptive equipment, either manual or electric, may expand the world of the child with CP and may foster independence not only in mobility, but also in other areas of function. Mobility, which offers a level of control over oneself and the environment, will improve the child's self-image and lead to other positive behavioral changes. Of course, this mobility also affords the opportunity for the child with CP to get into the same kinds of trouble and predicaments encountered by his or her peers with normal motor ability. Wheelchairs, tricycles, and scooters of different types can provide mobility, and their use should be considered early in the habilitative effort.

Lower Extremity Orthoses

The decision to use an orthosis and the choice of orthosis should be based on the physical therapist's assessment of ROM, foot alignment, voluntary control of movement in the lower extremity, and functional level of the child. Because the foot is intended to provide both stability and mobility, the effects of an orthosis on these two functions must be considered.

If the ankle and foot cannot be brought into a neutral position with the knee in extension in a non–weight-bearing position, an orthosis is contraindicated. The result of wearing an orthosis with a contracture at the ankle or foot will be that the child needs to compensate in another area of the foot to attain the range of motion needed for standing and ambulating. This compensation will cause hypermobility in the joints that are compensating, and will encourage continued hypomobility in the area of contracture and limitation.

A trial of serial casting may be used in an effort to reduce Achilles tendon contracture. Care must be exercised to lock the subtalar joint while applying the cast to gain dorsiflexion of the ankle, to ensure stretching of the gastrocnemius or soleus group, and to prevent hypermobility of the subtalar joint. Surgery is most likely needed if proper serial casting is unsuccessful after 2 to 3 weeks. Some of the orthoses commonly used for children with CP and their specific benefits are described.

Bivalved Short-Leg Cast (Inhibitive Cast)[76]

The primary goal of inhibitive casts and orthoses is to reduce the influence of abnormal tonic reflexes on the foot, ankle, and leg.[77] Short-leg casts can be made from fiberglass, plaster, or a combination of the two materials. The cast is bivalved so that it has an anterior and a posterior shell which are secured by webbed straps using Velcro or buckles. Tone-inhibiting casts should provide for hyperextension of the toes, pressure under the metatarsal heads, a stable ankle position, and deep tendon pressure along the calcaneal tendon.[77] The bottom of the cast is flat to facilitate standing, and it can be elevated at the toes distal to the metatarsal heads to provide for "roll-over" during ambulation. This cast may benefit the child who has strong plantar-flexion hypertonus and who also shows flexion of the knee during stance once the excessive tone is reduced. An example of an inhibitive cast is shown in Figure 4-23.

Knee-Ankle-Foot Orthosis

A knee-ankle-foot orthosis (KAFO) is rarely indicated for a child with CP.[78] It is too heavy and cumbersome for the child to use for ambulation without excessive effort and energy (Fig. 4-24). The child will typically demonstrate abnormal motor patterns and associated reactions with the increased effort required for ambulation. Well-fitting, molded ankle-foot orthoses will generally control the hips as well as the knees and feet, and should be considered before a KAFO is ordered.

Molded Ankle-Foot Orthosis

A molded ankle-foot-orthosis (MAFO) is indicated for control of the following:

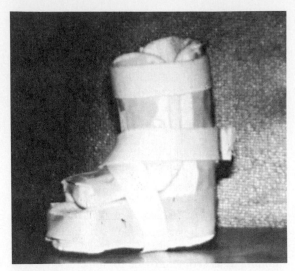

Figure 4-23. *An example of an inhibitive cast.*

1. A functional equinus position caused by gastrocnemius-soleus hypertonus that can be corrected with treatment
2. Genu recurvatum during stance phase that results from a functional, not structural, equinus position
3. Pes valgus associated with hypertonus in the gastrocnemius-soleus group.[79]

It may also be indicated to improve gait efficiency, as the application of the ankle-foot orthosis can decrease the energy demands of gait in children with spastic diplegic CP.[57]

Orthoses can be made by professional orthotists using high-temperature plastics molded over a plaster mold of the child's calf, ankle, and foot. Alternatively, they may be made by a therapist using low-temperature plastics molded over the child's lower leg and foot with the appropriate padding. Low-temperature plastics, such as Aquaplast, are indicated when the exact orthosis needed is not yet known, when the child is still small, when the child is just beginning weight-bearing activities and early ambulation, or when the feet are likely to grow rather quickly. These orthoses are easily modified to the child's needs. Trim lines are typically placed slightly anterior to the malleoli, particularly when hypertonus of the gastrocnemius-soleus group is

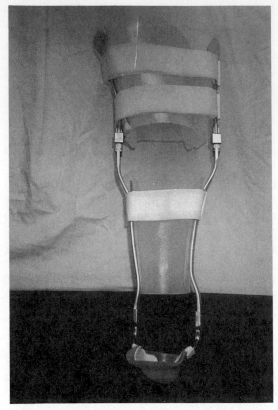

Figure 4-24. *A knee-ankle-foot orthosis. (Courtesy of Carlo Cocco, Cocco Brothers, Inc., Philadelphia, PA)*

present. The foot plate can end behind the metatarsal heads to allow roll-over during gait, or it can be extended to the end of the toes for increased support and inhibition of flexion and clawing of the toes, or it can be lifted slightly to decrease hypertonus (Fig. 4-25). When professional orthoses are made, a growth bar can be added initially for increased lower leg length with growth (Figs. 4-26 and 4-27).

Articulating Ankle-Foot Orthosis

A hinged ankle-foot orthosis (AFO), one with an ankle articulation, is indicated when free dorsiflexion is desired but the child continues to need a plantar-flexion stop. Middleton et al. found that the hinged AFO provides more natural ankle motion during stance phase, and greater symmetry of seg-

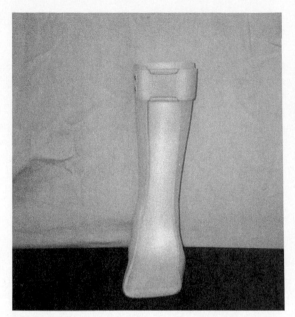

Figure 4-25. *A foot plate which is lifted slightly to decrease hypertonus. (Courtesy of Carlo Cocco, Cocco Brothers, Inc., Philadelphia, PA)*

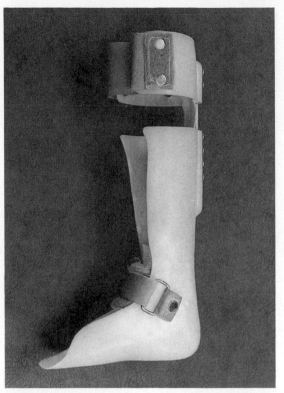

Figure 4-26. *Molded ankle-foot orthosis with growth bar. (Courtesy of Carlo Cocco, Cocco Brothers, Inc., Philadelphia, PA)*

mental lower extremity motion, than the rigid AFO's.[80] Such orthoses will inhibit plantar-flexion hypertonus while permitting free dorsiflexion, thus allowing the child increased ease in rising to stand and ambulating. They may also help to strengthen the muscles crossing the ankle, as unlike in the AFO, they are not held immobile (Fig. 4-28).

Anterior Shell Ankle-Foot Orthosis

An anterior shell AFO is indicated when knee extension cannot be maintained in stance during ambulation and excessive flexion of the ankle and knee is noted when the heel is in contact with the floor. Such orthoses are contraindicated when full knee extension cannot be achieved passively with the child in stance and the ankle and foot in neutral alignment.[76] The anterior shell can be molded over the trim lines of the MAFO so that there are two pieces to the orthotic, similar to the inhibitive casts. This arrangement assists in keeping the ankle in the orthosis in a child with excessive plantar-flexion

hypertonus as well. A floor-reaction brace is similar, as it has anterior support to prevent excessive ankle and knee flexion but is typically made in one piece. With a more flexible plastic, the orthosis can be molded in a single unit with a front opening for donning and doffing (Fig. 4-29.)

Supramalleolar Molded Orthosis

The supramalleolar molded orthosis (SMO) is indicated when ankle stability is critically important but limited tibial motion is desired. This orthosis provides less support than the MAFO and allows some tibia-over-foot motion during ambulation, but provides malleolar support by having the trimlines anterior and superior to the malleoli (Fig. 4-30).

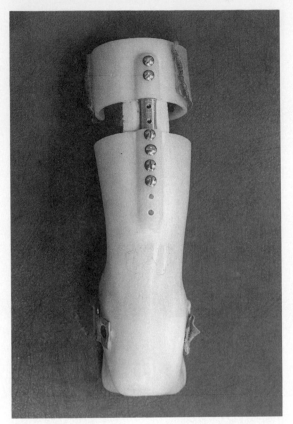

Figure 4-27. *Growth bar shown on orthosis. (Courtesy of Carlo Cocco, Cocco Brothers, Inc., Philadelphia, PA)*

Shoe Inserts

A variety of shoe inserts are available and they may be used for a number of reasons. They are indicated when there is dynamic control of the knee and ankle during gait, but assistance is required to maintain the calcaneous, subtalar, and midtarsal joints in neutral alignment. They are not helpful when the heel is held off the floor owing to hypertonus of the gastrocnemius-soleus group. The child's foot alignment, both in weight-bearing and non–weight-bearing positions, must be evaluated, as the heel cup can be designed for a specific problem. Trimlines can be anterior or inferior to either the medial or lateral malleoli, and the foot plate can be proximal or distal to the metatarsal heads (Fig. 4-31). Shoe inserts are made commercially, and they can also be made of low-temperature plastic in the clinic. They are sold under various names and are particularly popular with athletes. Some shoe companies make multiple, interchangeable inserts for their shoes, depending on the child's needs. Remember that the hindfoot must be well-aligned before the forefoot can be addressed with any orthotic.

High-Top Orthopedic Shoe/Phelps Short-Leg Brace

Phelps short-leg braces with high-top shoes have limited use in the management of ankle and foot problems in children with CP. The high-top shoe, even with a stiff heel counter, does not support or maintain the calcaneous in a neutral position. The child actually reshapes the shoe so that the foot is maintained in calcaneal eversion with subtalar and midtarsal joint malalignment. Adding a medial T-strap, secured around a Phelps short-leg brace, provides pressure against the medial aspect of the foot, but does not cause the changes in alignment needed in the rear part of the foot to move the subtalar joint out of pronation.

Neurosurgical Intervention for Children with Cerebral Palsy

Neurosurgical intervention, particularly selective dorsal rhizotomy, is not a new surgical approach to the treatment of children with CP. It is, however, a poorly understood procedure aimed at reducing the spasticity of children with CP.[81-84] Simply removing the spasticity does not, however, produce improved motor control. Patient selection is of the utmost importance, as only two groups of patients are appropriate candidates for selective dorsal rhizotomy. The first group includes patients who are functionally limited by spasticity but who have sufficient underlying voluntary power to maintain and eventually improve their functional abilities. Keen intelligence and motivation are also helpful characteristics. The second group includes nonambulatory

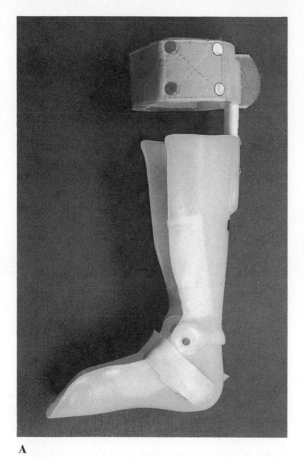 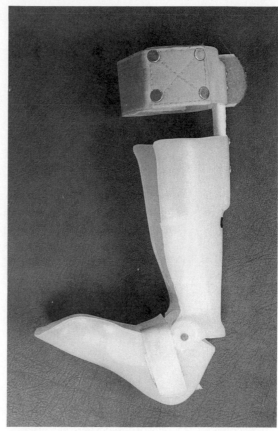

A   B

Figure 4-28. *A. An articulating molded ankle foot orthosis. B. An articulating molded ankle-foot ortho-sis in a position of dorsiflexion. (Courtesy of Carlo Cocco, Cocco Brothers, Inc., Philadelphia, PA)*

patients whose spasticity interferes with sitting, bathing, positioning, perineal care, classroom activities, and so on.[83,84]

The surgery is typically completed across segments L2-S2[81,83] or L2-S1,[84] and only a selected number of dorsal rootlets are sacrificed; those that appear to have the greatest influence on the spasticity and produce abnormal movement patterns. Intensive physical therapy is necessary after the surgery to address the weakness that underlies the spasticity.[81-84] The importance of strengthening and achieving improved motor control becomes apparent after the surgery.[82] There are varying approaches to physical therapy treatment after surgery. Abbott et al. advocate limiting the patient's active movements after surgery, outside of therapy, to avoid a return to the child's old patterns of limb use.[83] These researchers suggest that three components be included in the physical therapy program: (1) muscle stretching to gain joint mobility and range, (2) muscle strengthening to increase endurance, and (3) muscle reeducation to impart a better pattern of muscle use.[83] Giuliani advocates treatment aimed at strengthening the muscles and improving motor control because "treatment aimed at reducing tone and spasticity will not necessarily improve movement coordination."[82] Most recommend that therapy be continued for at least 6 to 12 months following surgery to allow optimal functional improvement.[81,83,84] Any necessary orthope-

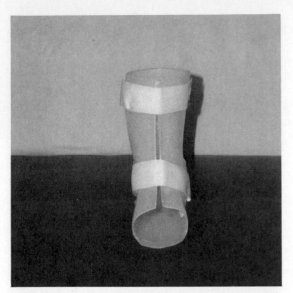

Figure 4-29. *Anterior shell ankle-foot orthosis, molded in a single unit with a front opening for donning and doffing. (Courtesy of Carlo Cocco, Cocco Brothers, Inc., Philadelphia, PA)*

dic procedures should be delayed until 6 to 12 months after surgery. There should be close cooperation between the neurosurgeon and the orthopedist.[84]

Another neurosurgical approach to the child with CP is to implant a spinal cord stimulator. This approach is also controversial, and can produce drastically different results in different children. A variety of electrodes are used. Waltz and co-workers, for instance, prefer four electrodes over two electrodes when working with the child with athetosis.[85] Optimal frequencies vary between less than 500 Hz[85] and 500 to 1450 Hz.[86] Placement of the electrodes is typically between C2 and C4, with the pattern and the polarity of the applied field being critical to achieving a satisfactory therapeutic result.[85] In the author's experience, once optimal settings have been achieved for the greatest reduction in spasticity and abnormal movement patterns, therapy is essential to address muscle strengthening, re-education, and acquisition of functional skills.

Orthopedic Surgery for Children with Cerebral Palsy

Limited function secondary to muscle contracture and bony deformity is a typical problem for children with a high degree of involvement with CP and for older children who have had limited previous therapeutic intervention. It is essential that any contemplated orthopedic surgery be discussed with and considered by the entire team working with the child, including the therapist and family. An understanding of abnormal development and movement compensations is critical for determining how surgery will likely impact the child's future function. As Green says, ". . . treating one problem without consideration of the others will result in unnecessary additional hospitalizations for subsequent operations. In addition, since each joint is intimately linked to another, surgical treatment of one joint problem may lead to worsening of an adjacent joint deformity unless it too is addressed. Thus, the surgical care of the lower extremities in spastic cerebral palsy requires that the entire patient be evaluated and all necessary surgical procedures be coordinated."[87] It is important that any neurosurgical intervention being considered be completed 6 to 12 months prior to orthopedic surgical intervention.[84] A reevaluation of the child's status will be necessary.

The common orthopedic problems that involve the lower extremities of children with CP are addressed in the following sections. General physical therapy interventions are also discussed. However, many surgeons have established their own postsurgical protocols, including the prescribed period of immobilization. Therefore, the information presented here should be used only as a guideline in planning and implementing a therapeutic program.

The Hip

Subluxation/Dislocation

Hips begin to migrate laterally, or to sublux, as a result of muscular imbalance. When left untreated, the hip may continue the migration until it is dislo-

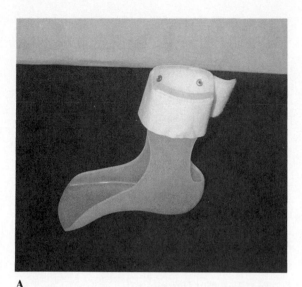

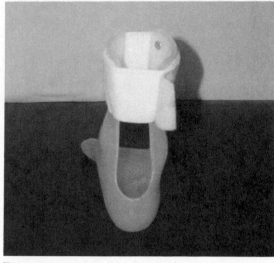

A   B

Figure 4-30. *A supramalleolar molded orthosis. A. Side view. B. Rear view. (Courtesy of Carlo Cocco, Cocco Brothers, Inc., Philadelphia, PA)*

cated. Gamble and co-workers maintain that this process occurs over a 6-year period and that there is a strong correlation between the stability of the hip and the ambulatory status of the patient.[88] Other causes of hip dislocation include persistent fetal femoral geometry, acetabular dysplasia, and flexion-adduction contractures.[88]

Conservative treatment options for the subluxated hip include passive muscle stretching of the

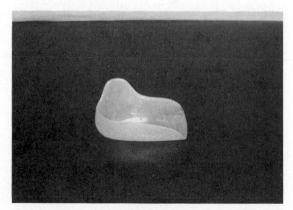

Figure 4-31. *An example of a shoe insert. (Courtesy of Carlo Cocco, Cocco Brothers, Inc., Philadelphia, PA)*

adductors and hip flexors and splinting of the hips in abduction (generally done at night while the child sleeps). With progression of the subluxation, surgery may become necessary, in which case tenotomies or myotomies are the treatments of choice. The effectiveness of muscle transfer is controversial.[88] Dislocated hips are a more serious problem for the child, as the hip may become painful, sitting may become more difficult, decubitus ulcers may be caused by asymmetrical weight bearing, nursing care may be made more difficult, and fractures are possible.[89,90] Various surgical interventions may be appropriate, including the following (listed in order of increasing complexity):

1. Soft tissue transfer and/or releases involving the adductors, iliopsoas muscle, or proximal hamstring[88,90–93]
2. Femoral osteotomy[88,90–92]
3. Pelvic osteotomies (iliac or Chiari)[88,90–92]
4. Resection of the femoral head and neck[88,92]
5. Arthrodesis and arthroplasty[88,91]

Treatment of each child must be individualized, and every surgeon has individual surgical preferences. The decision as to whether to operate at all in the child with severe involvement,[89] or whether to perform unilateral versus bilateral surgery,[95] is the surgeon's decision, ideally made after receiving input from the team members.

Postoperative management should include ROM exercise of the hips to maintain or increase the range, strengthening of muscles in an effort to achieve muscle balance around the hips, and proper positioning to prevent recurrence of the dislocation. The severity of the CP and the functional abilities of the child will dictate the treatment approach.

Adduction Deformity

Conservative management of the short adductors involves passive stretching and night-time bracing with the hips in as much abduction as possible. Proper positioning in a wheelchair is essential for maintaining the integrity of the hip joints. One indication for a more aggressive approach is when the ambulatory child has severe hypertonus of the adductors, which causes scissoring of the legs during ambulation. Scissoring of the lower extremities in the severely involved child will make sitting and perineal care difficult. Three typical surgical procedures are currently performed in such cases:

1. Adductor tenotomy[91,92]
2. Obturator neurectomy[90,91]
3. Posterior transfer of the adductors (with or without iliopsoas tenotomy)[91,92,96]

Postoperative treatment of the child includes continued stretching, strengthening of the muscles around the hips in order to achieve muscular balance, and functional training. Grogan et al. have developed a removable abductor bar so that therapy, including ambulation, can commence with long-leg casts on the child, and abduction can be maintained whenever the child is not in therapy.[97]

Flexion Deformity

Hip flexion contractures interfere with function in any upright position because full hip extension becomes impossible. Compensation occurs typically in the lumbar spine (increased lordosis) and the knees (increased flexion) so that body orientation in space can remain vertical. It is difficult to stretch the hip flexors because the pelvis tends to rock forward into anterior tilt while the lumbar spine hyperextends. For passive stretching to be effective, the pelvis must be stabilized in either a supine or prone position.

Surgical intervention usually includes soft tissue releases and can involve the iliopsoas muscle[90] or transection of the tensor fasciae latae muscle and aponeurosis and detachment of the heads of the rectus femoris.[91]

Physical therapy after surgery should include stretching into hip extension and strengthening of the hip extensors and abductors. Facilitation of functional skills should continue, with care taken to prevent a return to the child's previous compensatory patterns of movement.

Internal Rotation Deformity

Femoral anteversion, rather than muscular action, is a consistent deformity associated with exaggerated internal rotation during gait, as previously noted. Anteversion interferes with functional ambulation by tripping the child when the toe of one shoe gets caught behind the heel of the opposite shoe. A femoral derotation osteotomy, which may include medial hamstring release, is the standard surgery performed for this deformity.[87,90,91]

A longer period of immobilization is necessary for bony surgery than for soft tissue releases, and the child is likely to be unable to bear weight until the casts are removed. Rehabilitation is directed toward increasing ROM and strengthening the muscles around the hips. Unilateral hip surgery may result in leg length discrepancy, which must be considered during treatment and in consultation with the surgeon. Facilitation of functional skills is critically important to help the child learn new movement patterns and strengthen weakened muscles.

The Knee

Knee Flexion Deformity

Knee flexion deformity is often related to spastic, shortened hamstrings and can be secondary to a hip flexion deformity. Persistent flexion of the knee can lead to a contracture of the knee joint capsule and shortening of the sciatic nerve. Serial casting of the knees is a conservative approach to the deformity, that has been successful in some patients.[98] Soft splints applied at night for severe knee flexion deformities have proven to be both effective and inexpensive.[99] Hamstring lengthening is the most common surgical approach to knee flexion deformities.[87,90] Gage advocates lengthening the hamstrings and transferring the distal rectus femoris tendon to either the iliotibial band or the distal tendon of the semitendinosus.[100]

Postoperative management should include passive and active exercise into knee extension and strengthening of both knee extensors and flexors. Because the hamstrings cross the knee and hip joints, the therapist must also emphasize ROM and strengthening exercises for the hip musculature. Nightly use of knee extension splints should be considered to help maintain muscle length, especially in children who have difficulty learning new patterns of movement.

The Ankle and Foot

Equinus Deformity

Equinus, a very common foot deformity in children with CP, results from a muscular imbalance between the plantar flexors and dorsiflexors. It is manifested as toe-walking in the ambulatory child. Children with more severe involvement may have difficulty with foot placement on the pedals of the wheelchair, assisted stand-pivot transfers, and donning of shoes. Conservative management includes passive stretching, with care taken to "lock" the subtalar joint before stretching toward dorsiflexion. MAFOs can help maintain a neutral position at the ankle, but will not stretch the muscle group.

Achilles tendon lengthening is the most frequent surgical intervention for equinus deformity.[87,90,101] Strecker et al. have reported good results with a technique called heel cord advancement.[102] Overlengthening is the most common complication of surgery, and it results in a calcaneal gait or an increase in dorsiflexion during stance.[103] This gait is crouched in nature, with increased energy demands

and subsequent shortening of the muscles in the hips and knees.

Postoperative care typically involves an orthotic to maintain the surgically achieved range and to provide distal stability, thereby facilitating development of proximal strength and motor control. ROM through the ankle joint and strengthening for those with some voluntary control must always be emphasized.

Pes Valgus

Pes valgus is a deformity that includes eversion, plantar-flexion, and inclination of the calcaneous with abduction of the forefoot. These positions cause a medial prominence of the talus, which is commonly accompanied by callous formation on the skin. This deformity is usually flexible and can be corrected by reducing the subtalar joint and forefoot to a neutral position with the ankle plantar flexed. Three situations contribute to the deformity: (1) spastic peroneal muscles that change the axis of rotation of the subtalar joint to a more horizontal alignment and abduct the midfoot and forefoot; (2) gastrocnemius-soleus contracture causing plantar flexion of the calcaneous; and (3) persistent fetal medial deviation of the neck of the talus.[45]

Crawford and associates developed a procedure called staple arthroeriesis, which involves operative limitation of joint motion. It is used in children younger than 6 years of age to correct a pes valgus deformity until they are old enough to undergo arthrodesis. The authors have reported that the procedure, which involves driving a staple into the talus and calcaneous across the subtalar joint, works so well that, in many cases, additional surgery is not needed.[104] The most common of the later procedures that are performed include (1) the Grice extra-articular subtalar arthrodesis,[87,90,101,105,106] (2) peroneus brevis lengthening for less severe valgus,[101] and (3) triple arthrodesis for rigid deformities.[87]

The period of postsurgical immobilization varies greatly, depending upon the specific procedure and the surgeon's preference. An orthotic will almost always be used, and motion will either be significantly limited or eliminated. Long after surgery, the therapist may note joint hypermobility at sites proximal and distal to the arthrodesis, in which case special orthotics may be required.

Varus Deformity

Varus deformity is uncommon in children with CP. It results from imbalance between weak peroneal muscles and spastic posterior or anterior tibialis muscles.[87]

A variety of surgical procedures are performed for this deformity, including lengthening or splitting and transferring of either the posterior or anterior tibialis muscle.[87,90,107–109]

Therapeutic intervention should emphasize muscle reeducation, particularly when a muscle has been transferred; ROM exercise; strengthening; and facilitation of functional activities for which foot alignment is important (e.g., standing and gait). Each child should be evaluated for an orthotic with the recommendation discussed with the surgeon.

Home Management

A home management program is an essential part of the treatment plan for the child with CP. The home program should be designed to reinforce positions and movements that have been practiced in the physical therapy sessions, and it should be updated frequently. The therapist must consider the daily routine of the child and family when planning a home program. Exercise that is incorporated into the activities of daily living (ADLs) and play is more likely to be carried out than a separate, formal exercise regimen lasting 30 minutes. The therapist must also consider realistically the other non–child-related demands placed on the parents. Siblings, too, can be very valuable in assisting with the child's program and incorporating activities and exercise into an established routine. "The unique, spontaneous and competitive interaction of siblings offers increased incentives for functional independence."[110]

Therapeutic exercise for the baby is easily incorporated into daily care activities. Therapeutic handling aimed at normalizing tone and increasing movement can be done during routine activities, such as diapering, dressing, feeding, bathing, carrying, and lifting the baby from a supported position.

For the child who has an interest in other activities, a therapist might recommend taking up a musical instrument, therapeutic horseback riding, therapeutic aquatics, or any other activity that coincides with and reinforces the therapeutic goals of the child.

Consultation with the School

Communication between the therapist and the child's teacher is essential for appropriate and effective management and education of the child in the classroom. The therapist should obtain information from the teacher regarding the child's daily routine at school. With that information, joint planning for the child can result in an effective and efficient educational program.

The therapist must emphasize correct alignment while the child is sitting. Optimal height of a desk may contribute to postural control and, thus, to a greater degree of success with desktop activities. A learning position should be used, if possible, which stresses greater extension of the hip and knee. The result of keeping the child in a constantly flexed sitting position too long will likely be flexion contractures at the hip and knee. Periodic opportunity for movement, whether in physical education class or at the child's own negotiation, may also provide relief from the sitting position. There should be a sharing of the assistance and supervision required for quality of movement and safety. The physical education teacher should be informed of joint movement goals and specific types or patterns of movement that may either be deleterious or beneficial for the child. There should also be a review conducted with teachers for the purpose of and proper use of splints, braces, and other assistive or adaptive devices.

The occupational therapist and the speech-language pathologist will share information about the child's attention span, perceptual and cognitive deficits, and speech and language capabilities. This information, along with specific suggestions, should facilitate learning for the child.

Therapists should not expect teachers to handle children therapeutically for the purpose of obtaining postural control and automatic reactions. A more realistic expectation would be maintenance of correct alignment, relief from sitting, use of adaptive or assistive devices, and attention to issues regarding safety. The therapist must recognize the teacher as an important ally in the therapeutic arena. An extensive discussion of the role of the physical therapist in the schools can be found in Chapter 14.

Other Disciplines Involved in the Care of Children with Cerebral Palsy

Because CP is a developmental disability, it affects not only the child's posture, movement, and acquisition of motor skills, but also the development of perceptual skills, language, and cognition, as well as social-emotional growth. The child with CP must have a treatment program that considers the child as a "whole" person, not merely a combination of systems.

In addition to the child's individual needs, which may be great, the child must be seen as a member of a family unit. The impact of a disabled child on parents, siblings, and the extended family must be considered in treatment planning. Although families are often expected to carry out many of the treatment tasks at home, professionals must recognize that family members may need periodic relief or respite from the burden of care.

There must be a coordinated effort among the many disciplines involved in treating the child with CP. Medical care may include the services of a general pediatrician, neurologist, orthopedic surgeon, podiatrist, ophthalmologist, and physiatrist. Habilitation personnel may include the physical therapist,

occupational therapist, and speech and language pathologist. Promotion of cognitive and social-emotional growth may require the services of teachers and psychologists. Communication among these professionals is essential for coordinated management of care.

The occupational therapist works with postural control and movement primarily as a prerequisite for fine motor skills as they relate to self-help activities—feeding, dressing, bathing, play, and the development of perceptual skills. During the child's adolescent years, the occupational therapist becomes more involved with prevocational testing and training.

The speech and language pathologist is also involved with the acquisition of postural control and movement against gravity. Specific attention is paid to alignment of the head and trunk in order to promote optimal respiration in support of speech. The coordination of breathing with oral motor skills is necessary for feeding and, on a more differentiated level, for speech. A manual or electronic communication board may be indicated if oral speech is not a possibility. Manual sign language is rarely appropriate for children with CP, who often lack the fine finger control to sign successfully. In addition to the motor deficits, the child's acquisition of language concepts may be delayed.

The psychologist may be involved in formal psychological testing of the child with CP to identify cognitive strengths and deficits. The psychologist will then make recommendations for appropriate educational placement to best meet the child's needs. Psychological therapy may be indicated if behavioral or emotional problems interfere with the social and emotional growth of the child and the family.

The recreational therapist may be involved in identifying leisure interests, and may work with the child and family in the selection and pursuit of leisure activities. Identification of toys appropriate for the child's developmental level and movement capabilities may allow independent play for the child, and is among the responsibilities of the recreational therapist. Some commonly used toys may be converted so that they can be electrically operated by battery and remote control. A joystick or press plate control may be used depending on the child's level of fine motor skill.

Community recreation centers and schools often sponsor swimming, gymnastics, horseback riding, and dance programs in which children with disabilities may participate with their able-bodied peers. An important goal for recreational programs is to develop a positive self-image and high self-esteem by emphasizing activities in which a child *can* participate successfully.

A social worker may assist the family in locating services for the disabled child. The social worker can also play an important role in guiding and teaching family members to be advocates for the disabled family member. The disabled child, as a member of a larger family unit, will have a significant impact on that unit. The social worker can provide counseling and support for the family to help resolve issues of concern.

References

1. Nelson K. What proportion of cerebral palsy is related to birth asphyxia? *J Pediatr.* 1988;113:572–574.
2. Nelson K. Relationship of intrapartum and delivery room events to long-term neurologic outcome. *Clin Perinatol.* 1989;16:995–1007.
3. Niswander KR, Gordon M. The Collaborative Perinatal Project. In: *The Women and Their Pregnancies.* DHEW Publication no. 73–379, 1972.
4. Ellenberg JH, Nelson KB. Cluster of perinatal events identifying infants at high risk for death or disability. *J Pediatr.* 1988;113:546–552.
5. Melone PJ, Ernest JM, O'Shea MD, Klinipeter KL. Appropriateness of intrapartum fetal heart rate management and risk of cerebral palsy. *Am J Obstet Gynecol.* 1991;165:272–276.
6. Torfs CP, van den Berg B. Oechsli FW, Cummins S. Prenatal and perinatal factors in the etiology of cerebral palsy. *J Pediatr.* 1990;116:615–619.
7. Nelson KB, Ellenberg JH. The asymptomatic newborn and risk of cerebral palsy. *Am J Dis Child.* 1987;141:1333–1335.
8. Freeman JM, Nelson KB. Intrapartum asphyxia and cerebral palsy. *Pediatrics.* 1988; 82:240–249.
9. Naeye RL, Peter EC, Bartholemew M, Landis JR. Origins of cerebral palsy. *Am J Dis Child.* 1989;143: 1154–1161.
10. Skidmore MD, Rivers A, Hack M. Increased risk of cerebral palsy among very low birthweight infants with chronic lung disease. *Dev Med Child Neurol.* 1990;32:325–332.
11. Luthy DA, Shy KK, Strickland D, et al. Status of infants at birth and risk for adverse neonatal events and long-term sequelae. *Am J Obstet Gynecol.* 1987;157:676–679.
12. Graziani L, Stanley C. Intracranial hemorrhage and the preterm infant. *Intens Caring Unlim.* 1987;5: 6–7.
13. Graziani L, et al. Mechanical ventilation in preterm infants: Neurosonographic and developmental studies. In press.
14. Graziani L, Mitchell DG, Kornhauser M, et al. Neurodevelopment of preterm infants. Neonatal neurosonographic and serum bilirubin studies. *Pediatrics.* 1992;89:229–234.
15. Scherzer AL, Tscharnuter I. *Early Diagnosis and Therapy in Cerebral Palsy: A Primer on Infant Developmental Problems.* New York: Marcel Dekker; 1982.
16. Bobath B, Bobath K. *Motor Development in the Different Types of Cerebral Palsy.* London: William Heineman Medical Books; 1982.
17. Molnar GE, ed: *Pediatric Rehabilitation.* Baltimore: Williams and Wilkins; 1985.
18. Brett EM, ed: *Pediatric Neurology.* New York: Churchill and Livingstone; 1983.
19. Stanley FS, English DR. Prevalence and risk factors for cerebral palsy in a total population cohort of low

birthweight (<2000 grams) infants. *Dev Med Child Neurol.* 1986;28:559–568.

20. Staheli LT, Duncan WR, Schaefer E. Growth alterations in the hemiplegic child. *Clin Orthop.* 1968; 60:205–212.

21. Holt KS. *Growth Disturbances: Hemiplegic Cerebral Palsy in Children and Adults.* London: William Heinemann Medical Books; 1961. Clinics in Developmental Medicine, No 4.

22. Kitchen WH, Doyle LW, Ford GW, Richards AL, Lissenden JV, Boyle LW. Cerebral palsy in very low birthweight infants surviving to 2 years with modern perinatal intensive care. *Am J Perinatol.* 1987;4:29–35.

23. Pidcock FS, Graziani LJ, Stanley C, Mitchell DG, Merton D. Neurosonographic features of periventricular echodensities associated with cerebral palsy in preterm infants. *J Pediatr.* 1990;116:417–422.

24. Kilbride HW, Daily DK, Matriu I, Hubbard AM. Neurodevelopmental follow-up of infants with birthweight less than 801 grams with intracranial hemorrhage. *J Perinatol.* 1980;9:376–381.

25. Graham M, Livens MI, Trouna JQ, Rutter N. Prediction of cerebral palsy in very low birthweight infants: Prospective ultrasound study. Lancet. 1987; 2:593–506.

26. Tudehope DI, Masel J, Mohay H, et al. Neonatal cranial ultrasonography as predictor of 2 year outcome of very low birthweight infants. *Austral Pediatr J.* 1989;25: 66–71.

27. Allen MC, Capute AJ. Neonatal neurodevelopmental examination as a predictor of neuromotor outcome in premature infants. *Pediatrics.* 1989;83: 498–506.

28. Burns YR, O'Callaghan M, Tudehope DI. Early identification of cerebral palsy in high risk infants. *Austral Pediatr J.* 1989;25:215–219.

29. Harris SR. Early neuromotor predictors of cerebral palsy in low birthweight infants. *Dev Med Child Neurol.* 1987;29:508–519.

30. Harris SR. Movement analysis—An aid to diagnosis of cerebral palsy. *Phys Ther.* 1991;71:215–221.

31. Nelson KB, Ellenberg JH. Children who "outgrew" cerebral palsy. *Pediatrics.* 1982;69:529–535.

32. Bly L. Abnormal motor development. In: Slaton DS, ed: Proceedings of a conference on Development of Movement Infancy offered by the Division

of Physical Therapy, University North Carolina at Chapel Hill; May 18–22, 1980.

33. Bobath B. *Abnormal Postural Reflex Activity Caused by Brain Lesions.* 2nd ed. London: William Heinemann Medical Books; 1972.

34. Bobath B. The very early treatment of cerebral palsy. *Dev Med Child Neurol.* 1967;9:373–390.

35. Bobath K. *A Neurophysiological Basis for the Treatment of Cerebral Palsy.* Philadelphia: JB Lippincott; 1980.

36. Bobath B, Bobath K. An analysis of the development of standing and walking patterns in patients with cerebral palsy. *Physiotherapy.* 1962;48:3–12.

37. Cochrane CD. Joint mobilization principles: Considerations for use in the child with central nervous system dysfunction. *Phys Ther.* 1987;67:1105–1109.

38. Fiorentino MR. *Normal and Abnormal Development—The Influence of Primitive Reflexes on Motor Development.* Springfield, IL: Charles C Thomas; 1980.

39. Illingworth RS. *The Development of the Infant and Young Child.* 8th ed. New York: Churchill and Livingstone; 1983.

40. Levitt S. *Treatment of Cerebral Palsy and Motor Delay.* 2nd ed. Oxford, England: Blackwell Scientific Publishers, 1982.

41. Magnus R. Some Results of Studies in the Physiology of Posture. Cameron Prize Lectures, University of Edinburgh; May 1926.

42. Weisz S. Studies in equilibrium reaction. *J Nerv Mental Dis.* 1938;88:150–162.

43. Bly L. The components of normal movement during the first year of life. In: Slaton DS, ed. Proceedings of a conference on Development of Movement in Infancy offered by the University of North Carolina at Chapel Hill, Division of Physical Therapy, May 18–20, 1980.

44. Polgar G, Promadhat V. *Pulmonary Function Testing in Children.* Philadelphia: WB Saunders; 1971.

45. Bleck EE. *Orthopedic Management of Cerebral Palsy.* Philadelphia: WB Saunders; 1979.

46. Shands AR, Steele MK. Torsion of the femur. *J Bone Joint Surg* 1958;40A:803–816.

47. Michele AA. *Iliopsoas.* Springfield, IL: Charles C Thomas; 1962.

48. Beals RK. Developmental changes in the femur and acetabulum in spastic paraplegia and diplegia. *Dev Med Child Neurol.* 1969;11:303–313.

49. Jordan P. Evaluation and Treatment of Foot Disor-

ders. Presentation at the Neurodevelopmental Treatment Association Regional Conference, New York; May, 1984.

50. Calliet R. *Foot and Ankle Pain.* Philadelphia: FA Davis, 1970.

51. Burnett CN, Johnson EQ. Development of gait in childhood. Parts 1 and 2. *Dev Med Child Neurol.* 1971;13:196–215.

51a. Sutherland D, Olshen R, Cooper L, Woo SL. The development of mature gait. *J Bone Joint Surg* 1980;62A:336–353.

52. Mylebust BM. A review of myotatic reflexes and the development of motor control and gait in infants and children: A special communication. *Phys Ther.* 1990;70:188–203.

53. Thelen E, Cooke DW. Relationship between newborn stepping and later walking: A new interpretation. *Dev Med Child Neurol.* 1987;29:380–393.

54. Saunders JB, Inman VT, Eberhart HD. The major determinants in normal and pathological gait. *J Bone Joint Surg.* 1953;35A:543–558.

55. Watt JM, Robertson CM, Grace MG. Early prognosis for ambulation of neonatal intensive care survivors with cerebral palsy. *Dev Med Child Neurol.* 1989;31:766–773.

56. Hicks R, Durinick N, Gage JR. Differentiation of idiopathic toe-walking and cerebral palsy. *J Pediatr Orthop.* 1988;8:160–163.

57. Mossberg KA, Linton KA, Fricke K. Ankle-foot orthoses: Effect on energy expenditure of gait in spastic diplegic children. *Arch Phys Med Rehab.* 1990; 71:490–494.

58. Schafer RC. Clinical Biomechanics: Musculoskeletal Actions and Reactions. Baltimore: Williams and Wilkins; 1983.

59. Bly L. Neurodevelopmental Treatment Baby Course. Newark, NJ; January, 1982.

60. Bobath B: Neurodevelopmental Treatment Approach to Cerebral Palsy. Course notes, pp 3–12; June–August, 1978.

61. Finnie NR. *Handling the Young Cerebral Palsied Child at Home.* 2nd ed. New York: Dalton Publications, 1975.

62. Molnar GE. Rehabilitation in cerebral palsy. *West J Med.* 1991;154:569–572.

63. Binder H, Eng GD. Rehabilitation management of children with spastic diplegic cerebral palsy. *Arch Phys Med Rehabil.* 1989;70:482–489.

64. Fetters L. Measurement and treatment in cerebral palsy: An argument for a new approach (Review). *Phys Ther.* 1991;71:244–247.

65. Kluzik J, Fetters L, Coryell J. Quantification of control: A preliminary study of effects of neurodevelopmental treatment on reaching in children with spastic cerebral palsy. *Phys Ther.* 1990;70:65–78.

66. Kamm K, Thelen E, Jensen J. A dynamical systems approach to motor development. *Phys Ther.* 1990; 70:763–775.

67. Bergen AF, Colangelo C. Positioning the Client with Central Nervous System Deficits: The Wheelchair and Other Adapted Equipment. 2nd ed. Valhalla, NY: Valhalla Rehabilitation Publishers; 1985.

68. Myhr U, von Wendt L. Improvement of functional sitting position for children with cerebral palsy. *Dev Med Child Neurol.* 1991;33:246–256.

69. Rose J, Gamble JG, Medeiras J, Burgos A, Haskell WL. Energy cost of walking in normal children and in those with cerebral palsy: Comparison of heart rate and oxygen uptake. *J Pediatr Orthop.* 1989;9: 276–279.

70. Logan L, Byers-Hinkley K, Ciccone CD. Anterior versus posterior walkers: A gait analysis study. *Dev Med Child Neurol.* 1990;32:1044–1048.

71. Levangie PK, Chimera M, Johnston M, Robinson F, Wobeskya L. The effects of posterior rolling walkers on gait characteristics of children with spastic cerebral palsy. *Phys Occup Ther Pediatr.* 1989; 9:1–17.

72. Canadian Medical Association. Editorial. *Can Med Assn J* 1987;136:57.

73. Kauffman IB, Ridenour M. Influence of an infant walker on onset and quality of walking pattern of locomotion: An electromyographic investigation. *Percept Mot Skills.* 1977;45:1323–1329.

74. *Mothering* 46, Winter 1988.

75. Pronsati M. Baby walkers—Considering full price of convenience. *Adv Phys Ther.* May 18, 1992:7.

76. Sussman MD, Cusick B. Preliminary report: The role of short-leg, tone reducing casts as an adjunct to physical therapy of patients with cerebral palsy. *Johns Hopkins Med J.* 1979;145:112–114.

77. Hanson CJ, Jones LJ. Gait abnormalities and inhibitive casts in cerebral palsy: Literature review. *J Am Podiatr Med Assoc.* 1989;79:53–59.

78. Jones ET, Knapp DR. Assessment and management of the lower extremity in cerebral palsy. *Orthop Clin North Am.* 1987;18:725–738.

79. Cusick B. Tone-Reducing Casts as an Adjunct to the Treatment of Cerebral Palsy. Lecture notes, Philadelphia; May 19, 1981.

80. Middleton EA, Hurley GR, McIlwain JS. The role of rigid and hinged polypropylene ankle-foot orthoses in the management of cerebral palsy: A case study. *Prosthet Orthot Int.* 1988;12:129–135.

81. Peacock WJ, Stoudt LA. Functional outcomes following selective posterior rhizotomy in children with cerebral palsy. *J Neurosurg.* 1991;74:380–385.

82. Guiliani CA. Dorsal rhizotomy for children with cerebral palsy: Support for concept of motor control. *Phys Ther.* 1991;71:248–259.

83. Abbott R, Forem SL, Johann M. Selective posterior rhizotomy for the treatment of spasticity: A review. *Child Nerv Syst.* 1989;5:337–346.

84. Oppenheim W. Selective posterior rhizotomy for spastic cerebral palsy. A review. *Clin Orthop Rel Res.* 1990;253:20–29.

85. Waltz JM, Andreesen WH, Hunt DP. Spinal cord stimulation and motor disorders. *Pace-Pac Clin Electrophys.* 1987;10:180–204.

86. Hugenholtz H, Humphreys P, McIntyre WM, Sparoff RA, Steel K. Cervical spinal cord stimulation for spasticity in cerebral palsy. *Neurosurgery.* 1988;22:707–714.

87. Green NE. The orthopedic management of the ankle, foot, and knee in patients with cerebral palsy. Neuromuscular disease and deformities. Instructional Course Lectures. 1987;36:253–256.

88. Gamble JG, Rinsky LA, Bleck EE. Established hip dislocations in children with cerebral palsy. *Clin Orthop Rel Res.* 1990;253:90–99.

89. Pritchett JW. Treated and untreated unstable hips in severe cerebral palsy. *Dev Med Child Neurol* 1990; 32:3–6.

90. Jones ET, Knapp DR. Assessment and management of the lower extremity in cerebral palsy. *Orthop Clin North Am.* 1987;18:725–728.

91. Root L. Treatment of hip problems in cerebral palsy. Neuromuscular diseases and deformities. Instructional Course Lectures. 1987;36:237–252.

92. Osterkamp J, Caillouette JT, Hoffer MM. Chiari osteotomy in cerebral palsy. *J Pediatr Orthop.* 1988; 8:274–277.

93. Smith JT, Stevens PM. Combined adductor transfer, iliopsoas release, and proximal hamstring release in cerebral palsy. *J Pediatr Orthoped.* 1989;9:1–5.

94. McHale KA, Bagg M, Nason SS. Treatment of the chronically dislocated hip in adolescents with cerebral palsy with femoral head resection and subtrochanteric valgus osteotomy. *J Pediatr Orthop.* 1990;10:504–509.

95. Carr C, Gage JR. The fate of the non-operated hip in cerebral palsy. *J Pediatr Orthop.* 1987;7:262–267.

96. Aronson DD, Zak PJ, Lee CL, Bollinger RO, Lamont RL. Posterior transfer of the adductors in children who have cerebral palsy. *J Bone Joint Surg.* 1991;73A:59–65.

97. Grogan DP, Lundy MS, Ogden JA. A method for early postoperative mobilization of the cerebral palsy patient using a removable abduction bar. *J Pediatr Orthop.* 1987;7:338–340.

98. Phillips WE, Audet M. Use of serial casting in the management of knee joint contractures in an adolescent with cerebral palsy. *Phys Ther.* 1990;70:521–523.

99. Anderson JP, Snow B, Dorey FJ, Kabo JM. Efficacy of soft splints in reducing severe knee flexion contractures. *Dev Med Child Neurol.* 1988;30:502–508.

100. Gage JR. Surgical treatment of knee dysfunctional in cerebral palsy. *Clin Orthop Rel Res.* 1990; 253:45–54.

101. Fulford GE. Surgical management of ankle and foot deformities in cerebral palsy. *Clin Orthop Rel Res.* 1990;253:55–61.

102. Strecker WB, Via MW, Oliver SK, Schoenecker PL. Heelcord advancement for treatment of equinus deformity in cerebral palsy. *J Pediatr Orthop* 1990; 10:105–108.

103. Segal LS, Thomas GS, Mazur JM, Mauterer M. Calcaneal gait in spastic diplegia after heel cord lengthening: A study with gait analysis. *J Pediatr Orthop.* 1989;9:697–701.

104. Crawford AH, Kucharzyk D, Roy DR, Bilbo J. Subtalar stabilization of the planovalgus foot by staple arthroereisis in young children who have neuromuscular problems. *J Bone Joint Surg.* 1990;72A:840–845.

105. Drvaric DM, Schmitt EW, Nahams JM. The Grice extra-articular subtalar arthrodesis in the treatment of spastic hindfoot valgus deformity. *Dev Med Child Neurol.* 1989;31:665–669.

106. Guttman GG. Subtalar arthrodesis in children with cerebral palsy: Results using iliac bone plug. *Foot Ankle*. 1990;10:206–210.

107. Johnson WL, Lester EL. Transposition of the posterior tibial tendon. *Clin Orthop Rel Res*. 1989;245: 223–227.

108. Medina PA, Karpman RR, Yeung AT. Split posterior tibial tendon transfer for spastic equinovarus foot deformity. *Foot Ankle*. 1989;10:65–67.

109. Barnes MJ, Herring JA. Combined split anterior tibial tendon transfer and intramuscular lengthening of the posterior tibial tendon. *J Bone Joint Surg* 1991; 73A:734–738.

110. Craft MJ, Lakin JA, Oppliger RA, Clancy GM, Vanderlinden DW. Siblings as change agents for promoting the functional status of children with cerebral palsy. *Dev Med Child Neurol*. 1990;32:1049, 1057.

Pediatric Physical Therapy,
second edition, edited by Jan
Stephen Tecklin. J. B. Lippincott
Company, Philadelphia © 1994.

5

Elena Tappit-Emas

Spina Bifida

Incidence and Etiology

Spina bifida is a disability causing locomotor dysfunction in children that is second only to cerebral palsy in incidence. With an incidence in the United States that approaches 1 in every 1000 live births, spina bifida is the second most common birth defect after Down's syndrome. Studies examining the possible causes of spina bifida have evaluated genetic, environmental, and dietary factors that might affect its occurrence. No definitive cause, including chromosomal abnormalities, has yet been identified.[1,2]

Many factors may lead to spina bifida, and a genetic predisposition may be enhanced by the existence of numerous environmental factors. Low levels of maternal folic acid prior to conception has been implicated by several studies. Maternal use of valproic acid, an anticonvulsant, is also known to induce this defect in offspring. Recently, maternal hyperthermia caused by saunas, hot tub and electric blanket use, and maternal fevers during the first trimester of pregnancy were studied.[3] Only hot tubs showed any tendency to increase the risk of spina bifida.

A high occurrence (4.5 per 1000 births) is seen in families of Irish and Celtic heritage, but Japanese families show a low occurrence of only 0.3 per 1000 births. A changing pattern of occurrence has appeared in the United States. An increase in spina bifida has been seen in children born to Hispanic and African-American families, perhaps owing to environmental factors and pollution as populations have shifted to industrialized urban areas.[4] Families in which spina bifida is present have a 2% to 5% greater chance than the general population of having a second child with the disorder.

Prognosis

In previous decades, long-term survival of children with spina bifida was reported to range from as low as 1% without treatment to 50% with treatment. A survival rate of more than 90% is expected today with aggressive treatment of the spinal defect and associated problems. This chapter presents the primary problems and concerns for this population, including hydrocephalus, motor and sensory deficits in the lower extremities, and related issues of clinical significance.

The use of antibiotics to limit infection, starting in 1947, and the surgical insertion of ventricular shunts in 1960 to limit hydrocephalus were major advances in treatment. Recently, early and consistent use of intermittent clean catheterization to empty the bladder completely has dramatically improved the survival rate by controlling urinary tract infection and renal deterioration, both of which have been major causes of mortality. These measures, along with the practice of early back closure, continue to improve the survival of children with spina bifida. With this improved survival rate has come an increase in the number of severely affected children. However, there is also an increased number of less severely involved patients who would likely have not survived with earlier treatment protocols. Therefore, the full spectrum and complexity of this disability can now be appreciated. Clinicians now have the opportunity, unavailable in previous eras, to work with and learn a great deal from this heterogeneous group.[5,6]

Definitions

The terms myelomeningocele, meningomyelocele, spina bifida, spina bifida aperta, spina bifida cystica, spinal dysraphism, and myelodysplasia are synonymous. Spina bifida is a spinal defect usually diagnosed at birth by noting the presence of an external sac on the infant's back (Fig. 5-1). The sac contains meninges and spinal cord protruding through a dorsal defect in the vertebrae. This defect may occur at any point along the spine, but is most commonly located in the lumbar region. The sac may be covered by a transparent membrane that may have neural tissue attached to its inner surface, or the sac may be open with the neural tissue exposed. The lateral borders of the sac have bony Protrusions formed by the unfused neural arches of the vertebrae. The defect may be large, with many vertebrae involved, or it may be small, involving only one or two segments. The size of the lesion is not necessarily predictive of the child's functional deficit.[4,6,7]

Spina bifida occulta and myelocele are less severe anomalies associated with spina bifida. *Spina bifida occulta* is a condition involving nonfusion of the halves of the vertebral arches, but without disturbance of the underlying neural tissue. This lesion is most commonly located in the lumbar or sacral spine and is often an incidental finding when roentgenograms are taken for unrelated reasons. Spina bifida occulta may be distinguished externally by a midline tuft of hair, with or without an area of pigmentation on the overlying skin. Between 21% and 26% of parents of children with spina bifida cystica

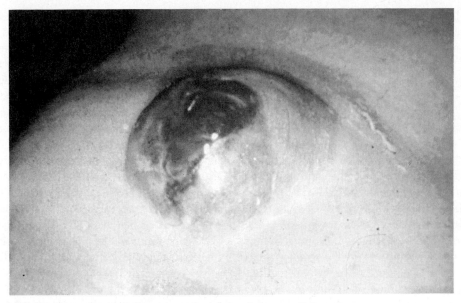

Figure 5-1. *Spina bifida defect in a newborn infant before surgical repair.*

have been found to have the occulta defect. Otherwise, spina bifida occulta has only a 4.5% to 8% incidence in the general population.[4,6,8] Neurologic and muscular dysfunction were previously thought to be absent in individuals with spina bifida occulta. However, recent work by Fidas et al. has revealed a high association of mild urinary tract disorders in these individuals.[9]

A *myelocele* is a protruding sac containing meninges and cerebrospinal fluid (CSF), but in this condition, the nerve roots and spinal cord remain intact and in their normal positions. Motor and sensory deficits, hydrocephalus, and other central nervous system (CNS) problems are not associated with a myelocele.[7]

Lipomeningocele, a superficial fatty mass in the low lumbar or sacral level, is another defect of the vertebrae which is usually included in this group of diagnoses. Neurologic deficits and hydrocephalus are not expected in patients with a lipomeningocele. However, there is a high incidence of decreased bowel and bladder function resulting from a tethered spinal cord in this population.[10,11]

Embryology

Spina bifida cystica, one of several neural tube defects, occurs early in the embryologic development of the CNS. Cells of the neural plate, which forms by day 18 of gestation, differentiate to create the neural tube and neural crest. The neural crest becomes the peripheral nervous system, including the cranial nerves, spinal nerves, autonomic nerves, and ganglia. The neural tube, which becomes the CNS, the brain, and the spinal cord, is open at both the cranial and caudal ends. The cranial end closes on approximately the 24th day of gestation. Failure to close results in a fatal condition called anencephaly. The caudal end of the neural tube closes on day 26 of gestation. Failure of closure or fusion at any point along the caudal border initiates spina bifida cystica or myelomeningocele. Common clinical signs of spina bifida cystica include absence of motor and sensory function (usually bilateral) below the level of the spinal defect and loss of neural control of bowel and bladder function. Unilateral motor and sensory loss has been reported. The pattern of loss may also be asymmetric. The functional deficits may be partial or complete, but they are almost always permanent.[6,12,13]

Hydrocephalus and the Chiari II Malformation

Hydrocephalus and the Arnold Chiari malformation are CNS abnormalities that are commonly associated with spina bifida. *Hydrocephalus* is an abnormal accumulation of CSF in the cranial vault. In individuals without spina bifida, hydrocephalus may be caused by overproduction of CSF, a failure in absorption of the fluid, or an obstruction in the normal flow of CSF through the brain structures and spinal cord. Obstruction by the Arnold Chiari malformation is considered to be the cause of hydrocephalus in most children with spina bifida. This malformation, also known as the *Chiari II malformation,* is a deformity of the cerebellum, medulla, and cervical spinal cord. The posterior cerebellum herniates downward through the foramen magnum, and brain stem structures are also displaced in a caudal direction. The CSF released from the fourth ventricle may face an obstruction by these abnormally situated structures, and its flow through the foramen magnum may be disrupted. Traction on the lower cranial nerves may also occur with this malformation. Studies using magnetic resonance imaging (MRI) have shown that most children with spina bifida have the Chiari II malformation. Among those with this malformation, the likelihood of hydrocephalus developing is greater than 90%.[14–17]

Theories related to the development of the Chiari II malformation are of interest. Previously, it was thought that the primary spinal defect acted as an anchor on the spinal cord, preventing it from sliding proximally within the spinal canal as the fetus grew. It was believed that this traction on the cord pulled down the attached brain stem structures into an abnormally low position. Hydrocephalus was thought to result solely from the hydrodynamic consequence of this blockage.[18] In 1989, a study by McLone and Knepper linked the occurrence of

spina bifida, the Chiari II malformation, and hydrocephalus.[19] These researchers postulated that a series of interrelated, time-dependent defects occur during the embryologic development of the primitive ventricular system, causing the Chiari II malformation and hydrocephalus. Their findings indicate that most affected children have small posterior fossae that are unable to accommodate the hind brain and brain stem structures. Therefore, neither downward traction nor downward pressure from hydrocephalus causes the malformation. Additionally, multiple anatomic anomalies are seen in the brain and cranium. Significantly, McLone and Knepper found that more than 25% of the neonates with spina bifida had head circumferences measuring below the 5th percentile.[19] These researchers have postulated that spina bifida results from mistimed steps in the development of the ventricular system initiated by failure of closure of the neural tube. This explanation has received widespread acceptance among both neuroanatomists and neurosurgeons. The explanation is of great interest to physical therapists who have speculated about the cause of CNS dysfunction in children with spina bifida. These children differ greatly from those with only hydrocephalus, with whom they are often compared. The McLone and Knepper theory begins to offer an anatomic rationale for the CNS abnormalities seen in many patients, and offers a viable basis for future investigation.[19]

Approximately 2% to 3% of children with spina bifida show significant effects of the Chiari II malformation on brain stem and cranial nerve function Display 5-1. Tracheostomy and gastrostomy may be life-saving measures for these symptoms, which are reported to resolve as the child grows and the brain matures. In severe cases of Chiari II malformation, significant upper extremity weakness and opisthotonic postures may be seen. Posterior fossa decompression and cervical laminectomy to relieve pressure on the brain stem and cervical spinal structures are accepted courses of treatment, but are associated with varying degrees of success. It is of interest that no correlation has been found between the severity of a child's symptoms and the degree of

Display 5-1
Symptoms Associated with Chiari II Malformation

Stridor—especially with inspiration
Apnea—when crying, or at night
Gastroesophageal reflux
Paralysis of vocal cords
Swallowing difficulty
Bronchial aspiration

hydrocephalus. In fact, no correlation has yet been found between the child's motor level and any other finding. Therefore, attempts to predict which children will have significant difficulties have been unsuccessful. Examination by MRI has revealed severe abnormalities in some children who are asymptomatic. There is speculation that brain stem auditory evoked potentials may provide some diagnostic assistance in the future. Physicians believe that there is much to learn at the microscopic level about this abnormality.[4,6,20–23]

Prenatal Testing and Diagnosis

Increasingly sophisticated prenatal testing has allowed the early diagnosis of spina bifida. Such testing provides information that allows families to make informed decisions about a pregnancy. For the family that chooses to bring their baby to term, appropriate and well-coordinated medical care can be arranged in anticipation of the birth.

Alpha-fetoprotein (AFP) is normally present in the developing fetus and is found in the amniotic fluid. AFP reaches its peak levels in the fetal serum and, subsequently, in the amniotic fluid from the 6th to the 14th week of gestation. After the 14th week, however, AFP continues to leak into the amniotic fluid through the exposed vascularity of the spina bifida defect. Abnormally high levels of AFP in the amniotic fluid provides strong evidence for a neural tube defect. Testing for AFP by amniocente-

sis and, more recently, in maternal blood samples, has been responsible for detection of approximately 89% of neural tube defects. Unfortunately, the tests used have the potential for both false-positive and false-negative results. Therefore, AFP results are routinely compared clinically with the results of ultrasonographic imaging.[6,14]

Improved ultrasound equipment and experienced technicians have enabled obstetricians to observe and document several cranial abnormalities that have a high correlation with spina bifida. Because a small back lesion on a neonate can be difficult or impossible to detect, clinicians are now using cranial signs as an indication of the abnormality. These clinical findings are then followed by ultrasonographic studies performed for the purpose of locating the back lesion.[24,25]

There has been speculation regarding the best method of obstetrical delivery when spina bifida is detected. A cesarean section may have a protective effect on the neural tissue of the back, thus improving the functional status of the child. Cesarean section also reduces the trauma to the exposed nerves of the back that would occur during vaginal delivery. Moreover, a cesarean delivery avoids the bacterial contamination of the neonate's open lesion associated with passage through the vaginal canal, thereby reducing the risk of meningitis. A cesarean section also avoids trauma to the back from a breech presentation, which could also affect the infant's neurologic function. Finally, back closure can be accomplished more rapidly following a scheduled cesarean section than after an unscheduled vaginal delivery.[26–30]

Management of the Neonate
General Philosophy of Treatment

Philosophies of treatment for the neonate with spina bifida vary throughout the world and among institutions within the United States. Because the back lesion was not universally thought to be life-threatening, institutions were free to develop their own protocols for the timing and intensity of treatment for these infants. However, the results of studies comparing various initial treatment regimens support the efficacy of early intervention. Immediate sterile care of the lesion to prevent infection is essential, and surgical closure of the back within 72 hours of birth is now the goal for most institutions.[4,6,31]

The objective of back surgery is to place the neural tissue into the vertebral canal, cover the spinal defect, and achieve a flat and watertight closure of the sac (Fig. 5-2). The open spine provides direct access to the spinal cord and brain. By preventing infection and its associated brain damage, the child's level of function, physical and cognitive, will be preserved. McLone and associates have shown that babies who suffer gram-negative ventriculitis are less adept intellectually than uninfected babies.[32] These findings are significant in that intellectual function was not significantly affected by either hydrocephalus or the level of paralysis.[4,31–33]

Although in many institutions children with spina bifida are treated aggressively with immediate back closure and rapid management of hydro-cephalus, some institutions practice selective treatment. That is, there will always be more aggressive management for those children who appear less involved. In these institutions, the care for the neonate with spina bifida will vary depending upon the level of lower extremity paralysis. Other factors influencing treatment decisions include the presence of accompanying abnormalities, such as hydrocephalus, kyphoscoliosis, and renal problems. Other institutions attempt to educate parents about their child's status and the implications of spina bifida on their lives. The parents may then act in a thoughtful manner in combination with the medical staff to choose a mutually acceptable course of action. During this period of education, which may last several hours or several weeks, the infant will usually be treated to maintain a stable condition and prevent infection.

This early period also provides time for the medical staff to gather information about the child's condition. This information is shared with the family so that discussion about hydrocephalus or orthopedic deformities, which require more involved early care, can begin. It is important to note that an accurate prediction of the child's potential is difficult in the early days. A vast number of variables will influence the child's condition and function in the coming years, so clinicians must be wary about presenting information about the child's future. An exception, of course, may be in the case of a severely impaired child with multiple congenital anomalies as well as spina bifida whose outcome is apparently bleak.[34–36]

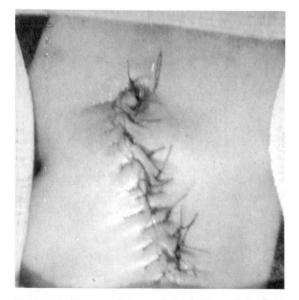

Figure 5-2. *The same defect as shown in Figure 5–1, after surgical repair.*

Preoperative Assessment

In many centers, the preoperative assessment is done by one physician experienced in the overall care of children with spina bifida. Consults are then requested for specific services necessary for each baby. More commonly, however, a team of experts will evaluate the baby and continue to monitor the child throughout the course of hospitalization. These professionals comprise the treatment team that will be involved in long-term care of the child.

The neurosurgeon is concerned initially with the location and extent of the infant's back lesion. Kyphoscoliosis presents a complication to back surgery and may lead to impaired wound healing because of excessive pressure over the suture site. Skin grafting is occasionally necessary to gain adequate skin coverage of a large lesion. Congenital scoliosis with accompanying fused ribs at the level of the back lesion usually predicts rapid progression of the scoliosis during the growth periods of childhood. The resultant effect of progressive scoliosis on pulmonary function may be life-threatening, even with bracing and surgical intervention.

A neonatologist or pediatrician may be consulted to assess the general health of the baby and to identify other congenital defects or cardiopulmonary dysfunction that may be present but that are unrelated to the spinal lesion.

The urologist will request urodynamic testing during the early neonatal period. However, immediate postnatal attention may not be indicated.

A comprehensive orthopedic evaluation may not be imperative, but the surgeon can offer insight into orthopedic problems that are present at birth. Difficulties that may be anticipated may also be discussed. Valuable information and education for the family and medical team can be provided as a result of early orthopedic intervention. Evaluation of the lower extremities and spinal alignment will help establish a plan of orthopedic care for the baby's first weeks of life. This plan of care can incorporate other appropriate staff for coordinated intervention.[4,6,36,37]

Management of Hydrocephalus

After back closure, 10% of affected infants recover, have the sutures removed, and leave the hospital without further complication. The remaining 90% will begin to develop hydrocephalus during the next several days or weeks. After back closure, the natural drain for CSF is unavailable and CSF pressure begins to rise in the cranium. Of the 90% who will develop hydrocephalus, approximately 25% are born with evidence of hydrocephalus and need

immediate shunt insertion. Studies show that an additional 55% will develop hydrocephalus within several days of birth. The remaining babies will need shunting within 6 months. The neurosurgeon carefully monitors changes in the baby's head circumference, and studies such as ultrasonography, computed tomography, or MRI, provide baseline information about the size of the lateral ventricles. Later comparisons can assist in determining the appropriate time for insertion of a shunt.

Changes in the baby's state often indicate increased intracranial pressure. As the enlarged ventricles cause the brain to expand within the flexible cranial vault of the infant, many symptoms are seen singularly or in combination. The two most common symptoms include *"sunsetting,"* a downward deviation of the eyes, and separation of the cranial sutures with a bulging anterior fontanelle.

The increasing fluid pressure may stabilize without surgery in some individuals, but it is impossible to predict when this will occur, how great the pressure will become, or how large the head will grow. Vital signs become depressed and respiratory arrest can occur when pressure on the brain stem structures becomes too great. Some individuals will survive without treatment for the hydrocephalus and become severely impaired.[4,5,36]

Surgical insertion of a shunt will relieve the signs and symptoms associated with increased intracranial pressure. The shunt is a thin, flexible tube that diverts CSF away from the lateral ventricles. It is secured at the proximal and distal ends and is radiopaque for easy location by radiographic studies. The ventriculoatrial (VA) shunt moves excess CSF from one lateral ventricle to the right atrium of the heart. Because infections of the system can lead to septicemia, ventriculitis, superior vena cava occlusion, and pulmonary emboli, this type of shunt is not used as commonly as in past years. The ventriculoperitoneal (VP) shunt is currently the preferred treatment for hydrocephalus. Although occlusion of this type of shunt may occur more easily than with the VA shunt, complications associated with the VP shunt are far less severe. As it exits the lateral ventricle, the shunt can be palpated distally along the neck, under the clavicle, and down the chest wall, just below the superficial fascia. The shunt inserts into the peritoneum where CSF is reabsorbed and the excess excreted[37,38] (Fig. 5-3).

Although shunt insertion is a common operation for most neurosurgical teams, it is yet another event for the infant who has already had at least one major procedure to close the back lesion. In order to spare the infant a second anesthesia, several centers have begun to perform simultaneous back closure and shunt insertion. Advocates of this approach also believe that healing of the back wound from the inside is compromised when the CSF pressure builds internally. With the double surgery, more rapid healing of the back wound is expected. Neither negative sequelae nor increased postoperative complications have been reported for the double procedure.[39,40]

After surgery, a plan for physical therapy, based upon the infant's condition, can be developed. The priority is for rapid healing, an uneventful recovery, and a speedy discharge to home. It is appropriate to wait at least 24 to 48 hours postoperatively before initiating physical therapy. In many cases, the ex-

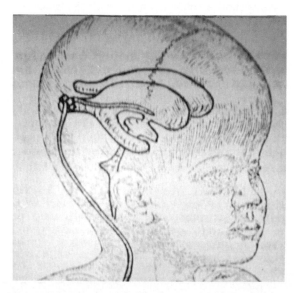

Figure 5-3. *Location of the lateral ventricles and placement of a ventriculoperitoneal shunt.*

tent of hydrocephalus prior to surgery will affect the decision about the baby's return to oral feeding, position changes, range of motion exercises, and normal handling in the upright position. Premature aggressive handling after surgery is not safe, particularly for the baby with a very large head circumference. Intracranial pressure can drop dramatically after shunt insertion, and vascular insult can occur if the baby is held upright prematurely.[36]

Physical Therapy for the Infant with Spina Bifida

Overview

Physical therapy can begin in the early preoperative period before back closure. Ideally, the therapist who provides the preoperative evaluation will continue treating the baby throughout the hospitalization. This same therapist can then provide long-term monitoring and education as the baby progresses to the outpatient department or specialty clinic. This staffing approach provides consistent support for parents during these early, difficult times. Also, the importance of staff continuity becomes increasingly important as the child grows and changes in function occur. The therapist with a good baseline of observations and documentation about the baby can be a valuable resource for the medical team. When a therapist has monitored the baby through the early period of care, the ability to detect subtle changes later is enhanced.[36]

Manual Muscle Testing

A manual muscle test by the physical therapist can provide objective information regarding the presence of active movement and the quantity of muscle power present in the baby's lower extremities (Display 5-2). Manual muscle testing should be performed before back surgery whenever possible. Testing is repeated approximately 10 days after surgery, then at six months, and yearly thereafter. The goal of these early testing sessions is to assist the medical staff in identifying the level of the back le-

> **Display 5-2.**
> *Information Provided By Manual Muscle Testing for Children with Spina Bifida*
>
> Baseline analysis for use in long-term comparisons
> Assessment of remaining muscle function
> Evaluation of muscular imbalance at each joint
> Prediction of the degree and character of existing deformity
> Prediction of potential for future deformity
> Assistance in determining the need for surgery and bracing

infant's position may be limited to lying prone or on the side. Although these positions make it difficult to test the hip rotators accurately, careful observation and palpation should allow for identification of most other muscle groups (Figs. 5-4 and 5-5).

A motor level is assigned according to the last intact nerve root found. Identification of this motor level allows consistency of communication among professionals involved with the baby. However, children assigned to the same motor level will vary widely in their muscle function, so it is very important to locate and grade each individual muscle as it becomes feasible.[41]

Extraneous factors may influence movement ability during the infant's first hours of life. The effects of maternal anesthesia, increased cerebral pressure from hydrocephalus, and general lethargy and fatigue from a difficult or long labor may depress spontaneous movements. Conversely, these same factors may render the baby hyperirritable when stimulated. Tickling the baby above the level of the lesion or around the neck and face is a stimulus to keep the baby moving. Movements of the extremities can be observed and contractions palpated

sion by assessing the lower extremity movement or lack thereof.[36]

Consideration must be given to positioning of the baby for the muscle test during the early stage of care. Depending on the status of the back lesion or surgical site and to protect the involved area, the

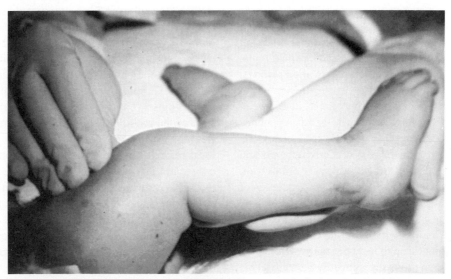

Figure 5-4. *Palpation and observation of the quadriceps muscle during a preoperative assessment of the function of the lower extremities.*

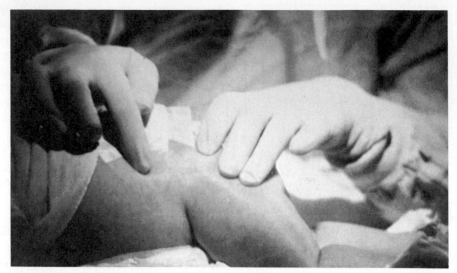

Figure 5-5. *Stimulation of the infant as a means of eliciting movement for testing the gluteus maximus and medius muscles.*

by stabilizing the limb proximally. Proper limb stabilization is necessary to avoid misinterpreting the origin of a movement. The principles for muscle testing in this population are much the same as for older patients. Gentle resistance to movement at one part of the leg may help increase the strength of a movement at a distal part of the limb. Allowing movement to occur at only one joint at a time will allow a more accurate interpretation. For example, holding the hip and knee firmly in either partial flexion or extension and preventing movement at those joints will enable the therapist to detect weak ankle motion that might otherwise have gone unnoticed. After locating each area of movement, the therapist must then assess the strength of the muscle responsible for the observed movement. Above all, patience and ingenuity will improve the accuracy of this measure of the baby's motor ability.[36,42]

The therapist should note whether or not muscles are functioning, which muscles are strong and can move a joint through its entire range, and which are weak and can move the joint only partially. This distinction will make determination of the motor level more precise. The ability to distinguish between active and reflexive movement, although sometimes difficult during the early period, can facilitate identification of the lesion level.[42]

Reflex movement is common in infants with thoracic paralysis. In these patients, there is no activity at the hip joint, but movement is noted distally at the knee or ankle. This movement, which looks like fasciculations of the muscle belly with a weak, continuous movement at the joint, may be seen when the baby is sleeping or when the other joints in that limb are not moving. The movement is usually observed in a flexor muscle and may be seen at the Achilles tendon in the form of plantar flexion. Reflex movements represent sparing of local reflex arcs. However, cortical control of the movement has been interrupted by the spinal defect. This reflex movement is of concern because of its involuntary nature and because it is unopposed by an active antagonist at the same joint. Therefore, this unchecked reflex activity can become a deforming force that often requires surgical intervention. The movement is often misleading to staff and family who may interpret the movement as a useful, functional motion. However, because the motion is not cortically initiated, it seldom has any functional value.[36]

Manual muscle testing grades can be modified until the child can be positioned appropriately for gravity and gravity-eliminated responses. Modification of testing procedures is also suggested until the child can follow verbal cues and be tested with resistance so as to increase the consistency and reliability of results. One successful method developed at Children's Memorial Hospital in Chicago uses an X to indicate the presence of strong movement, or O for an absent response, T for trace movement (when contraction is palpated but movement cannot be seen), and an R to indicate reflex movement. This scheme of grading, when combined with the existing scale of 0 through 5, or "absent" to "normal" classifications, provides significant information about the lower extremities.

This evaluation can help predict muscle imbalance and the consequential potential for deformity. If a deformity is present, early muscle testing can identify whether the cause of the limitation is passive, as a result of malpositioning in utero, or active, resulting from muscle imbalance around the joint. Distinguishing the cause of joint limitation is important for the orthopedic surgeon who may wish to operate early on the lower extremities. The surgeon will want to spare potentially useful muscle function and eliminate movement that will only be deforming in nature. If the stimulus for movement is questionable, the surgeon may choose to wait until the child is older and a more accurate evaluation is possible before deciding upon the type of surgery.[43]

Some centers have attempted to use electromyographic (EMG) studies to evaluate lower extremity innervation. EMG studies are interesting from an academic standpoint, but offer little functional information about the baby and are not widely regarded as valuable.

It is also of interest that poor correlation exists between early manual muscle testing and the child's future level of function. Future function depends upon strength of the lower extremity musculature, the child's total CNS function, motivation, intellectual capacity, and the family's capacity for long-term support and interest. These variables are only a few factors that can influence the functional potential of the growing child with spina bifida. They affect the child's success at using the movements present in the lower extremities. These concerns are addressed in greater detail in subsequent sections of this chapter.[44]

Results of early manual muscle tests can be compared with later tests in order to monitor the child's neuromuscular stability. It is a pleasant surprise to find increased movement or strength after back closure, but any decrease in movement must immediately be brought to the attention of the neurosurgeon. Deterioration of lower extremity motor function may indicate a surgical error, the development of hydromyelia, or a tethered spinal cord, each of which requires neurosurgical intervention.[45]

Range of Motion Assessment

Preliminary assessment of range of motion (ROM) can be performed prior to back closure. Normal neonates have flexion contractures of up to 30 degrees at the hips, 10 to 20 degrees at the knees, and ankle dorsiflexion of up to 40 or 50 degrees. Limitations in ROM in the baby with spina bifida should not be considered an indication for immediate and aggressive stretching. Early limitations of range require a safe plan of management for several weeks. When it becomes apparent that limitations will be both severe and long-lasting, a long-term plan can be developed which will likely include surgical correction.[46,47]

Several common limitations are seen in the neonate with spina bifida. Extreme tightness of the hip flexors is common in the child with motor level involvement at L-2 to L-3 or L-3 to L-4 owing to the presence of a strong iliopsoas with no opposing force offered from weak or absent hip extensors. Hamstrings, which exert a secondary hip extension force, are also lacking. Adductor tightness is also likely as a result of adductor innervation and the absence of the antagonist gluteus medius. If the baby has an insufficient range of hip flexion to tolerate prone positioning, the neurosurgeon and nursing staff must be informed in an effort to prevent possible fractures of the femur. Adapted prone positioning, with legs draped over a raised platform in the operating room, may be indicated during back closure. A modified prone or side-lying position postoperatively is generally safest. The physical therapist is often the first to note the need for special positioning following the preoperative assessment of range of motion.[48]

Dorsiflexion or a calcaneous deformity at the ankle is a common contracture seen at birth. The child with L-5 innervation has strong dorsiflexion, provided by the anterior tibialis and toe extensors, but weak or absent toe flexors and lack of plantar flexion from the gastrocnemius/soleus group. Plans may call for splinting the ankle at 90 degrees for optimal alignment during the early days in the hospital. In addition to splinting, gentle passive exercise often helps to reduce this deformity.

Provided that the baby is medically stable and the physician agrees, daily ROM exercise for the lower extremities can begin at bedside as early as the day after back closure. Although options are limited after surgery, prone and side-lying positions are adequate to perform all motions needed in the lower extremities at this time.[6,36,48]

Postoperative Physical Therapy

In order for the physical therapist to develop a complete and appropriate program for the infant who has undergone back closure and shunting, the results of both the neurologic and orthopedic evaluations must be considered. To be most effective, the therapist should also be sensitive to the state of the family members, who will have begun to visit their baby more regularly.

Communication

In most cases, parents of infants with spina bifida experience a very different and more difficult postpartum period than had been anticipated. Their baby was probably transferred to a tertiary care facility shortly after birth. Often, the needs of the recovering mother are superseded by the needs of the father and other family members to attend to the infant. Inaccurate information about spina bifida, in general, and their child, in particular, may further compromise family coping skills during this physically and emotionally difficult time. It has been reported that parents are often told by staff members that their child will be mentally retarded, will never walk, and will require institutionalization. These professionals, although well-intentioned, are not experienced in current methods of evaluation and treatment of children with spina bifida, and may only recall information from a previous era in which a bleak outlook for these babies was the norm rather than the exception. This misinformation causes many parents to become confused and frustrated, especially when the specialty team in the hospital presents apparently conflicting information. Communication between the therapist and other team members is important. All persons working with the infant must know and understand each other's findings. Information given to the family must be appropriate and consistent and should always be presented in a sensitive manner.[4]

Reflecting a positive and caring attitude during treatment sessions is an important objective for the physical therapist, as this approach may help to normalize the family's involvement with the infant. A home program can be taught to the family immediately. This is a constructive way for the therapist to begin interacting with family members and to facilitate their interaction with the infant. The therapist should encourage the family to observe and participate in the infant's care during hospitalization in order to prepare them for providing care at home. Waiting to educate the family until the last few days of hospitalization places increased stress on the family members, who must learn much from many people in a short time. An unexpectedly quick discharge may also leave no time for family education, which should be spread over the entire period of hospitalization, with follow-up sessions scheduled during outpatient or clinic visits.

Exercise

Passive ROM exercises should be brief, and should be performed only two or three times each day. The therapist can combine individual leg movements into patterns of movement so that the family need only learn three or four patterns for the home program. An example would be to combine flexion of the hip and knee of one leg, while holding the opposite leg in full extension. With the baby supine, both hips can be abducted at the same time, leaving only the foot and ankle to be done individually[36] (Figs. 5-6 and 5-7).

These ROM exercises are performed gently with the hands placed close to the joint being moved in order to use a short lever arm, thereby preventing unnecessary stress to soft tissue and joint structures. Several repetitions of each pattern, holding the joint briefly at the end of the range, should maintain and may increase ROM in joints with mild or moderate limitations. If severe limitations exist, exercise of the area affected may require additional time and repetitions. Aggressive stretching should be avoided, regardless of the severity of the joint limitation.

By participating in the educational process and exercise program during this early time, parents are encouraged to touch and move their baby's legs while being observed by the therapist. Opportunities to handle their baby with supervision can help alleviate concern that many families express about further injuring the infant. With the therapist's comforting and supportive words, the exercise program offers a valuable opportunity for positive parent-child interaction.

Passive ROM exercises must continue throughout the child's life. The goal is that the child will ultimately learn to perform the exercises independently. Passive exercise is often forgotten by therapists and parents as the child becomes more active, starts crawling, and therapy shifts to concentrate on gait training. Although many therapists consider the latter activities to be adequate to maintain range, regardless of the level of motor activity, only the innervated portions of the limb are being actively moved. If ROM exercises are discontinued,

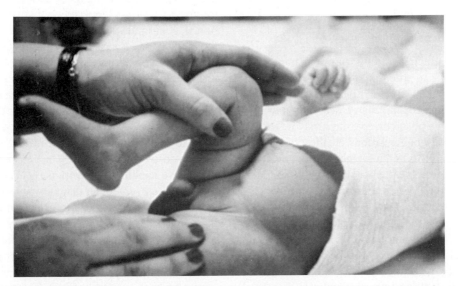

Figure 5-6. *Exercises for range of motion of the lower extremities. Full flexion of one hip and knee is combined with an extension of the opposite extremity.*

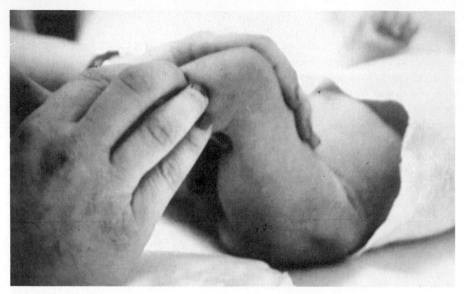

Figure 5-7. *Placement of the hand for a range of motion exercise of the knee. Note the use of a short lever arm.*

contractures will develop. For many children, contractures may develop over years, but for others, range is lost within a short time. With loss of range, function will also diminish.[6,14,36]

Positioning and Handling

The physical therapist often assumes responsibility for developing a program of positioning for the hospitalized baby. Although many positioning options are available as discharge nears, options during the first few postoperative days may be limited to prone or side-lying positions. As the child's medical status stabilizes and tolerance to movement improves, it is advisable to avoid leaving the child immobile for long periods. Handling and carrying strategies can be practiced by the therapist and then recommended to the parents. Finding a comfortable chair is most important and once seated, the therapist or family member can hold the child prone over the lap, rocking or swaying slowly side to side. This position is restful for the parent and provides novel movement for the infant. The baby may also enjoy

a slow walk around the hospital floor being held up and slightly over one of the parent's shoulders. This position gives the infant an opportunity to attempt to raise its head and look around. If a supine position is contraindicated, parents may gently cradle the infant prone across their forearms as they walk or sit. These positions will provide the family with a repertoire of acceptable handling methods when they come to visit their baby. Parents may feel less awkward if they do not need a nurse or therapist to hand them the baby on each visit. These positions are also nonthreatening for the infant, who needs time to recover and who will not respond well to aggressive handling of the trunk, head, or extremities. One must remember that the primary postoperative goals for such infants are uncomplicated healing of the back wound, speedy recovery from shunt insertion, and discharge from the hospital.[36]

Short periods of supine and supported upright sitting in the therapist's arms should not affect the course of back wound healing. A variety of positions helps to normalize the baby's experiences during waking hours, while eating, or quietly observing the surroundings. These short periods are also useful for the therapist, who can note the baby's responses to gravity in these positions, feel for changes in muscle tone, and observe any significant asymmetries, particularly through the shoulders and neck. Documenting this information will provide a useful baseline against which to compare later developmental findings.[4,6,36]

Families should first watch, then try to duplicate, the activities recommended for their baby. If a parent does not show some hesitation or anxiety upon first handling the baby, it may indicate a poor understanding of the baby's condition and may contribute to subsequent poor judgment in other areas of care. Even for families with experience raising other children, some level of fear or anxiety at first is a healthy sign.

The therapist can begin to "role release" as the hospitalization proceeds, delegating to the parents some ROM and handling activities. As this change in roles occurs, the therapist can begin to concentrate on other areas of the child's plan of care. At many hospitals, the therapist is asked to repeat the lower extremity manual muscle test prior to the infant's discharge.

The therapist can also observe the baby's state, noting changes secondary to hydrocephalus and shunt insertion, so as to provide additional baseline information which may help to identify a later shunt malfunction. When a malfunction occurs, in addition to the signs and symptoms presented in Table 5-1; a change in the baby's tone and responsiveness to movement may also be noted.

The family should be encouraged to be active in gathering information about their infant. They should be encouraged to play with and observe the baby, not only to foster positive interaction but also to aid the medical staff in assessing the infant's function. Interaction with the medical team becomes less frequent as the child grows and becomes increasingly medically stable. Observations by parents can help identify problems at an early stage so that appropriate medical care can be sought.

Table 5–1. *Signs and Symptoms of Shunt Malfunction*

Infants

Bulging fontanelle	High-pitched cry
Vomiting	Irritability
Change in appetite	Lethargy
"Sunset" sign of eyes	Seizures
Edema, redness along shunt tract	Excessive rate of growth of head circumference
	Thinning of skin over scalp

Toddlers

Vomiting	Lethargy
Irritability	Seizures
Headaches	New nystagmus
Edema, redness along shunt tract	New squint

School-Aged Children

Headaches	Vomiting
Lethargy	Seizures
Irritability	Decreased school performance
Edema, redness along shunt tract	Personality changes
Handwriting changes	Memory changes

Sensory Assessment

The physical therapist should perform a sensory assessment of the neonate with spina bifida. To gather information about possible sensory deficits, the therapist should try to ascertain areas of the infant's lower extremities that are sensitive or insensitive to touch. This sensory information, along with the results of muscle testing, can be used to accurately establish the level of the spinal lesion. One reason for the early assessment is to find the level of intact sensation so that the therapist can stimulate active motion. It is the novice clinician who strokes the plantar surface of the foot expecting to make the child move. This technique is successful only when the infant has intact sensation to the sacral nerve roots. Most infants with spina bifida have a higher level of insensitivity. The therapist may find that the level of motor function and sensation may not be similar in both legs. Early results of sensory testing may be inaccurate, depending upon the state of the infant. In addition, it may be difficult to accurately assess all sensory modalities in the newborn infant (light touch, deep pressure, temperature, etc.).

As sensory findings become more stable and reproducible, the information can be shared with the family, who must become educated about their child's skin anesthesia. Educating parents about skin care for the baby is often the shared responsibility of the nursing and therapy staffs. It is sometimes difficult for parents to understand the concept that their baby has areas of the lower body and legs that are insensitive to touch. The therapist can help the family discover this information on their own. Using a gentle touch, caress, or tickle, a family member can map out areas of responsiveness when the infant is awake but quiet. The therapist should not use a pin or other sharp object to demonstrate this testing. The baby's response to a pinprick is no more valid than its response to a gentle caress, and a sharp object may increase the parent's anxiety and concern about the baby's medical care.

Insensitive areas of the lower extremities require additional protection from use and abuse because the child will be unaware of injury to denervated areas. For example, families must always test the temperature of bathwater prior to immersing the child. The infant's legs and feet should always be protected while crawling. Prior to placing the infant on the floor to play, a search for hidden objects in the carpet may prevent an accidental injury from loose carpet tacks or a small toy. Socks or booties will also help to prevent problems when children begin to reach for and bite their toes, around the age of 6 to 8 months.

As the infant grows, skin insensitivity continues to be a problem. Application of new shoes or braces, for instance, requires vigilant attention to fit and avoidance of pressure areas will prevent sores or abrasions.

Normal sensation keeps the able-bodied person from sitting immobile for long periods. Intact sensory feedback causes these individuals to shift around frequently and change their weight distribu-

tion, thereby relieving pressure. Insensate persons, however, tend to develop skin problems secondary to sitting because they do not shift their weight, change their position, or relieve pressure. Similarly, able-bodied persons are able to adjust their gait to avoid abrasion when there is pressure from an ill-fitting shoe. Such readjustment does not occur with the child who has spina bifida, as areas of pressure are not perceived by the child with abnormal sensation. It is important, therefore, to introduce any new orthosis gradually. The orthotic should be worn for only a few hours each time, and the skin should be inspected to determine whether any pressure areas are present. When areas of redness consistently last for longer than 30 minutes, an adjustment of the orthosis is indicated. This plan for skin accommodation is best implemented over a weekend or in the evening, when the child has more time at home. It is best not to send the child for a full day of school with a new orthosis until proper fit is assured. Time spent addressing these issues initially may save the child from losing valuable time later as a result of immobility, serious infections, or additional hospitalizations.[6,14,36]

Care for the Young Child

Ongoing Concerns and Issues

After the initial medical care for the child with spina bifida, a plan of long-term care should be developed. Various approaches to continued care are seen throughout the United States, with many children seen by specialists located in one institution. Conversely, a primary care pediatrician may choose to refer the child to professionals in several locations as specific needs are identified. Professionals in the community who are affiliated with early intervention programs or private offices may provide care, but when care is divided among several sites, a new role may emerge for the parents. They may be forced to become case managers for their child to facilitate continuity of care and communication among the professionals. This added responsibility may present a large burden for many families and may result in less-than-optimal care for their children. It appears that, because of the multiple specialty areas involved in comprehensive care for children with spina bifida, care may be delivered best by experienced professionals who work together as a coordinated team. That is why many pediatric facilities attempt to organize an interdisciplinary clinic for children with spina bifida where several primary specialists can see the child on the same day. Families are encouraged to continue their child's care at a spina bifida specialty clinic if at all possible. With a team of specialists working together to complement one another, both the child and parents can benefit. Communication is facilitated and expedited with professionals in one location. Information can be shared to increase learning and maintain a current outlook. If problems are detected, the necessary personnel are present to address the concern without the need for another appointment. With consistency and coordination, trust in the professional staff can develop more easily, thereby enabling the family to be less stressed and potentially better able to cope with their child's needs.[4,6,36,49]

The child will need to return frequently to the clinic during the first year of care for evaluation by various specialists. The neurosurgeon will monitor the status of the back closure, hydrocephalus, and shunt (Display 5-3).[4,6] The orthopedist will evaluate limb flexibility, strength, and joint integrity. Splints and surgery are planned to prepare the child for standing (Display 5-4).[6,36] The urologist will monitor bowel and bladder function, assess renal status at regular intervals, and plan a course of care that includes intermittent catheterization and pharmacologic management (Display 5-5).[50,52] A bowel program that may involve periodic toileting, diet, medication, and biofeedback and behavior modification may be implemented to attain fecal continence.

As the child stabilizes in each of the specialty areas, visits to the clinic will become less frequent. It is not unusual for the child to be seen at 6-month intervals over several years and then yearly if there are no ongoing problems or major concerns. However, more frequent visits are necessary when a chronic problem requires close monitoring or treatment.

Developmental Difficulties

It has become apparent that CNS deficits exist in a number of children with spina bifida. In many cases, the effects of the deficits will have a negative impact upon gross motor, fine motor, perceptual motor, and cognitive function. The effects of these deficits can be more detrimental than the lower extremity paralysis or hydrocephalus that initially accompanies the condition. The Chiari II malformation has been identified and studied for several

---

Display 5-3.
Goals of Neurosurgical Care for Patients with Spina Bifida

Assess the location and size of the back defect
Perform closure of the back defect
Assess the extent of lower extremity paralysis
Assess and treat hydrocephalus
Monitor the function of the ventricular shunt
Monitor the patient for acute and chronic
   CNS abnormalities
Monitor the patient for CNS deterioration,
   tethered cord, and hydromyelia

Display 5-4.
Goals of Orthopedic Surgical Care for Patients with Spina Bifida

Prevent joint contracture
Correct musculoskeletal deformities
Prevent skin breakdown from structural
   malalignment
Provide resources to achieve best mobility
Monitor the patient for CNS deterioration,
   tethered cord, and hydromyelia

Display 5-5.
Goals of Urologic Care in Patients with Spina Bifida

Preserve renal function
Provide for adequate bladder emptying
Provide for urinary continence
Monitor the patient for CNS deterioration, tethered cord, and hydromyelia

---

decades, but only in recent years has there been mention of this malformation as it relates to CNS dysfunction. Using MRI, a more sophisticated imaging system than previously available, structural abnormalities have been identified visually. The specific extent of anatomic abnormalities and severity of the Chiari II can be determined by MRI. However, as previously noted, the clinical effects of the malformation in a particular child still cannot be predicted.

Up to 85% of children with spina bifida have low tone with minimal to moderate developmental delay. Delayed and abnormal head and trunk control, righting, and equilibrium responses are the most common difficulties. Eventually, these delays may be attributed to the Chiari II malformation, as children with only hydrocephalus do not exhibit movement problems with the same frequency or severity as those with both spina bifida and hydrocephalus.[6,36,53–55]

CNS problems are apparent early in the baby's life. Prolonged instability of the head and upper body is noted in the baby with spina bifida. When parents carry, lift, or move their young infant, the child with poor neck stability may retain the startle response longer than the normal infant. Often, parents compensate for this by supporting the baby's head in a manner that is more protective than usual so as not to elicit the startle response. This additional support begins a cycle in which the added support further limits the experiences and opportunities for motor behavior the baby receives. This limitation reduces the chances for the child to practice independent head control, and may never prolong the deficit.

The normal baby spends time in various positions from the beginning of life and experiences the effects of gravity upon the head and body. Normal infants will begin to stabilize their head over the shoulders in the supported upright position. This response is seen before the baby can lift its head from a prone or supine position. As the infant gains control of the head in space, a feedback mechanism develops between the baby and parent in which the baby communicates the need for support. Progressively less support is given and new ways to carry the infant are attempted as the baby's head becomes more stable. This development is most apparent when the baby is held upright in the parent's arms while being carried. At first, the parent's hand is placed behind the baby's head to prevent it from falling backward. Several weeks later, we see this supporting hand only when parents raise or lower the baby. In just a few additional months, no guarding of the head is required when the baby is upright.

In the infant with normal tone, there is physiologic stability of the head that is not present in the infant with hypotonus. Joint proprioception through the cervical spine and the normal stretch reflexes of the soft tissue structures of the neck permit the baby's head to fall slowly into gravity, with movement or position change, but only to a small degree. The infant can hold the head reasonably steady without much active participation.

The head of infants with low tone as a result of spina bifida will fall further forward or sideways before these stabilizing responses occur. The responses to gravity may be slow and weak. A mechanical disadvantage is added as the baby grows and the head becomes larger and heavier, and the task of head righting is made more difficult by the additional weight and weak musculature.

When the infant with spina bifida is placed in various positions and attempts to stabilize the head, compensatory patterns of movement may develop to provide some degree of success. Elevation of the shoulders is considered to be developmentally immature alignment for the infant who should have head stability by 4 months of age. This less mature method of head stabilization also interferes with the development of righting skills owing to inappropriate use of the neck musculature. Also, the upper arms are held stiffly at a time when the infant should be experimenting with and enjoying increased movement and abilities of the upper extremities.

Several months later, the child with insufficient trunk strength and stability to maintain the body upright against gravity may use the upper extremities as a prop while sitting. The shoulders remain elevated to provide stability for the head. The arms are held in internal rotation with scapular protraction. The forearms are pronated with wrist and hand flexion. Weight bearing on the hands is limited to the radial aspect. Without development of further head and trunk control, the child may remain stuck, unable to move into or out of sitting. To assist with positional changes, the motivated child may develop abnormal strategies for positional changes. These strategies are usually passive, involving little muscle activity from the neck and trunk, and thus do not help to improve the strength and coordination of the body. The child may throw the head to one side and collapse, or may lean forward over the legs to crawl out of the sitting position.

This pattern of propping is also seen when the baby attempts to lift the head and look around while in a prone position. Side-to-side weight shifting over the hands and arms will not occur. When the child lifts an arm to reach for a toy, the prop is removed, stability is lost, and the head drops. Even with experience, this pattern does not improve. The child may tilt the head to one side to perform a weight shift and to free one arm to reach, but the head cannot be maintained upright against gravity.

When an able-bodied baby lifts an arm to reach for an object, a weight shift to one side occurs. The head and chest remain elevated, and the trunk, neck, and lower extremity musculature actively stabilize the baby's position. The baby does not depend upon upper extremity support to lift the head. With weight shifting and movement in a prone position, the arms become more externally rotated while the forearms increase in supination with pressure across the ulnar surface of the hands. Increasing tactile stimulation across the hands helps to reduce the sensitivity of the grasp response. The normal upper extremity weight-bearing progression aids in the opening of the baby's flexed fingers and hands. Experiences in the prone position also provide considerable proprioception through the joints of the upper extremities. The child with spina bifida needs coordination and strength in the upper extremities to use assistive devices for ambulation and to perform paper and pencil tasks in school. With limited head and trunk stability as a problem, we must be alert for the infant who substitutes upper extremity support. Using the upper extremities in lieu of head and trunk support will limit the motor experiences of the arms and hands and may contribute to acquisition of abnormal truncal skills.

Paralysis of the lower extremities decreases the sensorimotor stimulation that the legs provide to the remainder of the body. Tactile, proprioceptive, and vestibular input is reduced secondary to the motor and sensory limitations of the legs. The degree to which this loss affects the individual depends on the movement and sensation available in the legs and the child's CNS status. If a child is able to explore the environment actively and independently he or she will gain knowledge about his or her body in relation to the environment. An intact baby has vast experiences, and learning is gleaned from many modalities. When movement and exploration are limited, learning is affected. Lower extremity paralysis, in combination with low tone and poor head control, makes movement difficult for many children with spina bifida, thereby decreasing the child's motivation to move. With negative reinforcements for movement, more sophisticated sensorimotor skills and learning will be hampered.

Therapists must appreciate the impact of these

impediments on learning in children with spina bifida. This information can be used to facilitate and encourage handling strategies that enhance more normal development and movement skills.[56–62]

Handling Strategies for Parents

Instructions for parents should begin before the child is discharged from the hospital and should continue until adequate and acceptable function is observed. Parents should be aggressive in their approach, but tempered by the medical status and age of their child. Teaching sessions should include verbal instruction as well as many opportunities for the parents to observe the therapist handling their baby.

Although parents and staff often focus upon the most conspicuous deficit—lower extremity paralysis—the physical therapist has the responsibility of also incorporating into the instructional program information that will promote the family's understanding of and development of gross, fine, and perceptual motor abilities above the waist. Gradual instruction can be offered based upon the status of the infant and the capacity of the family. Frequent gentle reminders can be given in early treatment sessions about the spinal defect and the CNS problems seen in some children. The family should be warned of potential problems, especially the child's difficulty in developing control of the head, neck, and trunk. The therapist may describe means of lessening or preventing such problems.

It is initially useful to teach the family to look for signs suggesting these additional difficulties. Hypotonus in the child may cause a delay in acquisition of antigravity head control in all directions.[53] Parents should not permit the baby to be held or positioned with the head at severe angles to the body. These positions will allow muscles and other soft tissues to overstretch. The infant who lacks active neck flexion will be asymmetrical in a supine position, and will have difficulty turning the head from side to side. Abnormal compensatory patterns of movement will be seen when the baby tries to move its head. The prone position, too, may lead to frustration if neck extensor strength is poor. As the infant tires of keeping the head turned to one side, it may begin to cry. In response, the parent may lift the baby or roll it into a different position. By responding in this manner, the parent unknowingly assumes responsibility for a motor skill that the child must master. Parents should be educated that their behavior can interfere with appropriate neck and trunk muscle development that is needed to lift the head correctly.

Literature on normal development indicates that infants acquire head stability in supported upright postures before they can lift their heads from prone or maintain midline control in supine. Gaining the ability to stabilize the head while upright facilitates strengthening of all the musculature needed to lift and control the head while prone or supine (Figs. 5-8 and 5-9). With these thoughts in mind, the therapist can recommend that parents offer their baby with spina bifida experience in all positions, with a strong emphasis on upright postures.[37,41,59]

Parents can be taught to carry their awake, alert child with the head unsupported to facilitate development of head control, but without allowing the head to fall suddenly in an uncontrolled manner, thereby eliciting a startle response. Holding the baby high on the shoulder rather than at the chest level also facilitates development of head control (Fig. 5-10). Another useful strategy is for the parents to sit at a table while holding the baby in a supported sitting position on the table at eye level. In this position, the parent can encourage visual play, and can provide experiences for independent head control. The infant could be held around the shoulders at first and then at chest level, depending on its balance ability.

Parents should be instructed to observe the infant for prolonged asymmetries or sensitivity to certain movements. The therapist should demonstrate good, symmetric alignment of the baby in various positions (Fig. 5-11).

Because of CNS deficits, children with spina

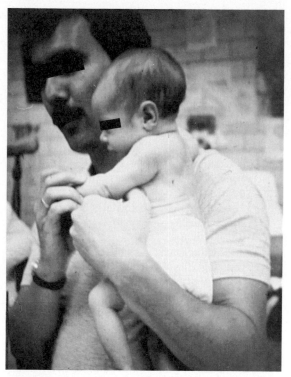

Figure 5-8. *Able-bodied infant at 6 weeks of age. The infant is stabilizing the head while in an upright position. Note the erect alignment of the thoracic spine in an infant with normal muscle tone.*

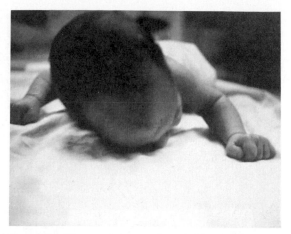

Figure 5-9. *The same infant as shown in Figure 5–8 is barely able to elevate the head to turn it from side to side in a prone position.*

ents develop an effective approach to management of their child. A comprehensive program will best provide the support and services for both parents and children.

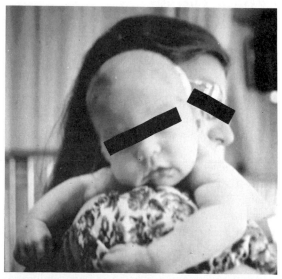

Figure 5-10. *Infant is being carried high on the adult's shoulder to stimulate independent movement of the head and an improved position of the upper extremities.*

bifida often require long-term therapeutic programs which may be unavailable or inconvenient to provide through the hospital. Early intervention programs in the community are recommended. Ideally, the community program should provide services for the family and child. The family often needs support and assistance once it leaves the secure environment of the hospital. This assistance is particularly important for the family in which there are other able-bodied children and for first-time parents. It is interesting to note that parents who are accustomed to the varying rates of development of previous children will deny or minimize the developmental delays of the child with spina bifida. Time and consistent input are required to help par-

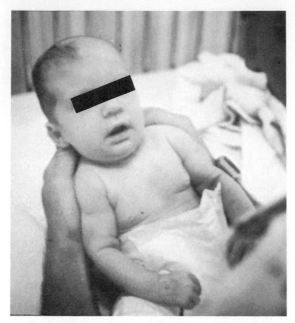

Figure 5-11. *This position is suggested for handling an infant in a supine position. Note the attempt to provide for a symmetric posture.*

Physical Therapy for the Growing Child

Developmental Concerns

A mutually acceptable long-range plan of care should be developed cooperatively by the physical therapist, neurosurgeon, orthopedic surgeon, and family. The plan for the young child with spina bifida is based largely upon objective findings from the physical therapist's evaluations. Repeated manual muscle tests and careful observation enables the therapist to identify the child's strengths and weaknesses in gross motor development and in movement of the child's lower extremities. Intervention can then be directed at specific needs within both areas of motor function (Display 5-6).

Children with spina bifida need to pursue activities that will improve righting and equilibrium responses of the head and trunk. When the therapist addresses these needs and sees improvement, there is a secondary benefit too. While stimulating the

---

Display 5-6.
Goals of Physical Therapy in Patients with Spina Bifida

Establish motor level of infant
Perform periodic muscle testing for comparison purposes
Instruct the patient and family in a home care program to help prevent deformity
Provide instruction to facilitate chronologic development
Assist in determining appropriate orthoses
Facilitate mobility program for ambulation or wheelchair use
Provide information regarding the patient's neurologic function to physicians
Monitor the patient for CNS deterioration, tethered cord, and hydromyelia

---

automatic balance responses against gravity in all positions, active responses in the lower extremities are noted. These responses serve as an important part of the child's exercise program.[36]

Sitting stimulates the child's balance, improves control of the head and trunk, increases the child's visual field, and provides an opportunity for many eye-hand experiences. Head righting and equilibrium responses can be tested by holding the child around the chest and slowly tilting him or her from side to side. The infant should respond by returning the head toward the midline. Next, the therapist brings the infant's body to midline and repeats the activity to the other side, to diagonal directions, and straight back. If no response occurs in any direction and the child's head hangs, or if the child becomes upset with the activity, the movement may have been too rapid or extended too far. A slower and less challenging tilt is used until a response is noted. As the child's responses to the stimuli become more brisk and strong, the angle of tilt can be increased. As the child improves, support can be moved to the chest or waist and the same activities repeated. During this work, the oblique abdominal and lower extremity musculature will contract in response to changes in the center of gravity, in an attempt to return the body to midline. As equilibrium responses are strengthened with this type of balance work, active hip flexion, hip adduction and abduction, knee extension, and ankle and foot movement can be elicited. It is interesting to note that children with poor upper body control and muscle strength in the lower extremities that has been graded as "trace" or "poor" by manual muscle testing often improve secondary to the effects of these head and trunk strengthening activities. Therefore, it is recommended that sessions of tilting last 10 or 15 minutes and that many repetitions be provided so as to enhance strengthening of all responses (Fig. 5-12).

Neck and thoracic extensor activity and strengthening are achieved when the child can hold a position of prone extension with the head and thorax held up against gravity without use of the upper extremities. Low back extensors, gluteals, quadri-

ceps, and plantar flexors will also contract if they are innervated. As the child is tilted from prone slowly to the side with its head erect, strengthening of the neck musculature and head righting and equilibrium reactions in prone will occur. This activity will also strengthen other trunk and lower extremity musculature. Hip abduction and extension may be seen with knee and ankle extension if those muscles are innervated.

Appropriate handling in the supine position can enhance the child's active head control in midline, thus decreasing the asymmetrical influence of gravity on the head. The supine position also facilitates bilateral upper extremity play and disassociation of body parts through rotation of the thorax on the lumbar spine, lumbar spine on the pelvis, and lower extremities on the pelvis. When the child holds its legs up and extends them to kick and play against gravity, muscles of the lower extremities, neck, and abdomen are strengthened. Neck and trunk flexors combine with the extensors to provide for good spinal alignment in sitting.

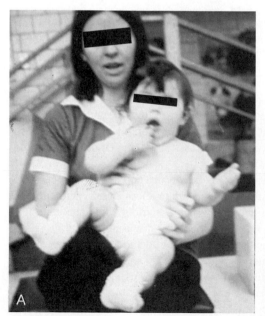 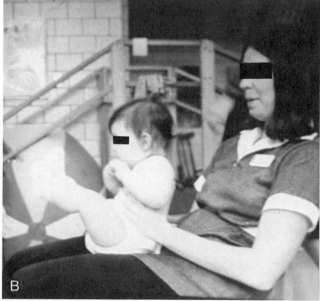

Figure 5-12. A *and* **B.** *Challenging the child's balance responses to elicit more sophisticated upper body abilities and strengthening of the lower extremities as they respond as well.*

An able-bodied infant, as early as 2 months of age, will bear weight on the lower extremities as a result of the positive support reaction. When this response is discovered by the parents, it usually is included in the repertoire of positions used in playing with and holding the child. A great deal of proprioceptive input is provided by weight bearing. Gravity acting on the body stimulates the joint surfaces in the neck, trunk, and lower extremities. This sensory input is important for body awareness and the perception of body in space. Standing also provides a novel perception of the relationship of the body to the immediate surroundings. When the child with spina bifida bears weight, contact between the femoral head and acetabulum and muscle contractions around the hip joint may help to stimulate acetabular development, thereby reducing the likelihood of hip joint dysplasia.

As the child grows, practice in standing will continue to challenge and improve body control and balance against gravity and will stimulate available muscles in the trunk and lower extremities to assist with a more independent stance. Families can be taught to assist their young child with brief periods of standing several times each day until the child can stand with less assistance, or until a standing device is provided (Fig. 5-13).[14,36]

Learning to push and pull with the arms to compensate for weakness in the trunk and neck may allow the child to roll, attain the four-point position, and, perhaps, to pull to a stand if lower extremity function is adequate. This progression, with its increased reliance on the arms, will ultimately lead to a higher level of bracing than the level of lesion might indicate, as well as use of an assistive device for the unstable body during gait. This higher level of bracing will limit the child's potential despite lower extremity movement. Therefore, for the child with spina bifida, it is not sufficient merely to identify that a developmental milestone has occurred. Rather, it is important to assess the movement, qualitatively, including such considerations as the child's ability to perform the movement against gravity, whether the movement is normal, and whether compensatory or abnormal patterns have

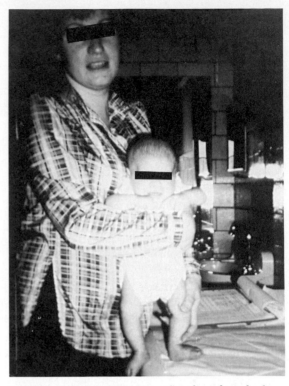

Figure 5-13. *Brief periods of standing throughout the day will help provide for well-aligned weight bearing in the child without fully innervated musculature of the lower extremities.*

developed. One can then identify patterns of movement to be enhanced or strengthened as foundations for future skills, as well as movements that should be avoided.[36]

These areas of concern can be incorporated into a safe and appropriate therapeutic regimen. The physical therapy plan should include activities performed in all positions, the use of gravity to challenge the child, and varied and changing movement stimuli to facilitate motor development. By providing these opportunities and experiences, there is an increased likelihood that the child's gross, fine, and perceptual motor abilities will be less affected, and that the gross motor potential will be commensurate with the motor level of the lower extremities.

Infant Devices

The issue of seats and various baby devices should be addressed by the therapist. The available literature on development is consistent in its insistence that all infants need to be active to acquire the strength and motor control necessary to move against gravity, attain erect sitting and standing postures, and walk. The infant must receive and integrate vast amounts of sensory and motor information to build a foundation of knowledge about his or her body and to develop the ability to function effectively within the environment. Infant walkers, jumper seats, swings, bouncer chairs, and the excessive use of infant car seats can have a negative impact on motor development and sensorimotor integration. These devices may further retard the development of the infant with spina bifida who is already at risk for motor delay. (Several of these concerns are explored in greater detail in Chapter 13.)

All infants must experience the upright sitting position because of its importance for learning. This position gives the child a new visual perspective of its surroundings and provides the first sensation of the effects of gravity, the weight of the head, and the work necessary to stabilize the head over the shoulders. However, to practice and gain confidence in these early skills, the infant must be stimulated by movement—for example, while being carried in a parent's arms. The experiences of random and varied weight shifting and tilting as the parent moves and walks are physiologically important as well. Bobbing and jerking movements of the head stimulate stretch reflexes in the joint receptors of the neck, producing muscle contractions that mark the infant's beginning attempts at head control. This stimulation is essential. However, many infant seating devices offer total support. This degree of support is unwise for the low-toned infant with spina bifida who is slow to develop head control. These infants need frequent sessions with activities that challenge the head, neck, and trunk. The infant should be actively moving and turning to see its surroundings and to appreciate gravity acting upon its body in different planes. To be passively entertained in seating devices allows little or no active participation in movement or in the learning process. The device passively entertains without offering any development benefits.

Consider the child who has sufficient lower extremity function to successfully move around the room in an infant walker. The child's position is often tilted to one side in the walker, with resultant poor alignment. Coordinated reciprocal movements are not necessary to gain momentum in this device, and weight bearing through the legs is often momentary and sporadic. A thrusting pattern is all that is necessary to propel the device. It is inappropriate to facilitate and strengthen these patterns because thrusting has no carryover for developing coordinated movements or providing stability to the lower extremities or trunk, both of which are vital components for ambulation and standing. Rather, infants should bear weight on their lower extremities while maintaining more normal, erect alignment of the trunk and upper body. In this way, much proprioceptive input is provided to the spine and legs. Parents who are concerned about the "weak" legs of their infant with spina bifida must be guided and encouraged to provide appropriate, active work for the child's whole body. When moving and playing, children use all parts of their body at once. A child who is excited by a bright object will move the arms and use the legs to lift and kick; these movements will help to strengthen the innervated musculature of the legs. Holding the infant in a standing position while offering adequate support will promote control of the upper body while offering stimulation in this upright posture.

Parents often prefer that their infant be allowed to spend short periods in infant seats or walkers because of the enjoyment afforded by the devices. Because most parents strive to keep their children happy and content, the time the infant spends in these devices often increases insidiously, further reducing the time spent moving actively around the floor. In assessing the use of such devices, one must also consider the life-style of the family. Many parents spend much time in the car, at the market or shopping center, and other places where the infant will be placed in a supported, seated position. When the time the infant spends sleeping and eating is added to this, it may become apparent that little time is spent in more therapeutic positions. However radical an approach, the therapist may find it best to totally discourage the use of these devices except, of course, in the case of an infant car seat while traveling.[14,36,55–58,63]

Orthotics

Introduction to Bracing

A discussion of orthotics is most logically approached by grouping the motor levels that require similar orthotic management. Thus, in this chapter, children with thoracic and L-1 to L-3 lesions are considered to have high-level paralysis, children with L-4 to L-5 lesions are considered to have low lumbar paralysis, and those with sacral lesions comprise the final group. Devices for early splinting, preambulation devices, and bracing for standing and ambulation will be discussed for each of the groups. Although the grouped motor levels have similarities, within each group are children with very different patterns of active musculature, strength, and function. Thus, one should remember that each child must be evaluated individually and, depending on the findings, a management plan developed. The information presented here may be useful for the therapist to consider and build upon with future experiences.[41]

Philosophies of Bracing

Many clinics have a bracing philosophy that establishes a pre-set plateau of maximum function for children with spina bifida. In addition, several publications have supported the concept that an ultimate level of mobility exists for children at each motor level. Such a philosophy advocates establishing reasonable expectations for each child because much time, effort, and expense can be spent on orthotic management. This philosophy of bracing is thought, by some, to be an efficient method that supports the notion that functional outcome is pre-

dicted by motor level. A clinic that follows this model would be reluctant to brace a child with a thoracic or high lumbar lesion after the early childhood years as the literature indicates that most adolescents with such lesions are mobile from a wheelchair, and have discarded the possibility of ambulation. However, recent research has acknowledged that a number of variables affect the ultimate level of performance of the child, of which lower extremity function is only one. CNS function, motivation, learning capacity, and desire for movement are also very important factors that should be considered when deciding whether to proceed with or terminate an ambulation program. From an ethical standpoint, one might question whether the plateau should be set by anyone other than the patient, with consideration of his or her capacity.

The middle ground may afford a more realistic view. Adopting this approach would mean that thoughts and concerns would be shared among the medical staff, the patient, and the family when establishing goals for bracing for ambulation. Because the patient's needs and abilities would constantly be changing, the goals established would also have to be flexible. Recent changes in medical care for children with spina bifida, as well as advances in orthotics technology, seem to warrant an ongoing analysis and a creative approach to help each child attain an optimal level of performance, regardless of motor level. Achievement of a particular level of function is as important for a child with a low-level lesion as it is for one with a high-level lesion.[14,36,64]

General Principles for Orthotics and Gait Training

Any discussion of bracing raises the fundamental question of whether the child should be braced high, with levels of bracing removed as motor control is mastered, or whether the child should be braced low, with sections added as the need dictates. Unfortunately, orthotic prescription is imprecise and it is a field that becomes refined with clinical experience. A brace that is applied to a moving, growing, changing child can be considered to be correct only for the period that that child remains exactly as he or she was when evaluated. This period will be shorter for the 2-year-old child than for the 10-year-old. This means that the 5- or 6-year-old youngster who is growing rapidly and is very active may require frequent brace revisions and repairs.

In order to make an appropriate brace selection, CNS function and the effects of CNS dysfunction on the child's ability to move must be considered. The orthopedic surgeon, physical therapist, and family should try to gather as much objective information about the child as possible prior to devising an orthotics program. The physical therapist should have spent time with the child and family, and should have an accurate impression of the child's motor ability. Asking parents about their perceptions of their child's motor function can provide insight into the way the family views the child. In this way, differences between at-home and clinic performance can also be identified. Parents can simply be asked to describe the ways in which the child likes to play, favorite positions, response to the upright position, degree of assistance needed to change positions, and how the child moves on the floor. (Keep in mind that it is not unusual for a parent to verbalize that the child seems not ready to be upright.) Many changes in bracing programs are based upon sound recommendations from parents working with the child at home.

Regardless of the brace ordered, families must be aware of whom to call and what action must be taken if the brace is inadequate or does not produce the desired result. They must also understand that the failure of or problems with the brace do not mean that they or their children are failures or are somehow inadequate. Families should be educated regarding both good and improper fit, when brace modification will be needed, and when it will be appropriate to add or subtract sections of the brace. With this knowledge, parents can contact the therapist or clinic with their findings so that necessary appointments can be made. Remember, changes involving increased support should not

be construed as failure, regression, or lack of progress.

Decisions to change the bracing level, unlock joints, or change an assistive device should be made in a thoughtful and considered manner. The child's attitude toward and readiness for gait training plays a large part in the timeliness of these decisions. We can aim for safe and functional ambulation by 5 or 6 years of age in preparation for mobility in school, but given the numerous tasks and skills to be mastered, 5 or 6 years is not a great deal of time to prepare. Parents and therapists may feel rushed when the child is almost ready to begin school, but sufficient time must be allowed for mastery of skills at one stage before progressing to the next. Some families are forceful when expressing their desire to have their child standing and ambulating as soon as possible. The responsible method of practice is to pace the progression of skills slowly to achieve the safest, most secure, and least stressful result for the child. In keeping with this measured approach, only one change at a time should be made to the orthosis or assistive device. Otherwise, it becomes difficult to ascertain which change produced the effects observed.

A well-defined orthotic program should begin as early as the child's first day of life. After the initial evaluation of the child, the physical therapist should discuss with the orthopedic surgeon the deformities present and those likely to occur secondary to muscle imbalance around a joint. The therapist and surgeon should then develop a plan of care, including the necessary orthotics, to address current and anticipated problems. Such an early orthotics program is designed to prepare the child for upright positioning at as close to the normal age as possible. Orthopedic surgery during the first year can be coordinated to achieve the goal of upright posture.[37,65]

Thoracic Level Paralysis

The child with no motor control below the thorax has flaccid lower extremities and is at risk for developing a frog-legged posture. This posture is common in immobile infants who remain in a supine position for long periods of time. The legs are abducted, externally rotated, and flexed at the hips and knees, with no active motion to counteract the effects of gravity. If left uncorrected, this frog-legged position will result in the muscles and other soft tissues become increasingly tight with time.

Prone positioning, daily ROM exercise, and gentle nighttime wrapping of the legs with elastic bandages into extension and abduction can prevent this deformity. Additional flexibility can be gained using these interventional strategies in areas where minimal to moderate tightness may already exist. As the child grows, a total body splint or total contact orthosis may be used during naps and throughout the night to prevent loss of motion. Proper fit of the orthosis will prevent limb movement that can lead to abrasions. Because the child also needs to work on control of the head and trunk, the first orthosis, adapted with wedged rubber soles, can be used for brief periods of standing. During these sessions of standing, the child can practice and become proficient in balance activities of increasing difficulty (Fig. 5-14). Prone lying in the splints is recommended to help avoid pressure over the bony prominences, such as the ischial tuberosities, sacrum, and calcaneous. Skin breakdown at these sites is common with persistent supine positioning. Inspection of the skin is essential after each session with the orthosis.

If the child has moderate to severe limitations in ROM, it is inappropriate to use the orthosis to force the limbs into better alignment. That type of problem will probably be managed best by surgical release of tight soft tissue structures, including the iliotibial band, hip external rotators, and knee flexors. The orthosis can be used after surgery to maintain the desired position and the newly achieved level of flexibility.

A total contact orthosis should always include a thoracolumbar section to stabilize the pelvis and lumbar spine to provide good alignment for the lower extremities. Lacking proper support of the trunk and pelvis, the child can flex the trunk later-

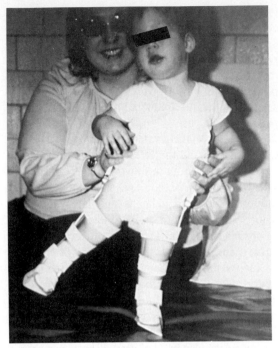

Figure 5-14. *A total contact orthosis with wedged soles may be used for standing and activities involving a shift in weight.*

ally when in the splint causing malalignment of the lower extremities with adduction of one hip and abduction of the other relative to the pelvis. A plantar-flexion deformity often develops in the child with total limb paralysis. Contractures involving the foot joints will make brace and shoe fit difficult; therefore, a total body orthosis should include a lower leg portion to hold the ankle in a neutral or plantigrade position for weight bearing.

For the older child with a high thoracic lesion who may spend most of the day without braces, a simple splint can be fabricated to maintain good foot position with the child seated in a wheelchair, thus allowing easy shoe fit. It might also be appropriate for such an individual to use a total body orthosis at night in order to decrease the flexion/abduction contracture that commonly occurs in individuals who sit all day.[6,36]

High Lumbar Paralysis

Children with a motor level from L-1 to L-3 will usually exhibit strong hip flexors and adductors but no other significant strength, either poor or fair, at the hips and knees. Such children generally benefit from use of a total body splint. The splint can maintain hip and knee extension with moderate abduction (30 degrees for both legs) if used during sleep. It can also serve as the child's first standing device.

Most children with high lumbar paralysis will require bracing to stand. Bracing is indicated to support the knees and ankles and provide medial-lateral stabilization at the hips and pelvis. A small number of children with this type of paralysis who have good balance and an intact CNS will ambulate without orthotic control at the hips and pelvis, but they will require bracing above the knees, as well as some type of assistive device. Hip subluxation and dislocation are common in children with high lumbar paralysis owing to significant muscle imbalance around the hip. There has been much discussion and debate regarding the optimal surgical approach for hip problems in such patients. The current consensus is that surgery to relocate the hip is not indicated. This approach avoids many postoperative complications, including a frozen, immobile joint, which may result from an open reduction procedure. This complication may compromise sitting and standing alignment, necessitating additional surgery. Redislocation is common owing to limited stabilization by dynamic forces around the hip. These issues have caused the orthopedic community to reevaluate their role with these children. Simple surgical release of soft tissue structures may be needed if active hip flexors and adductors have tightened to the point of restricting range. With unilateral dislocation, an asymmetric pelvis will result if the involved hip becomes limited in adduction and flexion. This asymmetric posture creates an uneven foundation for sitting and standing and interferes with proper fit and alignment of braces. Evaluation for a shoe lift will also be necessary for the child with unilateral dislocation in order to equalize leg lengths with the child upright. Aggressive procedures to relocate the hips are a thing of the past for these children.[6,36,65,66]

When hip dislocation occurs, therapists and parents must continue passive ROM exercises to ensure no additional loss of flexibility. The hips will usually tighten in flexion and adduction as a result of the abnormally positioned femur. There is often fear that additional damage will occur with ROM exercises, but this is seldom, if ever, the case. Rather, more harm is done by discontinuing the exercise.[6,36]

Orthotics for Children with High Paralysis

When children with T-12 to L-3 motor levels are almost 12 months old and exhibit adequate head control, they should be considered for upright positioning in the **A** frame (or the Toronto standing frame). This frame can be used for short standing sessions during the day in an attempt to duplicate the activities of able-bodied children who pull to a stand for short periods, but are predominantly mobile on the floor (Fig. 5-15). A schedule of upright positioning for 20 to 30 minutes four or five times each day seems manageable for most parents. Because the devices are free-standing, this represents the child's first opportunity to be upright for play without having hands-on assistance from a parent or using the upper extremities for support. Self-feeding and fine motor activities are ideal during this standing time. Parents should be instructed to challenge their child during the standing period by working on head-righting and balance skills. Slowly tilting the frame in one direction, watching for the child's righting response in the head and trunk, then repeating the tilt in another direction is a recommended activity for the first 5 to 10 minutes of each standing session. The frame should be tilted slowly and at a small angle, and all directions should be performed. Based upon the child's success, further strengthening of the responses and the musculature involved can be achieved by increasing the angle of tilting. Passive standing in front of

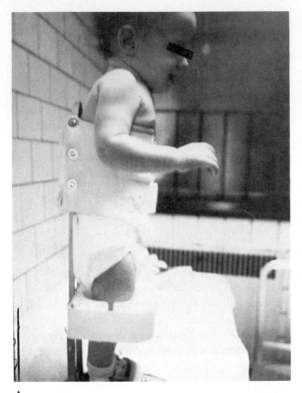
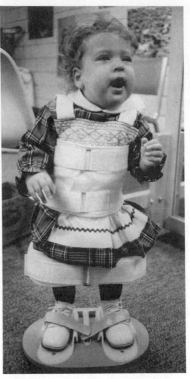

A   B

Figure 5-15. *Toronto A frame showing good alignment for standing. A. Side view. B. Front view.*

the television is not recommended, and unsupervised standing is not advisable because the child's wiggling body may cause the frame to topple.[14,36]

As the child progresses with developmental activities, such as rolling around the floor, getting into and out of a sitting position, and attempting to crawl, the child may show an intolerance for the lack of mobility of the standing frame. This indicates that the child is ready for bracing and ambulation training. Children with moderate to severe CNS deficits and delayed head and upper extremity function may continue to use the standing frames until they are unable to properly fit into the frames (at around 3 to 4 years of age). As the child outgrows the frame, the parapodium or Orlau swivel walker are orthotic options that will provide continued and valuable time in an upright posture while

providing adequate support to meet the needs of the child with significant motor delay. Regardless of the device, the child must continue a program of developmental and preambulation skills to improve function in the upper body, neck, trunk, and arms. While in the device, the child can learn to weight-shift, which will cause the device to move forward. The parapodium requires a walker or crutches for progression. The Orlau swivel walker has a ball-bearing plate at its base which allows the device to move forward on a level surface without assistive devices and with only a side-to-side swivel movement by the child. As skills improve, the child can begin ambulation training in either of the devices and may progress to another, less supportive orthosis.[36]

Until recently, the standard Hip-Knee-Ankle-

Foot orthosis (HKAFO) was the only option for the child with high paralysis. A thoracic corset could be added to the HKAFO for the child with limited trunk control,[67] but this resulted in an extremely immobile child with the potential for exercise ambulation only. Another more recent option—the Louisiana State University reciprocating gait orthosis (RGO)—has since been developed. The RGO uses a system of cables with a dual-action hip joint that flexes one lower extremity while maintaining the opposite hip in locked extension for a stable stance, thereby allowing a reciprocating pattern of gait. A properly fitted RGO provides stability at all lower extremity joints and supports the trunk and pelvis over the legs. Many children who have used the RGO and an assistive device have progressed to a more energy-efficient and safer gait pattern than was possible with the HKAFO. As a child's upper trunk stability improves, the RGO can be modified without decreasing the child's abilities. By retaining the cables and dual-action hip joints but removing the chest strap and thoracic uprights, the child can use the mechanism for an assisted reciprocating gait but with less restriction to the upper body.[68-71]

The isocentric RGO is a new device that eliminates the cable system but maintains the same function as the original RGO. Clinics using the original RGO are slowly switching to the new isocentric model when patients need their first brace, or when the patient's original RGO no longer fits and a new brace is required.[72]

With hip and knee joints locked, the child ambulating with either of these reciprocating braces and an assistive device performs a lateral weight shift onto one leg and leans slightly back at the shoulders to facilitate forward flexion of the unweighted lower extremity. Repeating the weight shift and leaning to the other side produces forward flexion of the opposite lower extremity. This gait pattern requires no active motor function in the lower extremities (Figs. 5-16 to 5-18).[70]

When using the standard HKAFO with pelvic band and locked hip joints, the child can learn a hop-to or swivel pattern of gait first, later mastering the swing-through pattern. The child with active

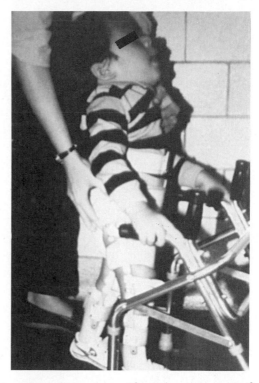

Figure 5-16. *Gait training with a reciprocating gait orthosis. A lateral weight shift with a slight tilt backward causes the unweighted leg to begin a swing phase.*

hip flexors can attempt to walk with one or both hip joints unlocked in a reciprocating gait pattern. With both hips unlocked, the child must avoid falling forward, which is made likely by the absence of functional low back extensors or gluteals. To maintain an erect posture, the child must hyperextend the lumbar spine and shift the center of gravity posteriorly. However, this set of skills requires that the child use both upper extremities to remain erect by pushing up on the walker or crutch handles (Fig. 5-19). When using a reciprocating pattern with the hip joints unlocked on the HKAFO, the pelvic band provides control of abduction/adduction and medial/lateral rotation of the lower extremities, motion the child is unable to control actively. For some children with a high lumbar lesion and an intact CNS, the pelvic band may be removed to allow further freedom with transfers and provide a faster

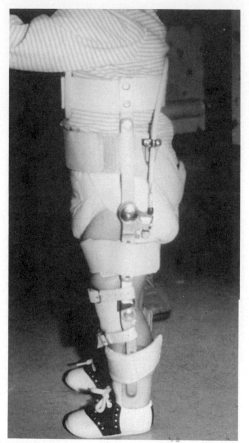

Figure 5-17. *Alignment and fit of an RGO with a thoracic strap and uprights, cable and dual action hip joints.*

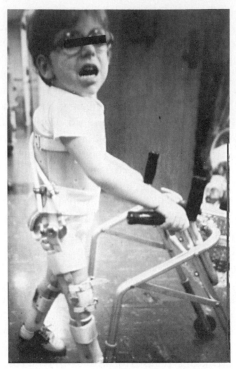

Figure 5-18. *A reciprocating gait orthosis, fit over a plastic body jacket, is used to manage scoliosis. Note the erect alignment in this child with paralysis at the level of T-8 to T- 100.*

swing-through gait pattern. Trunk stability and hyperextension of the lumbar spine are essential for a stable stance, and these factors make these children more closely resemble patients with traumatic paraplegia than those with a congenital disability.[64,65]

Regardless of the orthosis, most young children and their therapists find the rollator walker the most effective assistive device to begin gait training. With four points of stability and two wheels on the front, the rollator provides good support and the child does not have to lift the device to advance it, as occurs when progressing a standard walker. The use of parallel bars should be avoided initially during gait training because they provide too much stability and the child may develop patterns of pulling and leaning that will be dangerous when making the transition to a walker. Exceptions may be made, however, such as in cases when a child has extreme difficulty learning to use a walker. However, in these cases, the author has found that the child with difficulty has usually been braced too low (Table 5-2).

The decision to progress the child to either axillary or forearm crutches will depend upon the child's ability. The normal progression cannot be easily predicted or plotted, and a degree of experimentation is always necessary. A child wearing a body jacket to control scoliosis will often find axillary crutches difficult to use. Although axillary crutches encourage an upright position, they are

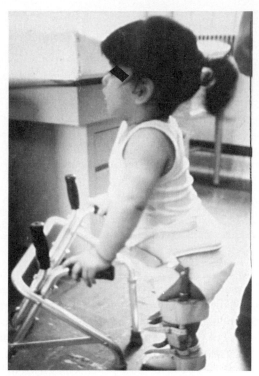

Figure 5-19. *Hip-knee-ankle-foot orthosis with hips unlocked. The child maintains balance with a hyperextended lumbar spine and support from a walker.*

best used for reciprocating or hop-to gait patterns. The swing-to and swing-through patterns are most safely and efficiently accomplished with forearm crutches. Over the years, however, the child may develop a tendency to lean forward onto the forearm crutches in a habitual posture, and this weight-bearing pattern may lead to an upper thoracic kyphosis with elevated and protracted scapulae. If kyphosis begins to develop, the therapist and family must work together with the child to maintain a flexible, erect thoracic spine and well-aligned shoulders. Prone lifts and shoulder external rotation with depression exercises, in both the prone and supine position, will help to strengthen the lower trapezius muscles, which may reduce the severity of the kyphosis.

As children with a high-level paralysis approach adolescence, many choose wheelchairs for mobility to achieve more competitive function with their peers. As transition to a wheelchair occurs, children who discard bracing usually spend little or no time standing. They will also experience the growth spurts and weight gains that are normal for all adolescents. Spending a full day in the wheelchair increases the likelihood of flexion contractures, which are very common in nonambulatory adolescents, and which can restrict proper wheelchair skills and activities. Therefore, children who

Table 5-2. *Ambulation Sequence: T-12 to L-3 Motor Level*

	CNS Status		
	Normal→Mild Deficit	*Mild→Moderate*	*Moderate→Severe*
Pre-ambulation orthosis	Toronto A Frame	Toronto A Frame	Toronto A Frame
Assess	Ambulation bracing at 15–24 months	Ambulation bracing at 15–24 months	Continue with A Frame
Ambulation orthosis	HKAFO, locked hips; rollator walker	RGO; thoracic uprights; rollator walker	Orlau swivel walker; no assistive device
Progress	As above, hips unlocked	RGO; remove uprights; rollator walker	RGO; thoracic uprights; rollator walker
Progress	As above, crutches	As above, crutches	
Progress	KAFO, pelvic band removed; crutches	Assess for further changes	Assess for further changes

HKAFO, hip–knee–ankle–foot orthosis; *KAFO,* knee–ankle–foot orthosis; *RGO,* reciprocating gait orthosis.

choose wheelchair mobility should also maintain a regimen of positioning and physical activity aimed at avoiding joint contractures and musculoskeletal deterioration. Prone positioning, standers, parapodiums, or braces can be used during prescribed therapy sessions at home or school. Swimming, wheelchair sports, wheelchair aerobics, and other activities that help to control weight and improve cardiovascular function may also be included in the activity regimen.

As with infants, consideration of upper extremity and trunk strength, coordination, and mobility is appropriate with the older children and young adults with spina bifida. Significant changes in size and weight can result in loss of strength, immobility, and, ultimately, diminished abilities.[6,36,64,65,67,73,74]

Low Lumbar Paralysis

Children with L-4 or L-5 motor function usually have strong hip flexors and adductors. Gluteus medius and tensor fascia lata may contribute to hip abduction, although the strength of these muscles may vary from "poor" to "good." Hip extension from the gluteus maximus is usually absent. These children are at risk for early hip dislocation or later progressive subluxation, depending upon the relative strengths of the muscles surrounding the hip joint. Inherent ligamentous laxity in the child with low tone also contributes to hip joint instability.

Manual muscle testing of the muscles around the knee usually shows strong quadriceps and medial hamstrings (semitendinosus and semimembranosus), but absent lateral hamstring function. Kicking and crawling during early childhood can produce an internal tibial torsion deformity owing to the unopposed pull on the tibia by the medial hamstrings. This imbalance in forces can cause a toeing-in posture during standing and gait, which is first seen as the child pulls to a stand and begins to cruise, then ambulate.

Careful manual muscle testing is crucial in children with these lower lesions because there is often great variation of motor ability at the ankle and foot

---

Display 5-7.
Common Foot Deformities in Patients with Spina Bifida

Pes calcaneous—calcaneovarus, calcaneovalgus
Talipes equinovarus—clubfoot
Pes equinus—flat foot
Convex pes valgus—rocker-bottom foot, vertical talus
Pes cavus—high arch with toe clawing
Ankle valgus

(Display 5-7). Anterior and posterior tibialis muscles, long and short toe extensors, peroneus longus and brevis muscles, and toe flexors may be functional, but the strength in these muscles may vary from "poor" to "normal." If significant imbalances in strength are found, these patients may need to be splinted at night to prevent a progressive loss of flexibility.

When dorsiflexors are stronger than plantar flexors, a calcaneous deformity may have been present at birth, or it may develop through early childhood. An exceptionally high arch—a pes cavus deformity—may be caused by the unopposed action of the anterior tibialis, which results in a foot with a reduced weight-bearing surface. The distribution of body weight is limited to the heel and ball of the foot. Bracing and shoe fit can be difficult, and surgery is often indicated to weaken or eliminate deforming forces and to realign the bones.

A calcaneovarus or calcaneovalgus foot may occur in children with low-level paralysis when there is an absence of the gastrocnemius/soleus muscle group. Various combinations of strengths and weaknesses in the musculature of the foot and ankle can produce abnormal foot alignment and abnormality of the weight-bearing surfaces of the foot. The orthopedic surgeon may consider muscle lengthening procedures and tendon transfers in an attempt to balance the dynamic forces around the joints.

Clubfoot (talipes equinovarus) is the most common foot deformity in children with spina bifida who have an L-4 or L-5 motor level (Fig. 5-20). Diagnosis and management of clubfoot has prompted extensive discussion by orthopedic surgeons. Many now suggest early taping and gentle manipulation, followed by application of a well- padded splint, rather than serial casting, which had been used extensively in recent years. This change in approach is a response to the problem of pressure over the bony prominences resulting from casting and the associated problems of irritation and skin breakdown. Clubfoot is often very resistant to conservative treatment, however, and surgical correction often provides improved distribution of weight-bearing and easier orthotic fit. Recurrence of clubfoot secondary to incomplete surgical correction is not uncommon, and may lead to irritation and skin breakdown from a brace or shoe. Gentle stretching exercises to maintain flexibility and a well-padded, properly fitting brace are important, although additional surgery to correct the deformity is almost inevitable. When tendon lengthening is used in lieu of

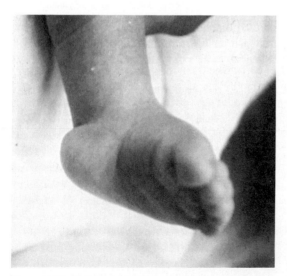

Figure 5-20. *Talipes equinovarus (clubfoot deformity) in a neonate.*

total excision of tendons to correct clubfoot, the deformity is more likely to recur. Since children with this level of motor paralysis will always need bracing to stabilize the ankle, tendon excision has no real negative impact on the child's brace level or ambulation potential. Initial surgical correction should be planned to correct the deformity completely in order to prevent additional procedures. Consistent stretching of the skin and soft tissue of the medial foot prior to clubfoot repair has been found to prevent wound dehiscence, a common complication resulting from the skin being stretched thin and taut to cover the longer, corrected foot following surgery.[6,36,74]

Debate continues regarding surgery for the child with unilateral or bilateral hip dislocation and an L4 to L5 motor level. When deciding upon a course of management, the surgeon must consider the child's total function, including lower extremity strength and developmental skills. Surgical correction may be avoided if high bracing and assistive devices are indicated by the pattern of lower extremity weakness. Surgery may also be avoided for the child with poor lower extremity strength and significant CNS involvement. Surgery may be indicated for the child with good motor control of the trunk and strong quadriceps. Active gluteus medius muscles make possible ambulation with low bracing without assistive devices, but some surgeons may choose to relocate this child's hips to prevent gait deviations that would otherwise require assistive devices. Surgery might also prevent later degenerative changes in the unstable hip that could cause pain around the hip joint in the child with normal sensation. However, other surgeons contend that bilateral dislocations should never be repaired surgically for fear that postoperative complications may diminish the child's potential for gait. Unilateral dislocation should be corrected only in the child with intact CNS function who has the potential for ambulation with short bracing, and who is unlikely to have gait deviations that require an assistive device.[37,74-76]

Children with L-4 to L-5 paralysis and significant CNS deficits are often unable to control their trunk in an upright position. This inability often conveys to the therapist the impression (often false) that a higher level of paralysis exists. The therapist and the family should continue their attempts to remediate the effects of the CNS deficit, including low tone and poor motor control, by improving coordination of the head, shoulders, and trunk. At around 3 years of age, the child may be working from a Toronto standing frame and, later, may use an RGO for gait training. Both devices offer a psychological and motivational boost for a child who has been slow to develop. If gait training is patient and thoughtful, there could be relatively easy success. Before the advent of the RGO, many children with poor trunk stability and low lumbar paralysis were fit with low bracing. These inappropriate orthotics and the ineffective attempts at gait training they caused resulted in frustration for children, parents, and therapists alike. The RGO seems to provide significant benefits to this group of children.[37,70]

The child with a lesion at L-4 to L-5 without any apparent CNS deficit can be provided with braces according to their lower extremity function (Table 5-3). Many of these children are able to pull to a stand or are attempting to stand by 10 to 12 months of age, and will not require a standing frame. If the child can control the knees while upright, use of an ankle-foot orthosis (AFO) can be initiated (Fig. 5-21). "Twister" cables, which provide a rotatory force, may be added later if rotation needs correction. Internal rotation, emanating from unequal forces behind the knee, is most common (Fig. 5-22). However, external rotation of both legs, or a combination of internal rotation of one leg and external rotation of the other leg, may occur. Twister cables can be adjusted to control any of these combinations, and are valuable in aligning the lower extremities during gait. The child may learn to control minimal rotational deviation and avoid later surgical correction. Twister cables may also assist in allowing the loose ligamentous structures at the knee

Table 5-3. *Orthotic Management for L-4 to L-5 and Sacral Motor Lesions*

	L-4 to L-5	Sacral
Muscles present	Hip flexors and adductors Quadriceps Medial hamstrings Anterior tibialis Some gluteus medius Some foot intrinsics	All, with possible exception of gluteus maximus, gastrocnemius-soleus group, ankle and foot intrinsics
Pre-ambulation orthotics	Toronto standing frame (some children may pull to stand, bypassing the frame, and begin with bracing*)	Usually none needed*
Ambulation bracing	RGO; KAFO with weak quadriceps; AFO with or without "twisters" if torsion is present*	AFO with weak gastrocnemius-soleus or crouched gait. Some need no bracing, but a shoe insert may help maintain proper foot alignment.
Assistive devices	Rollator walker or crutches. An independent gait is possible for some, usually with a gluteus medius lurch and lumbar lordosis.	Possibly a walker early on; most progress to an independent gait*
Expected functional level	Ambulatory in life unless increased body weight; flexion contractures; poor CNS status: further complications may reduce ambulatory status	Independent gait with moderate to minimal deviations based on patterns of weakness

*Control of upper body and CNS status may modify these levels.
RGO, reciprocating gait orthosis; **KAFO,** knee-ankle-foot orthosis; **AFO,** ankle-foot orthosis.

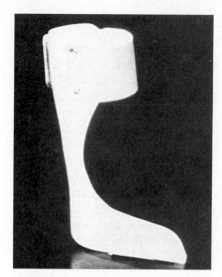

Figure 5-21. *A plastic ankle-foot orthosis is aligned at 90 degrees or at a neutral position.*

to tighten, thereby correcting some of the deviation. For children who retain the rotational deformity, surgery is usually recommended around the age of 6 years. The procedure should correct the bony malalignment and transfer the active medial hamstrings to a more midline orientation so that the deformity does not recur.

A knee-ankle-foot orthosis (KAFO) may be used for a child with weak quadriceps and difficulty maintaining either unilateral or bilateral knee extension when upright. A patellar pad will help maintain knee extension while reducing the pressure exerted across the thigh and tibial straps of the KAFO. This reduction in pressure decreases the probability of skin breakdown at those sites. Although a pad at the knee adds to the time spent donning and doffing the brace, it appears to be a valuable component that ensures a level of knee

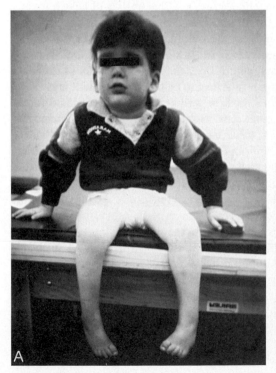
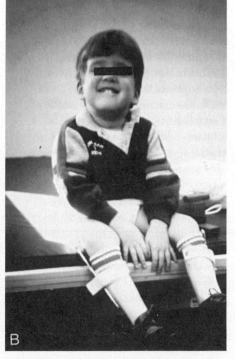

Figure 5-22. A and B. *A child with an L-4 to L-5 motor level and significant in-toeing is portrayed. Twister cables are attached to an ankle-foot orthosis to control rotation or torsion until surgery is indicated.*

extension that the more proximal and distal straps alone will not offer. If unilateral knee flexion is noted, the child should be examined prior to considering a KAFO in order to eliminate the possibility of a leg length discrepancy causing flexion of the longer limb during stance.[6,36]

Some clinics use a "floor reaction" or "anticrouch" orthosis for children who have difficulty attaining knee extension. This orthosis is an ankle-foot orthosis (AFO) with an anterior shell that facilitates knee extension at heel strike. The orthosis is theoretically sound and highly successful with other disabilities; however, almost perfect fit is needed to achieve the desired gait responses for the child with spina bifida. Problems of pressure across the anterior tibia have caused some centers to avoid this device. Regardless of the orthosis chosen, a careful assessment of the resulting gait pattern will indicate the likelihood of success or failure of a particular device.

The child with an L-4 or L-5 motor level is often able to begin ambulation after one or two sessions of gait training with a rollator walker. The family can continue working with the child at home after only a brief demonstration in the clinic. Crutch training for the young child is often more involved and lengthy, and clinicians believe that crutches may be ill-advised until the child reaches 4 or 5 years of age and has a good level of skill and self-confidence in the upright position. The child must also have a sufficient attention span to benefit, without stress, from the crutch training sessions. The child with L-4 to L-5 paralysis will often attempt independent, unassisted ambulation. The gait pattern usually includes a hyperlordotic lumbar spine and a side-to-side gluteus medius lurch. The degree of these deviations depends upon the strength of the hip extensors and abductors relative to the flexors and adductors. Gait will appear more normal when good back and abdominal strength can assist with alignment of the lumbar spine and pelvis.

Despite the high degree of activity in these children, ROM exercise remains important. A prone program is useful to counteract the hyperlordotic posture of the spine that occurs secondary to the anterior pelvic tilt with flexed hips during ambulation. Lying prone for prescribed periods during the day and through the night can minimize development of hip flexion contractures. Moderate to severe hip flexion contractures are the single most influential factor leading to the deterioration of ambulation skill in these children. Hip flexion contractures of 20 degrees or more in the child using AFOs and crutches will diminish gait velocity to 44% of normal. A 10 degree contracture reduces gait velocity to 65% of normal. Activity to maintain spinal mobility, to prevent a fixed lordotic spine, and supine and sitting activities to address abdominal muscle strength are also recommended for the long-term program at school and in the home.[37,74,75,77]

Sacral Level Paralysis

The child with sacral paralysis will have a greater degree of muscle function throughout the lower extremities than a child with spina bifida at any other motor level. In the former, muscular forces around the hips and knees are in better balance, with full or partial innervation of the hip extensors and lateral hamstrings, as well as muscles innervated from the lumbar roots. Stronger function of the gluteus medius, medial hamstrings, and quadriceps is expected in this population. The incidence of hip subluxation and dislocation is lower than at other motor levels. Significant hip flexion contractures should not develop, and abnormal torsions of the femur and tibia are not as prevalent as with lesions involving other levels. Because of the additional musculature available at the proximal joints, the gait pattern of the child with sacral innervation more closely resembles a normal gait.

Manual muscle testing demonstrates considerable variation in muscle function among children with lesions at this motor level. Variation is greatest at the foot and ankle, with the gastrocnemius/soleus being the major group that may still be weak. The toe flexors may be present and may provide some secondary ankle plantar flexion, but they are usually not strong enough to stabilize the ankle and totally replace a weak gastrocnemius/soleus. As a result, AFOs will be indicated for most of these children.

The child with sacral innervation may not need external support at the ankle if strong plantar flexors are present. Close observation, however, is necessary during childhood when there is rapid growth and changes in weight. The gastrocnemius/soleus group that is rated as having "poor" or "fair" function may adequately stabilize the tibia of a small child for proper standing and walking for short distances. As the child grows, the lever arm of the muscle will lengthen, often resulting in changes in muscle efficiency and alignment. The loss of mechanical advantage means that additional strength is needed for stabilization, but this may not be available. The gastrocnemius/soleus group controls the forward movement of the tibia over the foot as the stance phase of gait progresses from heel-strike. When strength is inadequate, a crouched gait may develop. Because the tibia is permitted to roll forward too far and too rapidly into excessive dorsiflexion, hip and knee flexion will result. The child should be observed walking during the physical therapy assessment. With strong gluteus medius and quadriceps muscles, the child may be able to stand erect, but without adequate gastrocnemius/soleus muscle function, excessive dorsiflexion and knee flexion will be noted during gait. Flexion contractures can develop if this posture is not remediated. Surgical lengthening of tight hamstrings will be necessary as a result of the changes noted above, and a once independent ambulator may need assistive devices for support. The child may develop limited ambulation capacity owing to the added energy needed for this type of gait. The crouched gait and its associated problems can be prevented simply by using an AFO when the child begins to walk. The child whose posture is maintained by an orthosis may choose to go for short periods without bracing (to a party or special event) without compromising future potential.[36]

The information now available from podiatric specialists indicates that this group of children may benefit from having molded shoe orthoses placed within the typically prescribed AFO. This arrangement may prevent many of the hindfoot and midfoot malalignments that can arise as the children grow older. Articulating ankle joints will permit limited dorsiflexion, which may be indicated for some children who are likely to benefit from the opportunity to use active musculature in the ankle and foot.[77]

The child with sacral innervation will commonly have some mild gait deviations. Compared to the child with a higher motor level, the child with sacral paralysis may appear not to need therapeutic intervention. However, benefits will likely be accrued from a program that will "fine tune" the gait. Thoracic and abdominal strengthening is recommended to address the oblique abdominals as well as the rectus abdominus. The child should also practice correct alignment of the shoulders, trunk, pelvis, and limbs during standing and ambulation. Tactile, verbal, and visual reinforcement can all be used to help the child learn and maintain proper posture for long periods of time. Children involved in a long-term program like this may still have an abnormal gait pattern but can, when they choose, assume a more correct alignment (e.g., at a party, entering a restaurant, or walking down the aisle for school graduation). Realistically, the therapist may not be able to offer the child options that more closely approximate normal movement. The more disabled patients often provide an overwhelming responsibility for a busy clinician. It is a true pleasure, however, to have the opportunity to work with children who can reach a high level of function. This process is also an educational experience. The therapist must observe closely to analyze subtle gait deviations and to deduce the areas of trunk and limb weakness that contribute to the deviation. Careful, critical observational skills benefit all patients (Fig. 5-23).

Compared to children with involvement at other motor levels, fewer children with sacral paralysis have hydrocephalus and require a shunt, and fewer exhibit pathologically low tone. Therefore, many of the CNS and biomechanical factors that negatively influence the child with spina bifida are not preva-

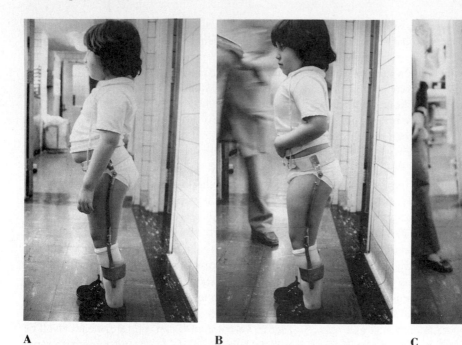

A   **B**   **C**

Figure 5-23. *Nine-year-old girl with an S-1 motor level. A. An independent gait has been achieved with ankle-foot orthoses and twisters. Note the poor alignment and low tone of the trunk, as well as the anterior pelvic tilt with hip flexion. B. Following a long-term program of active exercises for problem areas, she works hard to align the thorax and lumbar spine cortically and improve pelvic alignment. C. Increasing success with more correct posture.*

lent in children with low-level lesions. As a result, children with sacral paralysis who present with hip instability are treated aggressively if they appear to have the potential for unassisted gait.[4,36]

The use of preambulation devices may be unnecessary if the child acquires strong balance responses in the trunk and is developing a normal quality of movement. At between 10 and 15 months of age, the child may be pulling to stand independently, just as would a nondisabled child of that age. A foot splint, commonly worn at night to maintain alignment, may also be used during the day to stabilize a weak ankle for standing while awaiting definitive bracing.

For the child with CNS difficulties, it is important to follow the same course of therapy that would be prescribed for a child with a higher level lesion. The program can include activities that address flexion and extension strength against gravity through the head and trunk, and balance and equilibrium skills in all positions. The program should also include passive and active exercises for the lower extremities to prevent joint contractures.[36]

Casting After Orthopedic Surgery

Earlier in this chapter, various deformities commonly associated with different motor levels were mentioned, as were surgical procedures to correct these deformities. Following many procedures, the child is usually in some type of cast for a temporary period of immobilization to allow the surgical site to heal undisturbed. Casts should never be considered to be a benign treatment method for the child with spina bifida. Pressure and irritation of insensate skin are always risks for these children. Fractures, loss of joint flexibility, and loss of gross motor skills are commonly noted upon removal of the cast. Children with minimal CNS deficits may lose postural security and antigravity muscle strength during immobilization. It is troublesome to see children lose skills that they have worked long and hard to gain.

Most surgeons agree that children should be casted for the shortest possible time needed for adequate healing. Because of problems related to immobility, and to minimize hospitalizations, multiple anesthesias, and periods of immobility, surgeons try to plan several procedures that can be performed at one operative session. One should remember that periods of immobility are, nonetheless, necessary. Casting is an important part of the orthopedic program to reduce deformity and ultimately gain function. With some forethought and planning for the child and family, therapists can assist in making this period less of a problem.[36,78-80] Returning children as quickly as possible to their preoperative status, or to an improved status, is a postoperative objective for the therapist. Recommendations for treatment and management of the child can be discussed with the family before surgery in order to ensure that the child's needs are understood and adequate preparation is made. Most families experience a great deal of stress at this time, and the therapist may have to be available for several short sessions to accomplish all the necessary teaching.

Many children will be in hip spica casts following hip surgery. If surgery is performed for a unilateral problem, the full hip spica may still be used to stabilize the pelvis and opposite limb, thereby preventing movement and malalignment at the surgical site. With the surgeon's approval, prone positioning will help prevent pressure sores on the calcaneous, sacrum, and ischial tuberosity, and will challenge the child to lift and extend the head to watch television, read, or play. Prone positioning in a reclining wheelchair or scooter board can provide mobility if the child can use the upper extremities for propulsion; this also reduces the need for the child to be carried or moved around the house. Sim-

ilar prone positioning on a wagon for long walks outdoors may help the family survive this period with less anxiety because the child is occupied and happy. Some clever families have adapted hand trucks or dollies to safely stand and move their older, heavier child (Fig. 5-24). After several days, physicians may permit the child to stand, a position that can be maintained for long periods, especially during meals and for play. If the cast is asymmetric, towels propped under the feet will help to level the child. To ensure safety, it is necessary to lean the child on a chair, table, or sofa that will not move. In

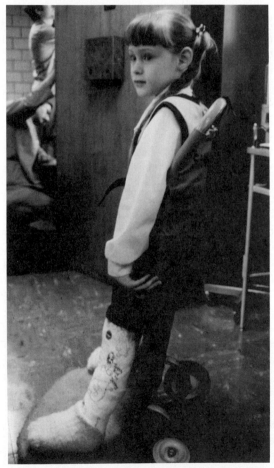

Figure 5-24. *A parent finds an imaginative and safe way of standing and moving their older child in a hip spica by adapting a commercially available hand truck.*

addition, it may be necessary for a family member to remain with the child to prevent falling. Families living in multilevel homes may have to prepare a temporary bedroom for the child on the first floor. An old mattress or a few thick blankets on the floor are usually comfortable. Instruction in strategies for safely lifting and turning the child while using good body mechanics will be appreciated by the family and the child, and are the responsibility of the physical therapist.

Regardless of the age of the child in a spica cast, daily exercise periods are important to prevent loss of neck and trunk strength and to maintain the automatic balance responses. Prone lifts, supine head lifts, standing and tilting for 15 to 20 minutes in all directions should be instituted several times each day. As the child attempts to maintain balance, muscles are working above and within the cast. This activity places stress on the bones of the lower extremities, thereby reducing demineralization and, possibly, the risk of a fracture when the cast is removed. Postural insecurity will also be reduced as vestibular and proprioceptive stimulation are provided by these challenging antigravity activities (Fig. 5-25).

In many clinics, the child is admitted for a period of intensive therapy aimed at ensuring the child's return to function following cast removal. Lower extremity ROM and strength are the immediate concerns, along with improvement in balance and the equilibrium responses of the neck and upper body, and a return to the child's former level of physical function. An increase in function can be achieved in a short period of time if the therapist properly targets all of the child's needs and does not address only lower extremity flexibility.

If the child has a high-level lesion, surgery was likely performed to gain passive flexibility for good limb alignment and brace fit. For such a child, a review of ROM exercises with the parents, an orthotic evaluation, and a review of activities to further improve upper body control may be all that is needed after cast removal. The child may then be monitored, until adequate function is achieved, through an outpatient clinic, community facility, or school physical therapy program.[36]

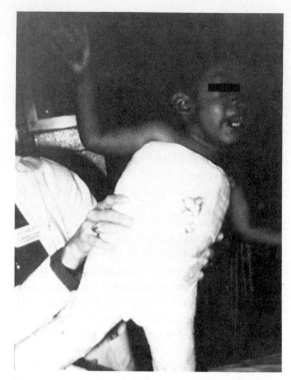

Figure 5-25. *Child with a hip spica cast after hip reduction surgery. Note how the child is both standing and being tilted. Standing, when the surgeon approves, about 10 days after surgery, is one aspect of the home care program.*

The child with a high-level lesion who demonstrates a significant loss of motion at the hip or knee is at risk for fracture. A brief hospitalization may be indicated to regain the lost mobility. The child might also be sent home in a bivalved cast, with a program of frequent ROM exercise and sedentary activities if the family is able to comply.[79,80]

Procedures to relocate or stabilize the hip joint in children with L-4 to L-5 lesions include simple tendon lengthening, femoral or pelvic osteotomy, or the more complex Lindseth procedure, which involves transfer of the external obliques. Candidates for the Lindseth procedure are those children with the potential for unassisted gait and an intact CNS. Admission to the hospital after cast removal following a Lindseth procedure may be necessary to ensure that joint mobility and balance skills are again safe and acceptable, and that the child is working toward ambulation without an assistive device.

A period of 6 to 12 weeks in a hip spica cast can reduce mobility in the lumbar spine and the lower extremities. Usually, it is difficult for the child to achieve a 90-degree angle at the hips when sitting because of tightness in the hamstrings and hip extensors after being in extension in the cast. Hip and low back tightness frequently causes abnormal alignment in sitting, with the child's pelvis rocked posteriorly, and a secondary thoracic spine kyphosis which requires remediation. Gentle activities are indicated to increase pelvic and hip mobility and strength. Active thoracic extension with active hip flexion and use of abdominal muscles will help in attaining and holding a 90-degree sitting alignment. Care should be taken to avoid placing the child in a sitting position until mobility is regained at the hips and spine.

Parents should be warned to prohibit their child from crawling after removal of a spica cast, because crawling requires hip and knee flexion exceeding 90 degrees. Hip rotation is also required as the child moves into and out of sitting and the four-point position. If the necessary flexibility and range is not present in these motions when the cast is removed, fractures may occur.[36]

Following surgery of the knees or ankles, children will have either long- or short-leg casts and the family will require instructions to avoid excessive supine positioning and sitting. These positions place pressure on the heels and will lead to skin breakdown. Flexion contractures and their associated deformities are a major concern. Sitting, crawling, and knee-walking with short leg casts will foster increased tightness of the hip and knee flexors. Information regarding alternative positions should be offered to avoid positions that encourage flexion. Prone-lying is the preferred position, and standing and ambulation are preferred activities, when feasible. Ambulation is achieved quickly when walkers, rather than crutches, are used as assistive devices during this temporary period. Lack of good balance through the trunk, poor proprioception, and possibly malaligned casts makes

crutch-training difficult. By comparison, instruction with a walker is usually a faster and safer choice. Strengthening exercises can be used for back, hip, and knee extensors, along with exercises for the trunk to help keep the child mobile during the period of casting. With such a program the child will also be likely to demonstrate a greater degree of readiness for returning to the previous, or an improved, level of function once the cast is removed.

Central Nervous System Deterioration

Throughout life, the individual with spina bifida, clinicians, and family members should be vigilant regarding any change in function that could indicate hydromyelia or a tethered spinal cord. These neurologic conditions can affect the patient's mobility, urologic function, activities of daily living (ADLs), and educational capacity. If diagnosed and treated in a timely fashion, the effects can be temporary. If left untreated, the symptoms can worsen and become permanent. Clinicians must be knowledgeable about these problems because their effects can be noted by the physical therapist during routine evaluations or reevaluations, manual muscle testing, or parent interview.[75]

Hydromyelia

Hall, Lindseth, and associates conducted a study of rapidly progressive scoliosis occurring in patients with spina bifida and found some children with excessive CSF migrating into the spinal cord.[81] Pockets of excess CSF indicated that normal CSF circulation was impaired. This collection of fluid down the spinal cord caused areas of pressure and necrosis of peripheral nerves, which resulted in the weakness that produced the rapidly progressive scoliosis. Other symptoms that have been found to be associated with hydromyelia include progressive upper extremity weakness and hypertonus. If the problem was caused by a shunt malfunction, one might expect enlarged ventricles, but computerized tomography (CT) scans have shown no such increase in the size of lateral ventricles. Nonetheless, revision of the VP shunt has produced improvement in the symptoms. In some centers, a percentage of affected children have required spinal shunting at the level of the fluid pockets to ensure that the excess fluid would be completely eliminated. Lindseth, an orthopedic surgeon, has become a strong advocate for further investigation of all cases of rapidly progressive scoliosis. He believes it is important to detect any CNS complication and not treat the scoliosis as a purely skeletal abnormality. Left untreated, the hydromyelia can cause continuing deterioration in upper and lower extremity function as the fluid collects along the spinal cord.[6,14,36,81,82]

Tethered Spinal Cord

At approximately 10 weeks' gestation, the vertebral column and spinal cord are the same length. Spinal nerves exit horizontally at their corresponding vertebrae. By 5 months' gestation, the vertebral column has grown more rapidly than the spinal cord, which at that time ends at S-1. At birth, the cord is at L-3, and by adulthood, the cord is at the L-1 to L-2 vertebral level.

A tethered spinal cord occurs when adhesions anchor the spinal cord at the site of the back lesion. The child is growing rapidly, but the cord is not free to slide upward, instead remaining bound at the level of the back defect. Excessive stretch to the spinal cord causes metabolic changes and ischemia of the neural tissue, with associated degeneration in muscle function. Rapidly progressive scoliosis, hypertonus in the lower extremities, and urologic dysfunction are attributed to tethering of the cord. Changes in the gait pattern may be seen in older children. Increased tone upon passive ROM and asymmetric changes in muscle testing results, together with areas of decreasing strength, should alert the therapist to the developing problem. Close examination by professionals and vigilance by parents can usually identify early functional changes associated with a tethered cord. When tethering is suspected, myelography is diagnostic. Subsequent neurosurgical release can free the cord, which can then migrate upward to the appropriate position. If the release is performed in a timely manner, irreversible neurologic damage can usually be prevented.[4,83–88]

Scoliosis

Hydromyelia and tethered cord should always be suspected if scoliosis develops in a child with a motor lesion below T-12. The child with thoracic paralysis does not have active trunk musculature to provide antigravity strength and is always at risk for scoliosis. However, a child with a lumbar or sacral lesion with full trunk muscle innervation should be evaluated when any curvature develops over a short time period. Clinics that provide surgical treatment for hydromyelia and tethered cord report a reduction in the overall occurrence of scoliosis requiring spinal fusion. Following untethering of the spine, there is a significant reduction, but no reports of total correction, in the severity of curvature.[82–84,88]

A group of children with spina bifida may develop scoliosis without evidence of a CNS problem. When scoliosis occurs and trunk alignment is poor, children will require additional upper extremity support to remain erect in sitting and standing. In sitting, the uneven pelvis causes pressure at areas of increased weight-bearing. Braces become ill-fitting, which can lead to deterioration of mobility, and changes in balance cause the gait to become more difficult. Propelling a wheelchair may become more strenuous because the child must work both to maintain an upright posture and to use the upper extremities effectively.

Spinal braces are useful for the child without trunk support, but surgical fusion is inevitable for most of these children. There are numerous methods for and preferred approaches to spinal fusion, and the periods of immobility and restrictions on daily activity vary with each. The type of instrumentation employed and the area and extent of the fusion will also influence these parameters.

If the fusion extends to the sacrum, pelvic mobility will diminish, and ambulatory ability will be affected. Gait analysis has shown greater excursion of movement at the pelvis in ambulatory children with spina bifida than in able-bodied children. Given this information, surgeons have been reluctant to fuse the sacral area of ambulatory children if this can be avoided. The upper extremity and trunk movement necessary for successful wheelchair propulsion are also limited if flexibility of the distal spine is diminished or absent.

The physical therapist must be concerned with postoperative activity level and resumption of mobility. Maintaining flexibility and strength in all extremities and preventing skin problems during this period of immobility must be a priority. When full activities are permitted, it is important to reassess the patient to determine whether function has been lost. Spinal fusion will influence the performance of many ADLs, new skills and adaptive strategies will need to be developed.[6,36]

Perceptual Motor and Cognitive Performance

The population of children with spina bifida represents a diverse and varied group. The children vary considerably in the problems that are present and their abilities, but therapists must be aware of possible difficulties that may affect the learning potential of their patients. This section provides a brief overview of the vast amount of information that is available on this topic (see the resources cited at the end of this chapter).

Great interest and concern has been expressed regarding the cognitive, sensory, and perceptual motor function of children with spina bifida. Studies have shown that the intelligence of this population is unrelated to motor level, severity of hydrocephalus prior to shunt insertion, or number of shunt revisions. Those complications that do influence intellect in this population include untimely treatment of hydrocephalus, cerebral infection, and other CNS problems.[4,32]

Intelligence testing for children with spina bifida places them within the normal range for most tests, but below the population mean. Willis and associates found test scores in this population to be particularly low in performance IQ, arithmetic achievement, and visual motor integration.[89] When the

children were retested at an older age, the arithmetic achievement and visual motor integration scores declined even further, but the reading and spelling abilities did not decline. These problems are thought to be attributable to a visual-perceptual-organizational deficit that influences the child's ability to solve mathematic and visual-spatial problems.[89]

Other studies have noted a high degree of attention deficit or distractibility in some children with spina bifida, these problems were especially profound in those who showed poor language development. These children had poor development of auditory figure-ground, which allows a child to recognize and to attend to relevant features in the auditory environment. A child with difficulty in this area may not be able to identify relevant auditory input and discard the irrelevant. Therefore, in a rich auditory environment, extraneous sounds distract the child from the assigned task. These children often do better in a quiet, secluded testing situation, but classroom performance for similar tasks was poor. Horn et al. found limited development of language comprehension in many of the children tested.[90] Individual vocabulary comprehension was normal, but comprehension of a story was poor. The children had difficulty identifying and retaining relevant features of the story and discarding the unimportant ones. Difficulty learning and memorizing lists of unrelated words has also been noted. However, memory for related facts was better, such as when answering questions about a short story.[90]

In the studies just mentioned, little information was available regarding the effects of early medical treatment for the child. Methods of treatment for hydrocephalus and ventricular infections were not delineated. Other factors that influence sensorimotor learning and testing outcome, including level of mobility and sensation in the trunk and lower extremity, were not mentioned. Therefore, it is difficult to determine precisely which factors may be responsible for the problems that influence learning. Decreased opportunity to develop manual skills has been thought to be a factor, as have the mobility limitations that affect the child's experiences with moving the body relative to stationary objects and manipulation and movement of those objects. Theoretical rationales for dysfunction include potential cerebellar damage from the Chiari II malformation. CNS damage affects the range, direction, force, and rate of voluntary movements and the manner in which movement is interpreted.

Any discussion of perceptual development should include problems of ocular function. Compared to the normal population, strabismus occurs six to eight times more frequently in those with spina bifida. Visual-spatial problems during manipulation activities have also been noted in some children with spina bifida. The lack of conjugate gaze influences spatial relationships, constancy of size, and development of normal visual perception for these children. Other, more frequent ocular problems in children with spina bifida include nystagmus, poor ocular motility, and other convergence defects. These abnormalities have been attributed to brain stem dysfunction, although there has been no correlation by MRI studies of the severity of the Chiari II malformation and these ocular defects.

The consensus is that children with spina bifida need a broad range of movement and learning experiences during the early years. Increased experiences in many areas may decrease the impact of any specific limitations. Testing with age-appropriate materials is critically important, and eliminating test items that include a motor component affords a more accurate and valid result[91-97] (Fig. 5-26).

Wheelchair Mobility

Much of this chapter has been devoted to bracing and ambulation issues, but some type of seated mobility must also be considered for the many children for whom this is appropriate and necessary. Any decision to use one of the many devices should include the patient, family, and professional staff involved with the child. It is appropriate first to determine the need for and proposed uses of seated mobility. Is it for recreation and peer group interaction, indoor or outdoor use, or for use at school or preschool? A first device might be a hand-propelled caster cart or star car ordered through a medical supply company. Many commercially available electric cars or motorcycles can be modified with a hand switch rather than the usual foot pedal. These devices are inexpensive and low to the ground, facilitating transfer to the floor or to a standing position. They are cosmetically appealing and are acceptable to disabled and able-bodied children alike.

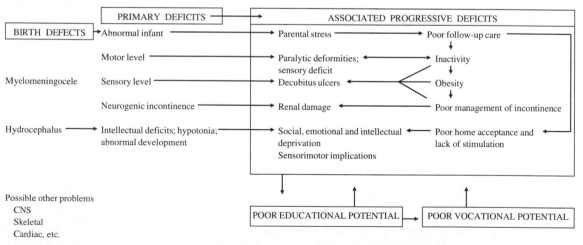

Figure 5-26. *Primary and progressive deficits in children with spina bifida. (Adapted from Syllabus of Instructional Courses, American Academy for Cerebral Palsy, 1974.)*

They can be fast and safe when used in the proper environment, and provide beneficial stimulation and opportunities for socialization. The child's upper extremity ability and the presence of abnormal tone can guide the therapist in selecting the correct device, whether manual or electric. Excessive upper extremity work to propel and maneuver a device may frustrate the child and produce unacceptable changes in tone. One study examined young children with otherwise poor mobility who used motorized chairs. Benefits noted included increased curiosity, initiative, motivation, communication, exploration, and interaction with objects in the environment. There were also significant decreases in dependency and in demanding and hostile behaviors.[98]

The family that needs a wheelchair so that their child can be included on trips out-of-doors can use a stroller until the child is 5 or 6 years of age. Strollers are available in larger sizes, and can be used in combination with ambulation. It is not unusual for an able-bodied child of that age to ride in a stroller for periods of time during a family outing.

A traditional wheelchair can be obtained prior to the child starting school. Safe transportation on the school bus is an issue. The therapist may have to research the method of transportation to be used. The smaller child can be carried onto the bus and secured in a regular seat. The child would then ambulate at school. Knowing which wheelchairs can be safely secured on the bus in a particular community will be helpful for the child who is not ready to ambulate (Fig. 5-27).

Other indications for a wheelchair include lack of efficient community mobility, resulting in limited cognitive and psychosocial experiences; marginally functional or unsafe ambulation; speed in ambulation that is inadequate to maintain a level consistent with peers and/or family; and increasing recreational activities.

The therapist should remember the increased risks for the child in a wheelchair. Scheduling time to use the chair and time out of the chair should be considered. The chance of abandonment of a gait program by a child with the potential of reaching a

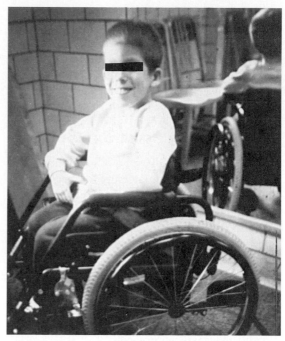

Figure 5-27. *A light-weight wheelchair is selected for long-distance use in the school and community. This child also uses a reciprocating gait orthosis for shorter distances in the home and school.*

high level of efficient ambulation is always a risk of wheelchair use. Flexion contractures of the hips and knees, pressure problems, and spinal deformity are other issues for the seated child. Therefore, the child should spend time both out of the chair and out of the seated position every day. Prone positioning, standing in a prone or a supine stander, and ambulation are options available for the child.

As the child matures and mobility needs change, an electric wheelchair or cart can provide added speed and efficiency. A motorized device, which will conserve energy, may be very important for the individual facing a full and hectic day at school or work.

Various wheelchair cushions may prevent or reduce the development of pressure sores. Several materials are available, including high-density foam, which can be modified for even weight distribution. Regardless of the cushion chosen, activities for pressure relief are the best means of preventing skin breakdown on the posterior thighs and buttocks and should be performed, without fail, throughout the day. Frequent wheelchair push-ups and out-of-chair time should be incorporated into the daily schedule to provide for regular pressure relief.[6,14,36,98–100]

The Adult with Spina Bifida

Care of the patient with spina bifida does not end with the move to an adult facility for medical care. Being aware of the abilities, problems, and concerns of the adult with spina bifida is helpful for the clinician specializing in pediatric care. By analyzing the aging process and its effect on the patient, the therapist may develop a perspective that will influence younger patients. Seeing the long-term effects of many surgical and other therapeutic interventions can provide insight into areas of weakness and can improve the approach to care by modifying existing management protocols.[101]

In a study of patients with spina bifida, Dias et al. found that 80% lived with parents or other relatives.[102] Half of those individuals were older than 30 years of age. Eighty-two percent had achieved some level of independence, whereas 6% were totally dependent. Seventeen patients had married and were living away from family members. The degree of independence was not related to the lesion level or degree of ambulation achieved.[102] Dunne and Shurtleff identified some common complaints of adults with spina bifida, including obesity, social incontinence, recurrent urinary tract in-fections, chronic decubiti, joint pain, hypertension, neurologic deterioration, and depression.[103] McLone and colleagues cited other problem areas affecting the adult with spina bifida, including job training, employment, and achieving psychological and physical independence from family.[104] These studies indicate that the adult population has multiple and varied needs that may best be met by a multidisciplinary team approach.

Conclusion

There are many approaches to treating children with spina bifida. The disability is a complex one that requires an understanding of the many systems that are affected by its presence. The information presented in this chapter provides a background for a better understanding of this birth defect. Depending upon the setting in which the physical therapist is employed, certain sections of the chapter may be more or less relevant. Concerns and strategies for intervention suggested throughout this chapter reflect a general philosophy that physical therapists must be knowledgeable and aware of all facets of the disability. The therapist should also be sensitive to the protocols and concerns of the other professionals treating the child. The true challenge to the physical therapist is to integrate these various perspectives into a creative treatment plan that produces the best result for each child. Combining experimentation and exploration, the therapist will discover new ideas for treatment that will help the child progress to his or her most productive and functional ability.

References

1. Morrisey RT. Spina bifida: A new rehabilitation problem. *Orthoped Clin North Am.* 1978;9:379–389.
2. Myers GJ. Myelomeningocele: The medical aspects. *Pediatr Clin North Am.* 1984;31:165–175.
3. Lunsky AM, Ulcicus M, Rothman KJ, Willett W, et al. Maternal heat exposure and neural tube defects. *J Am Med Assoc.* 1992;268:882–885.
4. McClone D. Neurosurgical management and operative closure for myelomeningocele. Presented at the

Annual Myelomeningocele Seminar; 1982; Chicago.

5. Scarff TB, Fronczak S. Myelomeningocele: A review and update. *Rehab Lit.* 1981;42:143–147.

6. Tachdjian MO. *Pediatric Orthopedics.* 2nd ed. Vol 3. Philadelphia: WB Saunders; 1990;1773–1880.

7. Behrman RC, Vaughn VC, eds. *Nelson's Textbook of Pediatrics.* 11th ed. Philadelphia: WB Saunders; 1979.

8. Wolraich M. The association of spina bifida occulta and myelomeningocele. Presented at the 2nd Symposium on Spina Bifida; 1984; Cincinnati, Ohio.

9. Fidas A, MacDonald HL, Elton RA, McInnes A, et al. Prevalence of spina bifida occulta in patients with functional disorders of the lower urinary tract and its relation to urodynamics and neurophysiological measurements. *Br Med J.* 1989;298:357–359.

10. D'Agasta SD, Banta JV, Gahm N. The fate of patients with lipomeningocele. Presented at the American Academy of Cerebral Palsy and Developmental Medicine (ACPDM); 1987; Boston.

11. Kanev PM, Lemire RJ, Loeser JD, Berger MS. Management and long-term follow-up review of children with lipomyelomeningocele. *J Neurosurg.* 1990;73: 48–52.

12. Moore KL. *The Developing Human: Clinically Oriented Embryology.* Philadelphia: WB Saunders; 1974.

13. Robbins SL. *Pathologic Basis of Disease.* Philadelphia: WB Saunders; 1974.

14. Umphred DA, ed. *Neurological Rehabilitation.* St. Louis: CV Mosby; 1985.

15. Sharrard WJ. Neuromotor evaluation of the newborn. In: *Symposium on Myelomeningocele.* St. Louis: CV Mosby; 1972.

16. Peach B. The Arnold-Chiari malformation. *Arch Neurol.* 1965;12:165.

17. Peach B. The Arnold-Chiari malformation. *Arch Neurol.* 1965;12:109.

18. McCullough DC. Arnold-Chiari malformation—Theories of development. Presented at the 2nd Symposium on Myelomeningocele; 1984; Cincinnati, OH.

19. McLone DG, Knepper PA. The cause of Chiari II malformation: A unified theory. *Ped Neurosci.* 1989;15:1–12.

20. Lutschg J, Meyer E, Jeanneret-Iseli C, Kaiser G. Brainstem auditory evoked potential in myelomeningocele. *Neuropediatrics.* 1985;16:202–204.

21. Hesz N, Wolraich M. Vocal cord paralysis and brainstem dysfunction in children with spina bifida. *Dev Med Child Neurol.* 1985;27:528–531.

22. Hoffman HJ, Hendrick EB, Humphreys RP, et al. Manifestations and management of Arnold-Chiari malformation in patients with myelomeningocele. *Child's Brain.* 1975;1: 255–259.

23. Staal MJ, Melhuizen-de Regt MJ, Hess J. Sudden death in hydrocephalic spina bifida aperta patients. *Ped Neurosci.* 1987;13:13–18.

24. Pilu G, Romero R, Reece A, Goldstein I, et al. Subnormal cerebellum in fetuses with spina bifida. *Am J Obstet Gynecol.* 1988;158:1052–1056.

25. Benacerraf BR, Stryker J, Frigotto FD. Abnormal ultrasound appearance of the cerebellum (banana sign): Indirect sign of spina bifida. *Pediatr Radiol.* 1989;171:151–153.

26. Thiagarajah S, Henke J, Hogge WA, Abbitt PL. Early diagnosis of spina bifida: The value of cranial ultrasound markers. *Obstet Gynecol.* 1990;76:54–57.

27. Bensen J, Dillard RG, Burton BK. Open spina bifida: Does cesarean section delivery improve prognosis? *Obstet Gynecol,* 1988;71:532–534.

28. Luthy DA, Wardinsky T, Shurtleff DB, Hollenbach KA, et al. Cesarean section before the onset of labor and subsequent motor function in infants with myelomeningocele diagnosed antenatally. *N Engl J Med.* 1991;324:662–666.

29. Shurtleff DB, Luthy DA, Benedetti TJ, Hickok DE, et al. Perinatal management, cesarean section and outcome in fetal spina bifida. Presented at the American Academy of Cerebral Palsy and Developmental Medicine; 1987; Boston.

30. Hogge WA, Dungan JS, Brooks MP, Dilks SA. Diagnosis and management of prenatally detected myelomeningocele: A preliminary report. *Am J Obstet Gynecol.* 1990;163:1061–1064.

31. Raimondi AJ, Soare P. Intellectual development in shunted hydrocephalic children. *Am J Dis Child.* 1974;127:664–671.

32. McLone DG, Czyzewski D, Raimondi AJ, et al. Central nervous system infections as a limiting factor in the intelligence of children with myelomeningocele. *Pediatrics.* 1982;70:338–342.

33. Ellenbogen RG, Goldmann DA, Winston KW. Group B streptococcal infections of the central nervous system in infants with myelomeningocele. *Surg Neurol.* 1988;29:237–242.

34. Banta J. Long-term ambulation in spina bifida. Presented at the American Academy of Cerebral Palsy and Developmental Medicine; Chicago; 1983.

35. Murdoch A. How valuable is muscle charting? *Physiotherapy.* 1980;66:221–223.

36. Schafer M, Dias L. *Myelomeningocele: Orthopedic Treatment.* Baltimore. Williams and Wilkins; 1983.

37. *An Introduction to Hydrocephalus.* Children's Memorial Hospital; Chicago, IL; 1982.

38. Raimondi AJ. Complications of ventriculoperitoneal shunting and a critical comparison of the 3-piece and 1-piece systems. *Child's Brain.* 1977;3:321–342.

39. Bell WO, Sumner TE, Volberg FM. The significance of ventriculomegaly in the newborn with myelodysplasia. *Child's Nervous System.* 1987;3:239–241.

40. Bell WO, Arbit E, Fraser R. One-stage myelomeningocele closure and ventriculo-peritoneal shunt placement. *Surg Neurol.* 1987;27:233–236.

41. Manning J. Facilitation of movement—the Bobath approach. *Physiotherapy.* 1972;58:403–408.

42. Daniels L, Williams M, Worthingham C. *Muscle Testing: Techniques of Manual Examination.* Philadelphia: WB Saunders; 1956.

43. Strach EH. Orthopedic care of children with myelomeningocele: A modern program of rehabilitation. *Br Med J.* 1967;3:791–794.

44. Asher M, Olson J. Factors affecting the ambulatory status of patients with spina bifida cystica. *J Bone Joint Surg.* 1983;65A:350–356.

45. Bunch W. Progressive neurological loss in myelomeningocele patients. Presented at the American Academy of Cerebral Palsy and Developmental Medicine Conference; San Diego; 1982.

46. Coon V, Donato G, Houser C, et al. Normal ranges of hip motion in infants. *Clin Orthop.* 1975;110:256–260.

47. Haas S. Normal ranges of hip motion in the newborn. *Clin Orthop Related Res.* 1973;91:114–118.

48. Dias L. Hip contractures in the child with spina bifida. Presented at the 2nd Symposium on Spina Bifida; 1984; Cincinnati, OH.

49. Banta JV, Lin R, Peterson M, et al. The team approach in the care of the child with myelomeningocele. *J Prosthet Orthot.* 1989;2:263–273.

50. Lie HR, Lagergren J, Rasmussen F, et al. Bowel and bladder control of children with myelomeningocele: A Nordic study. *Dev Med Child Neurol.* 1991;33:1053–1061.

51. Brem AS, Martin D, Callaghan J, et al. Long-term renal risk factors in children with myelomeningocele. *J Pediatr.* 1987;110:51–55.

52. Anagnostopoulos D, Joannides E, Kotsianos K. The urological management of patients with myelodysplasia. *Pediatr Surg Int.* 1988;3:347–350.

53. Wolf LS. Early motor development in children with myelomeningocele. Presented at the American Academy of Cerebral Palsy and Developmental Medicine; Washington DC; 1984.

54. Mazur JM. Hand function in patients with spina bifida cystica. *J Pediatr Orthop.* 1986;6:442–447.

55. Anderson P. Impairment of a motor skill in children with spina bifida cystica and hydrocephalus: An exploratory study. *Br J Psychol.* 1977;68:61–70.

56. Bobath B. Motor development, its effect on general development and application to the treatment of cerebral palsy. *Physiotherapy.* 1971;57:526–532.

57. Bobath B. The treatment of neuromuscular disorders by improving patterns of coordination. *Physiotherapy.* 1969;55:18–22.

58. Bobath B. The very early treatment of cerebral palsy. *Dev Med Child Neurol.* 1967;9:373–390.

59. Caplan F. *The First Twelve Months of Life.* New York: Grosset and Dunlap; 1973.

60. Turner A. Upper-limb function in children with myelomeningocele. *Dev Med Child Neurol.* 1986; 28:790–798.

61. Turner A. Hand function in children with myelomeningocele. *J Bone Joint Surg (Br).* 1985;67:268–272.

62. Agness PJ. Learning disabilities and the person with spina bifida. Presented at the Spina Bifida Association of America Meeting; 1980; Chicago.

63. Cronchman M. The effects of babywalkers on early locomotor development. *Dev Med Child Neurol.* 1986;28:757–761.

64. Charney EB, Melchionni JB, Smith DR. Community ambulation by children with myelomeningocele and high level paralysis. Presented at the American Academy of Cerebral Palsy and Developmental Medicine; San Francisco; 1989.

65. Beaty JH, Canale ST. Current concepts review. Orthopedic aspects of myelomeningocele. *J Bone Joint Surg (Am).* 1990;72:626–630.

66. Menelaus M. Hip dislocation: Concepts of treatment. Presented at the 2nd Symposium on Spina Bifida; 1984; Cincinnati, Ohio.

67. Stauffer ES, Hoffer M. Ambulation in thoracic paraplegia. *J Bone Joint Surg.* 1972; 54A:1336. Abstract.

68. Hoffer MM, Feiwell EE, Perry R; et al. Functional ambulation in patients with myelomeningocele. *J Bone Joint Surg* 1973;55A:137–148.

69. Yngve D, Douglas R, Roberts JM. The reciprocating gait orthosis in myelomeningocele. *J Pediatr Orthop.* 1984;4:304–310.

70. Dias L, Tappit-Emas E, Boot E. The reciprocating gait orthosis: The Children's Memorial experience. Presented at the American Academy of Developmental Medicine and Child Neurology; 1984; Washington DC.

71. Douglas R, Larson PF, D'Ambrosia R, et al. The LSU reciprocating gait orthosis. *Orthopedics.* 1983;6:834–839.

72. Center for Orthotics Design, Inc.

73. Williams L. Energy cost of walking and of wheelchair propulsion by children with myelodysplasia. *Dev Med Child Neurol.* 1983; 25:617–624.

74. McDonald CM, Jaffe KM, Mosca VS, et al. Ambulatory outcome of children with myelomeningocele: Effect of lower extremity muscle strength. *Dev Med Child Neurol.* 1991;33:482–490.

75. Schopler SA, Menelaus MB. Significance of the strength of the quadriceps muscles in children with myelomeningocele. *J Pediatr Orthop.* 1987;7:507–512.

76. Sherk HH, Uppal GS, Lane G, et al. Treatment versus nontreatment of hip dislocations in ambulatory patients with myelomeningocele. *Dev Med Child Neurol.* 1991;33:491–494.

77. Knutson LM, Clark DE. Orthotic devices for ambulation in children with cerebral palsy and myelomeningocele. *Phys Ther.* 1991;71:947–960.

78. Drummond D. Post-operative fractures in patients with myelomeningocele. *Dev Med Child Neurol.* 1981;23:147–150.

79. Rosenstein BD, Greene WB, Herrington RT, et al. Bone density in myelomeningocele: The effects of ambulatory status and other factors. *Dev Med Child Neurol.* 1987;29:486–494.

80. Lock TR, Aronson DD. Fractures in patients who have myelomeningocele. *J Bone Joint Surg (Am).* 1989;71:1153–1157.

81. Hall P, Lindseth R, Campbell R, et al. Scoliosis and hydrocephalus in myelomeningocele patients: The effect of ventricular shunting. *J Neurosurg.* 1979;50: 174–178.

82. Mazur JM, Menelaus MB. Neurologic status of spina bifida patients and the orthopedic surgeon. *Clin Orthop Rel Res.* 1991;264:54–64.

83. Banta J. The tethered cord in myelomeningocele: Should it be untethered? *Dev Med Child Neurol.* 1991;33:167–176.

84. McLaughlin TP, Banta JV, Gahn NH, Raycroft JF. Intraspinal rhizotomy and distal cordectomy in patients with myelomeningocele. *J Bone Joint Surg (Am).* 1986;68:88–94.

85. Mazur J, Stillwell A, Menelaus M. The significance of spasticity in the upper and lower limbs in myelomeningocele. *J Bone Joint Surg (Br).* 1986;68:213–217.

86. Flanagan RC, Russell DP, Walsh JW. Urologic aspects of tethered cord. *Urology.* 1989;33:80–82.

87. Kaplan WE, McLone DG, Richards I. The urological manifestation of the tethered spinal cord. *J Urol.* 1988;140:1285–1288.

88. Grief L, Stalmasek V. Tethered cord syndrome: A pediatric case study. *J Neurosci Nurs.* 1989;21:86–91.

89. Willis KE, Holmbeck GN, Dillon K, McLone DG. Intelligence and achievement in children with myelomeningocele. *J Pediatr Psychol.* 1990;15: 161–176.

90. Horn DG, Pugzles Lorch E, Lorch RF, Culatta B. Distractibility and vocabulary deficits in children with spina bifida and hydrocephalus. *Dev Med Child Neurol.* 1985;27:713–720.

91. Wolfe GA, Kennedy D, Brewer K, Jacobs RA. Visual perception and upper extremity function in children with spina bifida. Presented at the American Academy of Cerebral Palsy and Developmental Medicine; San Francisco; 1989.

92. Cull C, Wyke MA. Memory function of children with spina bifida and shunted hydrocephalus. *Dev Med Child Neurol.* 1984;26:177–183.

93. Mauk JE, Charney EB, Nambiar R, Diamond GR. Strabismus and spina bifida. Presented at the American Academy of Cerebral Palsy and Developmental Medicine; 1987.

94. Lennerstrand G, Gallo JE. Neuro-ophthalmological evaluation of patients with myelomeningocele and Chiari malformations. *Dev Med Child Neurol.* 1990;32:415–422.

95. Rothstein TB, Romano PE, Shoch D. Meningomyelocele. *Am J Ophthalmol.* 1974;77:690–693.

96. Horn DG, Lorch EP, Lorch RF, et al. Distractibility and vocabulary deficits in children with spina bifida and hydrocephalus. *Dev Med Child Neurol.* 1985; 27:713–720.

97. Ruff HA. The development of perception and recognition of objects. *Child Dev* 1980;51:981–992.

98. Butler C. Effects of powered mobility on self-initiated behaviors of very young children with locomotor disability. *Dev Med Child Neurol.* 1986;28:325–332.

99. DeLateur B, Berni R, Hangladarom T, et al. Wheelchair cushions designed to prevent pressure sores. *Arch Phys Med Rehabil.* 1976;57:129–135.

100. Fiewell E. Seating and cushions for spina bifida. Presented at the 2nd Symposium on Spina Bifida; 1984; Cincinnati, OH.

101. Borjeson MC, Lagergren JL. Life conditions of adolescents with myelomeningocele. *Dev Med Child Neurol.* 1990;32:698–706.

102. Dias LS, Fernandez AC, Swank M. Adults with spina bifida: A review of seventy-one patients. Presented at the American Academy of Cerebral Palsy and Developmental Medicine; Boston; 1987.

103. Dunne KB, Shurtleff DB. The medical status of adults with spina bifida. Presented at the American Academy of Cerebral Palsy and Developmental Medicine; 1987.

104. McLone DG. Spina bifida today: Problems adult face. *Semin Neurol.* 1989;9:169–175.

Bibliography

Williamson GG. *Children with Spina Bifida: Early Intervention and Pre-School Programming.* Baltimore: Brooks Publishers; 1987. (Family concerns and PT/OT interventional strategies)

Scherzer A, Tscharnuter I. *Early Diagnosis and Therapy in Cerebral Palsy.* New York: Marcel Dekker Inc.; 1982. (Handling strategies for young children)

Pediatric Physical Therapy,
second edition, edited by Jan
Stephen Tecklin. J. B. Lippincott
Company, Philadelphia © 1994.

6

Christine R. Morgan

Pediatric Oncology

For each of the common childhood cancers, the survival rate has increased over the past several decades. In the 1960s, for example, less than 20 percent of children with acute lymphoblastic leukemia survived for more than 5 years, whereas in the 1980s, more than 70 percent survived.[1] Along with the physical problems directly related to the oncologic diseases, the various forms of medical management cause side effects that often require intervention by several disciplines. Thus, increasing numbers of pediatric physical therapists will be treating these children, not only in acute care hospitals, but in rehabilitation, outpatient, home care,

and school settings as well. For these reasons, pediatric physical therapists need to be informed about the wide range of pediatric oncologic diseases, current medical management, and the resultant side effects of these treatments.

Treatment of children with cancer is performed at pediatric cancer centers throughout the United States. These centers enroll patients in clinical trials that are monitored by the National Cancer Institute to ensure consistency of treatment across the country. These cancer centers are often associated with one of two national groups: (1) the Children's Cancer Study Group (CCSG) and (2) the Pediatric Oncology Group (POG). Each of these groups meets biannually to review results of current studies and to develop plans for new treatment strategies.[2]

Incidence

Cancer is the chief cause of death by disease and the second leading cause of death overall, following trauma, in children ages 1 to 14 years. An estimated 7800 new cases of cancer in children occurred in the United States in 1991, with an estimated 1500 deaths, one third of which were attributable to leukemia.[3]

Etiology

The causes of childhood cancer are largely unknown. However, several environmental and genetic factors have been associated with an increased risk of cancer in children.[4,5] One environmental factor is *ionizing radiation*. Exposure to radiation in infancy and childhood can be the result of atomic bomb explosions, nuclear fallout or, more commonly, the use of irradiation for medical treatment.[6] Chemical agents, including some types of hormones and chemotherapeutic agents,[5] have also been implicated as carcinogens in humans.

Certain pediatric cancers may have both a hereditary and nonhereditary form, including Wilms' tumor and retinoblastoma. Also, certain hereditary diseases or chromosomal disorders, such as neurofibromatosis, which has an increased association with several forms of pediatric cancer, or Down's syndrome, which has an increased link to childhood leukemia,[5] may predispose children to cancer.

Signs and Symptoms

Common signs and symptoms of cancer in children can include fever, pain, a mass or swelling, bruising, pallor, headaches, neurologic changes, and visual disturbances.[3] Children may often be misdiagnosed initially, as these signs and symptoms are frequently seen in other common pediatric disorders.

Types of Cancers

Childhood cancers generally vary from those seen in adults. The most frequently seen cancers of adulthood involve the lung, breast, colon, and skin, whereas those in children most often include the leukemias, embryonal tumors, and sarcomas. Common types of pediatric cancers include the following:

- Leukemia
- Central nervous system (CNS) tumors
- Lymphomas
- Neuroblastoma
- Wilms' tumor
- Bone cancer
- Rhabdomyosarcoma
- Retinoblastoma

Leukemia

Leukemia is a malignant disease of the blood that originates in the bone marrow, the gel-like substance which fills the inner cavities of bones.[7] The marrow produces various blood components, including erythrocytes or red blood cells, thrombocytes or platelets, and leukocytes or white blood cells. In leukemia, undifferentiated or immature white blood cells, called blasts, tend to proliferate in the bone marrow. The accumulation of these nonfunctional cells eventually inhibits the production of normal blood cells, thus resulting in the typical signs and symptoms related to deficiencies of these cells (Table 6-1). Leukemia cells may also begin to invade various organs of the body, causing enlargement and dysfunction.[7]

Leukemia is the most common form of cancer in children, comprising approximately 2500 cases per year. There are two major types of leukemia in children; acute lymphoblastic leukemia (ALL) and acute myelogenous leukemia (AML). The ratio of occurrence of ALL to AML is 4:1.[8]

ALL, also called acute lymphocytic or acute lymphatic leukemia, is the most common form of pediatric leukemia. It is slightly more common in boys than in girls, and occurs more frequently in

Table 6-1. *Explanation of the Complete Blood Count (CBC)**

	Red Blood Cells (Erythrocytes)	White Blood Cells (Leukocytes)	Platelets (Thrombocytes)
Function	Contain hemoglobin which carries O_2 to the body and returns CO_2 to the lungs	Mobilize body's defense system against infection	Prevent and stop bleeding by clumping together to form a clot at the site of injury
Normal values	Hemoglobin: Infant/child, 12 g/dL Adult female, 12–16 g/dL Adult male, 13–18 g/dL	7000–11,000 (off chemotherapy) 1500–4000 (on chemotherapy)	150,000–400,000/mm^3
Name for low value	Anemia	Neutropenia	Thrombocytopenia
Low value	< 8 g/dL	ANC† <500	<20,000/mm^3
Signs and symptoms associated with low values	Fatigue, pale lips, pale skin, loss of appetite	No obvious signs	Bleeding gums, nose bleeds, increased bruising, petechiae

*Information adapted from Children's Hospital of Philadelphia Information for Parents Instructions for Home Management of a Child with Cancer
†Absolute neutrophil count

whites than in nonwhites.[9] The peak age of occurrence is 3 to 4 years.[8]

AML, also called acute granulocytic leukemia or acute nonlymphocytic leukemia, primarily affects adults, but is the second most common form of leukemia in children. Like ALL, AML also occurs slightly more frequently in males than in females,[8] and in whites more frequently than in nonwhites.[9] It is more common in teens than in children ages 1 to 10 years, although no peak age is evident.[10]

Chronic forms of leukemia, including chronic myelogenous leukemia (CML), also exist but are rare in the pediatric population.[8]

Symptoms of leukemia include fever, pallor, bone pain, lethargy, anorexia, and bleeding.[11] The diagnosis of leukemia in children is made initially on the basis of an abnormal complete blood count (CBC), and definitively by a bone marrow biopsy.

Initial treatment of leukemia is generally a 2- to 3-year process which includes the following stages:

- Induction Phase—An attempt to eradicate all malignant cells from the body
- Remission—An apparent disappearance of disease symptoms and abnormal cells in the bone marrow

- Consolidation/Maintenance Therapy—Continuation of treatment despite remission, as a significant number of undetectable cells may persist and could proliferate without further therapy

A relapse is a reappearance of leukemic cells in the bone marrow with a recurrence of all signs and symptoms.[7]

Generally, treatment protocols vary according to the type and severity of the leukemia, and may include any or all of the following:

- Combinations of chemotherapeutic agents
- Intrathecal injections of chemotherapeutic drugs into the CNS*
- CNS irradiation*

Bone marrow transplantation (BMT) may be performed if a compatible donor is available. BMT is generally performed after the first relapse in patients with ALL but, in those with AML, it may be performed as soon as the first remission is achieved since the prognosis is significantly poorer.[13]

*Specific treatment of the CNS may be necessary as many chemotherapeutic agents do not readily cross the blood-brain barrier.[12]

Brain Tumors

Brain tumors are the most common form of solid tumors in children, and the second most common form of pediatric cancer overall.[9,14] Brain tumors are occasionally congenital, occur most frequently in children ages 1 to 10 years of age, and are slightly more common in males than in females.[9] Signs and symptoms of brain tumors in children vary widely according to the size and location of the tumor. Common symptoms include headaches, nausea, vomiting, irritability, balance disturbances, ataxia, hemiparesis, and visual problems.[15,16]

Treatment of brain tumors may include surgical resection (if possible), including total resection or tumor debulking. Irradiation is also a primary treatment for CNS tumors, although it must be used cautiously in young children owing to the late effects of decreased IQ and learning problems seen in patients who have received cranial irradiation.[17] Chemotherapy may be utilized to treat CNS tumors, although its effectiveness is often significantly decreased owing to difficulty in crossing the blood–brain barrier.[12] Shunt placement may be necessitated by blockage of cerebrospinal fluid (CSF) flow by the tumor, which may result in increased intracranial pressure.[18] Prior to shunting, however, it is important to ensure that no malignant cells are present in the CSF as, otherwise, the procedure may increase the risk of spread to other parts of the body.

Some postoperative problems commonly associated with CNS tumors include limited range of motion of the neck, hemiparesis, ataxia or dysmetria, weakness, and speech and/or visual problems.

The most common pediatric brain tumors include:

- Medulloblastoma
- Astrocytoma
- Ependymoma
- Brain stem glioma
- Craniopharyngioma[18]

Medulloblastoma

Medulloblastomas comprise 10 to 20 percent of primary CNS tumors, occurring predominantly in the cerebellum.[15] Early signs are those of increased intracranial pressure[19] (see Table 6-2), as well as ataxia.[18] Treatment includes surgical resection (if possible), followed by irradiation, as medulloblastoma is very radiosensitive.[15] Metastases may occur throughout the meninges and involve areas outside the CNS.[19]

Astrocytoma

Two primary forms of astrocytomas occur in childhood, including cerebellar astrocytomas and supratentorial astrocytomas. Cerebellar astrocytomas comprise 10 to 20 percent of childhood CNS tumors,[18] with the most common symptoms being those associated with increased intracranial pressure, as well as ataxia. The primary treatment is surgery with the goal of total resection.[19]

Supratentorial astrocytomas comprise 35 percent of CNS tumors in childhood. Signs and symptoms of supratentorial astrocytomas include those related to increased intracranial pressure, as well as visual disturbances and seizures. Histologic subtypes of these tumors include fibrillary and pilocytic tumors, which are well-differentiated, as well as malignant anaplastic astrocytoma and glioblastoma multiforme, which are less differentiated, of a high grade, and very aggressive, widely

Table 6-2. *Symptoms of Increased Intracranial Pressure**

Classic traid
  Morning headaches
  Vomiting without nausea
  Diplopia or other visual disturbances
Subacute signs
  Declining academic performance
  Fatigue
  Personality changes
  Complaints of vague intermittent headaches
In infants and toddlers
  Irritability
  Anorexia
  Developmental delay

Adapted from Heideman RL, Packer RJ, et al. Tumors of the central nervous system. In: Pizzo PA, Poplack DG, eds. Principles and Practice of Pediatric Oncology. Philadelphia: JB Lippincott; 1989: 505–554.

invasive tumors.[18] The primary treatment of supratentorial astrocytomas is surgery, although total resection is frequently not possible owing to tumor location. Radiation therapy is also commonly utilized. Chemotherapy may be indicated for those patients with high grade tumors.[15]

Ependymomas

Ependymomas comprise 5 to 10 percent of primary CNS tumors,[18] occurring in the posterior fossa and cerebral hemispheres.[20] Initial signs and symptoms relate to increased intracranial pressure in posterior fossa ependymomas, and include seizures and focal cerebellar deficits in supratentorial tumors.[18] Treatment includes surgical resection, if possible, followed by irradiation.[15]

Brain Stem Gliomas

Brain stem gliomas comprise 10 to 20 percent of CNS tumors in children, with signs and symptoms that include progressive cranial nerve dysfunction and gait disorders.[18] The primary medical treatment for brain stem gliomas is irradiation because surgery is hazardous owing to tumor location and chemotherapy has not been found to be beneficial.[19] Treatment is generally palliative as the overall prognosis for these tumors is poor.[18]

Craniopharyngiomas

Craniopharyngiomas are histologically benign tumors that comprise 6 to 9 percent of primary childhood CNS tumors[18] and occur primarily in the midline suprasellar region.[15] Signs and symptoms of craniopharyngiomas include visual disturbances, headaches and vomiting, as well as endocrine disturbances.[19] Treatment of craniopharyngiomas includes total surgical resection, or subtotal resection with irradiation if total resection is not possible.[15]

Lymphomas

Hodgkin's disease and non-Hodgkin's lymphoma together comprise a heterogeneous group of malignant diseases arising from the lymphatic system.[20]

Hodgkin's Disease

Hodgkin's disease is a malignant disorder that arises primarily in peripheral lymph nodes.[20] It is most common in young adults in their 20s and 30s, and is more common in males than in females.[21] Initial symptoms of Hodgkin's disease include a painless swelling in the neck, groin, or axilla. Treatment generally includes radiation therapy and/or chemotherapy, depending on the extent of the disease.[20]

Non-Hodgkin's Lymphoma

Non-Hodgkin's lymphoma is a group of disorders that most frequently involve the abdomen and mediastinum.[20] These malignant disorders occur most commonly in children 7 to 11 years of age,[22] and in males more frequently than females.[21] Initial symptoms may include abdominal pain or swelling, swelling of the face and neck, or difficulty swallowing.[20] Treatment of non-Hodgkin's lymphoma includes irradiation and chemotherapy, used individually or in combination, depending on the location and extent of disease.[23]

Neuroblastoma

Neuroblastoma is a tumor that develops from neural crest cells. It may arise anywhere in the sympathetic nervous system, with the most common sites of origin being the adrenal glands or paraspinal ganglion.[24] Neuroblastoma occurs early in life, with 25 percent being diagnosed by 1 year of age and 75 percent by 5 years of age.[20] Males are affected slightly more frequently than females.[21] The initial symptoms of neuroblastoma vary according to the location of the tumor, but most commonly include pain, an abdominal mass, or persistent diarrhea. Total surgical resection offers the best chance for cure, although chemotherapy and irradiation are both utilized in cases of subtotal resection.[20] A significant feature of neuroblastoma is its ability to regress spontaneously in some cases.[4]

Wilms' Tumor

Wilms' tumor or nephroblastoma is a tumor that originates in the kidney and occurs in both hereditary and nonhereditary forms.[20] The hereditary form is autosomal dominant, may be bilateral or multifocal, and generally occurs at an earlier age than the nonhereditary form.[4] Wilms' tumor is most common in children from birth to 15 years of age,[20] with the peak age being 1 to 4 years of age.[9] Signs and symptoms of Wilms' tumor include an abdominal lump or mass, hematuria, fatigue, low-grade fever, or abdominal pain.[20] Certain developmental anomalies are associated with Wilms' tumor, including aniridia, hemihypertrophy, and genitourinary abnormalities.[4] Treatment for Wilms' tumor includes a radical nephrectomy with removal of surrounding tissue and lymph nodes, followed by chemotherapy and possible irradiation.[20]

Bone Tumors

The two most common forms of bone cancer in pediatrics include osteogenic sarcoma or osteosarcoma, and Ewing's sarcoma.[9]

Osteogenic Sarcoma

Osteogenic sarcoma, the most common form of bone cancer in children,[9] arises from the epiphyses of the long bones where active growth is occurring. The most common sites of disease are the long bones of the extremities, including the femur, humerus, and tibia.[25] Osteogenic sarcoma occurs most frequently in individuals 10 to 25 years of age, and affects males more frequently than females.[20] Symptoms include pain, swelling, and possible pathologic fracture.[4] Metastases, especially to the lungs, may arise rapidly.[25]

Treatment of osteogenic sarcoma generally includes amputation with excision of a wide margin of tissue above the proximal aspect of the tumor to ensure total disease removal. Types of lower extremity amputations performed for osteogenic sarcoma include above-knee (AK) or below-knee (BK) amputations, hip or knee disarticulations, or hemipelvectomy. A limb salvage procedure, involving removal of the tumor and surrounding tissue without severing of the limb, may be performed as an alternative to amputation in order to preserve limb function or improve cosmesis. Limb salvage procedures vary according to the extent of tissue involvement, but always include the resection of a wide margin of unaffected tissue around the tumor in order to prevent recurrence of the malignant lesion. Bone replacements used in limb salvage procedures may include cadaver allografts, as well as autologous or vascularized grafts. Metal endoprosthetic devices may also be utilized for bone and joint replacements.[26]

The decision to perform amputation versus a limb salvage procedure involves many factors, including the age and level of musculoskeletal development of the patient, the size and location of the tumor, the possibility of metastases, and the lifestyle and preference of the patient and family. Poor candidates for limb salvage procedures include those with distal tibial lesions or those with extensive proximal tibial lesions, as a wide margin of tissue is unavailable to excision.[26] No difference in survival rates has been found between the two procedures.[27,28]

Another surgical option for children with osteogenic sarcoma, primarily those with distal femoral tumors, is rotationplasty. In this procedure, the distal femur, knee joint, and proximal tibia and fibula are resected. The remaining portion of the distal lower extremity is then rotated longitudinally 180 degrees and the residual distal tibia is fused to the proximal femur. The reversed ankle joint is then able to act as the knee joint, with the foot encompassed in the prosthetic shank. The primary advantage of this procedure is the increase in residual limb length from an AK to a BK level, with a resultant increase in overall function.[29,30]

Radiation therapy has not been found to be effective in the treatment of osteogenic sarcoma, primarily because of the radioresistance of the tumor.[7,25]

Ewing's Sarcoma

Ewing's sarcoma is a tumor of the bone that arises most frequently in the bone shaft. It may originate from the long bones, such as the femur and humerus, but it may also be found in the ribs and pelvis as well. Ewing's sarcoma is seen primarily in individuals 10 to 25 years of age, most commonly affecting teens. Symptoms include pain or tenderness, swelling, fever, chills, and weakness. Common metastatic sites include the lungs and other bones. Because of the tumor's significant radioresponsivity, the treatment most frequently utilized for Ewing's sarcoma is irradiation. Chemotherapy may be utilized as well.[20]

Rhabdomyosarcoma

Rhabdomyosarcoma is a soft tissue tumor that arises from muscle cells. The most common sites of occurrence include the head and neck, pelvis, and extremities. Rhabdomyosarcoma is generally not a well-encapsulated tumor and may spread rapidly. It occurs most commonly in children ages 2 to 6 years, and more frequently in males than in females. The initial symptom of rhabdomyosarcoma is a noticeable mass. Treatment generally includes surgery, followed by irradiation and chemotherapy.[20]

Retinoblastoma

Retinoblastoma is a tumor of the eye that may or may not be hereditary. One-third of the cases are bilateral.[20] Retinoblastoma generally appears before the age of two,[4] and tends to remain localized for long periods before metastasizing.[20] Males and females are fairly equally affected by retinoblastoma.[21] Irradiation is the primary treatment for tumors that are diagnosed at an early stage. However, for tumors diagnosed later, removal of the eye may be necessary. Chemotherapy and/or irradiation may be used to treat metastases.[20]

Treatment

Medical Management

The primary forms of medical treatment utilized for children with cancer include surgery, chemotherapy, and irradiation. These treatments may be used individually or in combination, depending on the type of cancer and its location in the body.

Surgery

Surgery for children with solid tumors is performed to eradicate the tumor by removing as many cancerous and precancerous cells as possible. A wide margin of normal tissue along the tumor's edge may also be excised because of the possibility of transitional cells. Care is taken during tumor resection to remove the tumor as one mass, if possible, in order to prevent "seeding" of cancerous cells into normal tissue. If complete resection of the tumor is impossible, surgery may also be utilized for tumor debulking or diagnostic biopsy. Irradiation and/or chemotherapy may be used preoperatively to shrink a tumor, or postoperatively to treat residual tumor, metastases, or micrometastases.

Chemotherapy

Chemotherapeutic agents are chemical substances, used alone or in combination, to control or palliate cancer processes. These agents disrupt the reproductive capabilities of cancer cells, resulting in tumor death.[7] Different chemotherapy drugs affect cells in different stages of the cell cycle. Most chemotherapeutic agents do not readily cross the blood–brain barrier. Thus, unless injected intrathecally, these drugs have little effect on malignant cells in the CNS.[12] The major chemotherapeutic agents are grouped according to their effect on cell chemistry and include alkylating agents, antimetabolites, antitumor antibiotics, plant alkaloids, and corticosteroids.[31]

Goals of chemotherapy include:

- Preoperative shrinking of tumor
- Curative therapy
- Adjuvant therapy to treat residual tumor or metastases
- Palliative therapy for symptom relief

Chemotherapeutic drugs are administered by oral, intramuscular, intravenous, subcutaneous, or intrathecal methods.[20]

Irradiation

Radiation therapy is the directing of high energy electromagnetic emissions at a tumor in order to cause cell death. The ionizing radiation acts to disrupt the DNA of the cell, compromising the cell's reproductive capacity and causing the death of the tumor. The amount of radiation that may be utilized is limited by the patient's *radiation tolerance*, which is the ability of surrounding normal tissue to resist the effects of irradiation. Certain organs, such as the liver, kidney, and lung, have a poor radiation tolerance, whereas other organs, such as the brain and the extremities, are relatively radioresistant. To increase normal tissue tolerance, *fractionated treatments* may be administered, which involve the use of multiple, smaller doses of radiation as opposed to one large dose[7] (Fig. 6-1).

The goals of radiation therapy include the following:

- Reducing tumor size preoperatively
- Destroying residual tumor postoperatively
- Destroying tumor that is unable to be removed surgically
- Decreasing tumor size for palliative relief of symptoms

Side Effects of Chemotherapy and Radiation Therapy

When considering the mechanisms by which chemotherapy and irradiation work, it is evident that both treatments act to disable the reproductive capacity of rapidly growing cancer cells. However, since targeting only cancer cells is impossible, these treatments also affect normal, fast-growing cells, such as hair follicles, gastrointestinal tract cells, and bone marrow cells, resulting in side effects, such as alopecia, nausea and vomiting, and myelosuppression. Other common side effects of chemotherapy and irradiation include musculoskeletal, cardiovascular, and respiratory problems, as well as nervous system toxicity.[32]

Bone Marrow Transplantation

The high doses of chemotherapy and radiation required to kill cancerous cells also cause death of the bone marrow cells. Thus, new marrow cells unexposed to the powerful therapy must be provided. This is accomplished by harvesting healthy marrow from a histocompatible donor and transfusing it into the affected patient. The donor marrow then

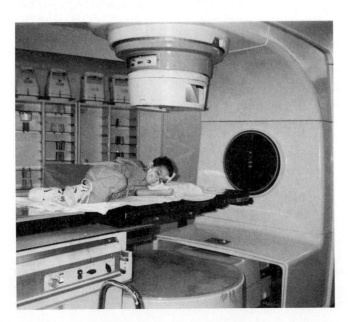

Figure 6-1. *Three-year-old child with a brain tumor positioned for radiation therapy.*

disseminates into the patient's bone and, unless rejected, begins to produce healthy blood cells once again.

The primary types of bone marrow transplants include:

- Autologous—using the patient's own marrow
- Allogeneic—using marrow from a histocompatible donor

In order to find a compatible donor for an allogeneic transplant, *human leukocyte antigen* (HLA) typing is performed to determine whether tissues from a donor, usually a sibling, will be accepted by the recipient. There is a one in four chance that two siblings will match perfectly.[13]

The entire transplantation process lasts a minimum of 6 to 8 weeks if minimal complications occur, and includes the following phases:

- Pretransplantation—begins approximately 10 days before the actual transplant, when preliminary total body irradiation (TBI) and chemotherapy are administered to eradicate residual disease and to immunosuppress the patient for the greatest opportunity for graft acceptance. The patient is placed in a sterile or laminar airflow (LAF) room at this time.
- Transplantation—donor marrow is harvested in the operating room (OR) through multiple aspirations from the anterior superior iliac spine (ASIS) and posterior superior iliac spine (PSIS). The marrow is filtered, treated, and then administered to the patient.[13]
- Posttransplantation—the patient remains in strict isolation until the graft has been accepted and the bone marrow begins to produce blood cells, thus enabling the patient to fight off infection. During this phase, supportive care is generally required, including multiple blood transfusions and antibiotics.

Numerous complications may occur during the transplantation process, including:

- Failure of engraftment/rejection
- Interstitial pneumonia
- Infection
- Hepatic veno-occlusive disease
- Drug treatment side effects[13]

Another major complication of bone marrow transplantation is graft-versus-host (GVH) disease, which may occur in allogeneic transplants when donor graft cells recognize the host tissue as foreign and react against it. The acute form of the disease generally occurs soon after transplantation and may include diarrhea, skin rash, and hepatic dysfunction. The extent of disease may be mild to life-threatening. Chronic GVH disease generally occurs 4 to 6 months posttransplant and is often a generalized multisystem disease which may have a profound effect on immune function and may lead to death.[33,34]

Physical Therapy Management

Chart Review

When initially consulted regarding a pediatric oncology patient, the physical therapist should conduct a thorough chart review prior to the physical therapy evaluation. Significant information obtained from the chart includes the type and location, as well as the stage, or extent of spread, of the disease. Although criteria vary with each form of cancer, general staging guidelines identify stage I as an area of localized disease that generally offers the best chance for cure; the stages progress through stage IV, which refers to widespread or metastatic disease and generally indicates a very poor prognosis.

Additional information obtained from the chart should include past and present medical management, such as surgical procedures, irradiation, and chemotherapy. For patients who have undergone surgical excision of a tumor, it is important to note the extent of the resection, as partial resection may indicate the need for further medical intervention. Ventriculoperitoneal shunt placement, as well as placement of a central line or indwelling catheter, used to withdraw blood or administer intravenous (IV) medications, are also significant factors in the past surgical history. For children undergoing radiation therapy, the duration of treatment is important to note. Similarly, for patients receiving chemotherapy, the types of drugs are significant, as many have side effects that impact on the child's physical status and treatment program.

For hospitalized patients, the results of the CBC should be listed daily in the chart. These blood cell counts are significant to physical therapists, as abnormal levels require modifications in the approach to the child as well as to the treatment program (see Table 6-1). A patient's nutritional status is also important to note because it may have an effect on the child's activity level and performance in therapy.

Physical Therapy Evaluation

While conducting the initial evaluation, the physical therapist must be aware that the child may not tolerate a lengthy initial session. Thus, the elements of the evaluation must be individually prioritized for each patient. Specific limitations should be considered, as they influence the child's overall function. Components of the physical therapy evaluation are detailed below, along with specific information and precautions for each of the areas as they relate to pediatric oncology.

A thorough musculoskeletal examination should be performed, including tests of range of motion (ROM), muscle strength, posture, sensation, and pain. When performing the ROM evaluation, particular attention should be given to cervical mobility in those children who have undergone brain tumor resection, as these patients tend to guard or restrict movement at the incision site because of fear and/or pain. Special consideration should be given to ROM of the involved extremity or residual limb of patients who have undergone limb salvage or amputation procedures. Hamstring and heelcord length may be limited in children who have been inactive or confined to bed for long periods of time. Limitations in joint ROM may also be present in areas where chemotherapeutic drug extravasation has occurred.

A general strength and sensory evaluation should be included in the physical therapy assessment. Caution should be used when providing resistance to evaluate strength in those patients who are thrombocytopenic owing to the potential for bruising as well as bleeding into a muscle or joint. Significant findings of the sensory evaluation may include asymmetry as seen with hemiparesis, or proximal versus distal discrepancies that may indicate peripheral neuropathy secondary to chemotherapy.

Deformities, such as scoliosis, kyphosis, and leg length discrepancies, may be detected during the postural evaluation, especially in those patients who have had epiphyseal damage as a result of radiation therapy.[32,35] Children with brain tumors may present with a lateral head tilt.

The pain assessment is an important component of the pediatric oncologic evaluation. Various methods of assessment may be utilized for different age groups according to the child's ability to identify and communicate feelings of pain. Examples of pain assessment methods/tools include the observation of pain-related behaviors in infants and toddlers, facial expression charts for younger children, and body-mapping or visual analogue scales for older children.[36]

The neurologic examination includes the assessment of muscle tone and reflexes, as well as balance and coordination skills, especially in those children with CNS involvement. Current theoretical models of sensory organization in balance testing are systems-mediated, incorporating visual, proprioceptive, and vestibular input. In patients with CNS involvement, it is important to distinguish among these systems, as the results will impact significantly on the treatment plan.[37] Visual assessment should also be performed to detect such problems as diplopia or visual field deficits. Facial paralysis may occur in patients with cranial nerve involvement.

The evaluation of gait and overall functional status is very significant for children with cancer. Common gait deviations include asymmetry secondary to hemiparesis, ataxia secondary to CNS/cerebellar effects, and high steppage resulting from peripheral neuropathy.[35] The functional assessment should also include evaluation of developmental skills in infants and toddlers, as well as transitional abilities and higher level gross motor skills in older children.

Finally, respiratory status and cardiovascular en-

durance should be evaluated, especially in those patients who have undergone irradiation to the mediastinum, as they have an increased risk for adverse
pulmonary effects.[32] Endurance may be significantly decreased in children who have been inactive or at bedrest for long periods of time.

When establishing goals for this patient population, it is important to consider the child's needs, as
well as those of the family. Physical therapy goals
for pediatric oncology patients may be:

- Preventative—avoiding disabling sequelae prior to
  their occurrence
- Restorative—maximizing motor return in patients
  with deficits
- Supportive—promoting the greatest level of functional independence possible when residual disease
  exists and progressive disability is anticipated
- Palliative—increasing or maintaining comfort and independence in patients with terminal disease.[38]

Physical therapy in pediatric oncologic patients
addresses not only the primary effects of the disease but also the side effects of medical interventions. The oncologic diseases most frequently requiring physical therapy intervention due to
primary effects include bone cancers (owing to amputation or limb salvage procedures) and CNS tumors (because of their neurologic sequelae).

Physical Therapy Intervention: Disease-Related Disability

Bone Cancer

If at all possible, children undergoing amputation or
limb salvage procedures for bone cancer should be referred to a physical therapist prior to surgery. The
preoperative physical therapy session(s) should include instruction in ambulation with assistive devices, as well as exercises to be initiated immediately postoperatively. The physical therapist should
also address postoperative expectations, providing
an introduction to prosthetics as well as an explanation of the components of the rehabilitative process.

Immediately following amputative surgery, an
initial prosthesis is placed on the residual limb in
the operating room. This prosthesis remains intact
for 6 to 8 weeks, assisting with the shaping of the
limb as well as providing a surface for immediate
weight-bearing. Gait training is generally initiated
1 to 2 days following surgery.[39]

After 6 to 8 weeks, the patient advances to a
temporary prosthesis, which is necessary because
frequent weight changes during postoperative chemotherapy may cause the volume of the residual
limb to fluctuate. To accommodate the changes in
size, varying thicknesses of lining material or
stump sox should be used as needed.[35] The physical
therapist should monitor the residual limb size
using circumferential measurements to determine
when stabilization has occurred. With stabilization,
the patient may then progress to a definitive prosthesis.[39]

Postoperative physical therapy management of
amputees includes ROM exercises, a limb positioning program, strengthening activities, as well as
gait training and postural exercises. The ROM program emphasizes stretching of the hip and knee
flexors, as these muscle groups are most likely to
develop contractures. The positioning program is
developed to reinforce the stretching, with particular emphasis on prone-lying for periods throughout
the day. Strengthening of all major muscle groups
of the residual limb should be performed, with particular attention to the abductors in patients with
AK amputations so as to avoid a Trendelenberg gait
pattern,[39] and to hip elevators and abdominals in
children with hip disarticulation so as to promote
pelvic tilt.[40] Gait training activities also include instruction in the use of the prosthesis and assistive
device, with the promotion of as normal a gait pattern as possible. Instruction in stair climbing and
falling activities should also be provided. Postural
exercises should focus on identifying the child's
center of gravity as well as maintaining a level pelvis in weight-bearing positions. In order to promote
independence, the child and family should be instructed in prosthetic mechanics and donning and
doffing the device.

For patients who have undergone limb salvage
procedures, the physical therapy program varies ac-

cording to the area, the amount of tissue resected, and the types of endoprosthetic devices utilized. All programs should include ROM and strengthening exercises for surrounding joints and musculature, as well as skin care techniques for the involved region to promote incisional healing and to prevent skin breakdown. Orthoses may also be required to provide limb support and increase joint stability, as well as to minimize pain.

Central Nervous System Tumors

The scope of physical therapy for children with CNS tumors is extremely broad owing to the great variety of signs and symptoms that may occur, depending on the size and location of the tumor and the medical treatments utilized.

Most patients with brain tumors will initially undergo surgical resection.[35] Physical therapists should be consulted 1 to 2 days postoperatively to initiate a bedside program of passive ROM and positioning. Some patients, especially those with abnormal muscle tone, may require foot and ankle splints to prevent plantar flexion contractures. A positioning program and splint schedule should be posted at the bedside for the nursing staff and other caregivers.

Patients may undergo intraoperative placement of a ventriculostomy to drain CSF externally following surgery. These children remain in the intensive care unit (ICU) at bedrest until the body is able to absorb the excess CSF independently, or until an internal shunt is placed. During this period of inactivity, active-assistive, active, or resistive exercises and passive stretching are performed to prevent further musculoskeletal sequelae while the child's movement and function are restricted.

Once the child becomes medically stable and the ventriculostomy, if present, has been removed, the head of the bed is elevated to increase the child's alertness and promote increased orientation to upright positioning. The head elevation may cause headaches, nausea, and dizziness, requiring gradual increases in upright angles. Once the child tolerates a more erect position, sitting in a reclining wheelchair may begin for increasing periods of time, with a gradual raising of the seat back toward a more upright position. During this period, the patient should be performing active neck ROM exercises in all planes and participating in active exercises and functional activities. Depending on the need for monitors or ventilators, the child may soon progress to treatment sessions in the physical therapy department. These sessions may include sitting balance, transitional, mobility, and progressive ambulation activities. In patients functioning at a more advanced level, higher level gross motor and coordination skills may be incorporated into the treatment program. Handling and facilitation should be utilized with infants and very young children to promote age-appropriate motor skills following normal developmental sequences.

Common neurologic sequelae of CNS tumors in both surgical and nonsurgical patients include hemiparesis, ataxia and dysmetria, balance disturbances, and visual problems. Children may also demonstrate cognitive sequelae, including poor judgment and attention to safety factors, as well as learning and motor planning deficits that impact on physical therapy treatment. Additional disorders, such as visual/perceptual problems, aphasia, dysarthria, and feeding/swallowing problems, may require input from other members of the rehabilitation team, including occupational and speech therapists (Fig. 6-2).

Physical therapy management of patients with hemiparesis as a result of a brain tumor should include activities to maintain the musculoskeletal status of the affected side, including passive ROM, positioning, and sensory education. Splinting may also be necessary to maintain or assist a joint and prevent deformity. Facilitation/inhibition techniques are utilized to promote motor recovery on the affected side. Functional skill instruction should be provided, including bed mobility, transitions, and ambulation. Once the patient reaches a plateau, compensatory strategies may be necessary if residual deficits persist. These strategies often include assistive devices, such as a walker with a platform attachment, cane, one-arm drive wheelchair, or orthosis. For patients with ataxia and dysmetria,

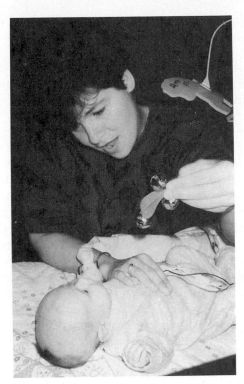

Figure 6-2. Sensory stimulation activities with a 6-week-old child who is status post brain tumor resection.

ties where displacements are unexpected as well as anticipated (Fig. 6-3). During feedforward activities, the patient is challenged to achieve the necessary postural set prior to performing a movement task or functional activity. The incorporation of functional tasks into balance activities may result in improved patient performance, as the child has a clearly defined goal around which to organize motor behavior. A variety of environmental contexts and varying surfaces should be incorporated into the treatment program to permit greater generalizability to normal environmental conditions. Balance beams, tilt boards, and "physioballs" are frequently utilized for the promotion of balance skills in children. Instruction in compensatory techniques should also be provided, such as avoiding ambulation in dark areas and on uneven surfaces until adequate balance skills have been acquired.

Visual problems, such as diplopia and hemianopsia, are common in patients with CNS tumors. Compensatory strategies may be utilized until the

physical therapy treatment should include activities that challenge the neuromuscular system. Provision of manual support, approximation, or resistance, as well as the addition of weights to the trunk or extremities, may provide increased proprioceptive feedback and improved proximal stability, resulting in an increased fluidity of distal movement. Weights and wheels may also be added to the walker to provide a fixed point of stability. Proprioceptive neuromuscular facilitation activities, such as rhythmic stabilization and slow-reversal-hold techniques, may be incorporated into the treatment session to promote increased stability.[40] The provision of verbal and visual feedback to the patient is a significant component of treatment activities with this patient population.

Balance disturbances may be addressed in both feedback and feedforward modes, including activi-

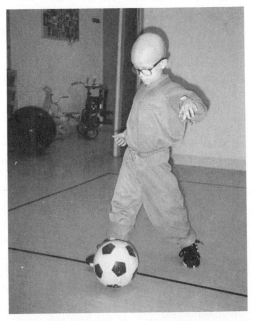

Figure 6-3. Kicking a ball emphasizes balance and coordination as well as distal motor control for a child with peripheral neuropathy.

disturbances resolve, including eye-patching for diplopia and increased visual scanning in patients with visual field deficits.

Physical Therapy Intervention: Medical Side Effects

Pediatric physical therapists may have only a limited role in minimizing the impact of some of the common side effects, such as alopecia, nausea and vomiting, and myelosuppression, caused by various cancer treatments. However, the role of the physical therapist is vital in the treatment of those children experiencing other problems secondary to disease and treatment side effects, such as musculoskeletal problems, cardiopulmonary effects, and neurotoxicity of medications.

Alopecia

The majority of children undergoing medical treatment for cancer will develop alopecia. Although younger children may not be concerned with this condition, older children and teens may be quite conscious of their physical appearance. Patients may elect to wear hats or wigs during treatment sessions. Physical therapists should work to promote a positive self-image in these patients, as well as to provide emotional support and reassurance that the hair loss is generally temporary.

Nausea and Vomiting

The effects of nausea and vomiting may cause a decrease in the child's ability or motivation to participate actively in a physical therapy program. The scheduling of treatment sessions at times during the day when these effects have subsided may increase participation in and compliance with therapeutic activities. A bedside program may also be developed for family members or other caregivers to carry out with the patient at times when side effects have decreased, such as in the evening.

Myelosuppression

Myelosuppression in pediatric oncology patients may be caused by many factors, including chemo-therapy, irradiation, infection, or bone marrow invasion by the malignant lesion. With chemotherapy, myelosuppression generally occurs within 10 to 14 days following drug administration. Medical management of immunosuppressed children may include multiple blood transfusions,[32] as well as isolation or sterile precautions.

When treating children who are myelosuppressed, the levels of each particular type of blood cell are important to note, as decreased levels of each may impact on the treatment session differently. Patients with *anemia*, a decreased percentage of red blood cells, will also have a decreased hemoglobin level, which affects the oxygenation of tissues and return of CO_2 to the lungs. These patients may exhibit fatigue, pallor, shortness of breath, loss of appetite, and decreased endurance.[7] Packed red blood cell transfusions may be necessary for relief of symptoms. Physical activity must be graded according to patient tolerance until blood levels return to normal. Children may require frequent rest periods during therapy sessions, and vital signs should be monitored. Patients with severe symptoms may require instruction in energy conservation techniques.[42]

Thrombocytopenia, a decrease in platelets, indicates a diminished ability of the blood to clot, resulting in an increased potential for bleeding or hemorrhage. Common signs of thrombocytopenia include bleeding gums, nosebleeds, bruising, or petechiae. Physical therapy guidelines for patients with thrombocytopenia, as developed at the Sloan Kettering Cancer Center, are included in Table 6-3. Patients may require transfusions for very low platelet levels or if active bleeding occurs.

Of the five types of white blood cells, the most significant indicator of the ability to fight infection is the neutrophil. The level of neutrophils in the body, the *absolute neutrophil count (ANC)*, is calculated by multiplying the total white blood cell count by the percentage of mature neutrophils.[42] A child with an ANC of less than 500 is considered to have *neutropenia*, which indicates a significantly impaired ability to fight infection. Guidelines for caregivers of children with neutropenia include

Table 6-3. *Physical Therapy Guidelines for Patients with Thrombocytopenia (as developed at the Sloan Kettering Cancer Center)*[41]

Thrombocyte Count	Appropriate Activity Level
30,000–50,000/mm^3	Active exercise only, no resistive exercise
20,000–30,000 mm^3	Gentle active or passive exercise only
<20,000 mm^3	Minimal exercises and essential activities of daily living (ADLs) only

strict adherence to sterile precautions as ordered by physicians, including the wearing of masks, gowns, gloves, and shoe covers. Frequent handwashing should be performed as well. Children with very low white blood cell levels may require bedside physical therapy treatment. Patients, if permitted to leave their rooms, may be required to wear a mask in hospital corridors and in the physical therapy department for their own protection. Neutropenic patients who are permitted in the physical therapy gym should be scheduled at those times when a minimal number of other patients are present in the treatment area. Physical therapists with infections of any type should not treat neutropenic patients. All precautions should be continued until neutrophil levels increase adequately to enable the patient to fight infection once again.

Musculoskeletal Sequelae

Multiple musculoskeletal problems may occur in pediatric oncologic patients as a result of disease and medical intervention. Although the most effective treatment is prevention, physical therapy management is generally symptomatic if problems occur.

ROM limitations may occur owing to the effects of bedrest, guarding of a joint because of pain, skin and soft tissue fibrosis from irradiation, or drug extravasation into or near a joint. Treatment of contractures includes a passive ROM/stretching pro-

gram, although because of the potential for bleeding, caution must be utilized with those patients who are thrombocytopenic. Equipment, including splints or serial casts, dynamic bracing, or continuous passive motion devices, may also be utilized for treatment of contractures.[35] In addition to the ROM program, in those patients with skin involvement, scar management techniques, such as compression dressings, may be indicated to minimize scarring effects.

Muscle weakness and atrophy are common in pediatric oncology patients, and may frequently be accompanied by a decrease in cardiovascular endurance as a result of inactivity or bedrest. The strengthening program may include isometrics as well as active-assistive, active, or resistive exercises. Cardiovascular fitness in children may be addressed with such activities as ball games, bicycle ergometry, progressive ambulation, or higher level gross motor activities, such as hopping, jumping, skipping, and running.

The treatment of pain in pediatric oncology patients is a complicated issue. Whereas physical therapy techniques, such as transcutaneous electrical nerve stimulation (TENS), massage, and superficial thermal agents, may be effective in treating pain of muscular origin,[35] disease-related pain in children is customarily managed medically with nonnarcotic or narcotic analgesics. The involvement of a pediatric pain team, which includes a physical therapist, is ideal for the pain management of children with cancer. Such teams are currently active in the several major pediatric treatment facilities in the United States.

Multiple skeletal sequelae may occur in children with cancer as a result of the disease and treatment effects. Bony instability may develop in patients who have undergone limb salvage procedures, as well as in children with metastatic bone disease. Treatment should include techniques to minimize stress on the bone, such as protective body mechanics, non–weight-bearing ambulation with an assistive device, and use of splints or bracing. Scoliosis, kyphosis, and leg length discrepancies may develop as late effects of cancer treatment.[32,35] Spinal deformities should be addressed with strengthening and mobility exercises for the trunk and associated musculature. Advanced deformities may require evaluation and intervention by an orthopedic physician. Leg length discrepancies may require the addition of a shoe lift or orthotic to prevent pelvic obliquity and permanent deformity. Postural exercises should be incorporated into the physical therapy program of all children with skeletal deformities.

Mobility or gait problems are common in this population owing to peripheral neuropathy, limb salvage and amputation procedures, and the effects of bedrest or bony abnormalities as described earlier. Progressive ambulation training should be utilized with these patients, including assistive devices and orthotics as needed.

Edema may occur as a result of an interruption in the lymphatic drainage system caused by tumor blockage or lymph node resection. Treatment should include gravity-assisted drainage using elevation, active muscle pumping and, if necessary, the use of compression garments.[35]

Equipment needs for these children may include wheelchairs and assistive devices for activities of daily living equipment (ADL), as well as prosthetics or orthotics.

Cardiopulmonary Effects

Multiple cardiac and pulmonary complications may result from the medical interventions used in children with cancer. Cardiomyopathy may be caused by the anthracyclines, a group of chemotherapeutic drugs that includes doxorubicin (Adriamycin) and daunorubicin. Similarly, pericarditis may result from irradiation of the mediastinum, and may occur acutely as well as months to years after treatment. Both disorders may eventually result in congestive heart failure.[32] Grading activity programs in accordance with patient tolerance, as well as frequent rest periods and close monitoring of vital signs, is indicated for these children. Instruction in energy conservation techniques may be provided to patients exhibiting significant cardiac insufficiency.

Chemotherapy and radiation therapy, as well as metastatic lung disease, may result in pulmonary compromise. Common pulmonary problems in children with cancer include pulmonary fibrosis and interstitial pneumonitis,[32] which lead to decreased chest wall mobility, dyspnea, and decreased exercise tolerance.[42] Physical therapy for these patients should incorporate respiratory activities to maintain lung expansion and chest wall mobility. Suggested activities include deep breathing exercises, incentive spirometry, pulmonary or breathing games, and cardiovascular conditioning activities.

Neurotoxicity

A common side effect of the chemotherapeutic vinca alkaloids, especially vincristine, is a progressive peripheral neuropathy[32] for which physical therapy is frequently indicated. Initial signs of vincristine neurotoxicity include loss of the Achilles tendon reflex, followed by paresthesias of the fingers and toes. Distal sensory loss may occur, accompanied by progressive distal weakness which initially affects wrist and finger extensors as well as ankle dorsiflexors. If the drug is continued at this point, generalized progressive weakness may follow, resulting in a significant decrease in overall function.

Once the drug is discontinued, reversal of the symptoms of neurotoxicity generally occurs fairly rapidly, beginning with the resolution of the paresthesias, followed by an increase in muscle strength. However, superficial sensory loss and depressed deep tendon reflexes may resolve more slowly, if at all. Overall, the symptoms of the neuropathy are largely reversible and cause minimal residual disability.[43]

Common initial physical sequelae of neurotoxicity include foot drop during ambulation, wrist drop, weak grasp, and decreased distal sensory feedback. Patients with more profound involvement may develop an inability to ambulate, with distal muscle weakness and atrophy.[44-46] An equinovarus deformity of the foot may develop owing to paralysis of the extensor muscles of the foot and ankle, which results in an unopposed flexor pull.[47]

The physical therapy program for patients with peripheral neuropathy should include ROM/ stretching as well as distal strengthening exercises. Orthotics, such as molded ankle-foot orthoses, (MAFOs), may be indicated to maintain adequate foot and ankle position and to support the foot during ambulation. Wrist splints may also be required to maintain and assist the distal upper extremity. Patients should be instructed in compensatory strategies for altered sensation, such as using caution on uneven surfaces and using visual rather than tactile and kinesthetic cues to maintain balance.[35] Instruction in skin care techniques such as closely monitoring bath water temperature and checking daily for signs of skin breakdown when using an orthotic, especially in areas of decreased sensation, must also be provided to patients and families. Patients with more advanced peripheral neuropathies may require instruction in the use of assistive devices for ambulation, such as walkers or canes. Severely affected patients may require wheelchairs and other ADL equipment.

As symptoms begin to resolve, more aggressive use of facilitation techniques, such as proprioceptive neuromuscular facilitation, should be incorporated into the physical therapy program, along with continued strengthening exercises. Serial casting or heelcord lengthening procedures may be necessary for fixed contractures of the ankle.

Physical Therapy Intervention: Bone Marrow Transplantation

Physical therapy treatment should be an integral part of a BMT admission because of the significant potential for pulmonary, musculoskeletal, and neurologic problems. Common problems include decreased ROM, weakness, pneumonia, deconditioning, and muscle atrophy. These sequelae may occur as a result of long periods of confinement in the LAF room, the patient's general inactivity level, and/or the various procedures and side effects of treatment. The LAF room provides for air exchange in a manner to provide an environment that is almost free of micro-organisms.

Physical therapists should be consulted upon admission of the child. Initial treatment goals are generally preventive, and may include:

1. Maintenance of joint ROM and prevention of contractures
2. Maintenance of muscle strength and prevention of atrophy
3. Promotion of pulmonary hygiene and prevention of pneumonia
4. Maintenance of balance, coordination, and endurance
5. Promotion of overall physical and emotional well-being[48]

When treating a patient in the LAF rooms, the physical therapist is required to follow specific sterile isolation precautions which generally include handwashing, followed by the donning of a mask, gown, gloves, hat, and shoe covers. All items taken into the room must be sterilized, making the use of physical therapy equipment difficult. Thus, creativity is important in the development of therapeutic activities for these patients. Manual forms of resistance are frequently utilized for strengthening. Balls and other smooth pieces of equipment may be cleaned with disinfectant and used, provided no Velcro or other potential sources of bacteria are present. Some facilities will permit cardiovascular training equipment, such as a stationary bicycle, to remain in the BMT unit permanently. Specific rules and regulations of individual facilities should be investigated and strictly followed by physical therapists for the sake of the patient's health and well-being.

The physical therapy treatment program for BMT patients should include ROM, strengthening, pulmonary exercises, as well as balance and coordination activities. The ROM activities should emphasize the stretching of hamstrings, heelcords, and hip flexors, which may become particularly tight owing to positioning and general inactivity. Strengthening may include active and resistive exercises. Resistance may be provided manually by the therapist or by utilizing the patient's own body weight. Examples of strengthening exercises include sit-ups, bridging, push-ups, arm circles, straight leg raises, and short arc quadriceps exercises. Awareness of the patient's platelet count prior to each session is extremely important, as stretching and resistive exercises may cause bleeding or hemorrhage in those patients who are thrombocytopenic. Activities, such as bicycling in the supine position, jumping jacks, or jogging in place, will help to maintain aerobic capacity and cardiopulmonary endurance. Balance and coordination may be addressed with one-foot balance activities; heel, toe, or line walking; as well as reaching and targeting games. Deep breathing exercises may be used to maintain aerobic capacity and chest wall mobility in an effort to prevent pneumonia and other pulmonary complications. Instruction in relaxation techniques may help children to deal better with anxiety, pain, and the effects of treatment. Motivating these children to be active at a time when they may be quite ill and depressed is a particularly challenging task for the pediatric physical therapist.[48]

Initial physical therapy treatment should also include the development of a bedside exercise and activity program to be posted in the LAF room. Instruction regarding the program components should be provided to the child and family early in the hospitalization course when the patient is feeling fairly well. Then, if the patient is unavailable for physical therapy treatment at certain times during the day because of other procedures or illness, these activities may be carried out with the child at a later time.

Physical Therapy Intervention: Terminal Disease

The pediatric physical therapist may be consulted to assist in the management of homebound children with terminal cancer. Treatment of these patients may include passive ROM exercises, pain management techniques, and positioning to prevent skin breakdown as well as to increase the patient's comfort. Family instruction in positioning, transfers, skin care, and exercises is also a vital component of the physical therapy program. Wheelchairs, hospital beds, pressure relief cushions and mattresses, ADL and assistive devices, as well as commodes and bathing equipment, may be required. Psychological and emotional support of the patient and family must also be provided owing to the extreme stress and devastation associated with the impending death of a child from cancer.

In summary, the physical therapist is an essential member of the pediatric oncology team, which generally also includes physicians, nurses, occupational therapists, speech therapists, social workers, nutritionists, and child life therapists. With this population, each team member must focus not only on the issues relevant to his or her own discipline, but must also address the whole child as well as the child's role within the family structure, school, and community. Thus, physical therapy for these patients must address not only the physical status of

---

Display 6-1.

Resource Agencies that Provide Literature, Brochures and Information for Professionals and Families

Agency	Means of Contact
The American Cancer Society	Contact local agencies
The Oncology Section of the American Physical Therapy Association (APTA)	1–800–999–APTA
The Association for Brain Tumor Research	1–312–268–5571
The National Cancer Institute	1–800–4–CANCER
The Candlelighter's Childhood Cancer Foundation	1–800–336–2223
The Leukemia Society of America	1–212–573–8484

the child, but also the social and emotional issues associated with the diagnosis of cancer in children.

Several excellent resource agencies provide literature to professionals, as well as brochures and information which may be shared with patients and their families. These agencies are listed in Display 6-1.

Display 6–2.
Case Study

M.B. is a white female who was diagnosed as having ALL in 1984 at 3 years of age. Initial treatment included a 2½-year chemotherapy protocol of vincristine, methotrexate, and Adriamycin. Following the completion of the protocol, remission was maintained for approximately 9 months, at which time M.B. suffered a relapse. A more intense treatment protocol was initiated, including CNS irradiation and chemotherapy. Concurrently, M.B.'s family underwent HLA testing to determine the availability of a compatible bone marrow donor.

At 7 years of age, M.B. underwent an allogeneic BMT using marrow donated from her 9-year-old brother. Following the transplant, she was confined to the LAF room for 7 weeks. The physical therapy department was consulted during this admission for maintenance of her general activity level and strength, as well as for prevention of contractures, skin breakdown, and pulmonary complications.

Subsequently, M.B. developed chronic GVH disease that severely affected her joints, necessitating consultation for home physical therapy services owing to pain, decreased ROM, and significantly impaired function. Treatment consisted of a stretching program, general strengthening and mobility activities, as well as progressive ambulation as improvement occurred. Equipment was also needed, including a wheelchair, walker, and MAFOs. Once M.B. became ambulatory, physical therapy was continued at an outpatient facility for gait training and promotion of higher level gross motor skills.

In October of 1990, M.B. developed a serious blood infection, prompting admission to an acute care facility and treatment with amphotericin. During this admission, an IV infiltration occurred, resulting in a large, open wound on the dorsum of M.B.'s left foot. Following skin grafting, M.B. was discharged to home, where she developed extreme pain attributable to graft rejection. She was readmitted and treated with hyperbaric oxygen twice a day for 2 weeks, then returned home to allow healing to occur. Physical therapy services were reinitiated in the home since M.B. was nonambulatory again. Treatment consisted of wound care and, later, scar management techniques, and ROM activities to the left foot, ankle, and other joints owing to the residual effects of GVH disease. General strengthening and mobility activities were also performed, along with ambulation training using a non–weight-bearing pattern with a walker, and later, progression to partial and then full weight-bearing for the left lower extremity.

M.B. is now 11 years old and is demonstrating no recurrence of her leukemia. She has, however, required heelcord releases as a result of the effects of her GVH disease. She remains mildly limited in her higher level gross motor skill ability, including running and jumping, owing to joint problems as well as scarring on her left foot. She has been able to return to school this year and otherwise remains healthy and active.

References

1. Silverburg E, Boring CC, Squires TS. Cancer statistics, 1990. *CA* 1990;40:9–26.
2. Bleyer WA. The impact of childhood cancer on the United States and the world. *CA* 1990;40(6); 355–367.
3. American Cancer Society: *Cancer Facts and Figures 1991*. Atlanta; American Cancer Society; 1991.
4. Nesbit ME. Clinical aspects and differential diagnosis of the child with suspected cancer. In: Pizzo PA, Poplack DG, eds. *Principles and Practice of Pediatric Oncology*. Philadelphia: JB Lippincott; 1989:83–92.
5. Pui C-H, Christ WM. Pediatric solid tumors. In: Holleb AI, Fink DJ, Murphy GP, eds. *American Cancer Society Textbook of Clinical Oncology*. Atlanta: American Cancer Society; 1991:453–480.
6. Kohn HI, Fry RJ. Radiation carcinogenesis. *N Engl J Med* 1984;310:504–511.
7. Link MP. Cancer in childhood. In: Bleck EE, Nagel DA, eds. *Physically Handicapped Children, A Medical Atlas for Teachers*. 2nd Ed. New York: Grune and Stratton; 1982.
8. Pui C-H, Rivera GK. Childhood leukemias. In: Holleb AI, Fink DJ, Murphy GP, eds. *American Cancer Society Textbook of Clinical Oncology*. Atlanta: American Cancer Society; 1991: 433–452.
9. Young JL, Ries LG, Silverberg E, et al. Cancer incidence, survival, and mortality for children younger than age 15 years. *Cancer* 1986;58:598–602.
10. Grier HE, Weinstein HJ. Acute nonlymphocytic leukemia. In: Pizzo PA, Poplack DG, eds. *Principles and Practice of Pediatric Oncology*. Philadelphia: JB Lippincott; 1989:367–382.
11. Pui C-H, Rivera G. Leukemia. In: Rudolph AM, Hoffman JI, eds. *Pediatrics*. 18th Ed. East Norwalk, CT: Appleton and Lange; 1987:1096–1104.
12. Vietti T, Bergamini RA. General aspects of chemotherapy. In: Sutow WW, Fernbach DJ, Vietti TJ, eds. *Clinical Pediatric Oncology*. St. Louis: CV Mosby; 1984:210–243.
13. Quinn, JJ. Bone marrow transplantation in the management of childhood cancer. *Pediatr Clin North Am* 1985;32:3.
14. Sutow, WW. General aspects of childhood cancer. In: Sutow WW, Fernbach DJ, Vietti TJ, eds. *Clinical Pediatric Oncology*. St. Louis: CV Mosby; 1984;1–13.
15. Association For Brain Tumor Research: *A Primer of Brain Tumors*, 4th Ed. Chicago: Association for Brain Tumor Research; 1988.
16. Blossom B, Barnhart L. Brain tumors. In: Umphred DA, ed. *Neurologic Rehabilitation*. St Louis: CV Mosby; 1985:442–451.
17. Duffner PK, Cohen ME, et al. Late effects of treatment on the intelligence of children with posterior fossa tumors. *Cancer* 1983;51:223–237.
18. Heideman RL, Packer RJ, et al. Tumors of the central nervous system. In: Pizzo PA, Poplack DG, eds. *Principles and Practice of Pediatric Oncology*. Philadelphia: JB Lippincott; 1989:505–554.
19. Eys JV. Malignant tumors of the central nervous system. In: Sutow WW, Fernbach DJ, Vietti TJ. *Clinical Pediatric Oncology*. St. Louis: CV Mosby; 1984.
20. U.S. Department of Health and Human Services: *Young People with Cancer*. Bethesda, MD: National Cancer Institute; 1991.
21. Young JL, Miller RW. Incidence of malignant tumors in U.S. children. *J Pediatr* 1975;86:2.
22. Murphy SB. Classification, staging and end results of treatment of childhood non-Hodgkin's lymphomas: Dissimilarities from lymphomas in adults. *Semin Oncol* 1980;7(3):332–339.
23. American Cancer Society. *Cancer Manual*. 7th Ed. Boston: American Cancer Society; 1986.
24. Hayes FA, Smith EI. Neuroblastoma. In: Pizzo PA, Poplack DG, eds. *Principles and Practice of Pediatric Oncology*. Philadelphia: JB Lippincott; 1989: 607–622.
25. Gahagan CA. Physical therapy management of patients with osteosarcoma. *Oncol Section Newslett* 1984;2(2)6–7.
26. Link MP, Eilber F. Osteosarcoma. In: Pizzo PA, Poplack DG, eds. *Principles and Practice of Pediatric Oncology*. Philadelphia: JB Lippincott; 1989:689–712.
27. Eilber FR, Morton DL. Limb-salvage for skeletal and soft tissue sarcomas. *Cancer* 1984;53:2579–2584.
28. Simon MA, Aschliman MA. Limb-salvage treatment versus amputation for osteosarcoma of the distal end of the femur. *Bone J Surg* 1986;68:9.

29. Jaffee N. Advances in the management of malignant bone tumors in children and adolescents. *Pediatr Clin North Am* 1985;32:3.

30. Murray MP, Jacobs PA. Functional performance after tibial rotationplasty. *J Bone Joint Surg* 1985; 67:3.

31. Cooper MR, Cooper MR. Principles of medical oncology. In: Holleb AI, Fink DJ, Murphy GP. *American Cancer Society Textbook of Clinical Oncology*. Atlanta: American Cancer Society; 1991:47–68.

32. Mulne AF, Koepke JC. Adverse effects of cancer therapy in children. *Pediatr Rev* 1985;6:9.

33. Lenorsky C, Feig SA. Bone marrow transplantation for children with cancer. *Pediatr Ann* 1983;12:6.

34. Ramsay NK. Bone marrow transplantation in pediatric oncology. In: Pizzo PA, Poplack DG, eds. *Principles and Practice of Pediatric Oncology*. Philadelphia: JB Lippincott; 1989:971–990.

35. Gerber LH, Binder H. Rehabilitation of the child with cancer. In: Pizzo PA, Poplack DG, eds. *Principles and Practice of Pediatric Oncology*. Philadelphia: JB Lippincott; 1989:957–970.

36. Shapiro, B. The management of pain in pediatrics. Lecture Notes, as presented to the Delaware Valley Pediatric Special Interest Group at Children's Hospital of Philadelphia. Philadelphia; January. 1990.

37. Nashner LM. Sensory, neuromuscular, and biomechanical contributions to human balance. Proceedings of the American Physical Therapy Association Forum, Nashville, TN: June 13–15, 1989.

38. Stanger M. Physical therapy intervention with pediatric oncologic amputees. Lecture, American Physical Therapy Association CSM. Orlando, FL, Feb., 1991.

39. Urbscheit, NL. Cerebellar dysfunction. In: Umphred DA, ed. *Neurological Rehabilitation*. St. Louis: CV Mosby; 1985:452–473.

40. Villaneuva R. Principles of total care—Rehabilitation. In: Sutow WW, Fernback DJ, Vietti TJ, eds. *Clinical Pediatric Oncology*. St. Louis: CV Mosby; 1984:319–331.

41. Iltis M. Cancer chemotherapy toxicity guidelines for the physical therapist. *Oncol Section Newslett* 1986; 4(3):5–7.

42. Rosenthal S, Kaufman S. Vincristine neuropathy. *Ann Intern Med* 1974;80:733–737.

43. Holland JF, Scharlau C, et al. Vincristine treatment of advanced cancer: A cooperative study of 392 cases. *Ca Res* 1973;33:1258–1264.

44. Allen JC. The effects of cancer therapy on the nervous system. *J Pediatr* 1978;93:(6):903–909.

45. Casey EB, Jellife AM. Vincristine neuropathy: Clinical and electrophysiological observations. *Brain* 1973;96:69–86.

46. Ryan JR, Emami A. Vincristine neurotoxicity with residual equinovarus deformity in children with adult leukemia. Cancer 1983;51:423–425.

47. James MC. Physical therapy for patients after bone marrow transplantation. Phys Ther 1987;67:6.

Pediatric Physical Therapy,
second edition, edited by Jan
Stephen Tecklin. J. B. Lippincott
Company, Philadelphia © 1994.

7

Laurie Grigsby de Linde

Rehabilitation of the Child with Burns

- **Epidemiology, Etiology, and Prognosis**
  Child Abuse and Neglect
  Prevention
- **Structure and Function of the Skin**
- **Classification of Burns**
  Depth
  Size
  Causative Agent
  Minor, Moderate, and Major
  Classifications
- **Scar Hypertrophy and Contracture**
- **Initial Treatment and Medical Management**
- **Wound Management**
  Dressing Change
  Hydrotherapy

- **Surgical Management**
  Skin Graft and Donor Site
  Cultured Epithelial Autografts and Dermal Substitutes
- **Role and Goals of the Therapist**
  The Emergent Phase
  The Acute Phase
  The Skin Graft Phase
  The Rehabilitation Phase
  The Reconstructive Phase
- **Psychosocial Issues**
  Support/Self-Help Groups
- **Outcomes**
  Functions of the Skin
  Growth and Physiological Functions
  Psychosocial and Behavioral Adaptation

The purpose of this chapter is to provide a basic description of pediatric burn care and to discuss the role of the therapist in the treatment of the child with burns—from the acute phase through the rehabilitation phase, with emphasis on the latter.

It frequently has been said that children are not small adults. Certainly, the treatment that is appropriate for adults with burn injuries is not necessarily applicable to children with these same injuries and vice versa. Moreover, the treatment for a 9-month-old baby may differ from that for a 3-year-old child, which, in turn, may be different from the approach used for a 10-year-old child. The discussion in this chapter concerning therapy generally is limited to children younger than 12 years of age because children 12 and older are physiologically more similar to adults.

The role of the therapist is broadly addressed.

The specific role of the therapist is defined, in part, by the individual setting, and also may be dependent upon the particular facility's medical and surgical techniques and approach.

Epidemiology, Etiology, and Prognosis

The exact number of burn injuries that occur each year in the United States is not known because there is no comprehensive system for gathering such data. However, estimates are based upon information collected by several voluntary registries and compiled by surveys. Each year, approximately 2.2 million people in the United States, or 1 in every 100, seek medical attention for burns or have 1 or more days of restricted activity because of a burn injury.[1] Most of these injuries occur at home and are treated on an outpatient basis.[2] Only about 3 percent of burn victims are hospitalized.[3] Approximately 5500 people die annually as the result of fires and burns.[4] Every year, approximately 440,000 children receive treatment for burns.[2] Preschoolers account for the highest age-specific incidence of burns and for 47 percent of all deaths in residential fires.[5] The leading cause of accidental death in the home for children ages 1 through 14 years is fires and burns.[6]

According to statistics compiled by the National Burn Information Exchange (NBIE),[6] scald burns are the most frequent type of burn injury for infants and toddlers, accounting for 72 percent of burns in this age group, whereas flame and contact burns represent 25 percent of the burn injuries for this group. A water temperature of 140°F can cause a deep partial-thickness to full-thickness burn in 3 seconds, and this same depth of injury can occur within 1 second when water is heated at 156°F.[7] Percolated coffee is 180°F, and hot grease or hot oil is approximately 400°F.[8] One can imagine in terms of pediatric development how scald injuries might easily occur, as children at these ages are learning to reach and grasp and to walk and climb.

According to the NBIE data, the frequency of scald burns is decreased to 54 percent by 2 to 4 years of age, whereas flame burns are increased to 34 percent. Most burn injuries in this age group occur as a result of play activities and include children beginning to experiment with matches and lighters. In the 5- to 12-year and 13- to 18-year age groups, flame burns are the most prevalent type of burn injury. In the former age group, children are most often burned by a fire near where they are playing or standing. Adolescents in the latter age group are often burned during a variety of activities, such as lighting fires, riding in or driving vehicles, and during cleaning or repair activities.

A greater number of boys than girls are burned in all age groups. Most burn incidents in very young children occur indoors while at home. As the age of the child increases, burn injuries tend to happen outdoors, both at and away from home. There is an increase in the number of vehicular and work-related burn injuries during adolescence. For all age groups, the kitchen is the most common place for burn injury. In younger children, this is followed by by the bathroom, whereas for older children, the yard is the next most likely site of injury.

The NBIE data indicate that persons 5 to 34 years of age have the best survival rates. Older children have a better survival rate than younger children, and the survival rate becomes progressively worse as age decreases. As one might expect, mortality increases with severity (extent and depth) of injury.

Child Abuse and Neglect

Ten percent of all physical child abuse is by burning.[9] Approximately 2 percent of all pediatric burns are intentional.[10] According to one source, child abuse or flagrant neglect accounts for 20 to 30 percent of all pediatric burn admissions.[11] Abuse or neglect may be suspected when one or more of the following is seen:

- The distribution of the burn injury is stocking-, sock-, or glove-like in configuration (Fig. 7-1), especially if it is bilateral, indicating that the child may have been dipped or placed into a hot liquid or the distribution is indicative of deliberate immersion.

- The story of how the burn happened is incompatible with the injury itself or with the child's developmental ability (or with the child's own report, if he or she is able to give one).
- The parent or caretaker delayed in seeking medical attention or there is a history of going to multiple emergency rooms or doctors when the child sustains injuries.
- Other injuries (such as bruises), old scars, and the like are present or the child appears to have been neglected (undernourished, immunizations not up-to-date, and so on).
- The parent or caretaker appears to be under the influence of drugs or alcohol or appears mentally unstable.
- There is a current or previous history of involvement of the family with child protective agencies.

Many states have laws requiring that certain professionals, including physical therapists and occupational therapists, report suspected cases of child abuse. However, such reporting is often done by another professional, such as a physician or social worker.

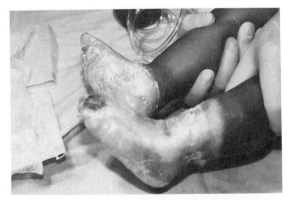

Figure 7-1. *Acute, circumferential, mostly full-thickness burns of both feet in a "sock" pattern, sustained by a child younger than 1 year of age. Child abuse was suspected. (Note: To help decrease pain and to limit the time of wound exposure, the topical antimicrobial agent has been applied to gauze instead of directly on the patient, and the dressing to be applied has been prepared prior to the old bandage being removed.)*

Prevention

Because of the high incidence and common pattern of distribution of types of burn injuries among children of various age groups, prevention efforts have been directed toward educating parents, children, and others as to how these injuries occur and how they can be prevented. Several suggestions for preventing pediatric burn injuries include the following:

- Lowering water heater temperature settings to 124° or lower
- Keeping cords to coffee pots and cups with hot liquids out of reach of young children
- Keeping young children in a safe place during food preparation and serving
- Turning pot handles toward the back of the stove and cooking on rear burners when possible.
- Supervising children in the bathtub and testing bathwater with a liquid crystal thermometer before placing the child in the tub
- Placing safety caps on electrical outlets
- Teaching children that matches are tools, not toys
- Teaching older children and adolescents about the dangers of high-voltage wires and about the dangers of and safe use of gasoline and other flammable liquids.

Additionally, other prevention efforts have focused on federal regulations mandating the use of flame-retardant fabrics and materials in such articles as children's sleepwear and mattresses to help decrease the number and severity of burns resulting from the ignition of these items. Current efforts are focused on the development of a safer child-resistant cigarette lighter design, a "fire-safe" cigarette standard, and eventual laws promoting the sale of such, and there are endeavors in some local communities to support legislation requiring that home water heaters have a maximum temperature setting.

Structure and Functions of the Skin

The skin, like the heart and lungs, is a vital organ of the body. In fact, it is the largest organ of the body, varying in thickness from 0.5 mm in the eyelids to 4 mm in the palms and soles.[12] The skin is composed of the more superficial and thinner (20 to 400 μ) layer, the epidermis, and of the deeper and thicker (440 to 2500 μ^{13}) layer, the dermis. In the basal layer of the epidermis are granules of melanin which give skin its color.[12] The dermis is vascular, and the epidermis, although avascular, has its deeper layers nourished by fluid from the dermis (Fig. 7-2).[12] Contained in the skin are sweat glands, hair follicles, sebaceous glands, and, on the fingers and toes, nails. Sensory nerves and sympathetic fibers to vessels, to arrector pili muscles, and to sweat glands abound in the skin.[12] The skin helps regulate body temperature, preserves body fluids, protects against infection (by serving as a barrier and also by having certain bactericidal abilities), protects against radiation, and acts as a barrier to help protect vital organs and other body structures against external objects and fluids. Because of nerve endings that sense touch, pain, and temperature, the skin aids in both protective and discriminatory sensation. The skin also assists in vitamin D production. The skin, along with its appendages, can help reveal an individual's race, age, sex, and health. Ridges in the skin on the fingertips gives each person a unique set of fingerprints. The skin on the face, with fluctuations in blood flow (e.g., blushing) and with the action of the underlying muscles, can express an individual's emotions.

Whenever the skin is significantly damaged or destroyed, these functions may become impaired. Because the skin is an organ, when the skin is damaged or destroyed, there are not only local but also systemic effects.

Classification of Burns

Burns can be classified by depth, by size (percentage of body surface area [BSA] burned), and by causative agent, or they can be classified as minor, moderate, or major for purposes of triage.

Depth

Burns can be classified according to the depth of skin damaged or destroyed (Fig. 7-3). They are

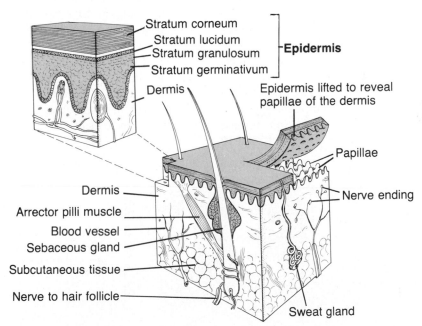

Figure 7-2. *Anatomy of the skin. (From Rosdahl CB. Textbook of Basic Nursing. 5th ed. Philadelphia: JB Lippincott; 1991; 117.)*

variously classified as partial-thickness burns (formerly known as first-degree and second-degree burns) or as full-thickness burns (previously referred to as third-degree burns). Partial-thickness burns can be either superficial or deep. Superficial partial-thickness burns involve the epidermis and the upper portion of the dermal papillae. They are painful, appear red, and frequently present with blisters. Superficial partial-thickness burns will heal in about 2 weeks or less without scarring.

Deep partial-thickness burns injure the dermis. They are waxy-white in appearance and are pliable. Such burns may be insensitive to light touch, but painful to deep pressure. If they become infected, dry out, or have impaired circulation, deep partial-thickness burns can convert to full-thickness wounds. Deep-partial thickness burns will heal spontaneously by epithelial cells from remaining dermal appendages, but the time required for healing may be 3 to 6 weeks or longer, and such burns heal with scar tissue that can hypertrophy and contract. Although deep partial-thickness burns will heal spontaneously without skin grafting, because of the prolonged healing time and frequently poor functional and cosmetic outcome, as well as other reasons listed later, many surgeons elect to excise and graft these wounds when possible and indicated.

Full-thickness burns, by definition, destroy the full thickness of the skin. Such burns can appear as cherry-red, white, or brown and leathery; and thrombosed veins may be visible. Hairs can be easily extracted owing to the death of hair follicles. Because the nerves have been destroyed, full-thickness burns are anesthetic to touch. (This does not mean that there is no pain associated with such burns. Activation of the nerves around the periphery of the burn, exposure of the wound to air by removal of dead tissue, or manipulation of the wound can cause extreme pain.[14]) Full-thickness burns will not heal without skin grafting. Even with skin grafting, such burns may result in scar contracture and hypertrophy. Electrical burns often damage muscle, nerve, and bone; histologically they resemble crush injuries. Treatment of these injuries often varies from that of other burns, and so will not be dealt with in this chapter.

The actual depth of injury may not be accurately or easily determined on the first day, even by the most experienced surgeon. Burn injuries frequently present with varying depths of involvement and are rarely of uniform depth; such factors as how the injury occurred, the thickness of body skin in the area of the burn, and whether or not the individual was wearing clothes all have a bearing on the depth of injury. The skin of infants and young children is thinner than that of adults, so, for example, a hot liquid that would cause a superficial, partial-thickness burn in an adult may cause a deeper injury in an infant or toddler. Knowing the depth of the burn is important in determining triage, resuscitation, wound care and closure, and prognosis.

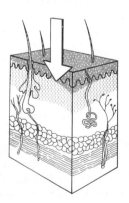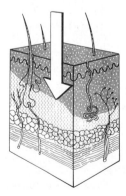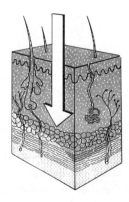

Figure 7-3. *Diagram of depth of burn: partial thickness, superficial (left); partial thickness, deep (center); full thickness (right).*

Size

Burns are also classified according to size or total percent of body surface area (TBSA) burned. The TBSA is counted as 100 percent. The palm of an individual's hand is estimated to be about 1 percent of the TBSA. Frequently, for adults, the "Rule of Nines" is used to calculate the TBSA burned. According to this rule, in an adult, the head represents 9 percent of the TBSA, each upper extremity counts as 9 percent, the trunk represents 36 percent, each lower extremity represents 18 percent, and the genitalia is assigned 1 percent. However, a child's head (especially that of a baby) is larger in proportion to the body than an adult's head is, and a child's lower extremities are smaller in proportion to the body than an adult's lower extremities are to the body. For example, the head of a baby who is younger than 1 year of age is counted as 18 percent, whereas each lower extremity represents 13.5 percent. Because of such differences, modified versions of the "Rule of Nines" are used to calculate the TBSA burned in children. One such pediatric burn extent assessment chart has been developed by Lund and Browder.[15] Estimating the TBSA burned is important in determining triage of the patient, figuring fluid resuscitation and nutritional needs, planning wound closure, and predicting prognosis.

Causative Agent

A third way of classifying burns is according to the causative agent or method: scald, contact, flash, flame, chemical, radiation, or electrical. Knowing the causative agent or method can be important in giving appropriate treatment. For example, if an individual sustains a chemical burn, knowing which chemical caused the burn is necessary in order to apply the correct antidote and in determining the need for copious water lavage, which would not necessarily be done for an electrical burn or for a flame burn.

Minor, Moderate, and Major Classifications

Burns also can be classified as minor, moderate, or major according to guidelines established by the American Burn Association (ABA) for purposes of triage. For example, a minor burn for an adult might be a partial-thickness burn involving less than 15 percent of the TBSA; such a patient could be treated as an outpatient. A minor burn for a child might be a partial-thickness burn involving less than 10 percent of the TBSA, but hospitalization might be considered for such a patient. The ABA recommends that an individual with a major burn be admitted or transferred to a burn center.

Burn Center

In 1990, the ABA published guidelines for the development and operation of burn centers,[16] defined as "a service system based in a hospital that has made the institutional commitment to meet the criteria specified in this guide."[16] Although these guidelines were not applied to the hospitals that responded to a survey to be included in the ABA's *Burn Care Resources in North America 1991–1992* directory, the directory lists 148 hospitals in the United States with burn services. Of these, at least 16 are exclusively pediatric facilities.

Burn Team

In its guidelines for burn centers, the ABA specifies which personnel should staff the burn center, as well as which specialists and personnel should be on call or available for consultation. (The criteria state that "Both physical and occupational therapy should be represented in the burn center staff.") Within the ABA guidelines, each burn center establishes its own burn team. Personnel who comprise the burn team and their specific roles may vary from institution to institution or according to the individual needs of a given patient or the particular phase of healing, although there generally is a core team. The pediatric burn team frequently includes a surgeon, nurse, occupational therapist, physical therapist, social worker, respiratory therapist, dietitian, child life therapist, hospital chaplain, discharge planner, various specialists (pediatrician, pulmonologist, psychiatrist, plastic surgeon, infection control specialist, etc.), and most importantly, the child and family. Because many children do not have a traditional nuclear family, it is often necessary to determine who, in the child's view, comprises the family.

Scar Hypertrophy and Contracture

As previously mentioned, there are two common, though often avoidable, sequelae of deep partial-thickness and full-thickness burns: scar hypertrophy and scar contracture. Scar hypertrophy and scar contracture can impede both physical and psychological functioning. *Scar hypertrophy* is a raised, thick, usually hard, often knotty-appearing, area of scar tissue (Fig 7-4). Scar hypertrophy results from an imbalance of collagen synthesis and collagen lysis. Hypertrophic scars are, at times, also called keloids, although some investigators distinguish between the two. Although debate persists concern-

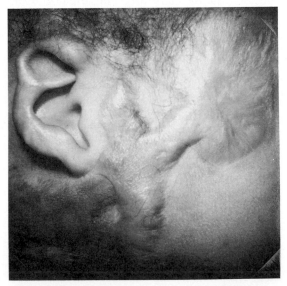

Figure 7-4. *Scar hypertrophy of a healed, ungrafted, deep, partial-thickness burn of the face.*

ing the distinction between hypertrophic scars and keloids, keloids are often considered to be the most severe degree of hypertrophic scarring.[17]

To determine which variables might be predictors for the development of hypertrophic scarring, one study considered such factors as the race and age of the patient, the location of the burn, and the length of time before the (ungrafted) burn was healed.[18] The investigation concluded that the length of time required to heal the burn was the most important indicator. Blacks in the study had a greater incidence of hypertrophic scarring than others if the burn took more than 10 to 14 days to heal. Burns of the chest, upper extremity, and foot were more likely to become hypertrophic than were burns in other anatomic areas, whereas burns of the hands, face, and neck were less likely to become hypertrophic than burns in other locations. The investigators attributed the increased incidence of hypertrophic scars in the presternal region of the chest, the back, and the deltoid region to wound tension. Another investigator[19] has also concurred that increased tension, which promotes collagen deposition and lessens collagen lysis, may contribute to the formation of hypertrophic scars, evidenced by the appearance of hypertrophic scars in areas of motion, such as the joints (Fig. 7-5). The authors of the first-mentioned study, citing other investigators,[20] also acknowledge that the depth of the wound is related to the incidence of hypertrophic scarring because burns of the reticulodermis are likely to heal with a hypertrophic scar, whereas more superficial burns involving the papillary dermis do not. However, these authors report that it is more accurate to quantify length of healing time rather than to estimate the depth of the wound subjectively. In the study, the age of the patient was not found to correlate with an increased incidence of hypertrophic scarring. However, others[21,22] have suggested that younger patients may have an increased incidence of hypertrophic scars compared to other age groups, probably because of an increased rate of collagen production.

Scar contracture is the pulling or shortening of scar tissue, which can result in the loss of joint mo-

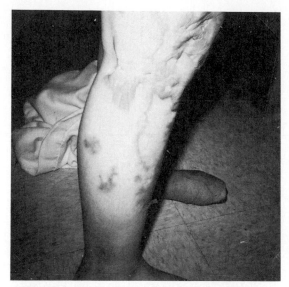

Figure 7-5. *Scar hypertrophy of a healed, ungrafted, deep, partial-thickness burn of the right lower extremity. Note the increased hypertrophic scarring around the knee joint, which may be the result of increased tension promoting collagen deposition and lessening collagen lysis.*

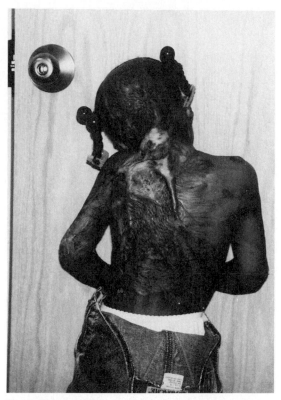

Figure 7-6. *Severe scar contracture and hypertrophy resulting not only in disfigurement and loss of motion, but also affecting posture and ambulation.*

tion or skin mobility. Contracture may be attributed to the action of myofibroblasts, which are cells that have contractile properties, that are found in the healing burn wound, and that can manipulate the spatial orientation of the newly synthesized collagen fibers.[17] Alternatively, fibroblasts, working as individual units, may produce the forces necessary for scar contracture.[23] Scar contracture that is not located over a joint can lead to disfigurement, especially if such a contracture involves the face. Scar contracture over a joint can lead to loss of joint range of motion (ROM) or posture and gait deviations (Fig. 7-6). Because of the contracting force of scar, which results in loss of skin mobility, a loss of joint ROM also can result from contracting scar tissue that is adjacent to, although not covering, a joint (see Fig 7-7). The scar will contract until it meets an equal or opposing force.[24] What is initially just loss of motion from contracting scar can, if left uncorrected, lead to a gradual shortening of joint capsules, muscles, tendons, and ligaments. A contracting scar in an adult may not cause any loss of

motion, whereas that same size scar in a small child may cause a loss of motion.[25]

The processes of scar contracture and scar hypertrophy begin almost as soon as the burn wound begins healing, although initially they may not be readily visible. Collagen accumulation in the wound has been noted to begin by 3 days after the injury.[26] There is a high rate of collagen synthesis in the wound,[27] and such activity returns to a normal pace by 6 to 12 months.[28] The scar is initially red because of an increased blood supply, but it fades over time. When the scar no longer is actively hypertrophying and contracting, it is said to be mature. The period of scar maturation for most children is approximately 12 to 18 months. For adults, this period may be shorter. While the scar is active, particularly during the first 6 months, the processes

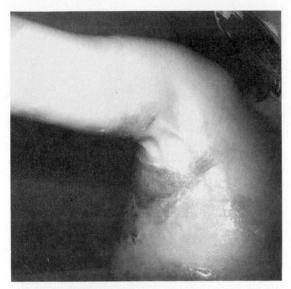

Figure 7-7. *Scar contracture of the axilla in a child who sustained deep partial-thickness and full-thickness burns to the trunk and upper extremity. Sheet-grafting has been performed. Although the axilla itself was spared, contracting scar on both sides of the joint has resulted in a loss of motion.*

of hypertrophy and contracture can be controlled or corrected by nonsurgical approaches, such as pressure, splinting, and ROM exercises, which will be discussed later. As scar maturation progresses, these treatments become less effective in altering scar. After the scar is mature, most nonsurgical treatments are no longer effective, and surgery, if indicated, may afford the only treatment alternative.

Initial Treatment and Medical Management

The initial treatment and medical management of the pediatric burn patient depend, in part, upon the depth, size, and location of the burn; the presence of other concomitant injuries, such as smoke inhalation; the age of the child; and the premorbid health of the child. The injury itself will trigger physiological responses which, in turn, will affect treatment requirements.

Establishing and maintaining an adequate airway and breathing are the first concerns when treating a thermally injured patient. If the patient has inhaled steam or noxious gases, intubation may be necessary because bronchospasm and upper airway edema[29] may develop, possibly resulting in airway obstruction within hours.[30] Oxygen is administered if the patient has inhaled high levels of carbon monoxide. The endotrachial tube may be removed once edema has subsided, usually within a few days.[30] Patients with more extensive airway or lung injuries will require sustained or more involved treatment.

When a patient's respiratory status is evaluated initially, cardiac hemodynamic status is also assessed, and the patient is examined for other injuries,[31] such as fractures and lacerations. Prophylactic tetanus toxoid (and sometimes benzathine penicillin) is administered to help prevent infections. A careful past medical history and a history of the burn incident are recorded. The wounds are evaluated, cleaned, and bandaged.

Because of the inflammatory process and increased capillary permeability in patients with deep partial-thickness or full-thickness burns, fluid leaves the blood and is dispersed into the interstitial spaces. Patients with burns of less than 10 to 20 percent of their TBSA, depending upon other considerations, may be able to compensate for this fluid shift physiologically through such measures as vasoconstriction and urine retention.[30] Patients with burns involving a greater percentage of TBSA will develop hypovolemic shock and can die if not treated. Replacement of the circulating fluid loss is termed fluid resuscitation. Fluids cannot be administered orally to patients with larger-area burns because of ileus (obstruction of the bowel), which occurs secondary to shock. Fluids, with electrolytes similar to serum, and colloid are given intravenously. Patients with smaller burns may be able to take fluids orally. However, children, in particular, may be unwilling to drink and, therefore, may require intravenous fluids. In a few days, with adequate fluid replacement, the fluid in the interstitial spaces returns to the intravascular spaces, and the patient will diurese, signaling successful fluid resuscitation.[30] After fluid resuscitation, the patient may still require the administration of fluids because fluid is also lost through the burn wound and because the patient may be unwilling or unable to take sufficient fluids orally.

A urinary catheter is placed in patients with large burns so as to monitor urine output during resuscitation. Patients with perineal burns may also require catheterization to keep bandages dry or to protect newly placed skin grafts during the skin graft phase.

Full-thickness burned skin is inelastic. Because of the body's response to injury and fluid resuscitation, the patient will become edematous. This is a systemic response that also occurs in the unburned parts of the body. In the case of circumferential burns of the extremities, the combination of inelastic skin and increasing edema can cause a tourniquet effect, resulting in compromised circulation to the distal extremities. If treatment is not initiated, ischemia and tissue damage or necrosis can occur. Monitoring of adequate circulation is usually accomplished by checking capillary refill in the fingers, by assessing the pulses through Doppler flowmetry, or, in the case of extremely deep burns, by measuring muscle compartment pressures.[32] When circulation is found to be compromised, an *escharotomy* is performed, which involves releasing the constricting inelastic burned skin by surgically incising it longitudinally down to subcutaneous fat on the midmedial and midlateral aspects of the limbs proximally to distally.[33] Escharotomy is usually performed within the first 24 to 48 hours of onset of the burn injury. Escharotomies may need to be performed on the chest to allow for adequate chest expansion and breathing in patients with deep circumferential burns of the trunk. When delayed escharotomy results in compartment syndrome, when deep burns involve muscle (as is often the case with electrical burn injuries), and when burns are accompanied by associated skeletal or soft tissue injury, the fascia will need to be released surgically,[33] a procedure termed a *fasciotomy*.

Initially, oral intake of fluids and food is prohib-ited in patients with larger burns in order to prevent the development of ileus. A nasogastric tube is inserted to empty the stomach to prevent vomiting and possible aspiration. Once bowel sounds return to normal, the patient can resume oral intake. In response to the burn injury, the patient is in a hypermetabolic state and caloric and nutritional requirements are greatly increased. Adequate nutrition is necessary to prevent wasting and to promote proper wound healing. The pediatric burn patient, because of the injury and a strange environment, may be unwilling to eat. The severity or location of the burns may make it difficult or impossible to eat. A patient with a larger burn may find it hard to consume the volume of food necessary to obtain sufficient calories. Additionally, the patient will be prohibited from eating on days when a surgical procedure is scheduled in the operating room. Because of such factors, the patient may receive a large portion of nutrition through enteral tube feedings or through peripheral vein infusions. Patients with smaller burns who are willing and able to eat may obtain all nutrition orally. When wound healing is complete, or following skin grafting procedures, if the patient is eating and drinking adequately, tube or parenteral feeds may be discontinued. The dietitian often instructs the parent in good nutritional practices prior to discharge.

A burn injury is one of the most painful events an individual can experience. In addition, the treatments administered, including some administered by the therapist, are themselves painful. Writing about the psychosocial care of the severely burned child, Knudson-Cooper and Thomas[14] cite the following research to plead for adequate pain management of burn patients. Studies have shown that medical professionals who treat burn patients underrate the patients' pain when compared with the patients' own estimates of their pain.[34,35] Additionally, the first-mentioned authors state that medical personnel generally accept that babies and children may experience pain differently than do adolescents and adults, although there is no reason for them to believe that babies and children feel less pain.[36,37] In some facilities, children may not receive medication for acute pain![38]

Pain management is essential for avoiding what would otherwise amount to torture and for enabling the patient to cooperate with treatment and to be involved in self-care. In addition to a variety of pharmacologic agents, relaxation techniques, hypnosis, and other methods of pain management can be employed effectively with children.[14] Besides specific medications and pain management techniques, the facility and each professional should have a treatment approach that has as a goal caring for the burn patient in a way that causes the least amount of pain. Some suggestions for minimizing patients' pain are made throughout the chapter.

Wound Management

The primary goals of wound management are to provide an optimal environment for wound healing, to provide a healthy tissue bed to receive a skin graft, and to protect healing tissue or a recently placed graft. Such goals are accomplished mainly through removing dead tissue, keeping the wound clean and minimizing bacterial invasion, preventing the wound or new skin graft from drying out, and protecting newly healing tissue or recent skin graft(s) from disruptive mechanical abrasion.

Dressing Changes

Many objectives of wound management are achieved through daily wound care and proper application and changing of bandages. Most burn patients will undergo bandage (also called dressing) changes at least daily. In some burn centers, therapists are responsible for or may assist with daily wound care for both inpatients and outpatients. (It may also be the case that the therapist, prior to or during performance of outpatient therapy, will need to change the patient's bandage.) During a dressing change, the old bandage is removed and the wound may be superficially debrided (nonviable tissue removed). At the same time, the wound is cleaned and examined, range of motion is quickly checked (or the patient may be briefly exercised by the therapist), and a topical antimicrobial agent and clean gauze bandages are applied. There are other wound dressings that may be used depending upon the extent and depth of injury, the phase of healing, and the protocol of a given burn center. For example, a biological dressing, such as human cadaver skin (allograft) or pigskin (xenograft), or a biosynthetic dressing, may be placed on the wound.

A review of pediatric burn deaths shows that sepsis is a major contributing factor and that the wound is the primary source of infection.[39] In a burn injury, the protective barrier of the skin is lost, and the burn wound becomes a host for bacteria. Topical antimicrobials play a vital role in helping to minimize bacterial colonization of the wound. Several topical antimicrobials may be employed depending upon the specific wound and the organisms to be controlled. Silver sulfadiazine is one of the most commonly used topical agents.

Dressings should not excessively inhibit motion. The thumb, for example, should not be wrapped into the palm, nor should bandages restrict chest expansion. However, bandages can be used to help position the patient. For example, during the emergent phase (see later section), bulky bandages can be used in place of splints to support the fingers and wrists in infants and toddlers.

Despite pain medication, the daily dressing change is undoubtedly one of the most painful experiences that the burn patient must endure. There are measures that can minimize the pain and trauma of this event. The patient should be adequately medicated prior to the dressing change. The patient's response to the dose received should be monitored and, when possible, the physician should adjust the dose or select a different medication accordingly. Bandages that stick to the wound not only cause pain upon removal, but if they are "ripped off," some of the newly healed tissue may also removed. When indicated, the bandage can be soaked off, or sterile water can be poured over the bandage to loosen it. Even very young children can participate in removing their dressings, which may help minimize pain and offer some sense of control and independence in a situation where they might otherwise feel helpless. Because some of the pain experienced during a dressing change is caused by exposure of the wound to air, such exposure time should be limited. Limiting the exposure time to air will help prevent the tissue from drying out and will also limit exposure to bacteria. To minimize the time required for a dressing change, bandages should be prepared ahead of time so that they may be quickly applied. Health care professionals who wish to observe the patient's wound should be present at the time of the dressing change so that the patient is not waiting with an undressed wound for them to arrive. Additionally, applying the topical antimicrobial agent to the gauze and then applying the gauze to the wound (instead of applying the topical agent directly to the wound and then applying the gauze) will also help to minimize pain during the dressing change.

Other measures may be helpful in minimizing pain and trauma during dressing changes in pediatric patients. Some of these include visualization and relaxation techniques, distraction techniques, and toys and music brought into the treatment room. If the parent desires, and if appropriate, the parent's presence during the dressing change can be beneficial for both the parent and the child. In some cases, however, children may cry more in the presence of a parent because they expect the parent to "rescue" them from the dressing change.

Hydrotherapy

Hydrotherapy is used in some burn centers as a part of wound management. The purpose of hydrotherapy is to help remove the old topical antimicrobial agent, to clean the wound, to help debride the wound (through the effect of the agitator), to increase circulation in order to promote wound healing, and to provide an environment for exercise. The drawbacks of hydrotherapy are that it can spread infection; it can increase the length of time required for a dressing change; it can increase cost (because of the additional personnel required to perform the procedure and clean the equipment); it can increase edema (especially if a limb is placed in a dependent position); and patients, particularly children, may find it to be more traumatic or painful than a dressing change without hydrotherapy, thus

making it an unsuitable environment for exercise. Because of the drawbacks of hydrotherapy, some burn centers limit its use to specific wounds or to certain phases of wound healing, or use hand-held showerheads to help clean the wound.

Surgical Management

One of the primary goals of the surgeon is to achieve permanent closure of the wound. Although there have been many advances in wound healing and surgical techniques in the past decade, an autograft is the most widely used method—and is considered to be the preferred permanent method—for wound closure. By definition, an autograft is a skin graft taken from and donated to the same individual. A detailed description of the autografting procedure is provided later in this chapter.

Because a superficial partial-thickness burn will heal in approximately 2 weeks with normal skin, the goals of the surgeon in such cases are to keep the wound free of infection, to provide adequate nutrition and fluids, and to manage pain until the wound is healed. Depending upon the size and location of the superficial partial-thickness burn, the age of the patient, and the ability of the parent, many of these burns can be treated on an outpatient basis.

A deep-partial thickness burn can heal without surgical intervention if adequate medical treatment and wound management are provided. However, as discussed earlier, depending upon the size of the wound, deep partial-thickness burns may take 3 to 6 weeks or longer to heal spontaneously. The surgeon may elect to graft the deep partial-thickness burn in a procedure called tangential excision and grafting. Such excision and grafting can be done within the first week of the burn injury and is ideally performed 2 to 5 days after the burn injury (termed *early excision and grafting*). Early excision and grafting may also apply to other wounds, particularly full-thickness wounds, which may be excised to fascia. Tangential excision and grafting of deep partial-thickness wounds during the first week shortens the patient's hospital stay, lessens pain, decreases the incidence of infection, improves cosmetic and functional outcome (by minimizing the amount of hypertrophic scar tissue development and scar contracture), and decreases the need for subsequent reconstructive procedures.[40,41]

There are drawbacks associated with early tangential excision and grafting of deep partial-thickness wounds, however, and not all patients are candidates for this procedure. Early excision and grafting of deep partial-thickness burns usually involves significant intraoperative blood loss that may require substantial transfusion; this may not be recommended for medically unstable patients or those with inhalation injury. When a burn involves a significant percentage of TBSA, and particularly when the burn area consists of both deep partial-thickness and full-thickness burns and there is a limited number of donor sites for skin grafts, excision and grafting of deep partial-thickness burns is generally delayed. This is because the full-thickness burns have to be grafted first. Deep partial-thickness burns can be grafted after the first 3 to 5 days. However, the later such wounds are grafted, the more likely the wound is to be colonized by bacteria, and some other benefits of early excision may be diminished.

Smaller deep partial-thickness burns that are to be grafted can be treated on an outpatient basis for several days until the patient is admitted to the hospital for grafting or until the surgeon determines that the wound is indeed deep partial-thickness and would be treated best by excision and grafting.

A full-thickness burn, by definition, destroys the full thickness of the skin. The only way for such burns to heal is for the dead tissue to be removed and a skin graft to be applied. ("Fourth-degree" burns, which involve subcutaneous fat, fascia, muscle, or bone, may also require local or regional flaps for definitive coverage.[42])

Skin Graft and Donor Site

A *skin graft* is a piece of skin that is surgically shaved from an unburned part of the patient's body (called the donor site) and placed on the burned area. Obviously, if a full-thickness piece of skin

from the unburned donor site were taken and placed on the burned area, the burn would heal, but a wound of similar dimensions to the burn would remain at the donor site. Therefore, only a partial- or split-thickness (approximately 0.008 inch thick[43]) piece of skin is taken. Some areas of the body are preferred donor sites because of the thickness, texture, or color of the skin, because they are areas that will heal well, and also because they are in a region not usually visible. Common preferred donor sites include the lateral thighs and buttocks. However, when these areas are burned, or in an extensively burned individual, almost any skin on the body can be used.

Before the skin graft can be placed, the burned, necrotic skin, called *eschar*, must be removed. This is usually accomplished surgically, but enzymatic debriders may also be used. Surgical excision usually extends down to a level of viable tissue. Excision can be effected immediately prior to placing the skin graft, or, depending upon the depth and extent of the wound, it may be accomplished earlier, in a separate operation. If a full-thickness wound is not grafted during the same procedure, granulation tissue will develop which will help prepare the site for grafting.

Once the patient has been anesthetized, the skin is shaved from the donor site with an electric knife—known as a dermatome—that has settings to adjust the thickness of skin excised. Removal of the skin that is to be used for grafting is called *harvesting*. The procedure is called a sheet graft when the skin is placed "as is" on the excised burned area (also known as the recipient or graft site) (Figs. 7-6, 7-8, and 7-9). Alternatively, the skin may be placed in a skin mesher prior to its application to the recipient site. The mesher cuts small slits in the graft, after which the graft is stretched or expanded prior to placement on the recipient site. Such a graft is known as an *expanded mesh graft* (Fig. 7-10). The main purpose of meshing is to allow a skin graft to cover a larger area than could otherwise be covered using a sheet graft. The amount of expansion achieved is expressed as a ratio of the expanded to the unexpanded size. For example, an expanded

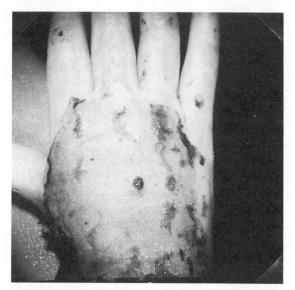

Figure 7-8. *Sheet graft of the dorsum of the hand (wrist to metacarpophalangeal joints) approximately 5 to 7 days after graft application. This patient can now be measured for commercially available, custom-fitting elastic pressure garments, and may be ready for light-pressure dressings worn over bandages.*

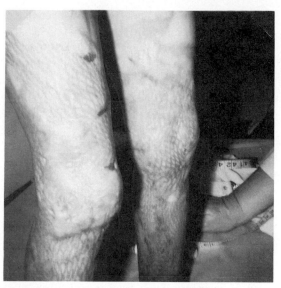

Figure 7-10. *Healed meshed grafts of the lower extremities. (Marks are soluble ink used in the measurement of this patient for custom-made pressure garments.)*

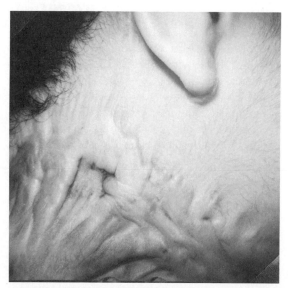

Figure 7-9. *Sheet graft of the neck. Note the hypertrophic scarring and contracture of the borders of the graft and of the healed, ungrafted areas. Note also the contracture under the graft.*

mesh graft that covers one and a half times its original or unmeshed size would be referred to as a 1.5:1 mesh graft. One advantage of a mesh graft is that compared to a sheet graft there is less likelihood that hematomas or serous fluid will collect under the graft, causing the graft to be nonadherent. A disadvantage of a mesh graft, particularly a large-ratio mesh graft, is that scarring occurs within the interstices or holes and such scarring can hypertrophy and contract. The permanent meshed pattern of the graft may also be cosmetically unattractive. Because sheet grafts provide a better cosmetic outcome with less contracture and hypertrophy, they are used on the face, neck, and hands, and are often preferred, when possible, for other functional areas of the body, such as the feet and the axillae.

The surgeon may secure the graft with surgical staples, stitches, or Steri-strips. The graft usually requires 4 to 7 days to become adherent or to "take." The grafted area is protected during this period by bulky dressings. If the graft site is over a joint, the joint is usually immobilized with a splint during this initial period, and exercise of the joint is discontinued for that same period. Movement or shearing forces can result in graft loss. Other factors that can contribute to graft loss or less-than-optimal graft take are infection, inadequate nutrition, or a poor graft bed.

The donor site itself is now a partial-thickness wound and is treated as such. The donor site will usually heal within 10 days to 2 weeks with normal skin, although it may be many months before the skin color appears normal. In some cases, there may be some permanent skin discoloration. Occasionally, a thicker graft is inadvertently, taken (remember that the skin of infants and young children is thinner than that of adults), and the donor site, because it is now deeper than a superficial partial-thickness wound, will heal with scar tissue. A donor site that heals with normal skin can be reused, if necessary. Such reuse is called *reharvesting*.

In the case of a burn involving a large percentage of TBSA, even when multiple donor sites are available, the surgeon may elect not to graft the entire burn at once because of the stress of surgery to the patient, particularly if the patient is already medically compromised or unstable. If the grafts do not take, not only is there still a large TBSA burn, but the donor sites are now additional wounds that must be healed, and the donor sites cannot be reused for about 10 days.

Cultured Epithelial Autografts and Dermal Substitutes

Several advances in wound healing and surgical techniques during the past decade have improved the outcome and increased survival of burn patients. Among these advances are two that have been shown to increase survival in massively burned individuals who lack sufficient donor sites: cultured epithelial autografts (or keratinocytes) and dermal substitutes.

In the case of cultured epithelial autografts, a small piece of unburned skin measuring approximately 1 inch in diameter is taken from the patient and grown in a laboratory. Within several weeks or less, there is enough skin to cover an entire body, and this skin can be grafted onto the patient from whom the original sample was taken. However, there are drawbacks and problems with cultured autografted skin. Wound closure must be delayed until the skin is grown, and the rate of graft take, depending upon the occurrence of graft site infection, varies from 15% to 80%.[44] Cultured skin grafts, lacking tensile strength, are fragile and easily cut or bruised.[45] Although dermal regeneration occurs below cultured epithelial autografts over 4 to 5 years, the skin lacks hair follicles and sweat glands. Sensory nerves and pigmentation are also absent.[45]

There are several dermal substitutes currently being evaluated. One substitute is an artificial dermis composed of a collagen mat which, when placed on an excised wound, allows vascularization and fibroblastic ingrowth.[46] Also being studied is the use of allografted skin, which, once the antigenic epidermis is removed, will accept the patient's cultured epithelial autograft.[47]

Role and Goals of the Therapist

The therapist plays a crucial role in the rehabilitation of the pediatric burn patient. The therapist's goals for the pediatric burn patient are to maintain or increase active and passive range of motion, manage soft tissue contours, maintain or increase strength and endurance, promote normal development and function, and inhibit loss of motion, deformity, hypertrophic scarring, and contracture. The therapist is involved in all phases of the burn injury from the acute through the rehabilitative and the reconstructive. The therapist is a member of the burn team and consults with other team members, including the patient and parents, when planning and executing treatment.

The role and goals of the therapist is discussed for each phase of recovery with emphasis on the rehabilitative phase. Although the primary focus is on the rehabilitative phase, rehabilitation essentially begins when the patient is admitted to the hospital, and the acute therapeutic intervention can affect the type, intensity, length, and outcome of rehabilitation.

The Emergent Phase

The emergent phase generally includes the first 48 to 72 hours after the burn injury. Whether the therapist works in a general hospital or in a burn center, it is advisable to have established a protocol with the surgery department dictating a consult upon the patient's admission if the patient has sustained deep or extensive burns. This arrangement ensures that the therapist is available and becomes involved as soon as necessary, and allows the therapist to become familiar with the patient's history and to evaluate, plan, and initiate treatment in a timely fashion.

Patient presentation during the emergent phase will depend upon the depth, extent, and location of the burn injury and upon any associated injuries, such as smoke inhalation. The patient may have extensive edema, be intubated, have undergone escharotomies, and have multiple bandaged areas, or the patient may have only a bandaged limb or chest with a burn of an as yet undetermined depth. Both the severity of the injury and the age of the child will affect the therapist's goals and specific treatment during this phase. The goals of the therapist during the emergent phase are to begin evaluation, set goals, and plan treatment. When indicated, the therapist may also be involved in controlling edema, beginning and maintaining motion and mobility, splinting and positioning, training in activities of daily living (ADL), and promoting normal development.

Evaluation, Goal Setting, and Treatment Planning

The evaluation process begins with a careful chart review. The physical therapist should next evaluate the patient during a dressing change to more closely examine the location, apparent depth, and extent of the burn wounds.

A generalized evaluation of ROM should be undertaken during the dressing change when bandages will not interfere with motion and when the

therapist can see the wounds. The patient may be edematous, which may limit full active and passive ROM. Because of young age, severity of injury, or pain, many children are unable to cooperate with ROM instructions. A goniometer cannot be allowed to touch an open wound, but it can be held about a half inch away from the patient during the evaluation. During the emergent phase, however, it is usually more practical to "eyeball" ROM, which should not be forced by the therapist.

Based on information from the chart and that obtained during a general examination, the therapist can then establish general long-term and short-term goals and begin treatment planning and execution. One goal is continued evaluation and monitoring of the patient. Evaluation is an ongoing process, and as changes occur in the patient's status or as the depth of wound or the surgical plan becomes known, the therapist's goals and treatment will be affected.

Splinting and Positioning

The purpose of splinting and positioning during this 48- to 72-hour period is to help control edema, provide support for edematous extremities, and inhibit contracture and loss of motion. It is often not necessary to splint children at this time except in the case of older children and adolescents and those who are extensively burned. The therapist should initiate positioning in bed. If the patient is able to get out of bed, the therapist should provide for proper bedside positioning.

An extremity or part of an extremity may be edematous even if it is not burned. Unlike adults, most children do not have long-term problems with edema. Edematous extremities may be elevated on pillows at heart level. Splints to support the wrist in a neutral position or slight extension and splints to position the ankles in approximately a neutral position may be provided for older children with burns in these areas. If necessary, bulky bandages can be used to provide support for younger children and infants.

There is an axiom that states that the position of comfort—flexion—is the position of contracture for burn patients. Patients are thus splinted or positioned to counteract contracting forces. As mentioned previously, it is often not necessary to splint children during the emergent phase, although the therapist, upon a surgeon's order, may elect to begin splinting and positioning children with severe burns or older children and adolescents later in this phase. The neck should be positioned in a neutral position or slight extension. Pillows under the head are prohibited because they promote cervical flexion. A splint can be used to position the neck, but it may be easier during this phase to use a roll under the shoulders. The shoulders should be positioned in approximately 90 degrees of abduction and in slight protraction. Again, during this phase, splints can be used or the position can be achieved using pillows under the arms. The limbs should be positioned in extension, with the ankles and wrists in a neutral position. To protect the extensor mechanism, as well as to prevent contracture, the proper position for a burned hand is for the metacarpophalangeal joints to be flexed, the interphalangeal joints to be extended, and the thumb to be placed in palmar abduction. (The exception to this is the patient with solely palmar burns, in which case the fingers are positioned in full extension and the thumb is placed in radial abduction.) Smaller joints in the hand may be difficult to position correctly because of edema and should never be forced into the ideal position. Splints or bulky bandages that approximate the desired position can be used to position the hand during the emergent phase if necessary.

If splints are used during this phase, they should be applied over the dressings and secured with Kerlix or Kling* bandaging because, with emerging edema, straps on splints could cause a tourniquet effect, and elastic wraps also could compromise circulation. The splint can be worn for 24 hours with removal for exercise or activities as desired. In any case, splints should be removed periodically and checked by the nursing and therapy staff for proper application, and circulation of the

distal extremities should be monitored to ensure that the splint is not too tight. Written instructions regarding proper splinting should be provided for the nursing staff.

Range of Motion

Active ROM exercises during the emergent phase help to control edema and initiate early motion. Muscle contraction serves as a pumping mechanism to aid venous and lymphatic return.[48] It is not necessary to move younger children during this time, but the therapist may begin gentle active ROM exercises in older children and adolescents. Active ROM may be limited by edema. As stated previously ROM exercises should be performed during dressing changes when the bandages do not restrict motion, the therapist can see the limitations in motion resulting from edema, the wound can be viewed, and the patient has received pain medication. Passive ROM should not be performed during this period.

Activities of Daily Living and Development

Depending upon the age of patient, the severity and location of burn, and the patient's mentation, the therapist may introduce several ADL and developmental activities. When appropriate, the therapist should teach bed mobility and transfers.

The Acute Phase

The acute phase extends from the emergent period until skin grafting or wound closure. The goals of the physical therapist are to maintain ROM, inhibit contracture, and promote function and normal development. Generally during this phase, edema subsides, the depth of the wound becomes evident, and the surgeon plans skin grafting or another course of treatment. The therapist should continue to observe the healing wound at regular intervals.

Splinting and Positioning

The purpose of splinting and positioning during the acute phase is to maintain or increase ROM by counteracting the force of contracting tissue. As

---

*Johnson & Johnson, New Brunswick, NJ

previously discussed, flexion, the position of comfort, is the position of contracture, so patients are positioned to counteract contracting forces. Patients with burns of the neck are splinted in neutral to slight extension, avoiding lateral flexion and rotation, and pillows are prohibited. (Care also should be taken to position the patient to avoid pressure on burned ears, which can result in chondritis.) Shoulders are positioned in approximately 90 degrees of abduction and slight protraction. Elbows and knees are splinted in extension. In the case of deep dorsal burns of the hand, correct positioning is necessary to prevent boutonnière deformities. A boutonnière deformity (hyperextension of the metacarpophalangeal [MCP] joint, flexion of the proximal interphalangeal [PIP] joint, and hyperextension of the distal interphalangeal [DIP] joint) occurs when the central slip of the extensor tendon to the proximal interphalangeal [PIP] joint ruptures and the lateral bands slide volarly. To help prevent such a deformity, as well as to inhibit contractures, the hand is positioned with the wrist extended 15 to 20 degrees, the metacarpophalangeal joints are flexed approximately 60 to 70 degrees, the interphalangeal joints are extended, and the thumb is abducted (Fig. 7-11). However, especially with younger children, this precise hand position may not be achieved, and should never be forced. The hips should be positioned in extension and abducted 15 degrees, and the ankles should be positioned in neutral. The therapist may also need to splint the mouths of patients with deep facial burns in order to inhibit the development of microstomia.

In general, unburned parts do not need to be splinted or positioned except as they affect the position of burned areas. The therapist should continually monitor ROM, especially in unburned joints in older patients and in patients who are hospitalized for long periods and in whom loss of motion may result from prolonged immobilization. In some cases, it may be necessary to apply foot splints to unburned feet to inhibit footdrop.

If the patient was splinted during the emergent phase, the splint may need to be adjusted in the acute phase to accommodate the changes that result from decreased edema. This process may be less

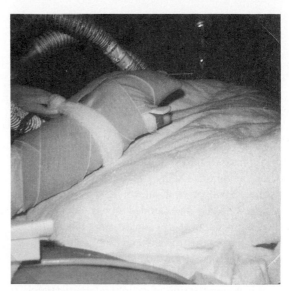

Figure 7-11. *A hand splint is used during the acute phase to help maintain range of motion, inhibit contracture, and protect tendons and joints. Elastic bandages are used during this phase to secure splints. Elevation of the extremity may be helpful in decreasing any residual edema.*

painful to the patient if the therapist adjusts or makes such splints immediately following the dressing change while the patient still has the benefit of recent pain medication. The splint can be applied with elastic wraps during this phase unless significant early edema persists. The splint-wearing schedule will depend upon the individual patient. Some patients will wear the splint continually except during dressing changes, during specific activities and exercises, or during periodic evaluation of fit and circulation. Other patients may require splinting only at night. Each patient's schedule may change during the course of the acute phase. One way to determine an adequate splinting schedule is to see how much motion the patient loses when the splint has been off for a specified period.

Although patients must be positioned properly to prevent contractures, their position in bed should be changed periodically over a 24-hour period to help prevent decubiti. The use of special beds or mattresses, designed to decrease pressure over bony prominences and reduce the pressure and shearing forces that might disrupt healing tissue or recent grafts, may be beneficial.

Cardiopulmonary status is also a factor to consider in determining appropriate positioning, particularly in patients who have sustained an inhalation injury or who, because of their injuries, will be at bedrest or hospitalized for a prolonged period. Elevating the head of the bed or placing the patient in a chair at scheduled times may help to maximize lung position and chest expansion and maintain or increase endurance. (The therapist should be cautioned, however, that elevating the head of the patient's bed for an extended time can contribute to hip flexion contractures if care is not taken to avoid such contractures through measures such as position changes and ROM exercises.)

Another concern when positioning the burn patient is the prevention of peripheral nerve stretch or compression injuries that can be caused by improper positioning.[49] For example, patients with medial thigh burns or a swollen scrotum, or those who are tall, may assume a position of externally rotated hips, flexed knees, and inverted ankles, which can result in footdrop secondary to peroneal nerve palsy.[49]

Range of Motion

During the acute phase, the purposes of ROM exercises and activities are to maintain or increase ROM by counteracting the contracting forces of healing tissue; to maintain joint motion, tendon gliding, and muscle activity; and to improve circulation. Because edema is resolving, limitations in ROM caused by edema should be decreasing, although during the early part of this phase, some restrictions in motion from edema may persist. During the acute phase, ROM may be limited by inelastic eschar or by contracting tissue. Just as during the emergent phase, ROM exercises should be performed during the dressing change. Once the extent of ROM is known, appropriate exercises can be done at the patient's bedside or incorporated into play activities.

In general, passive ROM exercises should be avoided. However, when children are unable to co-operate because of their injuries or their young age, *gentle* passive ROM, to the limits of resistance by the tissue, can be done. Passive ROM beyond such resistance can damage healing tissue. When possible, passive ROM exercise can be performed by the therapist in the operating room—while the patient is anesthetized—prior to any surgical procedure. When performed under these conditions such ROM exercises are painless, and the therapist is able to ascertain the true limits of motion.

Although maintaining ROM is a primary goal, the author cautions against excessive and aggressive ROM exercise. Overaggressive exercises may damage newly healing tissue and may cause pain that traumatizes the patient and leads to a decreased level of cooperation during the rehabilitation phase. Some infants, toddlers, and younger children who are not extensively burned and who undergo early excision and grafting will be hospitalized only briefly, and may not require daily ROM. Their joints, even if immobilized for several weeks, may not necessarily become stiff, and splinting may help to maintain motion. However, the patient's ROM must be closely monitored.

Exposed Tendons and Joints

At some point during the acute or early rehabilitation phase, patients with deep burns may present with exposed tendons or joints. Areas where the tendon or joint are superficial, or where the skin covering them is thin, are common sites for such exposure. Examples of such locations are the dorsum of the hand, particularly over the proximal interphalangeal joints; the posterior elbow; the dorsum of the foot; and the ankle. If the exposed tendon or the exposed joint and periarticular structures appear to be healthy and intact, and depending upon the location of the exposure, the therapist, under the direction of the surgeon, may still perform or ask the patient to perform supervised ROM exercises. In cases in which the tendon or joint appears to be fragile or necrotic, or the tendon has ruptured, or the joint and/or periarticular structures are damaged, exercises to the joint must be discontinued, the joint may need to be immobilized, and exercises to the adjacent joints may have to be discontinued or modified or special exercise techniques may need to be employed. The exposed tendons or joints also need to be protected from drying out.

Activities of Daily Living and Development

During the acute phase, depending on the age of the child and the severity of the injury, the patient may have difficulty with ADLs or may be dependent upon the nursing staff for help with ADLs as a result of treatment. Pain, bulky bandages, and splints may discourage the patient from engaging in such activities. As much as possible, the patient should participate in ADLs and assist with self-care. Splints that inhibit specified ADLs (e.g., self-feeding) should be removed to allow the patient to participate in such activities, after which they can be immediately reapplied. When indicated and appropriate, special ADL equipment (such as built-up handles on eating utensils) can be provided and the patient can be taught necessary techniques, such as transfers.

During the acute phase, patients without lower extremity burns may ambulate. However, because of pain, bandages, or upper extremity splints, such patients may require assistive devices or supervision. Patients with burns of the lower extremity which are not extensive or deep also may ambulate after application of supportive elastic wraps over dressings. However, it may not be necessary to force such early ambulation.

Age-appropriate toys, activities, music, and videos should be supplied according to individual needs, and interaction with other children should be facilitated. Most pediatric facilities have a playroom or employ a child life therapist who interacts with the patient in the unit or at the bedside.

The Skin Graft Phase

The goals of the therapist during the skin graft phase are to help protect the newly grafted area, to maintain motion in the nongrafted joints, and to initiate or finalize discharge planning. The grafted part is usually immobilized for 5 to 7 days until the graft is adherent. Depending upon the extent of the burn, the patient may undergo several skin grafting procedures.

Splinting and Positioning

If the area that has been grafted is over a joint, the joint is usually immobilized with a splint. Besides immobilizing the joint, the splint also maintains the joint in an anticontracture position during this time. If the therapist has not already splinted the joint in an area to be grafted prior to skin grafting, the therapist now should fabricate a splint that the surgeon can apply in the operating room after the grafting procedure. Alternatively, the surgeon may construct a plaster splint in the operating room. Such construction in the operating room may ensure a more accurate fit over bulky bandages and may be more cost-effective if the splint is to be used only during the skin graft phase.

Range of Motion

Although the grafted joint cannot be moved during this period, unburned or burned but nongrafted joints may still be moved. If the unburned or nongrafted area is directly adjacent to a fresh graft, the therapist should seek the surgeon's approval prior to initiating ROM exercises or other activities that might disrupt the new graft. The patient probably will experience pain or discomfort from the donor site, which may interfere with full active ROM.

Discharge Planning

Discharge plans should be finalized by the time of the last skin grafting procedure. However, discharge planning really should begin as soon as the patient has been evaluated and a treatment plan has been proposed. Although each patient should be treated individually and the course for some burn patients is unknown, many such patients follow a predictable course of treatment and have a predictable length of hospital stay. Discharge planning should be a team process, and it is helpful to have a member of the discharge planning department on the burn team.

Ongoing discussion about hospital discharge from the time of admission is encouraging for both the family and the patient, may help them prepare for the patient's eventual return to home, and allows them to be a part of the planning process. Judgment must be exercised during the acute phase in determining what information to share with the family and when.

The therapist should evaluate the patient's needs and the available resources when planning for discharge. Consideration should be given to the type and frequency of therapy necessary and the need for pressure garments or equipment. Additionally, the therapist should consider where the patient lives, the availability of local rehabilitation facilities, whether the local facility and discharging institution will jointly follow the patient and how, what the patient's insurance will cover, and the level of family support, and the family's ability to follow through with treatment. Another factor to be considered in discharge planning for school-aged patients is school reentry.[14]

Discharge Teaching

Just as with discharge planning, discharge teaching should begin as soon as the patient has been evaluated and a treatment plan has been proposed. Of course, the exact information that the family and patient will need cannot be predicted or provided from the outset, but the process of instructing them about therapy and involving them in patient care can begin at admission when appropriate. This approach also allows learning to occur over time, and helps the family prepare for eventual discharge. When the patient is ready to be discharged, the topics to be included in the therapist's discharge teaching plan may include skin care, scarring, use and application of pressure garments, ROM, splints, and ADLs or developmental activities.

Teaching methods and instruments can include verbal instructions, demonstrations, written instructions, and/or videos. The family and patient should have ample time and opportunity to review with the therapist the information presented and to practice specific skills, such as applying pressure dressings

and garments or splints. The information discussed and the skills demonstrated should be reinforced and expanded upon during outpatient visits.

The Rehabilitation Phase

The rehabilitation phase extends from the time of graft adherence—or, for deep partial-thickness burns that are not grafted, from wound closure—until scar maturation. The period of scar maturation for most children is 12 to 18 months after graft adherence or wound closure, with the scar generally being most active during the first 6 months. The goals of the physical therapist during this phase are to achieve mobility and weight-bearing; to maintain or increase ROM; to promote formation of a flat, soft, smooth, pliable scar; to increase strength and endurance; to achieve independence in ADLs; to facilitate normal development and participation in age-appropriate activities; and to facilitate the patient's return to home and school.

Initially, the patient may still have bandages in places to cover small open wounds; these wounds should heal in 1 to 2 weeks, although a few patients have wounds that persist or recur far beyond this period. Some patients have no open wounds, but may subsequently develop open areas as a result of scratching or friction in areas of fragile skin. (Wounds, particularly deep wounds or those located over joints, which persist or recur over an extended term may be a sign that the patient has insufficient skin coverage and will require further grafting.) The donor sites may not be healed during the first week after graft adherence.

Weight-Bearing and Ambulation

Patients who have undergone grafting in areas other than the lower extremities can begin weight-bearing on the first postoperative day (if medically stable and with a physician's order). Because the thighs and buttocks are frequently used for donor sites, however, these patients may experience pain or discomfort upon weight-bearing, ambulation, or movement. They will frequently stand or ambulate with their trunk, hips, and knees flexed. Because of pain in the donor or graft site, weakness, and their standing posture or gait pattern, these patients may be unsteady and may initially require support or assistive devices. Selecting the appropriate support may be complicated if the grafted site is on the axilla or hand.

Depending upon the child's age, medical status, and the size, location, and depth of lower extremity burns, weight-bearing and ambulation or preparation for these activities in the patient with newly grafted lower extremity burns are usually initiated 5 to 7 days after grafting. However, on the first day after grafting, the patient can be out of bed in a chair or wheelchair with the legs elevated and the knees and feet properly positioned. A sequence of steps often leads to independent ambulation. Again, depending upon the age, medical status, and extent of the injury, the sequence may take from 1 or 2 days to 1 or 2 weeks to complete. Prior to being placed in a dependent position, the recently grafted lower extremity should be wrapped with elastic bandages or a tubular elastic stocking (e.g., Tubigrip*) should be applied. (However, donor sites on the legs are not usually wrapped.) Such wrapping provides support to prevent blood pooling in the newly adherent graft, which could lead to hemorrhaging of fragile new capillaries and damage to the new graft. Elastic support also helps to diminish associated pain, itching, and the dark purple color that results when the lower extremity is placed in a dependent position without elastic support. (Even with adequate support, some of these signs and symptoms may be present to a lesser degree.)

The sequence of steps leading to independent ambulation may begin with leg-dangling. On the fifth to seventh day after graft placement, with elastic support applied, the patient may dangle the legs for brief periods while sitting in bed, in a chair or wheelchair, or on an elevated mat. Next, the patient may attempt weight-bearing with assistance for brief periods, then advance to ambulating with assistance, and finally progress to independent ambu-

---

Seton Products, Ltd., Tubiton House, Olham, Lancashire, England.

lation. Weight-bearing and ambulation often will increase ROM, particularly if the patient has limitations in ankle dorsiflexion.

Skin Care

Daily bathing with a mild soap is recommended to remove dead skin cells and old lotion in order to prevent them from clogging pores. Newly healed tissue or recently adherent grafts are fragile and should be protected from mechanical abrasion. Such areas will become more durable over time. Newly healed tissue and grafts also should be protected from chemicals, such as household cleaners, and from the sun.

PRURITIS (ITCHING). Skin grafts and scar tissue can itch severely during the first year following injury. Such itching can be agonizing and disruptive to the patient's normal activities, particularly sleeping. Scratching can cause open wounds because recently adherent grafts or newly healed tissue is fragile. Itching may be the result of increased histamine, and may be aggravated by dry skin. (Scar tissue and skin grafts do not have the same number of functioning sweat glands[50] and may also lack the number of sebaceous glands that are present in normal skin.) The doctor may prescribe an oral antipruritic. Keeping the skin well lubricated by applying lotions once or more daily can also diminish itching, and cool baths or compresses may also provide relief.[51]

MASSAGE. Massage of scar tissue and skin grafts helps to maintain motion by freeing restrictive bands and increasing circulation.[52] Massage may also be helpful in decreasing itching. Initially, only gentle massage should be employed, because the newly healed tissue is often too fragile to tolerate much friction. Many children enjoy massage because it decreases itching, but other children find massage painful and will not sit still for such treatment. Although all patients should have scar tissue and skin grafts lubricated by thoroughly rubbing in lotions—preferably twice each day—the therapist may select particular areas of concern for massage and may also instruct the parent in massage of these areas. Massage should be done prior to specific ROM exercises, especially passive ROM exercises.

Scar Evaluation

There is no universally accepted and practical instrument used to measure scars. However, scar evaluation is important for determining the need for and efficacy of treatment. Several tools or methods that measure one or more aspects of scar have been proposed. Some methods involve the use of tonometry and ultrasonography to measure scar firmness and pliability,[53] the use of tonometry to measure pliability and tension so as to quantify the course of cicatrization and evaluate the efficacy of therapy;[54] the use of laser Doppler flowmetry to study microcirculation in burn scars in order to assess scar maturity,[55] and the use of an elastometer to measure elastic properties of scar so as to objectively document scar response to treatment or scar maturity.[56] The Vancouver Burn Scar Assessment[57] is one instrument that therapists helped to develop which appears to be gaining acceptance by therapists. This particular method of assessment is a visual scale that rates scar pigmentation, vascularity, pliability, and height.

The therapist should periodically document scar changes, particularly as they relate to treatment. Periodic photographs of the scar can also be useful. Besides evaluating scar in healed wounds and grafts, the therapist also should evaluate the donor site for any signs of scarring.

Application of Pressure

Pressure is used to make or keep scars flat, soft, smooth, and pliable. Although controlled studies are sparse concerning the ability of pressure to prevent scar hypertrophy, and although the exact mechanism of pressure in controlling scar is not known, pressure appears to be clinically effective and is widely used in the United States. Generally, the pressure applied should equal or exceed capillary pressure. For pressure to be therapeutic, it should be applied early, and pressure garments should be worn continuously for the duration of scar maturation. Moreover, the pressure applied should be both conforming and adequate.

EARLY APPLICATION OF PRESSURE GARMENTS. Because the processes of scar hypertrophy and contracture begin almost as soon as the wound begins healing, pressure to control scarring should begin early. Pressure can be applied once grafts are adherent, or when deep partial-thickness wounds are healed so that there are openings no larger than the size of a quarter. Besides controlling scars, pressure in this early stage can provide support to recently adherent grafts or to newly healed tissue. The patient can then be measured for commercially available, custom-made pressure garments. However, because the pressure in such garments and the shearing forces exerted at the time of application is too strong for recently adherent grafts or newly healed scar tissue, the garments cannot be applied for several weeks.

In the interim lighter pressure can be applied, with gradual progression to stronger pressure over a period of a few weeks. For example, during the first week after graft adherence (about 1 to 2 weeks following graft placement) or during the first week after wound closure, the therapist can use one layer of a tubular elastic stockinette (Fig. 7-12) such as Tubigrip* or Elastic-net+, to fashion shirts and shorts to be applied on the extremities and trunk.

Fit. Tubular elastic stockinettes come in various widths ranging from approximately 4 cm to 32 cm. The manufacturer may provide a measuring tape or furnish printed guidelines to help the therapist select the appropriate size, however the therapist must exercise sound judgment in choosing the best size. Tubular elastic stockinette is too loose if it bags or does not cling to the patient, and it is too tight if it is constrictive, leaves deep indentations on the skin, or restricts circulation. In some cases, one size may be applied on the forearm, whereas a

---

*Seton Products, Ltd., Tubiton House, Oldham, Lancashire, England.

+The Jobst Institute, Inc., Box 653, Toledo, OH 43697.

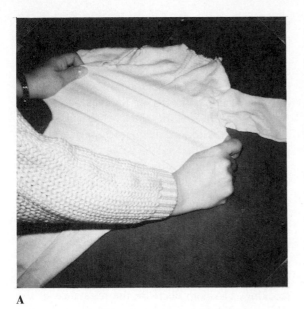
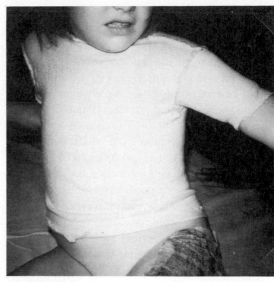

A B

Figure 7-12. (A) *Shirt constructed of tubular elastic stockinette.* (B) *A child who is approximately 1 week post–skin-graft application to a burned left chest and shoulder is wearing a shirt constructed of tubular elastic stockinette. The shirt is worn over a light dressing. The left thigh was the donor site.*

larger size may be needed for the upper arm. In the case of the lower extremity, three different sizes may need to be used.

Application. Before application, any open areas should be covered with a light dressing. Because the friction of application or the shearing forces exerted during movement could cause blisters or even small wounds, fragile-appearing areas also should be dressed with a light bandage. When the tubular elastic stockinette is being applied, it should be lifted over any dressings and gently placed. This technique helps to avoid dislodging the dressings, applying friction over open areas or fragile tissue, and causing possible pain. At least one manufacturer of tubular elastic stockinette supplies applicators. The most distal pieces are applied first. For example, in a patient with burns of the buttocks and lower extremity, the piece for the foot would be applied first, followed by the piece for the calf, the piece for the thigh, and finally application of the shorts in that order. Elastic stockinette pieces

should also be removed in a precise order, using the reverse pattern. This method of application avoids dislodging of bandages and friction that might lead to blisters, and helps to minimize pain. When pieces of various sizes are used on an extremity, each piece should overlap the next by approximately $1\frac{1}{2}$ inches. Such overlap ensures that, during movement, individual pieces will not become separated from other pieces, thereby avoiding both the uncovering of these areas and also swelling of the uncovered areas secondary to increased pressure on each side. Wrinkles and bunching in the tubular elastic stockinette should be smoothed.

By the second week after graft adherence or wound closure, the pressure can be increased by doubling the tubular elastic stockinette and the shirts and shorts made by the therapist. (The elastic stockinette garments provided by the manufacturer should not be doubled.) Several manufacturers of custom-made pressure garments also carry prefabricated, noncustom, pediatric pressure garments that are made of a lighter material and exert a lighter pressure, and these may be able to be introduced at that time.

The temporary or interim pressure garments should be worn about 22 hours per day. They should be removed for dressing changes, bathing, skin care, and specified exercises or activities.

LATER APPLICATION OF COMMERCIALLY AVAILABLE, CUSTOM-MADE ELASTIC PRESSURE GARMENTS. By the third week after graft adherence or wound closure, the patient is usually ready for commercially available, custom-made pressure garments which should have been ordered and received from the manufacturer by that time. At least five or six companies manufacture custom-fitted elastic pressure garments in the United States, including the Jobst Institute, Inc. (Box 653, Toledo, OH 43697), Bio-Concepts (2424 East University Dr., Phoenix, AZ 85034), Barton-Carey Medical Products (PO Box 421, Perrysburg, OH 43551), Gottfried Medical, Inc. (PO Box 8966, Toledo, OH 43623) and Medical Z (709 South Lane St., Seattle, WA 98104). Depending upon the company selected, there are a variety of fabric materials and colors, measuring systems, designs, and options available; a span of prices; and a range of services provided (for example, a company representative who will measure and fit patients instead of the therapist performing the activity).

Fit. Because a garment is custom-made and designed to apply a specific amount of pressure over a given area, it should fit snugly. It is too loose if it can be easily pinched or if it bags or bunches. The garment can be sewn tighter by the therapist, but the patient should be remeasured. The garment is too tight if there is distal swelling, coldness, discoloration, or, if the patient is old enough to complain, paresthesias. It is too tight if deep red marks which take longer than 20 minutes to fade are left on the skin from the pressure garment or if there is skin breakdown caused by a seam. The therapist can make small (approximately $\frac{1}{4}$ inch) cuts in the garment to provide a temporary adjustment, but, again, the patient should be remeasured. A second pressure garment should be ordered as soon as the patient is fitted with the first.

Application. There are several methods of application, and the parent and patient will find one that is easiest for them. One method is to apply the garment as is: glove directly on the hand, arm in the sleeve of a shirt, foot into the leotard, and so forth. Another way is to turn the garment inside out and then apply it so that, as it is being donned, it is on right side out. Either way, the garment should not be pulled or yanked, because such pulling, if repeated often, can lead to overstretching and can cause a distortion of the garment and lessening of the pressure that the garment is designed to apply. Rather, the garment should be inched on. One technique to ease application of a leotard is to first apply sheer knee-high stockings. The use of such stockings can help decrease the resistance of the skin to application of the leotard and generally does not interfere with the pressure. A similar method can be employed for the upper extremity.

A pressure garment can also be applied over dressings if there are still wounds or if there are wounds that have been created by a patient's scratching. The garment can be lifted over the dressing, or a small piece of elastic stockinette can be used to help hold the dressing in place when applying the pressure garment.

Wearing Schedule. The garment is recommended for wearing approximately 22 hours per day. It should be removed daily for bathing and skin care. Even if the parent does not bathe the child daily, we recommend that the pressure garment be removed, the healed area washed, and lotion applied. Patients with wounds also must have dressings changed at least once each day. Depending upon the patient, the garment may be removed one or two other times a day for additional lubrication to the scar or graft. The garment also should be removed if there are specified exercises recommended by the therapist, as the garment can impede movement. Moreover, the therapist should be able to observe the part being exercised to determine whether scar is limiting motion and, in the case of passive ROM exercises, to avoid overstretching.

Because the pressure garments can impede motion and diminish sensation, children younger than 2 years of age who are wearing pressure garments, such as gloves, may need to have the garment off for brief intervals during the day to experience more normal sensation and movement. Other than the parameters described earlier, children can engage in almost any activity, including swimming, while wearing the pressure garment. Pressure garments should be worn until scar maturation, which, for most children, is within 12 to 18 months.

The patient should have at least two sets of custom-fitting elastic pressure garments so that one set can be washed while the other is being worn. In some cases, three sets are recommended because of the increased wear and tear that certain garments, such as chinstraps and gloves, undergo. Initially, the patient usually receives only one set; the second set is then ordered when it is determined that the first set fits appropriately. At this time, the patient should wear the first set as much as possible, and only wear the temporary pressure garments when the custom-made one is being laundered. Once the patient has two sets of custom-fitting elastic pressure garments, temporary pressure garments should no longer be used. Because the child is growing and because the garments eventually wear out, they should be replaced every 2 to 3 months. Over time, a garment can lose much elasticity, thereby reducing pressure, while appearing to fit well. Because several weeks may elapse between the time the patient is measured and the actual fitting, the therapist should not wait unit the garment appears to be too small or too worn before measuring the patient for a new custom-made pressure garment.

Each manufacturer recommends daily laundering of pressure garments. However, washing machines and dryers, heat, and strong detergents can break down the elasticity in the garment, thereby diminishing the pressure provided. Even hand-washing the garments contributes to the breakdown of elasticity. Because of this problem and because many young children do not perspire as adults do, this author recommends washing pressure garments only when necessary or just laundering part of the garment (the feet of a leotard, for example). The approach will vary from patient to patient and from garment to garment (e.g., socks may need more frequent laundering than a shirt). Perspiration, petroleum-based lotions, activity, and ozone are other factors that may contribute to the breakdown of elasticity in the garment.

ENSURING ADEQUATE, CONFORMING PRESSURE. A child may have received a well-fitting pressure garment (and have worn temporary or interim pressure garments prior to that) and have been compliant with its use, and the therapist still may note scar hypertrophy and contracture a week or more later. Why? Although a garment is designed to apply a specific amount of pressure, the pressure garment itself has no pressure in it. However, once applied, depending upon the body surface, material, and fit, as well as other conditions, the garment will generate pressure.

Several factors affect the actual pressure being applied, including characteristics of body surface and movement. Characteristics of body surface that affect pressure are *contour* (concave versus convex surfaces), *resistance* (hard versus soft surfaces), and *surfaces with or without an opposing force.* The therapist should be aware of and anticipate the effects of these characteristics, as well as those of movement.

Contour (concave versus convex surfaces). Although custom-made pressure garments usually fit well over convex surfaces of the body, such as the forearm or calf, they tend to bridge over concave areas, such as the palm of the hand, between the scapulae, and so on. In the latter case, the garments provide little, if any, pressure over such areas.

Resistance (hard versus soft surfaces.) Pressure is more easily achieved over harder surfaces of the body than over softer ones. Harder surfaces of the body (e.g., muscular or bony surfaces, such as the anterior calf) provide greater resistance than do softer surfaces of the body (such as the stomach or the thigh). For example, one can depress a finger almost an inch into the thigh of a child before significant resistance is met.

Opposing Force. In order for pressure to be applied, there must be an opposing force. For example, a pressure garment over the volar aspect of the forearm helps to provide the opposing force for the garment over the dorsal surface of the forearm. Some areas of the body provide little, if any, opposing force when a pressure garment is applied. Examples of such sites include the shoulder and digit web spaces. Additionally, the amount of pressure being applied may tend to diminish distally.

Movement. At any given moment, movement can change the amount of pressure being applied by a garment. Muscle contractions and joint movement can change the contour and hardness of body surface areas and the amount of stretch or laxity in a pressure garment. For example, in one study,[58] a pressure sensor was placed on the dorsum of a hand under a Bio-Concept pressure glove. When the fingers were extended, the sensor gave a reading of 19 mm Hg. With the fingers flexed, the sensor demonstrated 45 mm Hg.

Inserts. Because of the factors just mentioned, it may be necessary to use inserts to compensate for inadequate pressure provided by pressure garments over certain areas of the body. An *insert* is material that is worn underneath the pressure garment over a specific area and that applies (along with the pressure garment) additional pressure over that area. Many materials can be used as inserts, including Polycushion* (Smith & Nephew Rolyan, Inc. PO Box 555, Menomonee Falls, WI 53052–0555), Aliplast 4E (molded) (Alimed Inc., 297 High Street, Dedham, MA 02026–9135), Otoform K (Dreze, Inc., Unna, Germany), and others, or a combination. The materials used will depend upon the specific area of the body and the patient's tolerance, as well as the scar's response to the material, the age of the scar, and when the material is being worn. Otoform K works well over the toes because it molds (forms) into the webbed spaces and contours of the toes. Aliplast 4E (of various thicknesses) molds well over the shoulder, but because Aliplast is semirigid, it may buckle during movement and actually lift pressure off part of the shoulder. Because of this effect, a less rigid (though perhaps not as strong) insert, such as Polycushion, may be used during the day, with Aliplast being used at night.

OTHER METHODS OF APPLYING PRESSURE. Pressure garments are the most common way to apply pressure on scar, but other methods may be as or more effective and have other benefits, such as being easier to apply or less expensive. For example, with a small, localized burn of an extremity, two layers of a snugly fitting tubular elastic stockinette and an insert may be as effective, more comfortable, less costly, and easier to apply than a pressure garment. When a splint is used for a palmar burn, it may be more effective to wear no glove underneath. If the splint is formed well and secured by Coban,* the splint, besides fitting more accurately without the glove, can provide conforming pressure because it is secured with the Coban.

The transparent plastic facemask was introduced in 1979 by Rivers et al.[59] as an alternative to the elastic facemask to control facial scarring (see Fig 7-15). As its name implies, the transparent facemask is a piece of hard, transparent plastic in the form of a custom-fitting facemask secured to the face by means of straps. The mask is constructed by forming heated plastic over a modified positive mold of the patient's face. The positive mold is made from a negative mold (an impression) of the patient's face. Although an impression may be made of an adult's face when the patient is awake (as described by Rivers et al.), in children, it is advisable to obtain an impression while they are anesthetized. The impression procedure may be scheduled, if possible, when the patient is going to the operating room for debridement and/or grafting of areas other than the face and neck.

The advantages of the transparent facemask versus the elastic facemask are as follows:

- The mask can be constructed and applied to the patient within 24 hours. (There is no waiting for the elastic garment to return from the manufacturer.)
- The therapist can see exactly where pressure is being adequately applied by observing blanching of the

---

3M Medical-Surgical Division, St. Paul, MN.

scar. The transparent mask can be adjusted accordingly by the therapist to increase or decrease pressure in specific areas.

- The patient's face is visible to other people and is not covered by an opaque mask.
- The transparent mask usually does not require the construction and exact placement of inserts.
- The transparent facemask may cause fewer problems with head growth and malocclusion than the elastic mask.

There are also several disadvantages of the transparent facemask, including the following:

- The cost of construction (therapist's time and possible operating room costs if the impression is taken under anesthesia and the patient is not undergoing another procedure) for the transparent mask may exceed the cost of an elastic mask.
- Although both types of mask often have to be replaced as the child grows and the mask wears out, the cost of a new transparent mask is probably greater.
- The transparent facemask, which is not a commercial device, is available in fewer locations than the elastic mask.
- The plastic used to construct the transparent mask is rigid, permits little movement of the facial muscles, and often limits mandible motion.
- The transparent mask may not cover as many areas on the head as the elastic mask. (However, the transparent mask can be used with a chinstrap or alternated with an elastic mask.)
- Perspiration is increased underneath the transparent mask, and plastic may be more uncomfortable than elastic.

PROBLEM SOLVING WITH PRESSURE GARMENTS AND INSERTS. Although the application of pressure may be effective in helping to flatten, soften, and smooth scars, potential problems, drawbacks, and difficulties are associated with this approach. The garments are porous, but they can still be uncomfortable, especially in the summer. A small number of children are allergic to the materials in the pressure garment. This may be remedied somewhat by applying a close-fitting garment of another fabric underneath the pressure garment. As discussed earlier, there may also be problems associated with too tight a fit. As also previously discussed, although the patient can engage in most any activity while wearing the garment, the garment can interfere with movement and sensation. Moreover, such garments may interfere with normal ADLs and, in small children, with toilet training, as a leotard or brief is usually too tight for toddlers to pull down and up without assistance. Also, the elastic chinstrap or facemask may cause snoring or interruptions in normal sleep.

The elastic chinstrap may also cause at least a temporary recession of the mandible,[60] and it, in combination with a neck conformer, may cause increased proclination of maxillary and mandibular incisors.[61] The elastic facemask may impede head growth in very young children[62] and may cause abnormal recession of mandibular growth.[63] Both the elastic facemask and the plastic facemask may affect facial growth.[61] Elastic shirts may cause regressed skeletal growth of the thoracic cage,[63] and elastic gloves may cause narrowing of the palmar arch.[63] However, the burn injury and/or the acute or reconstructive therapy, as well as the grafted skin and scar tissue, may also contribute to these problems.[62–64] When the facemask or elastic chinstrap is used, the child's head growth, facial growth, and dentition should be monitored.

There are several areas of the body where it is difficult to achieve or apply adequate pressure. For example, it is troublesome to apply pressure in the perineum. It is also difficult to apply sufficient pressure over the perineum and the buttocks if the child is in diapers.

Inserts also may cause problems or difficulties. Because most inserts are nonporous, perspiration will be increased in the areas covered by the inserts. Besides causing discomfort, the increased perspiration can lead to a rash or skin maceration, or to skin breakdown because of increased friction. There are several solutions to such problems. One is to remove the insert frequently. Another solution is to apply a layer of stockinette or gauze underneath the insert. If skin breakdown occurs, the area can be bandaged and the pressure garment can still be worn. Occasionally, the insert can still be worn over a bandage.

With normal movement, inserts may slip from their desired location. Children may also intentionally dislodge inserts or remove them.

Splinting

The purpose of splinting during the rehabilitation phase is to maintain or increase ROM (Fig 7–13). This is accomplished by providing an equal and opposing force to that of the contracting scar, by inhibiting contracture, and by maintaining tissue length. If the patient was splinted during the acute phase, the splint may no longer fit because the patient no longer has bulky bandages.

SCHEDULE. The splinting schedule will vary according to the patient's immediate potential for contracture and loss of motion. Such potential should decrease gradually over several months as the scar matures. If a patient loses a significant amount of motion when a splint is off for 2 hours, that patient will, at least initially, require a rigorous splinting schedule. Such a schedule may require the splint to be worn continually except for specified periods (lasting less than 2 hours each) of exercise, activity, and ADLs. Other patients may require splinting only for short periods during the day and then at night, or perhaps just at night. As the scar matures, the active force of the contracting scar should decrease, and the need for the splint should also decrease.

APPLICATION. Splints are worn over pressure garments. Exceptions to this rule occur when a splint both positions and provides pressure, or when a precise fit would be difficult to achieve and maintain in the presence of a pressure garment, as may happen with a small hand. In the former case, the splint would be worn directly against the skin. In the latter case, the splint may be alternated with a glove; alternatively, pressure could be applied to the dorsum by means of a sponge, and both sponge and splint would be secured by a pressure wrap. Elastic bandages are preferable to straps for securing splints in place and helping to maintain splint conformity. Elastic bandages also provide pressure that can help soften, smooth, and flatten scar; they can also give a slight dynamic quality to a static splint. Coban is very effective in securing pediatric splints and has the additional benefit of being difficult for the child to remove.

During this phase, splints should be custom-made for a child and should fit well. A secure fit helps to position the specific joint(s) correctly in addition to providing conforming pressure to the scar.

CASTING. Casting may be used during both the acute and rehabilitation phases to maintain position in pediatric patients when a splint position is difficult to sustain. For example, it may be preferable to immobilize the MCP joints in flexion while allowing active use of the distal joints.[65] Serial casting is effective in correcting contractures in both pediatric and adult burn patients in whom other methods of regaining motion have failed, in noncompliant patients,[66–68] in patients whose splints easily slip or are removed, or in those for whom other methods, such as dynamic splinting, cannot be used.[68] Serial casting can eliminate or delay the need for reconstructive surgery.[67] Once motion is regained through serial casting, it needs to be maintained through continued casting or splinting and ROM exercise. Depending upon the particular patient and the phase of healing, casts made of either plaster or synthetic materials may be used.

Range of Motion

The purpose of ROM exercises and activities during the rehabilitation phase is to help maintain or increase ROM by helping to maintain scar elasticity and elongation and by opposing the force of contracting scar. ROM exercises and activities during this phase also help to maintain muscle balance.

EVALUATION. Pressure garments should be removed for both evaluation of ROM and performance of ROM exercises. The garments can inhibit active and passive ROM, and when the garments are off, the therapist can observe the scar to see if

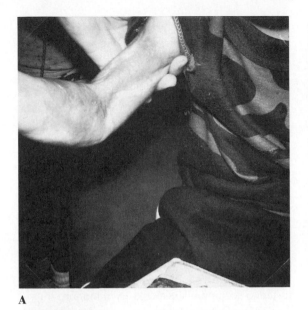

A

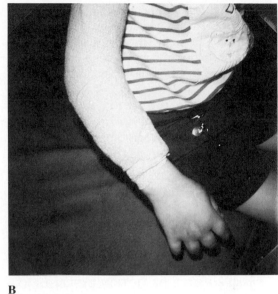

B

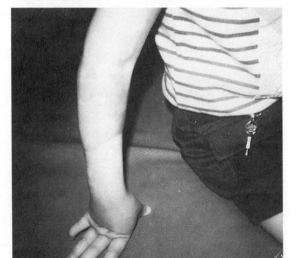

C

Figure 7-13. *Nonsurgical correction of scar contracture through splinting and pressure. (A) Scar contracture causing loss of full elbow extension. (B) A splint has been constructed and applied to the anterior surface under a Coban wrap. (C) Note the increased joint motion and flatter, smoother scar approximately 24 hours later.*

limitations in motion are caused by inelastic scar tissue.

As with other disorders, goniometry is the preferred method of evaluating ROM in children. When evaluating ROM during the rehabilitation phase, the therapist should evaluate active and pas-

sive ROM of individual joints, as well as total active and total passive motion across several joints. It is possible, for example, for a child to have full active and passive shoulder flexion with the elbow in flexion, but, because of contracting scar, have limitations in shoulder flexion with the elbow in extension. The therapist should also observe the quality of movement and how the motion is performed. For example, a child with burns of the anterior chest will frequently ambulate with protracted shoulders and limited trunk rotation.

ACTIVE RANGE OF MOTION EXERCISES AND ACTIVITIES. Prior to starting active ROM exercises, it is helpful for the therapist to lubricate and massage the scar tissue over and around the joint or area to be exercised. With younger children especially, it is useful to incorporate enjoyable activities which require the ROM desired. Basketball, for example, is a good activity for achieving shoulder flexion, whereas bicycles or tricycles facilitate hip and knee flexion and extension.

PASSIVE RANGE OF MOTION EXERCISES AND ACTIVITIES. Too often, children with burns have been traumatized by too aggressive or excessive passive ROM exercise. Judgment and experience are required to determine which patients are candidates for passive ROM and to learn how to perform passive ROM exercises for this population. If there is a limitation in passive ROM, before initiating passive ROM exercises, the therapist should attempt to increase motion through changes in the splinting or pressure program. Motion may be lost because the splint was off for too long a period or was incorrectly applied. Also, some joints with limited extension, particularly the knees and elbows, are amenable to serial splinting. It is difficult for the therapist (and painful for the patient) to stretch hard scar tissue. Softening the scar by increasing the pressure may yield an increase in ROM without the performance of passive ROM exercises. For example, before instituting a passive ROM program to gain shoulder abduction in a child with a burn of the anterior axilla, the therapist should first try to soften the scar in that location by increasing the applied pressure with the addition of an insert. When the scar is softened, the ROM may automatically increase.

It is particularly useful to lubricate and massage scar prior to performing passive ROM exercises, as dry skin may crack when it is stretched, and massage may soften tissue and facilitate passive ROM. The therapist may stretch the entire band of scar (multi-joint), or the scar over a single joint. The therapist may begin by stretching just to the point of slight resistance and maintaining that stretch until resistance is no longer felt. The therapist should stretch the scar until it blanches. If at least slight blanching does not occur, the therapist may not be stretching sufficiently to increase motion. Overstretching, on the other hand, causes unnecessary pain, and the therapist can tear or damage tissue which could then trigger an inflammatory response leading to increased local scarring. Gains in passive ROM should be incorporated into active ROM exercises or functional activities (Fig. 7-14) and maintained through splinting. The splint should be adjusted to accommodate increases in motion.

Passive ROM activities also can be employed, including, for example, placing a child prone or supine over a bolster or ball.

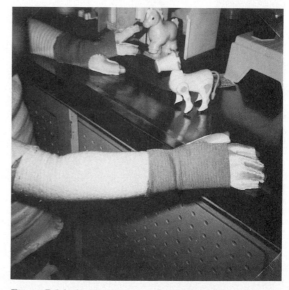

Figure 7-14. *Age-appropriate play activities facilitate active range of motion. This child is between 1 and 2 weeks post-graft application and is wearing tubular elastic stockinette and interim pressure gloves constructed of swimsuit lycra.*

Passive ROM exercises may be contraindicated if there is a substantial wound over a joint, the healing of which may be impeded by stretching. Also, some scars may be too mature to achieve a significant gain in motion from passive ROM exercises.

There are several modalities, such as paraffin and continuous passive ROM machines, which can be effective in helping to increase range of motion. These are discussed in the section entitled "Therapeutic Modalities."

Activities of Daily Living

Children with small burns often return to age-level functional independence within 1 to 2 weeks of hospital discharge with little or no ADL therapy. Children with more severe burns may have difficulty with ADLs because of the persistence of open wounds, decreased ROM or interference from pressure garments and splints. ADL problems may also be related to altered or diminished sensation.[69] The therapist should provide assistive devices and ADL training when necessary, while also trying to ameliorate factors that may interfere with functional independence, such as decreased ROM.

Strength and Cardiovascular Adaptation

Patients who are hospitalized for prolonged periods commonly lose muscle mass and cardiovascular endurance. This loss may be particularly obvious in the burn patient who is in a catabolic state during the acute phase. Most children with smaller burns appear to have little trouble and take little time resuming preburn activities that require age-level strength and endurance. However, during the early rehabilitation phase, children with larger burns may tire easily. Such patients initially may require strengthening and cardiovascular exercises. These activities must be planned according to the age-appropriate needs of the child, the specific areas burned, and the strengthening and cardiovascular training devices available. Nevertheless, few studies have been done on the pediatric burn patient. One study that involved treadmill stress-testing of pediatric burn patients[70] found that patients who were 1 or more years past the burn injury had an endurance of approximately 3 minutes (one stage) longer than did those patients who were still in the first year after their burn injury. Values for each year after 1 year showed little change. Patients sustaining burns of greater than 40% of their TBSA who underwent fascial excision (instead of tangential excision) or had inhalation injury, or both, showed diminished performance in the first year. After the first year, however, regardless of such complications, all pediatric burn patients tested were able to maximize their recovery, except that the performance of those patients who had sustained inhalation injury never equaled those without inhalation injury.

Therapeutic Modalities

Although there has been documented use of some modalities with adults who have been burned, there have been few reports of the use of therapeutic modalities for children with burn injuries. Moreover, several modalities are not recommended for use with children. For example, ultrasound can be used in burned adults to help increase ROM,[71] but ultrasound in children may be contraindicated when used around the epiphysis. There are, however, several modalities that are commonly utilized for burned adults which can also be used with certain children.

PARAFFIN AND SUSTAINED STRETCH TREATMENTS. Paraffin and sustained stretch treatments may increase collagen extensibility, increase skin pliability, decrease joint discomfort, and increase joint ROM.[72] Because of burn patients' decreased skin tolerance to heat and increased sensitivity to heat, and, particularly in the case of children, their fear of hot liquids, the paraffin is cooled before application. (Patients with a particular intolerance for or fear of heat, decreased sensation, or open wounds or fragile skin are not candidates for paraffin and sustained stretch treatments.) The paraffin is combined with mineral oil and the temperature is lowered to 115°F[73] or lower. The joint can be stretched either with the aid of a splint or held manually, and then dipped into the paraffin. The paraffin also can be painted on,[74] or coarse mesh gauze can be dipped into the paraffin and applied to the joint, after which gentle long stretch and active exercises can be performed.[73]

CONTINUOUS PASSIVE MOTION. Continuous passive motion (CPM) machines are gaining wide acceptance for use with burn patients.[75] They can be used during both the acute and rehabilitation phases. Although their use with burned adults has been studied and documented,[76,77] most machines do not fit small children. Some of the models, however, may be suitable for older children and adolescents. One group of researchers,[76] in discussing the use of CPM with patients sustaining hand burns, postulated that the patients who may benefit the most from CPM are those with burns involving multiple kinetic areas (the idea being that the CPM machine could be applied to one limb while the therapist worked on another), comatose patients, and patients who display limited active motion because of pain, anxiety, or edema. Such factors might also apply to the use of CPM with patients who have burns on other areas of the body. Although CPM may provide an additional, useful, therapeutic tool, many of the machines do not take the joint through the full ROM.

Other Therapeutic Approaches

SILICONE GEL. Topical silicone gel sheets have been used on hypertrophic scars in Europe since the mid-1980s. One controlled study[78] performed in the United States reported significant gains in ROM in patients with elbow contractures who were treated with both silicone gel and exercise compared to those who were treated with exercise alone. Another controlled study[79] that used silicone gel sheets to treat hypertrophic scars in adults documented improvement in one or more items of scar texture, color, thickness, durability, pruritis, and (where applicable) ROM assessed during clinical evaluation; and there was an increase in scar elasticity as measured by objective elastometry. In those patients whose scars showed improvement, the silicone gel

sheets were worn for at least 12 hours per day for 4 weeks; further improvement was noted after a second 4-week period. The mechanism of action of the silicone gel sheets remains unknown, and the gel sheets appear to work with or without the use of pressure to secure them in place.

Certain problems are associated with silicone gel sheets, including rashes and skin maceration.[79] A report of the use of silicone gel sheets on scars in pediatric patients[80] revealed another significant problem—poor durability of the gel sheets in active children which, in turn, increased the cost of the treatment.

MYOFASCIAL RELEASE. No studies have been done concerning the use of myofascial release in burn patients. However, therapists trained in myofascial release have begun to employ this technique in burn patients in whom the depth and extent of injury have produced scar problems that may be amenable to myofascial release.

HIPPOTHERAPY. Hippotherapy, or therapeutic horseback riding, has been used with children who have burn injuries. Riding therapy may increase ROM and strength and improve dexterity while providing an exciting activity that may also enhance the burned child's self-esteem and self-confidence.[81]

SWIMMING. Therapeutic swimming can also be useful in the treatment of burned children. The goal of such therapy is to provide a recreational activity designed to increase strength, endurance, and ROM in a medium that may decrease pain.

Developmental Considerations

The effects of burn injury on child development have received sparse investigation. A recent study[82] of 12 pediatric burn patients who were tested with the Denver Developmental Screening Test revealed delays in 6 of the subjects. The most severely injured showed the most significant delays. Although most of the delays were in the gross motor sector, delays also were noted in the fine motor-adaptive and personal-social sections of the test for five of the children. None of the subjects showed delays in the language category of the test. These researchers concluded that parents should be apprised of possible developmental delays, and that rehabilitation professionals should include the attainment of developmental goals in their treatment plans. Other than severity of injury, the study did not specifically identify the factors that may have contributed to the delays. A limitation of the study is that it was done early in the child's recovery, so it is not known how long these delays persist.

It is not uncommon for hospitalized children to regress developmentally. This is one reason why they should be encouraged to assist with or participate in their own care and ADLs, and should be involved in age-appropriate play and activities when possible. Despite such involvement and activities, to execute necessary treatment, facilitate care, ease the child's pain, and because of the child's injury, certain procedures must be performed which, along with the physical and emotional trauma, separation from family, and relative dependency, contribute to regression. For example, toddlers who have just mastered toilet training may be returned to diapers, and those who had finally been weaned from the bottle may be put back on it. When the child is discharged, the parent may complain that the child has lost mastery of abilities that the parent worked hard to help the child achieve. Such delays appear to be temporary, and earlier skills are usually regained when the child returns home and resumes his or her prior activities.

A developmental evaluation during the acute phase may not yield a true picture of the child's developmental status because of temporary regression or because of pain or a decreased ability to cooperate. The rehabilitation phase may be the preferred time frame for a developmental evaluation and specific remediation. Children who are victims of abuse or neglect may also be developmentally delayed, although it is possible that such delays may have preceded the burn injury.

As previously discussed, treatment during the rehabilitation phase also may interfere with execution of and acquisition of age-level skills. Sensation and movement may be limited by pressure garments. Splints may hinder motion and thus thwart independence in ADLs. Because the child may not be able to don and doff a pressure garment independently, the acquisition of toileting skills may be delayed or the child may require assistance.

Returning to School

If the burned child is school-aged, planning for school reentry should begin early during the child's hospitalization. Maintaining contact with the teacher and classmates through cards, phone calls, videos, and when possible, visits, helps the child focus on the goal of returning to school and facilitates reentry. Some hospital settings allow for tutoring. Children who were burned 1 or more years before entering school also may benefit from a school reentry program, particularly if the burns were extensive.

The purpose of the school re-entry program is to facilitate the child's physical, social, and emotional return to school by increasing the knowledge and understanding possessed by the teacher, classmates and other staff and students as to what happened to the burned child. Additional information provided may include reasons for the child's appearance and an explanation of care items, such as pressure garments and splints. The re-entry program can also provide increased support for the child (e.g., decreasing the child's fear and increasing self-esteem by describing the child as a hero), practical information for the school staff concerning the patient's splints and pressure garments, and information about the child's ADL needs, such as writing, mobility around the school, and use of the bathroom.

A variety of school re-entry programs can be employed, and the physical therapist can play an integral role in a school re-entry program. Some of these programs incorporate puppet shows, games, videos, and visits to the school by hospital professionals. Topics that might be included in a reentry program cover:

- What exactly happened to the burned child and information about the hospitalization
- Burn prevention and first-aid
- The noncontagious nature of burns
- The use of pressure garments or splints
- Scars
- The impropriety of teasing or staring
- The fact that the burned child is still the same child despite his or her different appearance
- The ability of the burned child to engage in most or all of preburn activities
- What classmates can do to help

It may be preferable to have the burned child and family present during the program.

The burn unit's therapist should work in conjunction with the school therapist to determine the patient's needs in school and to confer about the therapy program. The therapist also should provide information to the teacher and the school nurse concerning the application of and schedule for splints or pressure garments, ADL concerns, and handling of potential problems.

Burn Camp

Just as there are camps for children with various diseases or disabilities (e.g., diabetes camp, spina bifida camp, etc.), there also are more than a dozen burn camps in North America that offer a variety of programs for children who have sustained burn injuries. Several of these camps are coordinated or staffed by therapists, or therapists are encouraged to attend the camp to help with programs or to assist campers. The purpose of most of the camps is to provide a safe, recreational environment in which children with burns can interact with one another, build self-esteem, learn new skills, and have fun.

Cosmetics

Corrective cosmetics are used on burned adults and may also be of use in certain adolescents and children. Some patients may require hair pieces or prosthetic ears. At least one medical center[83] takes a more comprehensive approach, not only teaching make-up application but also providing instruction in color and fashion analysis and psychosocial skills.

The Reconstructive Phase

Once scars are mature, they usually do not respond to nonsurgical approaches to correct hypertrophy and contracture, and surgery may offer the only remedy. Burn patients may also require surgery because the type of wound closure accomplished in the acute phase may have resulted in a less-than-optimal cosmetic or functional outcome. A child may be discharged from therapy with full ROM only to develop a contracture later because the scar tissue and grafted skin did not keep pace with growth. Moreover, some reconstructive procedures yield better results when performed at certain times or ages. Children are evaluated regularly as they grow and mature to determine the need for reconstructive surgery.

Reconstructive surgery often is delayed until after scar maturation except in cases in which, for example, a contracture resulting in loss of motion cannot be corrected by nonsurgical approaches. After reconstructive surgical procedures, patients may require therapy similar to that described for the rehabilitation phase. In many cases, however, the course of therapy is often shorter and its intensity decreased.

Psychosocial Issues

Whether the burn is large or small, it can trigger short-term or long-term difficulties for both the child and family. Although many burn injuries are accidental, the parents of the child feel tremendous guilt nonetheless. Often, one parent will blame the other for the incident. Because a parent feels guilty, proper discipline for the burned child may not be maintained once the child is at home. Usually, the entire family will be affected in one way or another by the injury. Siblings of the burned child may feel neglected or resent the "extra attention" the burned child is receiving. The incident may place a burden on the family's finances. Carrying out the necessary daily treatment at home and keeping appointments at the hospital may also be stressful. Certainly, the burned child also has many issues with which to contend. For example, the child may have to endure staring or teasing, and may feel angry about the injury happening and the treatment required.

The therapist should be aware of these feelings and reactions, and should provide encouragement and support. When indicated, the therapist should involve or alert professionals who can help the patient and family.

There are a number of self-help and support groups for burn survivors and their families that provide a range of services. Among these is The Phoenix Society, Inc. (11 Rust Hill Road, Levittown, PA 19056; 215–946–BURN or 1–800–888–BURN), which will supply a list of local chapters or other self-help organizations upon request.

Outcomes

Functions of the Skin

As stated earlier, whenever the skin is significantly damaged or destroyed, the functions of the skin may be impaired. Several functions, such as protection against infection and regulation of body fluids and electrolytes, are primarily disturbed during the acute phase. Other functions, such as temperature regulation, can be impaired both during the acute phase and, at times, after healing. Other functions of the skin may be permanently impaired. Normal skin color may be lost. Skin grafts tend to be hyperpigmented, whereas scar tissue lacks pigment. These color changes are permanent. (However, some partial-thickness burns may heal with skin which is hypopigmented or depigmented, and such pigment changes may be improved by surgery.[84]) No hair will grow in areas where hair follicles are destroyed. Although the cosmetic function of hair can be restored through surgical procedures, such as tissue expansion of the scalp, when suffi-

---

Display 7-1.
Professional Organizations and Resources

The American Burn Association
   1–800–548–BURN
Periodicals
Journal of Burn Care & Rehabilitation (official publication of the American Burn Association) St. Louis, MO, Mosby-Year Book, Inc.
Burns (the journal of the International Society for Burn Injuries) Oxford, U.K., Butterworth-Heinemann, Ltd.

---

cient hair remains, there exists no practical answer for major hair losses on the limbs, trunk, and other areas. Nails are frequently damaged or destroyed in deep burns of the hands and feet. Injury or destruction of the sebaceous and sweat glands can lead to dry skin that requires frequent external lubrication. Scar tissue and skin grafts are not as durable as normal skin. A scar at maximum strength may be only 70 percent as strong as intact skin.[85] Often, the same scrapes and bumps that normal skin can withstand cause tissue breakdown in scarred and grafted skin.

Heat intolerance because of decreased sweating in scarred areas can be a problem in patients with deep partial-thickness and full-thickness burns involving a large percentage of TBSA. A study[50] of sweating in patients with healed burns revealed a decreased number of sweat glands in hypertrophic scar tissue, but the remaining sweat glands in burned areas were more hyperactive than those in normal skin.

Investigations of sensation in grafted skin and healed burns have yielded contradictory results, and there are few studies involving children. One study[86] of sensory loss over grafted areas of burned adults demonstrated diminished or absent sensation, as well as complaints of increased sensitivity to ambient cold, although the decrease in sensation rarely contributed to the subject's long-term impairment rating. The depth of injury appeared to be the best predictor of altered sensation. One researcher[87] concluded that the same graft type can show various degrees of innervation depending upon the depth and extent of injury, healing complications, and the amount of scar tissue.

An inquiry[69] of tactile function in burned children found that points or areas tested on the burned side had altered and often diminished sensation when compared with the corresponding unburned side, and that 60% of the subjects had one or more ADL problems related to altered tactile sensation. However, the researchers believed that all of the children appeared to have adjusted well to their tactile skills or problems. One investigator[88] conducted sensory evaluations and histologic studies of the tactile functions in eight adults who had received free full-thickness grafts to the palmar area and digits as infants and who were periodically evaluated over a period of up to 19 years. Nerve endings and fibers were found to be clustered around hair roots, and no encapsulated receptors were found in the grafts, yet with the exception of hyperesthesia, sensation was rated as good. It was concluded that specific sensory organs need not be present for sensation, and that normal sensations can develop after grafting in early childhood before awareness of sensations are firm.

Although scar tissue tends to become more pliable as it matures, it does not have the same elastic properties as normal skin. Thus, some patients with significant facial scarring may actually appear younger than their age because of the increased tautness of scar tissue and grafted skin. However, this same tautness often gives a mask-like appearance which does not yield to the normal nuances of facial expression.

Growth and Physiological Functions

Longitudinal studies[89] of burned children who underwent excisional therapy have revealed that growth delays and nutritional dysfunction, bone growth abnormalities, and physiological dysfunc-

tion, including alterations in cardiopulmonary, renal, audiologic, and immunologic function, can occur. Most of these problems occurred in children with burns over greater than 40 percent of their TBSA. Some of these deficits were temporary, whereas others appeared to be permanent.

Psychological and Behavioral Adaptation

Most studies on adjustment after burn injury have focused on quite severely injured patients, and not all investigators have been in agreement. As one might expect, children with burn injuries and their families have problems, but research indicates that the long-term adjustment for most of these children is good, suggesting that those with less severe injuries also have positive adjustments.

A study[90] of young adult survivors of severe childhood burn injury revealed that, although some survivors had significant indicators of psychological disturbances, most did not evidence psychopathology more often that did a normal group, and data indicated that they were typical of other people in their age group. A follow-up inquiry[91] concluded that positive psychological adjustment was predicted by increased family cohesion, independence, and increased expressiveness within the family. Intelligence was not a factor, and length of time after injury was a factor only during the first 2 years.

A study[92] of burn-disfigured children of primary-school age who had sustained burns over greater than 80% of their TBSA revealed that all of the children presented with pervasive developmental regression, accompanied by phobias, nightmares, and various other symptoms such as enuresis or encopresis. However, by the fifth year following the injury all of them, except one who had premorbid deficits had returned to an average level of progressive personality development. Even the one with premorbid deficits was found to be progressing well within his limitations. The researchers pointed to the parent(s) as being a fundamental factor in facilitating positive self-image in the child and in beginning and preserving the skill of active mastery in the child.

Another study[93] compared perception of body

image in children with burns (ages 5 to 15 years) 5 years after the injury with that of a control group of children without burns. No differences between the two groups were noted. Another investigation[94] of body image, self-esteem, and depression among burn-injured adolescents and young adults showed that those who perceived greater social support from family and particularly from friends had a more positive body image, greater self-esteem, and less depression than did those who perceived less support. The study found females to be more depressed than males. Surprisingly, the percentage of TBSA burned, the location of the burn, and the number of years elapsed since the injury were not found to be significant factors in this investigation.

Although the predominantly positive adjustment of those with larger burns would appear to augur well for individuals who have sustained burns involving a smaller percentage of TBSA, the exception to a favorable adjustment for those with smaller TBSA burns may be those with "hidden burns." One paper[95] reported on a group of individuals, predominantly women, who had been burned as children. The burns were primarily small and could be hidden by clothing. This group rarely exposed their scars, most were unmarried, and expressed unhappiness. As children, they were encouraged to hide their scars to avoid taunting; consequently, they grew up believing that the scars were "bad." The author of the paper recommended that burn care providers educate parents of newly burned children about the possible long-term negative effects of encouraging children to hide their scars.

Acknowledgments

Thanks to God for the privilege of working with children with burns and their families. Thanks to these children and their families for all they have taught me.

Thanks to Anne Putnam for all her practical help and support with this chapter. Thanks to my husband, Jorn, for his patience and support during the many hours I spent writing.

L. deLinde

References

1. Annual Survey. National Health Interview, 1985.
2. Peate WF. Outpatient management of burns. *Am Family Physician.* 1992;45:1321
3. National Hospital Discharge Survey, 1990.
4. Estimates, Peter Brigham, Burn Foundation of Philadelphia, 1992.
5. McLoughlin E, McGuire A. The causes, cost, and prevention of childhood burn injuries. *Am J Dis Child.* 1990;144:677–683.
6. East MK, Jones CA, Feller I, et al. Epidemiology of burns in children. In: Carvajal HF, Parks DH, eds. *Burns in Children: Pediatric Burn Management.* Chicago, IL: Year Book Medical Publishers, Inc.; 1988:3–10.
7. Moritz AR, Henriques FC. Studies of thermal injury. II. The relative importance of time and surface temperature in burns. *Am J Pathol* 1947;23:695.
8. Grube BJ, Heimbach DM, Williamson JC. Management of pediatric burns. In: Morray JP, ed. *Pediatric Intensive Care.* Norwalk, CT: Appleton & Lange; 1987:471–506.
9. Heath GA, Gayton WF, Hardesty VA. Childhood firesetting. *Can Psychiatr Assoc J.* 1976;21:229–237.
10. Epidemiology of burns in children—WHO: Victim types, 1964–1984 (n=18,764). Ann Arbor, MI. National Burn Information Exchange, June, 1985.
11. Bailey WC, ed. *Pediatric Burns.* Chicago, IL: Year Book Medical Publishers; 1979:68.
12. Lockhart RD, Hamilton GF, Fyfe FW. *Anatomy of the Human Body.* Philadelphia: JB Lippincott; 1969.
13. Moncrief JA. Grafting. In: Artz CP, Moncrief JA, Pruitt BA, eds. *Burns: A Team Approach.* Philadelphia: WB Saunders; 1979:275.
14. Knudson-Cooper M, Thomas CM. Psychosocial care

of the severely burned child. In: Carvajal HF, Parks DH, eds. *Burns in Children: Pediatric Burn Management.* Chicago, IL: Year Book Medical Publishers, Inc.; 1988:345–362.

15. Lund CC, Browder NC. The estimation of areas of burns. *Surg Gynecol Obstet.* 1944;79:352.

16. American Burn Association. Hospital and prehospital resources for optimal care of patients with burn injury: Guidelines for development and operation of burn centers. *J Burn Care Rehabil.* 1990; 11:98–104.

17. Linares HA. Hypertrophic healing: Controversies and etiopathogenic review. In: Carvajal HF, Parks DH, eds. *Burns in Children: Pediatric Burn Management.* Chicago, IL: Year Book Medical Publishers, Inc.; 1988:309.

18. Deitch EA, Wheelahan TM, Rose MP, et al. Hypertrophic burn scars: Analysis of variables. *J Trauma.* 1983;23:895–898.

19. Hunt TK. Fundamentals of wound management in surgery-wound healing: Disorders of repair. South Plainfield, NJ: Chirurgecom, Inc.; 1976.

20. Parks DH, Evans EB, Larson DL. Prevention and correction of deformity after severe burns. *Surg Clin North Am.* 1978;58:1279–1289.

21. Ketchum LD. Hypertrophic scars and keloids. *Clin Plast Surg.* 1977;4:301–310.

22. Peacock EE, Madden JW, Trier WC. Biological basis for the treatment of keloids and hypertrophic scars. *South Med J.* 1970;63:755.

23. Ehrlich HP. Do myofibroblasts produce the contractile forces which organize connective tissue matrixes (Abstract). American Burn Association Meeting; Seattle, WA, 1988.

24. Larson D, Huang T, Linares H, et al. Prevention and treatment of scar contracture. In: Artz CP, Moncrief JA, Pruitt BA, eds. *Burns: A Team Approach.* Philadelphia: WB Saunders; 1979:467–468.

25. Hulnick SJ (St. Christopher's Hospital for Children, Philadelphia, PA). Personal communication, 1988.

26. Clark RAF. Cutaneous tissue repair: Basic biologic considerations. Part I. *J Am Acad Dermatol.* 1985;13:702.

27. Diegelmann RF, Rothkopf LC, Cohen LK. Measurement of collagen biosynthesis during wound healing. *J Surg Res.* 1975;19:239–243.

28. Barnes MJ, Morton LF, Bennett RC, Bailey AJ. Studies on collagen synthesis in the mature dermal scar in the guinea pig. *Biochem Soc Symposium.* 1975;3:917–920.

29. Phillips AW, Cope O. The revelation of respiratory tract damage as a principal killer of the burned patient. *Ann Surg.* 1962;155:1.

30. Jones CA, Feller I, Richards KE. Nursing care of the burned child. In: Bailey WC, ed. *Pediatric Burns.* Chicago, IL: Year Book Medical Publishers; 1979:67–106.

31. Carvajal HF. Resuscitation of the burned child. In: Carvajal HF, Parks DH, eds. *Burns in Children: Pediatric Burn Management.* Chicago, IL: Year Book Medical Publishers, Inc.: 1988:78.

32. Robson MC, Burns BF, Smith DJ. Acute management of the burned patient. *Plast Reconstr Surg.* 1992;89:1158.

33. Zuker RM. Initial management of the burn wound. In: Carvajal HF, Parks DH, eds. *Burns in Children: Pediatric Burn Management.* Chicago, IL: Year Book Medical Publishers, Inc.; 1988:99–105.

34. Heidrich G, Perry S, Armand R. Nursing staff attitudes about burn pain. *J Burn Care Rehabil.* 1981;2:259–261.

35. Perry S, Heidrich G, Ramos E: Assessment of pain by burn patients. *J Burn Care Rehabil.* 1981;2:322–326.

36. Eland JM, Anderson JE. The experience of pain in children. In: Jacox A, ed. *A Source Book for Nurses and Other Health Professionals.* Boston: Little Brown & Co.; 1977:453–473.

37. Wagner M. Pain and nursing care associated with burns. In: Jacox A, ed. *Pain: A Source Book for Nurses and Other Health Professionals.* Boston: Little Brown & Co.; 1977:391–403.

38. Perry S, Heidrich G. Management of pain during debridement: A survey of U.S. burn units. *Pain.* 1982;13:267–280.

39. Linares HA. Autopsy findings in burned children. In: Carvajal HF, Parks DH, eds. *Burns in Children: Pediatric Burn Management.* Chicago, IL: Year Book Medical Publishers, Inc.; 1988:288,289.

40. Engrav LH, Heimbach DM, Reus JL, et al. Early excision and grafting vs nonoperative treatment of burns of indeterminant depth: A randomized prospective study. *J Trauma.* 1983;23:1001–1004.

41. Heimbach DM. Early burn excision and grafting. *Surg Clin North Am.* 1987;67:93–107.

42. Carvajal HF. Burn injuries. In: Behrman RE, ed. *Nelson Textbook of Pediatrics.* Philadelphia: WB Saunders Harcourt Brace Jovanovich, Inc.; 1992:233.

43. Parks DH, Wainwright DJ. The surgical management

of burns. In: Carvajal HF, Parks DH, eds. *Burns in Children: Pediatric Burn Management.* Chicago, IL: Year Book Medical Publishers, Inc.; 1988: 158,166.

44. Interview with Heimbach DM. Early excision and grafting: Clinical implications. *Boots Burn Management Rep.* 1992;1:8.

45. Egan M. Cultured skin grafts: Preserving lives, challenging therapists. *OT Week.* 1992;6:14.

46. Heimbach D, Luterman A, Burke J, et al. Artificial dermis for major burns: A multi-center randomized clinical trial. *Ann Surg.* 1988;208:67–73.

47. Cuono CB, Langdon R, Birchall N, et al. Composite autologous-allogeneic skin replacement: Development and clinical application. *Plast Reconstr Surg.* 1987;80:626.

48. Beasley RW. Secondary repair of burned hands. *Clin Plast Surg.* 1981;8:141.

49. Helm PA. Neuromuscular considerations. In: Fisher SV, Helm PA, eds. *Comprehensive Rehabilitation of Burns.* Baltimore: Williams & Wilkins; 1984:235–241.

50. Cadwallader C, Helm P. Sweat gland distribution in healed severe burns: Quantitative topical distribution and qualitative function (Abstract). American Burn Association Meeting; San Francisco, 1984.

51. Bell L, McAdams T, Morgan R, et al. Pruritis in burns: A descriptive study. *J Burn Care Rehabil.* 1988;9:306.

52. Cyriax JH. Clinical application of massage. In: Licht, S, ed. *Massage, Manipulation, and Traction.* New Haven, CT: Elizabeth Licht Publisher; 1960.

53. Katz SM, Frank DH, Leopold GG, Wachtel TL. Objective measurement of hypertrophic burn scar: A preliminary study of tonometry and ultrasonography. *Ann Plast Surg.* 1985;14:121–127.

54. Esposito G, Ziccardi P, Scioli M, et al. The use of a modified tonometer in burn scar therapy. *J Burn Care Rehabil.* 1990;11:86–90.

55. Leung KS, Sher A, Clark JA, et al. Microcirculation in hypertrophic scars after burn injury. *J Burn Care Rehabil.* 1989;10:436–444.

56. Bartell TH, Monafo WW, Mustoe TA. A new instrument for serial measurements of elasticity in hypertrophic scar. *J Burn Care Rehabil.* 1988;9:657–660.

57. Sullivan T, Smith J, Kermode J, et al. Rating the burn scar. *J Burn Care Rehabil.* 1990;11:256–260.

58. Reichenbacher F (Bio-Concepts, Inc., Phoenix, AZ). Personal communication, 1988.

59. Rivers EA, Strate RG, Solem LD. The transparent facemask. *Am J Occup Ther.* 1979;33:109–113.

60. Parks DH (Shriners Burns Institute, Galveston, TX). Personal communication, 1982.

61. Fricke N, Dutcher K, Omnell L, et al. Effects of pressure garment wear on facial and dental development (Abstract). American Burn Association Meeting, Salt Lake City, UT. 1992.

62. Grigsby L. The use of the facemask with children. Fifth Annual Meeting of the Mid-Atlantic Association of Burn Care Facilities; Philadelphia, 1982.

63. Leung KS, Cheng JCY, Ma GFY, et al. Complications of pressure therapy for post-burn hypertrophic scars. *Burns.* 1984;10:434–438.

64. McCauley RL, Fairleigh JF, Robson MC, Herndon DN. Effects of facial burns on facial growth in children: Preliminary report (Abstract). American Burn Association Meeting; Baltimore, 1991.

65. Flesch P. Casting the young and the restless (Abstract). American Burn Association Meeting; Orlando, FL, 1985.

66. Jordan MH, Lewis MS, Wiegand LT, Leman CJ. Dynamic plaster casting for burn scar contracture—An alternative to surgery (Abstract). American Burn Association Meeting; San Francisco, 1984.

67. Bennett GB, Helm P, Purdue GF, Hunt JL. Serial casting: A method for treating burn contractures. *J Burn Care Rehabil.* 1989;10:543–545.

68. Ridgway CL, Daugherty MB, Warden GD. Serial casting as a technique to correct burn scar contractures: A case report. *J Burn Care Rehabil.* 1991;12:67–72.

69. Stap L, Brock R, Zissermann L. The tactile functions of burned children. *J Burn Care Rehabil.* 1983;4:291–302.

70. McElroy K, Alvarado MI, Rutan R, et al. Cardiovascular adaptation: Exercise stress-testing the pediatric burn patient, a continuation (Abstract). American Burn Association Meeting; Salt Lake City, UT, 1992.

71. Bierman W. Ultrasound in the treatment of scars. *Arch Phys Med Rehabil.* 1954;35:209.

72. Head M, Helm P. Paraffin and sustained stretching in the treatment of burn contractures. *Burns.* 1977; 4:136.

73. Gross J, Stafford S. Modified method for application of paraffin wax for treatment of burn scar. *J Burn Care Rehabil.* 1984;5:394.

74. Johnson CL. Physical therapists as scar modifiers. *Phys Ther.* 1984;64:1383.

75. Covey MH. Application of CPM devices with burn patients. *J Burn Care Rehabil.* 1988;9:496–497.

76. Covey MH, Dutcher K, Marvin JA, Heimbach DM. Efficacy of continuous passive motion (CPM) devices with hand burns. *J Burn Care Rehabil.* 1988;9:397–400.

77. McAllister LP, Salazar CA. Case report on the use of CPM on an electrical burn. *J Burn Care Rehabil.* 1988;9:401.

78. Wessling N, Ehleben CM, Chapman V, et al. Evidence that a silicone wound dressing increases range of motion of limbs after contractures (Abstract). American Burn Association Meeting; Orlando, FL, 1985.

79. Ahn ST, Monafo WW, Mustoe TA. Topical silicone gel: A new treatment for hypertrophic scars. *Surgery.* 1989;106:781–787.

80. Brown M, Zuker R, Gibbons M. Experience with silastic gel sheeting in pediatric scarring (Abstract). American Burn Association Meeting; Salt Lake City, UT, 1992.

81. Tatum C (Pegasus Riding Academy, Inc., Philadelphia, PA). Personal correspondence, 1989.

82. Moore M, Alvarado MI, Rutan R, et al. Developmental screening: A measure of functional ability (Abstract). American Burn Association Meeting; Salt Lake City, UT, 1992.

83. Kammerer-Quayle, B. Personal Image Center at Rancho Los Amigos Medical Center, Downey, CA.

84. Kahn AM, Cohen MJ, Kaplan L. Treatment of depigmentation resulting from burn injuries. *J Burn Care Rehabil.* 1991;12:468–473.

85. Levenson SM, Geever EG, Crawley LV, et al. The healing of rat skin wounds. *Ann Surg.* 1965;161:293–308.

86. Ward RS, Saffle JR, Schnebly A, et al. Sensory loss over grafted areas in patients with burns. *J Burn Care Rehabil.* 1989;10:536–538.

87. Ponten B. Grafted skin: Observations on innervation and other qualities. *Acta Chir Scand [suppl].* 1960;257.

88. Matev IB. Tactile gnosis in free skin grafts in the hand. *Br J Plast Surg.* 1980;33:434–439.

89. Individual studies with multiple and often different investigators, Shriners Burns Institute, University of Texas Medical Branch, Galveston, TX. Reviewed by Robson MC: Burn injuries involving the "whole person." Rehabilitation and reconstruction of the burn patient (symposium notebook). American Burn Association Meeting; Salt Lake City, UT, 1992.

90. Blakeney P, Herndon DN, Desai MH, et al. Long-term psychosocial adjustment following burn injury. *J Burn Care Rehabil.* 1988;9:661–665.

91. Blakeney P, Portman S, Rutan R. Familial values as factors influencing long-term psychological adjustment of children after severe burn injury. *J Burn Care Rehabil.* 1990;11:472–475.

92. Beard SA, Herndon DN, Desai M. Adaptation of self-image in burn-disfigured children. *J Burn Care Rehabil.* 1989;10:550–554.

93. Jessee PO, Strickland MP, Leeper JD, Wales P. Perception of body image in children with burns, five years after burn injury. *J Burn Care Rehabil.* 1992;13:33–38.

94. Orr DA, Reznikoff M, Smith GM. Body image, self-esteem, and depression in burn-injured adolescents and young adults. *J Burn Care Rehabil.* 1989;10:454–461.

95. Breslau AJ. What can be learned from long-term follow-up of burn patients (unpublished data). Psychosocial Interest Group, American Burn Association Meeting; Baltimore, MD; 1991.

Bibliography

Carnes RW, Sollecito WA, Salisbury RE. Evaporative water loss from healed burn wounds. *J Burn Care Rehabil* 1981;2:239–247.

Compton CC, Gill JM, Bradford DA, et al. Skin regenerated from cultured epithelial autografts on full thickness burn wounds from 6 days to 5 years after grafting. *Lab Invest* 1989;60:600–612.

Morris SE, Saffle JR. Utilization of full thickness skin grafting in treatment of hand burns (abstract). American Burn Association Meeting; Baltimore, MD, 1991.

Schwanholt C, Greenhalgh DG, Warden GD. A comparison of full-thickness versus split-thickness autografts for the coverage of deep palm burns in the very young pediatric patient. *J Burn Care Rehabil* 1993;14:29–33.

Pediatric Physical Therapy,
second edition, edited by Jan
Stephen Tecklin. J. B. Lippincott
Company, Philadelphia © 1994.

8

Jan Stephen Tecklin

Pulmonary Disorders in Infants and Children and Their Physical Therapy Management

- **Characteristics of Children's Lungs**
- **Growth and Development of the Lungs**
- **Predisposition to Respiratory Failure**
- **Physical Therapy Assessment of Children with Respiratory Disorders**
  Assessment
  Chart Review
  Physical Examination
  Auscultation
- **Physical Therapy Treatment of Children with Respiratory Disorders**
  Removal of Secretions
  Breathing Exercises and Retraining
  Physical Development
- **Atelectasis**
  Medical Information
  Physical Therapy Evaluation

Physical Therapy Management
- **Respiratory Muscle Weakness**
  Medical Information
  Physical Therapy Evaluation
  Physical Therapy Management
- **Asthma**
  Medical Information
  Medical Management
  Physical Therapy Evaluation
  Physical Therapy Management
- **Cystic Fibrosis**
  Medical Information
  Medical Management
  Physical Therapy Evaluation
  Physical Therapy Management
- **Summary**

Health professionals have the general misconception that respiratory disorders and chronic pulmonary diseases are mainly adult problems. Nonetheless, statistics show that respiratory disease in infants and children is a major problem that accounts for a large share of childhood mortality and morbidity. Mortality statistics show that approxi- mately 30% of all deaths in term infants and 50% to 75% of deaths in premature infants in the United States are either caused by or are closely related to respiratory disease.[1] The morbidity statistics are staggering. Asthma alone is responsible for 10.1 million additional days missed from school when compared to days missed by children without asthma. Children with asthma are about nine times more likely to be unable to conduct their major activities of living when compared to all children without asthma.[2] Acute respiratory infections in children from 1 to 14 years of age are responsible for three to eight illnesses per year per child in both developed and developing nations.[1] Asthma resulted in 12.9 million contacts with physicians and 200,000 hospitalizations in 1988.[2] In the United States, 10% to 20% of children younger than 17 years of age have been reported to have a chronic respiratory problem. Of those, one fourth have chronic bronchitis, and one fifth have asthma.[3] These statistics may seem surprising, but not to the health professional who spends a great deal of time treating children with primary pulmonary diseases or respiratory problems secondary to other conditions.

Initially, this chapter provides background information that will enable readers to understand more completely the fragility of the neonatal and pediatric respiratory system, the process of development of that system, and the need for aggressive treatment of disorders of the system. These introductory topics include characteristics of children's lungs, growth and development of the respiratory tract, and predisposition to acute respiratory failure in children and infants. An overview of assessment and treatment by the physical therapist of pulmonary disorders in infants and children is then given. Medical information and a discussion of the physical therapy evaluation and management of four major respiratory problems of children—atelectasis, respiratory muscle weakness, asthma, and cystic fibrosis (CF)—are then presented, followed by questions about future research.

Characteristics of Children's Lungs

Waring[4] described seven unique characteristics of children's lungs that have an impact on the development of lung disease:

1. *Single Cause.* In children, unlike adults, most respiratory signs and symptoms can be explained by a single cause.

2. *Obligatory Miniaturization.* Airflow is related to the cross-sectional area of the airway. The cross section is related geometrically to the airway diameter. As the diameter decreases, the cross section decreases geometrically rather than linearly. As a result, a small obstruction will cause a massive reduction in the cross-sectional area of the lumen in a child's airway. Croup and bronchiolitis, which affect the subglottic trachea and bronchioles, respectively, are caused by edema resulting from infection within those airways. These diseases, which involve severe obstruction of the airways, are seldom, if ever, seen in older children or adults.

In addition to the ease of airway obstruction, the small size of the child's airway results in different physiologic requirements. Infants and small children, whose distal bronchiolar diameter is 1 mm, have a small cross-sectional area that causes a high resistance to airflow. The result of this high resistance, although normal, is greater work of breathing for the child.[5] When the increased likelihood of an obstruction is combined with the increased work of breathing, it becomes obvious why a child's small airways predispose him or her to severe illness.

3. *Interrelationship of Disease and Growth.* The 25 million pulmonary alveoli that are normally present at birth increase until the child is approximately 10 years of age, at which time the adult complement of 300 million alveoli should be present. Diseases that either interfere with the development of the lungs or destroy existing alveoli will decrease the potential number of alveoli in an adult.[6] The deficit in alveolar development reduces the pulmonary reserve and may predispose the child to lung disease during adulthood.

4. *Immunologic Innocence.* Once the transplacentally supplied antibodies from the mother are exhausted at 3 to 4 months of age, the infant is defenseless against many infectious microorganisms. The infant's antibodies are developed through periodic exposure to, or infection with, microorganisms.[7]

5. *High Genetic Impact.* Several of the childhood diseases with a major pulmonary component are transmitted genetically. The inheritance pattern may be recessive or dominant. CF is a primary example of a disease with clearly identified genetic factors that ultimately affect the lungs. Asthma has some genetic components, but they are ill-defined, and environment may play an important role in asthma.[8]

6. *Indiscreet Host Curiosity.* Small children explore their environment by placing objects in their mouths. This behavior may cause aspiration of foreign objects into the airway, or aspiration of toxic chemicals (e.g., furniture polish, turpentine, and kerosene).

7. *Diagnostic Imperviousness.* Three factors make the diagnosis of childhood pulmonary conditions difficult. A child younger than 5 years of age usually cannot perform pulmonary function tests. Second, because of the small size of their airway, the diagnostic tools commonly used in adults are too large for use in infants. Finally, many people have a psychological or emotional barrier to inflicting pain on children, even when the pain of a blood test or a lung biopsy could yield important information for diagnosing or curing a severe disease.

Growth and Development of the Lungs

A brief review of the major periods of lung development is useful in discussing obligatory miniaturization and the interrelationship between disease and growth, and it will provide insight into some unique aspects of the growth (in number) of pulmonary alveoli.

The earliest sign of lung development occurs during the embryologic period, 24 to 26 days after conception. Endodermal tissue of the primitive foregut expands into an anterior lung pouch when the embryo is 4 mm long. During this separation of the trachea and esophagus, aberrations in development may lead to one of several configurations of tracheoesophageal fistulae. Four days later, the lung pouch differentiates into right and left sides. Mesenchymal cellular tissue surrounding the developing lung buds will later differentiate to become muscle, connective tissue, and cartilage within the bronchial walls. Noncellular tissue will provide the elastic and collagen fibers that support the lung structures.[9]

The lung buds continue to grow and subdivide into smaller airways during the 5th to 16th week of gestation (i.e., the pseudoglandular period). Bronchial epithelium lines the primitive airways, and there is a burst of growth between the 10th and 14th week. Mucus-secreting glands and supportive cartilage appear late in the pseudoglandular period and continue their growth through the canalicular period. Branching and subdivision produces 8 to 32 bronchial generations, with the greatest number of divisions occurring in those lung areas that are most distant from the hilum, or root of the lungs.[9] The bronchial tree is complete from the glottis to the terminal bronchioles by the beginning of the canalicular period.

The major events that mark the 16th to 24th week (i.e., the canalicular period) are thinning and flattening of the bronchial epithelium and the appearance of capillaries. The capillaries, which protrude into the epithelium, provide close proximity of the blood supply to the airways. Thinning of the epithelium and capillarization provides the apparatus—the air–blood interface—for respiration. Gas exchange can take place by the end of the canalicular period.[9]

At approximately 25 weeks, the energy of the developing lung begins to form outpouchings of the terminal bronchioles to produce the pulmonary alveoli. This "terminal sac" or "alveolar" period continues until 8 to 10 years of age. A terminal bronchiole will branch into many alveolar pockets or ducts. These ducts are in continued proximity to the tiny capillaries formed during the canalicular period. Once sufficient numbers of alveolar/capillary units are present, life may be sustained, provided that the biochemical substance surfactant is present within the alveoli.[9]

Surfactant is a phospholipid material secreted by Type II cells that line the pulmonary alveoli. Surfactant reduces surface tension within the alveolus, thus allowing inflation of the alveolus with smaller pressures, and less work by the infant than would be needed to inflate a surfactant-deficient alveolus. Surfactant appears at its mature chemical level at approximately 34 weeks of gestation and indicates maturity of the lung by allowing the maintenance of continuous respiration.[10]

After birth, there is a continued subdivision of the alveolar ducts to form alveolar sacs (i.e., the true alveoli). The vasculature continues to parallel the growth in alveoli by branching and multiplying until alveolar growth ceases. From the 25 million alveoli present at birth, there is a 12-fold increase by 8 to 10 years, at which time the adult complement of approximately 300 million is achieved. Destructive processes within the period of alveolar multiplication may limit the potential for development of the adult number of pulmonary alveoli.[11]

Predisposition to Respiratory Failure

The following information is presented to describe more fully several mechanisms of acute respiratory failure and its rapid development in children and infants. Although acute respiratory failure is not a disease, it is often the final common pathway for many diseases that damage the developing respiratory system.

From the mortality data previously cited, it should be obvious that respiratory failure in infants and children is not uncommon. Several structural and metabolic factors in the pediatric population, although entirely normal, predispose them to acute respiratory failure. Respiratory failure can be defined as a condition in which impairment of gas exchange within the lungs poses an immediate threat to life. Downes and associates state that clinical signs and arterial blood gas determinations should be used to monitor infants and children for the development of acute respiratory failure.[12] The arterial blood gas levels compatible with respiratory failure are 75 mm Hg of carbon dioxide and 100 mm Hg of oxygen when the patient is receiving an inspired oxygen concentration of 100%. Respiratory failure exists when either of these arterial levels is reached in the presence of any of the following clinical signs—decreased or absent inspiratory breaths sounds, severe inspiratory retractions with accessory muscle use, cyanosis with inspiration of 40% oxygen, depressed consciousness and response to pain, and poor skeletal muscle tone.[12]

The most important general factor predisposing infants and children to acute respiratory failure is their high incidence of respiratory tract infections.

During the first several years of life, when immunologic defenses are developing, the child is at risk for infections. This risk, which increases as the environment of the toddler expands, probably peaks in the early school years when the child is bombarded with various infectious agents transmitted by classmates, teachers, and other personnel.[13] A recent study by Haskins and Lotch indicates that children in day care centers have an increased incidence of acute respiratory illnesses.[14] As the number of children in day care programs increases, we can expect an increase in the incidence of respiratory infections in the preschool age group.

Two major structural factors—airway size and poor mechanical advantage for the respiratory muscles—contribute to respiratory failure in a young child. The diameter of the tracheal lumen in a 1-year-old child is smaller than the diameter of a lead pencil. More than 85% of the child's peripheral bronchioles are smaller than 1 mm in diameter. A small amount of mucus, bronchospasm, or edema can not only effectively occlude the peripheral airways, but may also obstruct the larger, more proximal bronchi. With sufficient airway blockage, respiratory failure may quickly ensue.

The second major structural issue predisposing children to respiratory failure involves five items that cumulatively cause poor mechanical advantage to the respiratory bellows of the child's thorax:

1. Type I fatigue-resistant muscle fibers are not present in adult proportions in the diaphragm or other ventilatory muscles of the infant until 8 months of age.[15] This lack of fatigue-resistant fibers allows the infant's respiratory muscles to tire quickly, causing alveolar hypoventilation that may lead to respiratory failure.
2. Poor development of the abdominal muscles, used for coughing, renders the infant's airway susceptible to obstruction by mucus.
3. Horizontal alignment of the infant's rib cage and the round (rather than oval) configuration of the chest provide poor mechanical advantage to the intercostal and accessory muscles of respiration. These muscles lift the ribs and sternum to increase thoracic diameter and lung volume.

4. Sternal retractions often occur with intensified inspiratory effects. The lack of rigidity of the costosternal cartilage results in sternal retractions or indrawing that can functionally imitate a flail chest. Intense inspiratory effort may paradoxically decrease the thoracic volume when these substernal retractions occur. The child's ventilation is thus further compromised and hypoventilation occurs.

5. The baby's position may affect diaphragmatic excursion. The infant who is in a supine position works harder to ventilate because the abdominal viscera may impede full descent of the diaphragm.

A third important issue for the physical therapist is respiratory metabolism. The high metabolic rate of the child causes increased consumption of oxygen, increased heat loss, and increased water loss secondary to a faster respiratory rate. The range of normal respiratory rates for children is shown in Table 8-1.

In addition to having muscle fibers that are susceptible to early fatigue, the young child or infant has a poor muscle fuel supply. Glycogen supply in the muscle tissue is small in the infant, and is depleted quickly when muscular activity is increased, which occurs during respiratory distress.[16]

The aforementioned general, structural, and metabolic factors, although developmentally and chronologically normal and appropriate, may combine to render the young respiratory tract fragile and prone to failure during periods of stress, which are commonly seen in respiratory diseases.

Physical Therapy Assessment of Children with Respiratory Disorders

Chart Review

A review of the medical chart and chest roentgenograms, if available, should be the first aspects of the physical therapy assessment of a child. A chart review should provide information regarding the child's medical history; the clinical course of the child's current illness, including signs and symptoms and their precipitating factors; any previous treatment for the illness; and a referral for physical therapy. In addition to the written information found in the chart, physicians and nurses can often provide invaluable and immediate information regarding the child's current state. The chest roentgenograms are useful in identifying specific areas of the lung or thorax that may be affected by the illness. A complete roentgenographic interpretation is beyond the scope of physical therapy practice.

Physical Examination

Careful examination of the infant or child with respiratory distress can offer useful information. The younger the patient, the more the therapist may need to rely on careful observation, because the neonate cannot participate actively in a chest assessment. An age-appropriate description of the activities that the therapist will be performing should precede the actual physical examination.

General Appearance

The therapist should note the state of consciousness of the child and the level to which the child can cooperate with simple commands. Obvious skeletal abnormalities, peripheral edema, wounds, scars, and abnormal postures should all be considered. The therapist should also note the various pieces of

Table 8-1. *Range of Normal Respiratory Rates for Children**

Age (Yrs)	Mean Respiratory Rate (Range)
1	28 (18–40)
2	25 (19–35)
3	23 (18–32)
4	22 (18–29)
5	21 (17–27)
6	20 (17–25)
8	19 (15–23)
10	18 (15–22)
12	18 (14–21)
14	17 (13–21)
16	17 (12–20)

*Adapted from Waring WW. The history and physical examination. In: Kendig EL, Chernick V, eds: Disorders of the Respiratory Tract in Children. Philadelphia. WB Saunders; 1977:83.

apparatus that are being used (e.g., mechanical ventilator, oxygen hood or mask, intravenous or arterial lines).

Head and Neck

There are two common signs of respiratory distress in the infant or young child. *Nasal flaring* is probably a reflex to attempt to widen the nasal airway, thus decreasing resistance to airflow during periods of distress. *Head bobbing* that coincides with the respiratory cycle may be the result of attempts to use the accessory muscles of inspiration by an infant who has inadequate strength to fix the head and neck. Other signs that are commonly observed in the area of the head and neck include cyanosis, pallor, and audible expiratory grunting, particularly in the infant.

Evaluation of the Unmoving Chest

In this portion of the physical examination, the shape and symmetry of the thorax are noted, as are any unusual characteristics of the skin, including rashes, scars, and incisions. The thorax in the infant is more rounded in configuration than the thorax of an adult. The anteroposterior diameter of the thorax in the infant is likely to be equal to its transverse diameter, whereas in the adult's thorax, there is usually a much greater transverse diameter. Congenital defects that may be seen include pectus excavatum (or funnel chest); pectus carinatum (or pigeon-breast); barrel-chest, which is usually associated with hyperinflation of the lungs; and the thoracic deformity that is associated with scoliosis. Muscle development of the thorax should also be examined for symmetry and for the presence of hypertrophy of the accessory muscles, which suggests chronic dyspnea.

Evaluation of the Moving Chest

Determination of the respiratory rate is the first item assessed when evaluating the moving chest. Counting of respirations should be done inconspicuously, often when counting the pulse rate. As previously noted in Table 8-1, the younger the patient, the greater the normal resting respiratory rate. Regularity of breathing is a major item for evaluation, particularly in the neonate and in children with neuromuscular disorders. Short periods of apnea are not particularly unusual and may be referred to as periodic breathing in the neonate. True apnea exists when apneic periods exceed 20 seconds. Apnea can be associated with respiratory distress, sepsis, and central nervous system (CNS) hemorrhage. In addition to the rate and regularity, the ratio of inspiration to expiration (I:E) should be determined. This I:E ratio is usually approximately 1:2. Infants and children with obstructive airway disease, such as asthma and bronchiolitis, may have a marked increase in expiratory time; as a result, their I:E ratio may become 1:4 or 1:5. Synchronous motion of the abdomen and thorax should be observed. On inspiration, both thoracic expansion and abdominal bulging should be noted. When this synchrony is lost, a "seesaw" motion of thoracic expansion with abdominal in-drawing occurs on inspiration, with the opposite movements being noted on expiration. The presence of retractions of the chest wall should be noted. Retractions, or in-drawing, may occur in suprasternal, substernal, subcostal, or intercostal areas. Retractions, seen more frequently in pediatric patients, occur as a result of the compliant thorax of the infant and young child. During respiratory distress, the muscles of either inspiration or expiration, or both, place sufficient pull on the thorax to cause an in-drawing in several areas. When retractions are severe, they may reduce effective inspiration.

Evaluation of Coughing and Sneezing

Infants probably use sneezing more than coughing as both a protective and a clearance mechanism for the airway. Older infants and children must be able to cough effectively to clear secretions or other debris from their airway. It is important to determine the ability to cough in a child with neuromuscular disease who may be at risk for retention of secretion and aspiration of feedings.

Auscultation

Auscultation—listening to the lungs with a stethoscope—is a useful method of assessment. The stethoscope used for auscultation of the infant and young child is a smaller version of that used for adults (Fig. 8-1). The therapist should warm the stethoscope before using it, and depending on the age of the child, the therapist may show how it is used by demonstrating on a child's doll or on a puppet. Because of the proximity to the thoracic surface of the child's airways, as well as the thin chest wall in the young child and infant, sounds are easily transmitted and anatomic specificity may be reduced. A particular sound, therefore, although heard in one area of the thorax, may not correspond to the lung segment directly below the area in which the sound is heard. As a result, auscultation, particularly in the neonate or premature neonate, may not be as precise as in the older child or adult. Nonetheless, the therapist should attempt to ascertain the presence of normal and abnormal breath sounds throughout the lung fields. The therapist should also try to identify adventitious sounds, such as wheezes, crackles, rhonchi, rubs, and crunches. Stridor, a crowing sound associated with upper airway obstruction, and expiratory grunting, associated with airway collapse in the infant, are often audible without auscultation. Because of the ease of

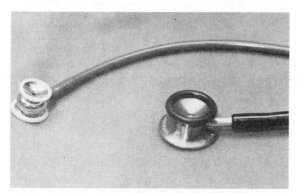

Figure 8-1. *Two sizes of pediatric stethoscopes. (Reproduced by permission from Irwin S, Tecklin JS. Cardiopulmonary Physical Therapy. St. Louis: CV Mosby; 1985.)*

transmission of sound through the infant's thorax, the therapist should attempt to correlate auscultatory findings with roentgenographic changes and other physical findings before instituting treatment.

Palpation

Palpation of the thorax in an infant or child is usually limited to examination of the trachea, which will indicate the position of the mediastinum. Palpation to identify subcutaneous emphysema and other gross findings, such as edema, may also be useful. As the child grows, the therapist may palpate to examine chest expansion and its symmetry, as well as the presence of bony lesions, such as rib fractures.

Other Assessments

Although this chapter deals with disorders of the pulmonary system, the therapist must consider all systems when assessing a child. Developmental assessment is often necessary for a child who has experienced periodic or chronic episodes of hypoxemia, as often occur with pulmonary disorders. Inadequate oxygenation for a period of time may cause minor or major CNS deficit, resulting in a developmental delay. (Normal development and tests of development are discussed in Chapters 1 and 2 of this text.) Various postural abnormalities can be the result of, or can cause, respiratory disorders. Scoliosis with a primary curvature of greater than 60 degrees will usually result in thoracic restriction and a decrease in lung volumes, as will severe pectus excavatum. Some chronic lung diseases, such as severe asthma and CF, lead to hyperinflated, barreled chest with abducted and protracted scapulae. These possibilities must be considered in the assessment of the child with pulmonary disorders. Common orthopedic disorders, some of which have respiratory complications, are discussed in Chapter 9. Finally, an assessment of the family's knowledge and ability to participate in the child's care are important when planning discharge from the hospital, as many pediatric pulmonary disorders are chronic, and will require continuing and effective care at home.

Physical Therapy of Children with Respiratory Disorders

Physical therapy for the infant or child with a pulmonary disorder can be categorized into three general areas:

1. Removal of secretions, either by traditional bronchial hygiene methods or contemporary techniques
2. Breathing exercises and retraining
3. Physical reconditioning

Of course, the degree to which these three areas are used will depend not only on the disease process(es), but also on the age of the child and his or her level of ability and cooperation. Neonates and infants will be treated almost exclusively with traditional bronchial hygiene procedures. Some breathing games and activities can be incorporated into the regimen when the child becomes a toddler. As the child grows older, exercises for breathing retraining and physical and postural reconditioning can be included in the program.

Removal of Secretions

Removal of secretions from the child's airway is the main goal of bronchial hygiene. Of all types of physical therapy treatment for patients with respiratory problems, bronchial hygiene has been most extensively studied and its efficacy is widely accepted. Bronchial hygiene includes both traditional methods—positioning for gravity-assisted drainage of the airways, manual techniques for loosening secretions, and removal of secretions by coughing and suctioning of the airway—and contemporary techniques, involving huffing, forced expiratory technique, and positive expiratory pressure.

Traditional Bronchial Hygiene

POSITIONING FOR GRAVITY-ASSISTED DRAINAGE. Using a working knowledge of bronchopulmonary segment anatomy, the therapist can position the infant or child to drain areas of the lung in which se-

cretions are found during the assessment. The positions place the segment or lobe of lung to be drained uppermost, with the bronchus supplying that lung area in as close to an inverted position as possible. In adults and older children, specific positioning for segmental drainage often involves the use of treatment tables or tilting beds. In infants and young children, the therapist's lap and shoulder serve as the "treatment table." The baby can be held and comforted while in each of the 12 drainage positions (Fig. 8-2). When the child reaches 2 or 3 years of age, the transition may be made from lap to treatment table, but many therapists and parents will continue to use the lap for children up to 4 or 5 years of age. Because most families do not have a hospital bed or tilt-table at home, other methods can be used for proper positioning (Fig. 8-3).

MANUAL TECHNIQUES OF PERCUSSION AND VIBRATIONS. The manual techniques of percussion and vibration are used to loosen or dislodge secretions from the bronchial wall, thus allowing easier removal when the child coughs, sneezes, or undergoes airway aspiration with a suction catheter. Although some major differences exist, the techniques used are similar to those performed on adults. One of the major differences is the amount of force used for either percussion or vibration. Common sense should dictate that minimal amounts of force should be used on the thorax of a premature infant who weighs 1 to 2 kg or less. Increased amounts of percussion and vibration force can be safely applied as the infant grows and as the bones and muscles of the thorax become stronger.

As with adults, the percussion and vibration should be applied to the area of thorax that corresponds to the lung and airways in which secretions are present. Another difference in the pediatric group is that a therapist's percussing or vibrating hand often covers the entire thorax. Other implements have been suggested for percussion and vibration in the infant as a result of this discrepancy in size. Several items used for percussion are shown in Figure 8-4, and different hand configurations for percussion of the infant are shown in Figures 8-5 to

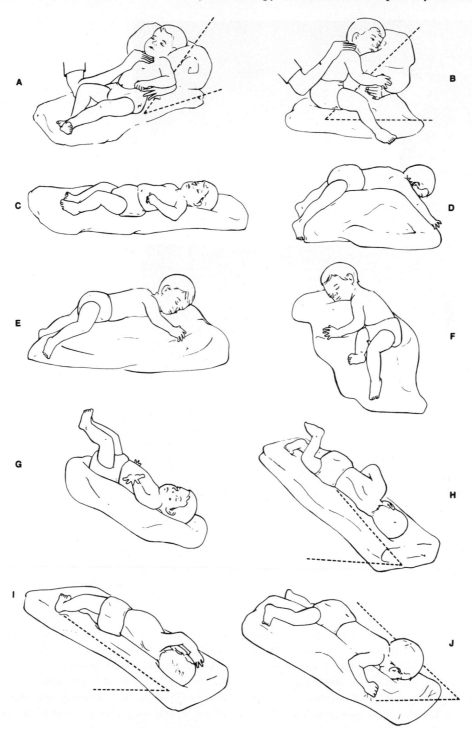

Figure 8-2. *Ten positions for postural drainage (H and I demonstrate lying on the right and left sides). (Reproduced by permission from Irwin S, Tecklin JS. Cardiopulmonary Physical Therapy. St. Louis: CV Mosby; 1985.)*

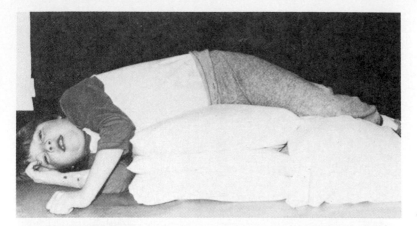

A

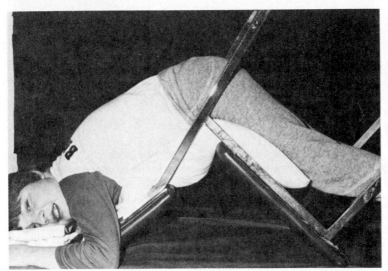

Figure 8-3. *Positioning methods for bronchial drainage at home using bed pillows* (A); *a desk chair* (B); *a stack of magazines with a bed pillow* (C); *and a bean-bag chair* (D). *(Reproduced by permission from Irwin S, Tecklin JS. Cardiopulmonary Physical Therapy. St. Louis: CV Mosby; 1985.)*

B

8-9. Crane has identified the following contraindications for chest percussion in the neonate: a significant drop in transcutaneous (or arterial) oxygen level during percussion, rib fracture or other thoracic trauma, and hemoptysis.[17] Crane also identified various conditions in which percussion should be used carefully in a child, including poor condition of the infant's skin, coagulopathy, osteoporosis or rickets, cardiac arrhythmias, apnea and bradycardia, increased irritability during treatment, subcutaneous emphysema, and subependymal or in-

traventricular hemorrhage.[17] Vibration, which may be used in addition to or in place of percussion, is a less vigorous technique than percussion. There are few true contraindications to vibration with the exception of hemoptysis and reduced oxygenation during treatment. Because vibration is usually done during the expiratory phase of breathing, and because the infant with respiratory disease often has a rate of 40 or more breaths per minutes, it is difficult to coordinate manual vibration with the expiratory phase of breathing. Some persons use various bat-

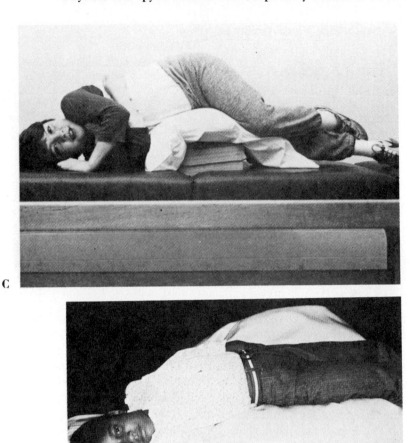

Figure 8-3. *Continued*

tery-powered vibrators that can be held against the infant's thorax during expiration and then quickly removed during inspiration. The modifications and precautions for both percussion and vibration become fewer as the infant grows, and treatment begins to more closely parallel that used for an adult.

COUGHING AND SUCTIONING. Infants and young children will seldom cough on request. Tod-

dlers and school-aged children have the language skill to understand the request for coughing, but will often choose not to cough. Imaginative means, including story telling, coloring games, and nursery rhymes, have been suggested to entice young children to cooperate.[18] In addition, the author has found that by prompting these young children to either laugh or cry (preferably the former), a useful and productive cough can often be elicited. Exter-

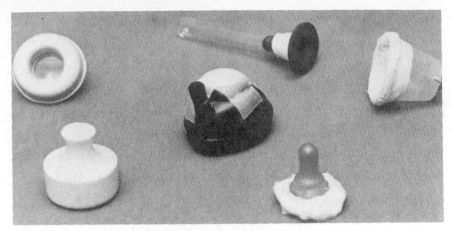

Figure 8-4. *Commercially available and adaptable devices for percussion. (Reproduced by permission from Irwin S, Tecklin JS. Cardiopulmonary Physical Therapy. St. Louis: CV Mosby; 1985.)*

nal stimulation of the trachea ("tracheal tickling") using a circular or vibratory motion of the fingers against the trachea as it courses below the sternal notch may be another useful technique for removing loosened secretions (Fig. 8-10). However, given the relative small size and fragility of the structures involved with this technique, great care must be employed to avoid injury. Coughing is par-

ticularly difficult for the child who has undergone thoracic surgery. Splinting the incision with the hands or with a doll or stuffed animal pressed close to the child's chest promotes the development of an effective cough (Fig. 8-11).

Airway aspiration by suctioning is often needed, particularly in the neonate, to remove secretions. Suctioning must always be done carefully because

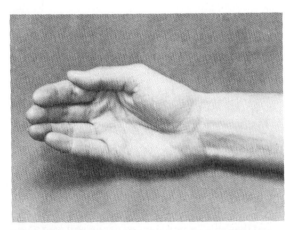

Figure 8-5. *Fully cupped hand for percussion. (Reproduced by permission from Irwin S, Tecklin JS. Cardiopulmonary Physical Therapy. St. Louis: CV Mosby; 1985.)*

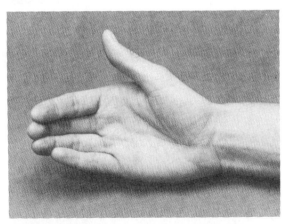

Figure 8-6. *Four fingers cupped for percussion. (Reproduced by permission from Irwin S, Tecklin JS: Cardiopulmonary Physical Therapy. St. Louis: CV Mosby; 1985.)*

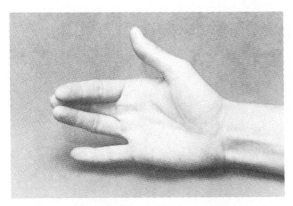

Figure 8-7. *Three fingers cupped for percussion with the middle finger "tented" (anterior view). (Reproduced by permission from Irwin S, Tecklin JS.* Cardiopulmonary Physical Therapy. *St. Louis: CV Mosby; 1985.)*

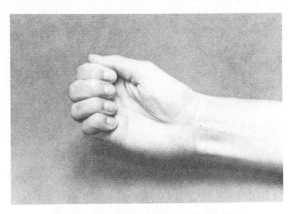

Figure 8-9. *Thenar and hypothenar surfaces for percussion. (Reproduced by permission from Irwin S, Tecklin JS.* Cardiopulmonary Physical Therapy. *St. Louis: CV Mosby; 1985.)*

it has significant risks, even when performed under the best circumstances. Crane has detailed a protocol for endotracheal aspiration.[17]

Contemporary Approaches to Bronchial Hygiene

During the 1980s, several new approaches to bronchial hygiene were developed. Various breathing maneuvers used to loosen and transport mucus were the common feature of these approaches. In

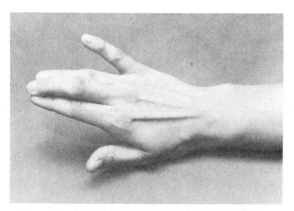

Figure 8-8. *Three fingers cupped for percussion with the middle finger "tented" (posterior view). (Reproduced by permission from Irwin S, Tecklin JS.* Cardiopulmonary Physical Therapy. *St. Louis: CV Mosby; 1985.)*

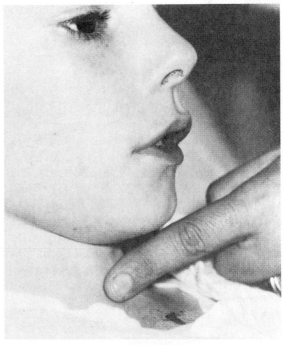

Figure 8-10. *Placement of the finger for the tracheal "tickle" maneuver. (Reproduced by permission from Irwin S, Tecklin JS.* Cardiopulmonary Physical Therapy. *St. Louis: CV Mosby; 1985.)*

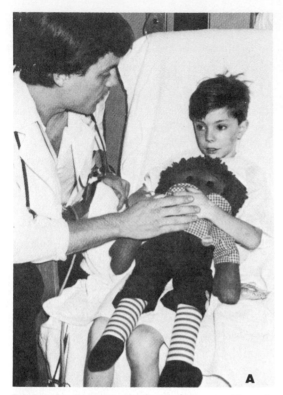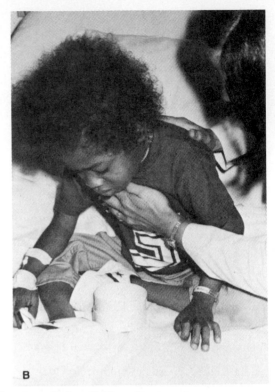

Figure 8-11. A. *Incisional splinting during coughing using a favorite stuffed toy.* B. *Manual compression over the midsternum to facilitate expectoration of sputum. (Reproduced by permission from Irwin S, Tecklin JS.* Cardiopulmonary Physical Therapy. *St. Louis: CV Mosby; 1985.)*

addition, these new techniques were all designed to obviate the need for an individual other than the patient to perform traditional manual techniques of percussion and vibration. These approaches were developed primarily for children and young adults with CF, although they are appropriate for all individuals with chronic lung disease that produces copious sputum.

AUTOGENIC DRAINAGE. This approach was introduced by Dab and Alexander, who describe autogenic drainage as follows:[19,20]

1. The child sits in an upright, or sitting position.
2. The child takes deep breaths at a "normal or relatively slow rhythm."

3. Secretions will move upwards as a result of the breathing.
4. When secretions reach the trachea, they are expelled with either a gentle cough or slightly forced expiration.

The authors recommend that slightly forced expiration be used because of their belief that the high transmural pressures that develop during coughing effectively cause airway collapse, thereby rendering the coughing effort ineffective.[19,20]

FORCED EXPIRATORY TECHNIQUE. The forced expiratory technique (FET) was developed in New Zealand, but was popularized in the late 1970s and into the 1980s by Pryor, Webber, Hodson, and Batten, all from Brompton Hospital in London.[21] As with autogenic drainage, the primary benefit derived from FET is that it can be performed without an assistant. Because the Brompton group has expressed great concern about what they believed to be misinterpretations of their original description,[22] their description of FET is provided here in a direct quotation from their original article.

> The forced expiratory technique (FET) consists of one or two huffs (forced expirations), from mid-lung volume to low lung volume, followed by a period of relaxed, controlled diaphragmatic breathing. Bronchial secretions mobilized to the upper airways are then expectorated and the process is repeated until minimal bronchial clearance is obtained. The patient can reinforce the forced expiration by self compression of the chest wall using a brisk adduction movement of the upper arm.[21]

In a subsequent article that attempts to clarify the various components of FET, the authors place particular emphasis on huffing to low lung volumes in an effort to clear peripheral secretions. In addition, the phrase "from mid-lung volume" has been clarified to mean taking a medium-sized breath prior to initiating the huffing. The authors recommend that patients use FET while in gravity-assisted positions, and further suggest that pauses for breathing control and periods of relaxation are part of the overall technique.[22]

POSITIVE EXPIRATORY PRESSURE (PEP) MASK. This technique employs an anesthesia face mask fitted with a one-way expiratory valve capable of offering variable levels of resistance. The resistance generates positive pressure within the airways, which appears to stabilize smaller airways, thereby preventing their collapse. By preventing airway collapse, distal air-trapping is reduced, and, more importantly, secretion removal is enhanced. Following a period of positive pressure breathing through the mask, perhaps with the child in a gravity-assisted drainage position,[23] FET and directed coughing can be used to expel secretions mobilized by mask breathing.

Breathing Exercises and Retraining

Because many of the commonly used breathing exercises require voluntary participation by the child, the classical methods for teaching improved diaphragmatic descent, increased thoracic expansion, and pursed lip breathing may not be useful in the infant or young child. DeCesare suggests using neurophysiologic techniques, such as applying a quick stretch to the thorax to facilitate contraction of the diaphragm and intercostal muscles, to increase inspiration for the baby or young child.[18]

The toddler can participate in games that require deep breathing and control of breathing. Asking the child to breathe in time to music or to the beat of a metronome can present the skill of paced breathing. Blowing bubbles from a bubble wand or blowing a pinwheel will help to emphasize increased control and prolonged expiration, which may be useful for the child with obstructive disease. Blow bottles may be useful as a means of strengthening the respiratory muscles. The bottles can be set up for inspiration or expiration, and various target levels of water transfer can be set for the child. Numerous types of incentive spirometers are also useful for enhancing deep inspiration after either medical or surgical diseases. Incentive spirometry has been studied extensively and is generally considered to be a useful adjunct to postoperative pulmonary care and a means of strengthening respiratory muscles.[24,25] Improving ventilation to the lower lobes by using diaphragmatic breathing and lateral costal expansion also helps to reduce postoperative pulmonary complications.[24]

Participation in breathing exercises usually improves as the child grows older. When appropriate, the therapist may use manual contact to teach diaphragmatic breathing, lateral costal expansion, and segmental expansion. Depending on the findings from the assessment of the moving chest, the therapist will choose one or more of these types of breathing exercises. The older child with severe, perennial asthma and the child with CF will often exhibit many of the same characteristics as adults with chronic obstructive pulmonary disease

(COPD). Paced diaphragmatic breathing may be very useful for these children and young adults. Reduced expenditure of energy is one of the major benefits of diaphragmatic breathing. Because exercise intolerance becomes a problem for children with asthma and CF, diaphragmatic breathing may improve the child's ability to walk, climb stairs, and perform other vigorous physical activities. Pursed-lip breathing may also be useful for breath control in the child with chronic lung disease. Relaxation exercise for the child with asthma is often suggested as a means of reducing breathlessness. Although there is no scientific evidence of any change in the pulmonary function of these children with relaxation exercise, there is strong anecdotal evidence of a reduction in the anxiety associated with dyspnea.

Physical Development

Activities to improve physical function in the infant or child with a pulmonary disorder may begin in the neonatal nursery. When possible, physical therapy treatments should be done with the infant removed from the isolette or warming bed. The handling and tactile stimulation provided by the bronchial hygiene session may be helpful adjuncts to the sensorimotor development of the infant, who may spend great amounts of time in a supine position. Of course, this type of movement is not always possible, particularly for the critically ill baby. As the pulmonary condition improves, the infant should begin to receive, in addition to respiratory physical therapy, appropriate intervention to assess and, if necessary, to treat delays in motor development. Chapter 3, devoted to the high-risk infant, describes an approach to this type of child.

Physical Training

Children with asthma and CF and those with respiratory disease secondary to neuromuscular or musculoskeletal problems represent two distinct groups for whom physical training is important. A case example of each group follows in this chapter. Programs of physical training usually include exercises to improve strength and range of motion (ROM), posture, and endurance.

Strength training is helpful in both groups of children. Children with severe asthma and moderately advanced CF are often limited in strength owing to inactivity and chronic or periodic hypoxemia. Darbee and Cerny advocate a strengthening program involving isotonic resistive exercise performed at a high number of repetitions rather than high levels of resistance.[26] They also believe that exercise should stress the shoulder girdle and thoracic musculature as a means of facilitating the respiratory pump.[26] Although data are sparse, one must assume that improving strength in these children will decrease their physical inactivity and disability. The group of children with neuromuscular disease, such as myopathy or spinal muscle atrophy, and musculoskeletal disease, such as juvenile rheumatoid arthritis, will have weakness that prohibits their full participation in normal childhood activities. A carefully planned, judiciously administered strengthening program should help both groups.

Decreased ROM is more commonly a problem for the neuromuscular/musculoskeletal group than for those with asthma and CF. When thoracic motion is considered as a part of ROM, however, then the children with asthma and CF have been found to have decreases similar to those occurring in children who have undergone recent thoracic surgery. This surgical group will have reduced thoracic motion after surgery and are at risk for both loss of shoulder motion and development of scoliosis. Exercises for deep breathing, thoracic expansion, segmental expansion, and upper extremity function can help to either prevent loss of motion or to regain motion that has been lost.

Strengthening of respiratory musculature has been scrutinized in recent years. Just as other skeletal muscles respond to training for both endurance and strength, the muscles of inspiration and expiration will respond similarly. Studies of groups of children with chronic obstructive disease and groups with specific respiratory muscle weakness have shown that significant improvement in respiratory muscle function accompanies breathing activities aimed at either endurance or strength, or both.[27] Inspiratory muscle training and strengthening have resulted in improvement in numerous physiological indices; however, the clinical or functional benefits have been defined less completely. Nonetheless, inspiratory muscle strengthening and endurance training should be considered if weakness is suspected in the vital respiratory pump. Expiratory muscle strengthening may benefit exercise tolerance and surely should enhance the force of expiratory maneuvers, including coughing. As with inspiratory muscle training, expiratory muscle training lacks completely persuasive clinical study. These exercises are described in the following discussion regarding respiratory muscle weakness.

The child with chronic lung disease will benefit from participation in a program of cardiovascular training or conditioning. Because of the tendency for running to precipitate exercise-induced bronchospasm in children with asthma, this group of young patients seems to respond much better to swimming programs. Children and young adults with CF participate throughout the United States in organized walking or jogging groups. The popularity of these groups can be traced to Dr. David Orenstein, who first popularized jogging for children with CF and who then studied the benefits for those children.[28] Darbee and Cerny provide an exceptionally complete description of exercise testing and training for children with lung dysfunction.[26]

Regardless of the specific exercise or physical reconditioning program, and regardless of the pediatric pulmonary problem, there is a major role for the physical therapist in treating children with lung disease.

The next section of this chapter describes four common disorders of the respiratory tract in children and their physical therapy evaluation and treatment.

Atelectasis

Atelectasis, or incomplete expansion of a lung or a portion thereof, was first described by Laennec in 1819.[29] Primary atelectasis occurs in the neonate as a result of pulmonary immaturity, and also can occur at any age as a result of inadequate respiratory effort. Secondary atelectasis occurs when gas in a lung segment is reabsorbed without subsequent refilling of that segment. The most common causes of secondary atelectasis include bronchial obstruction, abnormal pressure on the lung tissue, and removal of pulmonary surfactant by disease or trauma.[30]

Primary atelectasis in small areas of the newborn lung is a common finding during the first few days of life. The sick neonate with poor respiratory effort and generalized weakness may not fully expand all areas of the lung for several weeks. Major areas of secondary atelectasis may be the result of abnormal thoracic content causing external compression of the lung tissue or the airways. Among the most common causes of lung compression in young children are an enlarged heart or great vessels, congenital or acquired lung cysts, diaphragmatic hernia, and congenital lobar emphysema. The most common type of atelectasis seen by the physical therapist is caused by airway obstruction secondary to secretion of mucus or other debris, including meconium, amniotic content, foreign bodies, and aspirated gastrointestinal content. In critical care units, a misplaced endotracheal tube often causes a large area of atelectasis.

Medical Information

Signs and symptoms of atelectasis depend on the degree of involvement of the lungs. Common findings include decreased chest wall excursion of the affected hemithorax, tachypnea, and inspiratory retractions, as well as cyanosis if the atelectasis is large. The trachea will deviate toward the involved lung because of volume loss, and a dull percussion note, which indicates an airless lung, will be present. By auscultation, breath sounds will be reduced or absent. The roentgenogram will often demonstrate a sharply demarcated area of consolidation, although patchy areas of atelectasis are not uncommon in acute respiratory tract infection.

Medical management of obstructive atelectasis is directed toward the removal of the obstructing material or structure. When the atelectasis is associated with an acute infection, therapy that cures the infection will often eradicate the atelectasis. Good hydration will decrease the viscosity of the mucus. Postural drainage with chest percussion, vibration, and coughing, followed by deep inhalations, will help remove mucus, and a bronchodilator may widen the bronchus, thus allowing air past the obstruction. When an obstruction is caused by a neoplasm or other structure that occludes the airway or exerts pressure over the lung parenchyma, surgical removal of the item may be indicated. Endobronchial aspiration using a suction catheter may help to remove airway debris, and repositioning of a poorly placed endotracheal tube may correct atelectasis. If none of these more conservative measures is successful, bronchoscopy, using either a rigid or a flexible bronchoscope with administration of general or local anesthesia, is indicated to remove the intraluminal mucus or debris.[31]

Prognosis is usually good if the underlying disease process is not life-threatening and if the duration of the atelectasis has not been prolonged. Permanent damage to the bronchial architecture can occur with delayed or incomplete resolution of atelectasis. Pulmonary fibrosis and bronchiectasis are the most common sequelae of obstructive atelectasis.[31]

Physical Therapy Evaluation

A thorough review of the patient's chart is necessary to fully understand the pathophysiology of the condition and to identify the type of atelectasis (primary or secondary). The treatment for each type will include similar efforts to increase respiratory effort, but only secondary atelectasis requires bronchial hygiene procedures.

Review of the roentgenographic findings will identify the position of the atelectasis. The therapist should use the roentgenogram as a clinical tool when treating a patient with atelectasis. Lateral and posteroanterior exposures provide a three-dimensional view of the lung fields. The patient's chest and breathing should be noted. A large atelectasis narrows the rib interspaces and decreases excursion of the involved hemithorax. The muscular pattern of respiration should be noted—diaphragmatic versus accessory—and the patient's respiratory rate should be determined.

Palpation may indicate a shift of the trachea toward the atelectasis owing to volume loss in the lung. The airless lung has a dull percussion note that helps the therapist locate the atelectasis. Auscultatory findings will vary. The most frequent change is a diminution of breath sounds in the involved area. Complete obstruction of a large or main bronchus may result in complete absence of breath sounds. With patchy or incomplete atelectasis, crackles may be heard for the first of several deep breaths; however, with subsequent deep breaths, the alveoli may open and the crackles may decrease.

Other considerations in evaluating the child include the following:

- Mobility—Has the child been at bedrest for an extended time?
- Pain—Can the child take a deep breath and cough effectively?
- Cough—Can the child cough, and does he or she have sufficient strength or neurologic competence?

Physical Therapy Management

Several studies strongly support physical therapy procedures for the prevention of postoperative atelectasis in adult surgical patients. Therapeutic methods used in these studies included bronchial drainage, percussion, vibration, deep breathing,[32,33] maximal inspiratory efforts,[34] and electrical stimulation of the thorax with direct current.[35] The success of each treatment regimen was unequivocal. (The difference between adults and children in terms of airway cross section and strength of coughing has been previously discussed.)

Finer and associates found a significant decrease in the incidence of postextubation atelectasis in infants who were treated with bronchial drainage, vibration, and oral suctioning when compared to a similar control group treated only with bronchial drainage.[36] Atelectasis after extubation occurs commonly in infants, and is presumably caused by excessive bronchial secretions.

These studies have not evaluated the treatment of atelectasis; however, they have evaluated its prevention, which is the best treatment. Burrington and Cotton have reported the successful use of bronchial drainage, percussion, and coughing, preceded by inhalation of a bronchodilator, in 28 children who had aspirated a foreign body.[37] Of this group, 24 children coughed out the object after physical therapy. Although atelectasis is not always present with a foreign body in the airway, it is a common radiologic finding. When atelectasis is caused by aspirated material, physical methods can remove the material and relieve the atelectasis.[37]

Controlled studies of physical therapy for the treatment of atelectasis have not been published. The development of a rational approach to treatment should be based on the type and cause of the atelectasis. The methods used in the aforementioned studies are often included in the treatment of a child with atelectasis.

Postoperative atelectasis is a combination of primary and secondary atelectasis. Secretions are more abundant owing to irritation of the airway by the anesthetic gases and tube manipulations. With incisional pain, and with the generalized weakness that accompanies thoracic or abdominal surgery, the child has a less effective cough and the volume of inspirations is decreased. Deep breathing to achieve maximal inspiration will often be sufficient to resolve small areas of atelectasis. These efforts should be initiated early in the postoperative period—in the recovery room if possible—to prevent atelectasis. Coaching the child to breathe deeply, splinting the incision to reduce pain, and using proprioceptive techniques to facilitate the inspiratory musculature can help the child increase the depth of respiration. Positioning the patient to drain the major lung fields and percussion/vibration followed by attempts to cough will aid in the prevention of pulmonary complications. Incentive spirometers, used as a breathing game, will stimulate deeper inhalations. Percussion and coughing become critical components of the treatment if the patient develops atelectasis despite preventive measures. Aggressive percussion of the chest over the atelectasis and splinted coughing will work to mechanically dislodge and clear the obstructing mucus. Treatment often includes endotracheal suctioning to remove accumulated mucus and to further stimulate coughing. Early ambulation of the patient after surgery and the resultant stress on the respiratory system helps to mobilize secretions by causing the patient to breathe deeply.

Children with medical chest conditions develop atelectasis as a result of retained secretions. These children will find coughing and maximal inspirations easier to do because there is no incisional pain. Liberal and more aggressive use of chest percussion in these nonsurgical patients is helpful. Bronchial drainage with localized percussion will often dislodge the obstructing secretions, and coughing will clear the airway. Many physicians suggest aerosol inhalation, both to moisten the secretions and to deliver a bronchodilator. The rationale for these procedures of inhalation is that moist secretions will drain more easily from a bronchus that is maximally dilated. Data exist to support both of these methods as an adjunct to physical therapy.[38]

The use of autogenic drainage, FET, and POP should be considered for obstructive atelectosis.

Primary atelectasis caused by respiratory muscle weakness can be resolved by deep breathing and strengthening of the respiratory muscles.

Respiratory Muscle Weakness

Respiratory muscle weakness in children, as in adults, may be the result of a disorder affecting any link in the chain of neuromuscular events that produce a contraction of the respiratory muscles. Weakness or paresis of the respiratory muscles may be either mild and transient or severe and irreversible. The underlying pathologic process is the primary determinant of the duration and severity of the weakness. The physical therapist should develop a therapeutic regimen to treat the muscle weakness and to prevent or treat the resultant pulmonary symptoms within the limitations imposed by the disorder.

In the past decade, a growing population of ventilator-dependent children has arisen as a result of improved technology and care for acute and chronic ventilatory failure. These children, too, require physical therapy for problems associated with respiratory pump failure and for the delay in motor skill development caused by reliance upon the mechanical ventilator.

Medical Information

Diffuse pathology of the CNS (e.g., viral encephalitis or barbiturate intoxication) may lead to respiratory failure by paralyzing the voluntary and involuntary portions of the respiratory muscles. Abnormal neural control mechanisms and reflexes may ablate or reduce the physiologic response to chemical and mechanical stimuli. These stimuli may occur within the lungs, the brain stem, the blood, and cerebrospinal fluid (CSF). Examples of childhood disorders that result in a reduced response to respiratory stimuli are familial dysautonomia, sleep apnea, and obesity-hypoventilation syndrome. Lesions affecting the medullary centers that generate the inspiratory drive may cause marked changes in ventilatory patterns.

Spinal cord lesions above the C-4 level may result in total ventilatory paralysis. Because the phrenic nerve, which innervates the diaphragm, leaves the spinal cord at the C-4 level, a lesion above that level will affect all muscles of respiration. Injury to the high-thoracic or low-cervical cord often results in decreased lung volume and reduced chest wall compliance. Coughing will be inadequate if the abdominal muscles are paralyzed. These factors may cause respiratory insufficiency that may progress to respiratory failure. Acute respiratory care and long-term rehabilitation are essential components of a treatment plan for the child with a spinal cord lesion or injury.

Diseases affecting the efferent portion of the neuromuscular system are not uncommon in children. The progressive loss of anterior horn cells seen in Werdnig-Hoffmann syndrome leads to paralysis and early death secondary to respiratory failure. The result of acute polyneuritis (Guillain-Barré syndrome) is often respiratory paralysis. When this syndrome is fatal, it is usually attributable to respiratory failure. Because recovery from Guillain-Barré syndrome is often complete, the respiratory weakness must be treated aggressively and should include acute and long-term rehabilitation measures.

Degenerative diseases of the muscle (e.g., Duchenne myopathy) are characterized by progressive deterioration of pulmonary function. Adequate arterial oxygen and carbon dioxide values are maintained only through active efforts. Death is usually the direct result of respiratory failure, which often follows the development of pneumonia.

The thoracic cage normally provides for adequate function of the respiratory musculature. Abnormalities of the thorax, such as idiopathic scoliosis, scoliosis secondary to neuromuscular disease, and other specific congenital abnormalities, may result in a loss of mechanical advantage of the respiratory muscles.

The examples just mentioned can cause respiratory muscle weakness or mechanical disadvantage. They may also lead to the requirement for long-term management by mechanical ventilation. Mallory and Stilwell identify the physical therapist as a member of the typical team of caregivers for these technology-dependent children.[39] In addition, of the seven rehabilitation goals they have identified for the ventilator-dependent child, six are directly related to physical therapy knowledge, skills, and scope of practice. These seven goals include the following:

1. Increase in muscle strength
2. Increase in attention and cognition
3. Decrease in spasticity
4. Increase in chest wall movement
5. Accessory muscle breathing while upright
6. Diaphragmatic breathing
7. Assisted cough

All goals, with the possible exception of the second one, are direct benefits derived from physical therapy.[39]

Physical Therapy Evaluation

The parameters assessed in a comprehensive physical therapy evaluation for a child with respiratory muscle weakness are breathing pattern, respiratory muscle strength, chest and shoulder mobility, and airway clearance. In addition, when appropriate, the therapist should evaluate sensorimotor development.

Determining the breathing pattern is a major part of the evaluation. Minute ventilation—the product of the respiratory rate and the tidal volume—determines the arterial $PaCO_2$. The respiratory rate can be counted for 30 seconds or 1 minute, remembering that the child's normal respiratory rate at rest varies with age (a younger child will have a higher rate).[40] Tidal volume can be easily measured with a spirometer or a Wright respirometer used at the bedside. As with respiratory rate, tidal volume varies depending on the child's height. A taller child has a larger predicted tidal volume.[40] The pattern and symmetry of muscular effort must be ascertained. Is the child using primarily the diaphragm, intercostal muscles, accessory muscles, or glossopharyngeal muscles? Is the muscular pattern similar for each hemithorax?

The therapist has several methods available for evaluating respiratory muscle strength, including measurement of lung volumes, maximal static inspiratory and expiratory pressures, and electromyography. The first two methods are simple and inexpensive, but require the child's full cooperation. With normal lung tissue and without loss of elastic recoil, decreased inspiratory capacity or expiratory reserve volume suggest weakness of the inspiratory or expiratory musculature, respectively.[41] Respiratory failure may be imminent when the vital capacity declines to approximately 30% of predicted values. Maximal inspiratory and expiratory pressures are another good index of respiratory muscles. These pressures can be measured with appropriate pressure manometers, and measurements can be repeated as often as necessary.[42]

Evaluation of the mobility of the chest wall includes determining expansion of the chest wall in anteroposterior, transverse, and vertical directions during inspiration. Thoracic dimensions are determined during inspiration and expiration to document chest motion. ROM in the spine and the shoulder girdle should be examined, including glenohumeral, acromioclavicular, and sternoclavicular joints. Decreased motion at any one of these joints may result in reduced thoracic expansion.

Auscultation of the lungs of a child with respiratory weakness will serve several functions. Decreased breath sounds will help identify areas that are poorly ventilated. Lung areas with decreased or absent sounds may correlate with decreased chest motion or muscular effort. Breath sounds are the most reliable clinical tool for assuring good ventilation. Breath sounds can help the therapist evaluate the need for bronchial hygiene. If rhonchi and wheezes are heard, bronchial drainage and removal of secretions are probably necessary. Breath sounds may indicate the resolution or progression of pulmonary complications, such as pneumonia or atelectasis, and the therapist may choose to modify treatment accordingly.

The therapist should evaluate the child's cough. Integral components of a cough are sufficient active inspiration and coordinated closure of the glottis, followed by sudden contraction of the abdominal muscles to markedly increase intrathoracic pressure. With neuromuscular dysfunction, the child may lack any or all cough-related skills. Evaluation of inspiratory effort, glottis closure, and abdominal muscle strength is important in assessing coughing. The child must also coordinate the three components into an effective, sputum-producing effort.

Overall strength, mobility, and coordination, as well as the developmental level of the child, must be evaluated to plan a realistic rehabilitation program. A child who can actively locomote in some manner is less likely to suffer pulmonary complications and may improve pulmonary function as a byproduct of the rehabilitative effort. An aggressive therapeutic regimen is necessary, both to provide early mobility and to strengthen the respiratory musculature, thus improving ventilatory function.[43]

Evaluation of oral motor function—swallowing

and feeding—often requires an interdisciplinary effort by physicians, physical therapists, occupational therapists, speech pathologists, other therapists, and nurses. Swallowing must be evaluated for two reasons: eating is the best way for a child to thrive nutritionally, and aspiration of feedings is a major cause of respiratory problems in developmentally delayed and neurologically impaired children.[44] A discussion of aspiration and swallowing function is beyond the scope of this chapter, but a good general overview can be found in Farber's text.[45]

Physical Therapy Management

Physical rehabilitation for the child with neurologic impairment should include an exercise program to improve or maintain respiratory function. The exercises should strengthen inspiratory and expiratory muscles, especially the abdominal muscles that are necessary for effective coughing. A traditional method of "strengthening" the diaphragm by using abdominal weights has not withstood rigorous scientific evaluation.[46] More physiologically appropriate methods of improving inspiratory muscle strength and endurance may include resistive breathing,[47] use of incentive spirometers,[48] and maximal sustainable ventilatory capacity.[49] A battery of breathing exercises has improved spirometric values in children with Duchenne myopathy[50] and in children with cerebral palsy.[51] In addition, active and resistive exercises for the neck will strengthen the accessory muscles of inspiration (i.e., the sternocleidomastoid muscles and scalene muscles). Although accessory muscle use increases the energy cost of breathing, the accessory muscles may provide increased inspiratory volume to prevent respiratory insufficiency in the child with neuromuscular disease. Active and resistive exercises for strengthening of the abdomen, which may help develop a strong, effective cough, are well known by physical therapists. Many clinical aspects of respiratory muscle training have been discussed by Watts,[52] Adkins,[53] and Warren.[54]

Improving the pattern of breathing of a child with neuromuscular disease may provide two major benefits. First, in improved ratio of alveolar ventilation to dead space ventilation occurs when a slower, deeper pattern of breathing replaces a fast and shallow mode. The therapist may have the child attempt a slower and deeper pattern of breathing using various clinical cues, including counting, a metronome, or a spirogram. Care must be taken to avoid a deep breath which, owing to increased elastic resistance of the lung parenchyma at high volumes, may increase the work of breathing and negate the presumed improvement. Avoiding inefficient or counterproductive muscular effort is the second major benefit of changing the pattern of breathing. A child with respiratory distress may appropriately use the accessory muscles to aid inspiration and may use the abdominal muscles to enhance full expiration. This muscular pattern, however, can become habitual. If the diaphragm provides adequate ventilation, unnecessary muscular effort is exerted if the child continues to use the accessory muscles. Various training methods have been suggested, including relaxation exercises and neurosensory techniques, but no scientific data support these endeavors, nor do they suggest that short-term changes in muscular patterns during the therapeutic session have a residual effect or replace the inefficient patterns.

Although the importance of maintaining or improving mobility of the thorax in children has been identified and related treatment plans have been outlined,[52–54] no controlled studies of the techniques have been conducted. Active breathing exercises to improve thoracic mobility have been suggested for localized areas or for the entire chest. Manual stretching of the chest wall has been advocated but has not been tested. It is known that adults with decreased thoracic mobility have increased lung compliance and improved oxygenation for several hours after the use of incentive spirometers and positive pressure breathing.[55] It seems logical that a child, whose chest wall is normally more compliant than that of an adult, should also benefit from these two methods. Active or passive exercise to improve shoulder girdle mobility in children with paralysis may also improve thoracic excursion. Clinical studies must be undertaken to justify the time-consuming procedures used in the name of respiratory exercises.

Skill at coughing is important because of the smaller airway cross section in children and the predisposition to airway obstruction. Children with muscular weakness often lack an effective cough. Efforts to improve the cough usually involve strengthening of the abdominal muscles. Using sit-ups and straight leg raising has been discouraged because these activities primarily involve the rectus abdominus rather than the strong compressors of the abdominal wall (i.e., the transversalis and oblique muscles).[52] The use of expulsive maneuvers, such as blow-bottles or forced expiratory trials, seems to offer more kinesiologically appropriate means of strengthening the cough musculature. Other traditional methods of instruction in coughing rely on a "double cough," "huffing" on expiration, and external stimulation (irritation) of the trachea to elicit a cough.

Because many children with respiratory weakness and general inactivity accumulate secretions, bronchial drainage techniques are an important part of the home treatment program. If the parent suspects an increase in secretions as a result of a respiratory tract infection, the use of positioning for gravity drainage and chest vibration or percussion may prevent the development of pneumonia or atelectasis. Oral or nasal suctioning may be necessary to maintain a clear airway if a child cannot cough well and if secretions are voluminous. Parents should be trained in aspiration techniques and should have proper suctioning equipment in the home.

Despite many articles and textbooks that describe detailed physical therapy programs for patients with neuromuscular weakness of the chest, there is a dearth of well-substantiated clinical research to support many of the suggested treatment procedures.

Asthma

There are many definitions of asthma, all with some features in common, but none agreed upon universally. A recent panel of the National Heart Lung and Blood Institute proposed the following definition: "Asthma is a lung disease with the following characteristics: (1) airway obstruction that is reversible (but not completely so in some patients) either spontaneously or with treatment; (2) airway inflammation; and (3) increased airway responsiveness to a variety of stimuli."[56] It is now generally recognized that chronic airway inflammation and associated changes are largely responsible for the airway obstruction and increased responsiveness of the airways in children with asthma.[57]

Medical Information

Asthma is among the most prevalent of all chronic disorders, afflicting more than 10 million people in the United States, 3.2 million of whom are children. Although the mortality associated with childhood asthma is low, recent data suggest an increase during the 1980s.[58,59] There is enormous morbidity associated with the condition, as denoted by days lost from school, hospitalizations, and health care costs. Asthma in children is characterized by several factors. Boys seem to predominate over girls by as much as a 2:1 ratio, although this number is not firm. Exercise-induced asthma is common in children, with a reported prevalence of more than 90%.[60] Children with asthma are often allergic, with the inhaled allergen triggering a type 1 immunoglobin E (IgE)-mediated response. Symptoms may also be provoked by viral infections and emotional problems. Finally, the increasing mortality and continuing high morbidity associated with childhood asthma are attributable, in part, to a growing problem with asthma in the inner city populations.[61]

The physiologic changes responsible for the signs and symptoms of asthma are thought to be initiated by the release of one or more chemical mediators from the mast cells and eosinophils within the airways. These inflammatory mediators—histamine, prostaglandin D_2, leukotriene C_4, and others—stimulate a response that increases bronchial smooth muscle contraction, causes mucous secretions from the goblet cells of the bronchial epithelium, and may result in edema of the bronchial wall. The result of all three processes is often an obstruction of the airways. As airway obstruction progresses, expiratory airflow decreases, lung volumes and airway resistance increase, airway conductance decreases, and ventilation/perfusion inequality leads to arterial hypoxemia.

A fascinating aspect of asthma in children is the exercise-induced component. With strenuous exercise for a period of time, usually for more than 5 minutes, a child can develop many manifestations of asthma (e.g., dyspnea, wheezing, and airway obstruction) that may reverse spontaneously or with treatment. This exercise component is important to the physical therapist who is developing a conditioning program to increase exercise tolerance in the child with asthma. The response can be controlled by having the child using appropriate oral or inhalation medications prior to the exercise bout.

Medical Management

The medical management of children with asthma can be divided into three major categories: acute management, long-term management, and treatment of status asthmaticus. Two major drugs are used to reverse the acute severe bronchospasm for which a child is brought to the emergency room. The preferred drug is epinephrine, a sympathetic nervous system stimulator that is injected subcutaneously. The dosage may be repeated twice in 1 hour if relief does not follow the initial dose.[62] In addition to epinephrine, intravenous administration of aminophylline is often begun. (The mechanism of action for aminophylline within the immunologic system is beyond the scope of this chapter.[63]) In addition to these medications, the patient may inhale a nebulized solution of another sympathomimetic drug. The inhalation procedure deposits within the obstructed airways drugs that cause almost immediate bronchodilation. The child may also receive fluids and supplemental oxygen. In recent years, with the evidence that acute and chronic inflammation play a large role in asthma, the administration of anti-inflammatory medications, primarily corticosteroids delivered by oral and nebulized routes has also become standard treatment.

A child whose asthma is refractory to the aforementioned treatment regimen is considered to have status asthmaticus, or intractable asthma, and is often admitted to an intensive care unit. Administration of aminophylline and sympathetic stimulants is continued and corticosteroids are prescribed, although their effect is delayed for several hours. The child must be intubated and placed on ventilatory assistance if repeated arterial blood gas samples indicate respiratory failure. Although a serious step, mechanical ventilation will support the child while the severe intractable bronchospasm diminishes. Many acute care units use an asthma scoring system that is semiquantitative and may be helpful in following the course of status asthmaticus.[64]

The long-term medical management of asthma has several components: pharmacologic, environmental, and immunologic. The pharmacologic agents used may include sympathomimetic agents delivered orally or by aerosol; oral preparations of theophylline (methylxanthines); anti-inflammatory agents, including inhaled and oral corticosteroids; and cromolyn sodium, delivered by inhalation. Control of environmental factors plays a major role in asthma therapy. A dust-free environment for the child is imperative, and special air-filtration units may be required for the child's room. Removal of pets from the home, avoidance of tobacco smoke, and careful selection of foods to which the child is not sensitive are also major aspects of environmental control. If the youngster chooses to be active in athletics, care must be taken either to avoid levels of activity that may provoke bronchospasm or to use appropriate medication before engaging in asthma-inducing levels of physical exertion.

Another method of long-term therapy for allergic asthma is hyposensitization (allergy shots). Once allergens are identified by skin testing, extracts of these allergens are given in gradually increasing strengths by way of periodic injections. The rationale is that the child's immunologic system will respond to the minute doses of allergen by producing circulating antibodies. Once sufficient levels of antibodies are developed, environmental exposure to the allergen (e.g., pollen or food) will result in no symptoms of asthma because the acquired antibodies will alleviate the allergic response of the child.

Physical Therapy Evaluation

As with medical care, physical therapy evaluation and management of children with asthma is largely based on the clinical situation at the time (i.e., whether the child is in an acute, subacute, or chronic stage of the disease). The child with status asthmaticus will generally not tolerate well any maneuvers aimed at either bronchial hygiene or physical training. A notable exception is when the patient is intubated and mechanically ventilated.

Thy physical therapist's evaluation of a child on a ventilator should include auscultation in an effort to identify secretions and poorly inflated areas of lung. Evaluation of the child's position in bed and initial assessment of shoulder ROM are appropriate. An evaluation of the asthmatic patient in the subacute phases (i.e., when the severe bronchospasm has responded to medication) should include several parameters. The therapist must identify, through auscultation, where bronchial secretions have accumulated and if areas of the lungs are poorly ventilated. The pattern of ventilation and use of accessory muscles should be noted. Measurements of the thorax, including thoracic index, should be made during inspiration and expiration to determine chest mobility. Shoulder-girdle ROM should also be measured. Several or all of these evaluated items will be abnormal. The therapist must reevaluate these items with each treatment until the ROM, thoracic index, breath sounds, and pattern of breathing are normal.

A long-term rehabilitation plan for the child with asthma must also examine exercise tolerance, strength, and posture. Exercise tolerance may be evaluated by semiquantitative measures in the physical therapy department or by sophisticated testing in an exercise laboratory. Heart rate during a particular work load and time of recovery to resting heart rate are useful and simple indices of fitness or exercise tolerance.[65] Quantitative strength measurement of major muscle groups can be made with equipment that is readily available in the physical therapy department. Posture can be evaluated using a grid system.[66]

Physical Therapy Management

There is little, if any, rationale for physical therapy in the child with status asthmaticus. Status asthmaticus renders a child too dyspneic, anxious, scared, and physically unable to cooperate with the therapist for bronchial hygiene, breathing retraining, posture and ROM evaluation, or any rehabilitative endeavors. Bronchial drainage with chest percussion, vibration, and coughing should be used when the status asthmaticus begins to abate and the patient can tolerate these physical maneuvers. An exception to this approach is when the child is intubated for mechanical ventilation, in which case the child should undergo bronchial drainage, percussion, vibration, and suctioning if secretions are problematic.

When the severe bronchospasm begins to wane, accumulated secretions are often encountered in the previously narrowed airways. Aggressive bronchial hygiene is imperative during this subacute stage. Secretions that are not removed quickly predispose the patient to atelectasis and bronchial infection. Bronchial drainage with chest percussion and vibration is indicated within the limits of the youngster's tolerance and endurance. Secretion volume, color, consistency, and the child's vital signs before, during, and after treatment should be recorded.

In the long-term care of asthmatic children, intermittent bronchial hygiene treatments may be useful, but they are not used routinely as in other conditions, such as CF. Parents must know the drainage positions and manual techniques in order to treat the child at home. Parents should use bronchial drainage at the first sign of a respiratory infection or increased mucous production. The only reported study of the effects of drainage and percussion in children with asthma involved 21 outpatients. These children, who had mild to moderate asthma, were divided into a treatment group and a control group. The mean FEV_1 for the treatment group increased by 10.5% 30 minutes after therapy. The control group had a slight decrease in mean FEV_1 during the same period. The difference in mean FEV_1 values was significant at the 0.05 level.[67] Breathing training combined with relaxation techniques has been suggested for improvement of respiratory patterns in children with asthma. Several rationales for the use of slow, deep diaphragmatic breathing have been given. The work of breathing can be decreased by slowing the respiratory rate and by decreasing the ratio of dead space ventilation to minute ventilation. Increased diaphragmatic excursion also improves regional ventilation to the lower lobes in persons with architecturally normal lungs.[24] Because many small areas of atelectasis are present in the lower lobes, diaphragmatic breathing to improve lower lobe ventilation may be beneficial in asthma.

As a result of greatly increased residual volume and decreased expiratory reserve volume, the child with asthma often develops a shallow, rapid respiratory pattern that uses the accessory muscle of inspiration. Expiratory obstruction may cause expiration, which is usually passive, to become active through abdominal muscle and internal intercostal contraction. The therapist should teach the child to decrease use of the accessory muscles once the residual volume diminishes and expiratory flow improves. Continued use of this abnormal pattern of breathing is energy-depleting and inappropriate when an improvement in symptoms occurs. Jacobson's relaxation techniques have been used to decrease accessory and abdominal muscle use while increasing diaphragmatic excursion.[68] Relaxation techniques have also been advocated to reduce the anxiety and physical stress associated with an episode of asthma. Many anecdotal and verbal reports lend subjective support to the benefits of relaxation techniques in patients with asthma, but controlled studies are lacking. The effects of deep inspiratory and expiratory efforts in asthmatic patients was reported by Gayrard and associates, who found that deep, slow inspiration from functional residual capacity to total lung capacity yielded an immediate increase of 71% in airway resistance.[69] A similar, but weaker, response occurred with deep expiration. The patient's efforts toward deep, slow breathing must, therefore, be initiated carefully because a maximal effort can result in decreased airway function.[69] Nasal breathing, which warms and humidifies inspired air, has been advocated for patients with asthma who show exercise-induced bronchospasm.[70] Based on the role of heat exchange within the airways, warmed humidified air may provide an easy, cost-free method of reducing the bronchospasm that follows stressful exercise in children with asthma.[71]

Physical rehabilitation to improve endurance, work capacity, and strength are major goals in the long-term management of asthmatic children. Children with chronic asthma are often less physically fit than their normal peers. Exercise-induced bronchospasm may preclude a child with asthma from participating in vigorous exercise and the child may, therefore, be unable to respond to physical demands.[72] Appropriate medication before vigorous exercise may attenuate the bronchospastic response and the child can derive both the enjoyment and benefits of exercise. A formal physical training program should be preceded by qualitative or, preferably, quantitative evaluation of the child's response to strenuous exercise. The initial evaluation determines the level of exercise needed to improve strength and endurance and is a baseline against which the results of subsequent studies can be compared to determine improvement or deterioration. Among the more commonly used methods of training are free running, treadmill running, bicycle ergometry, and swimming.

Two controlled studies of swimming training in children with asthma showed similar results. Sly and associates assigned children to either a treatment group or a control group.[73] The treatment group participated in a swimming program for 2 hours three times a week for 13 weeks. Although no changes were recorded in pulmonary function or basic personality traits, a marked decrease in wheezing days was noted in the treatment group.

The mean number of days of wheezing for the treatment group was 31.3 during the 13 weeks before the training program; this figure declined to 5.7 days of wheezing during the swimming program. A similar control group of asthmatic children had a mean of 10.1 and 13.2 days wheezing, respectively, before and during the 3-week control period.[73]

Fitch and associates conducted a study of the results obtained with a 5-month swimming program in 46 asthmatic children compared to a control group of 10 children.[74] Included in the testing parameters were asthma score (based on wheeze, cough, and sputum), physical work capacity at a heart rate of 170, drug score (based on the amount of medication), FEV_1 levels, and response to an exercise challenge on a treadmill. A marked improvement in asthma score, drug score, and physical work capacity followed the training period. A concomitant improvement in posture was noted. No change was reported in FEV_1 or the severity of exercise-induced asthma. The authors concluded that swimming is an eminently effective method of physical training in asthmatic children.[74] Other aspects of physical therapy management for asthmatic children in terms of posture improvement and shoulder girdle and chest wall mobility exercises have been well described.[52,54,66]

Cochrane and Clarke recently reported the results of a 3-month medically supervised indoor training study of 36 patients with asthma, aged 16 to 40 years.[75] Although the age range largely exceeds childhood, the results are worth discussing. Training included an optimal duration and frequency of 30 minutes three times per week, with the target heart rate at 75% predicted maximum. The training sessions were varied to include cycling, jogging, and aerobics. Each session was preceded by a warm-up and followed by a cool-down, including light calisthenics and stretching. Changes in physiological parameters were compared to those in nontraining control group of patients with asthma. There were numerous improvements noted in cardiovascular, respiratory, and metabolic function in the training group, but not in the control group. Breathlessness was reduced during work levels corresponding to many activities of daily living (ADLs). There was no change in disease severity between the groups. There can be little doubt of the potential for physical training in individuals with asthma, but strong motivation and good compliance are important factors for the success of an exercise program for children with asthma.[75]

In addition to generalized physical training, a recent double-blind study showed that specific inspiratory muscle training over a 6-month period improved inspiratory muscle strength and decreased asthma symptoms, related hospitalizations, emergency room contacts, absence from school, and medication consumption.[76]

Cystic Fibrosis

Medical Information

CF is the most common lethal genetic disorder affecting white people. It is estimated to occur in 1 of every 1600 to 2000 births, and has a carrier rate of approximately 1 in 20 persons. CF is a generalized disorder of the exocrine glands, which, in its fully manifested state, produces high sweat electrolyte concentrations, pancreatic enzyme deficiency, and chronic suppurative pulmonary disease. The clinical presentation of CF varies, but usually includes combinations of productive cough, abnormally frequent and large stools, failure to thrive, recurrent pneumonias, rectal prolapse, nasal polyposis, and clubbing of the digits. Because of its variable presentation, CF is often misdiagnosed as asthma, allergy, celiac disease, and chronic diarrhea. The well-informed health professional should consider CF when any of these symptoms are encountered.

The gene for CF, inherited in a Mendelian recessive pattern, was recently identified on the long arm of chromosome 7.[77,78] In addition, the major mutation responsible for CF has been defined, leading to improved and more accurate testing and counseling.[79] When two carriers have a child, there is a 25% chance that the child will have CF, a 50% chance that the child is a carrier of the gene, and a 25% chance that the child will be completely free from the CF gene. Testing for the carrier or heterozygous state is now possible, as is prenatal testing. However, because of numerous factors, neither of these approaches has become standard procedure.

The incidence in white people has been mentioned. Although CF is much less common in the black population, it occurs in 1 in 17,000 births among African-Americans.[1] Cystic fibrosis is rare in the oriental population. The course of the disease, like its presentation, is variable. Although severe lung and gastrointestinal disease can be fatal for children with CF, survival rates have improved steadily over the last 25 years. For example, approximately 40% of individuals with CF survive to an age of 30 years and beyond.[1] Reports of large numbers of adults with CF have been published in several journals.[80–82]

The pulmonary disease associated with CF causes the greatest mortality. Pulmonary involvement in CF begins with the production and retention of thick, viscid secretions within the bronchioles. These secretions provide a medium in which bacterial pathogens flourish. The resultant infections produce more secretions and additional obstruction, and a vicious cycle is begun. The earliest pathologic changes may be reversed with aggressive treatment. With continued reinfection, bronchiolitis and bronchitis progress to bronchiolectasis and bronchiectasis. The latter two processes, which are irreversible, destroy elements within the walls of the airways.

In addition to these destructive processes, hyperplasia of mucus-secreting glands and cells occur within the lungs. Large quantities of thick, purulent mucus are produced, causing the airway obstruction that is common in CF. If the obstruction is partial, a ball-valve process may result in hyperaeration of the lung distal to the obstruction. Complete airway obstruction results in absorption atelectasis distal to the obstruction. Small areas of hyperaeration and atelectasis often exist in adjacent areas, and present a honeycomb pattern on a chest roentgenogram. The rapidity of pulmonary progression and success of treatment play major roles in determining the survival of a child with CF.

Pulmonary complications often include lobar atelectasis, bronchiectasis, pneumothorax, hemoptysis, pulmonary hypertension, and cor pulmonale. These problems have been discussed at length by others.[83–85]

Medical Management

Management of CF is directed toward decreasing airway obstruction and pulmonary infection, replacing pancreatic enzymes to help reverse the nutritional deficiency, and providing appropriate psychosocial and emotional support to the child and family. Control of pulmonary infection is the major therapeutic objective. Sputum culture and sensitivity tests to identify pathogens and determine appropriate antimicrobial drugs enable the physician to plan a rational course of medications. The most common bacteria causing infections in patients with CF are *Staphylococcus aureus* and *Pseudomonas aeruginosa*. Antimicrobial agents may be given orally or parenterally. There is no oral preparation available to combat the Pseudomonas species, so intravenous administration of the anti-pseudomonas drugs is necessary.

Reduction of airway obstruction is the most time-consuming aspect of comprehensive treatment for CF. Reduction of sputum viscosity by aerosolized or oral medications is thought to enhance physical efforts to loosen and drain mucus from the airways. Physical therapy is a major part of the care.

Replacement of pancreatic enzymes is essential for the 85% of patients with pancreatic dysfunction. Traditionally the recommended diet for patients with CF has included high-protein, high-carbohydrate, and low-fat foods. With more effective pancreatic preparations, many children have liberalized their intake of fat. Despite apparent control of pancreatic insufficiency with enzymes, patients with CF may need up to 50% more calories than their age- and weight-matched peers. Continually underweight children, or those who experience weight loss with a progression of disease, may benefit from commercial dietary supplements. Supplements must be chosen carefully and added to the diet. A nutritionist's counseling is necessary.

Psychosocial and emotional support for patients with CF and their families is the responsibility of all professionals who work with this population. Issues that must be confronted include chronic life-shortening illness, genetic disease, cost of drugs and care, time-consuming treatments, death of a child, denial, and guilt. Other issues emerge as patients reach adulthood: marriage, occupations, and dependence on others for treatment. A counselor or social worker plays a major role on the CF team, and several publications have addressed the psychosocial aspects of the management of CF.[86,87]

A nationwide network of centers is dedicated to the treatment of CF. These centers are sponsored by the Cystic Fibrosis Foundation (CFF) and can reach almost every population center in the United States. The CFF sponsors research projects, fellowships, conferences, fund raising, and other activities in its mandated task of providing the best care for children and adults with CF.

Physical Therapy Evaluation

Physical therapy evaluation for the child with CF is similar to the evaluation for the other disorders discussed in this chapter. Emphasis in CF must be placed on the obstruction by bronchial secretion that causes the numerous pulmonary problems and complications.

Auscultation for secretions must be done with the expectation of finding many areas with sonorous wheezes, harsh breath sounds, and crackles (all abnormal breath sounds). The sounds may not change for several days in a patient with advanced disease, and auscultation on an intermittent, rather than daily, basis may be helpful.

A determination of the child's ability to cough and raise secretions is crucial. An acutely ill child with CF who cannot cough effectively risks further deterioration in airway function. The roentgenogram is useful in identifying specific pockets or patches of advanced destruction of the lung. Many therapists believe that the three-dimensional view of the lungs afforded by posteroanterior and lateral chest films provides specific information to help direct treatment.

Qualitative and quantitative evaluation of exercise tolerance provides a basis for planning an exercise reconditioning program at a level appropriate to the child's tolerance. An evaluation of the child's muscular pattern of breathing may be accomplished by observation or by palpation.

Mobility of the chest wall should be determined for several reasons. A noncompliant thorax increases the work of breathing. Children with CF often have hyperinflated lungs, and so the chest wall may appear barrelled and fixed. If chest wall changes occur, the child may have difficulty developing the necessary pressures and flow rates to cough effectively or to increase ventilation during physical stress. Thoracic index, thoracic girth, and rib motion should be determined during full inspiration and full expiration.

Evaluation of the child's posture is essential to identify early changes caused by the hyperaeration and chronic coughing that accompany CF (Fig. 8-12). The thorax assumes a barrel-shape, with an increase in the normal thoracic kyphosis. Scapular protraction also becomes evident. With the anatomic changes in the upper thorax that accompany hyperaeration, range of motion of the shoulder girdle must be measured. A comprehensive evaluation should include those postural items that may affect both function and cosmesis.

Physical Therapy Management

Conventional Physical Therapy

The major role of physical therapy for the child with CF is in the aggressive use of bronchial drainage, chest percussion, vibration, and suctioning (if necessary). Treatment should be generalized because mucus is produced in most areas of the lungs. If specific segments have more advanced disease or exhibit increased production of mucus, emphasis

A   B   C

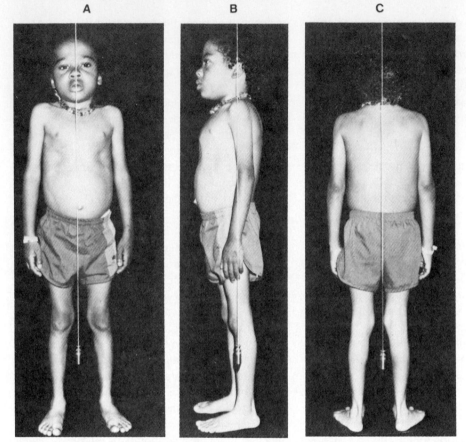

Figure 8-12. *Postural abnormalities in a child with cystic fibrosis. A. Anterior view. Notice that the shoulders are held high, especially on the right. This posture appears to offer better mechanical advantage to the accessory muscles for breathing. The lower ribs are flared, and the thorax appears barreled and elongated because of the hyperinflation of the lungs. A full postural evaluation might reveal other, less obvious abnormalities. B. Lateral view. The thoracic kyphosis and barreled chest seen here are common findings in children with obstructive pulmonary disease and hyperinflation of the lungs. C. Posterior view. The shoulders appear high with a protraction of the scapulae. Notice the enlargement of the thorax in relation to the rest of this patient's body. Pronated feet are also noticeable. (Reproduced by permission from Irwin S, Tecklin JS. Cardiopulmonary Physical Therapy. St. Louis: CV Mosby; 1985.)*

for treatment should center on these segments. Early studies of conventional bronchial drainage, percussion, and vibration in CF have helped to document their efficacy. Lorin and Denning, for instance have demonstrated that twice the amount of sputum per cough and per treatment was obtained when a combined treatment regimen of gravity drainage, percussion, and vibration was compared with cough alone.[88] Tecklin and Holsclaw have documented improvement in forced vital capacity and peak expiratory flow rate after bronchial drainage, percussion, and vibration in 26 children with CF.[89] Weller and colleagues have also reported increased peak expiratory flow rates after conventional treatment.[90] Feldman and associates have demonstrated remarkable improvement in flow rates at low lung volumes 45 minutes after treatment in nine patients with CF.[91] In Feldman's study, the isovolume flow rate near 25% of forced vital capacity increased from baseline by 70% 45 minutes after treatment.[91] These changes in small airway flow rates are consistent with the results of Motoyama.[92]

Desmond and co-workers employed a crossover design to determine whether pulmonary function decreased over a 3-week period during which physical therapy was withheld. There was a statistically significant decrease in flow rates that was reflective of small airway function, forced expiratory flow ($FEF_{25\%-75\%}$) and Vmax60 (total lung capacity [TLC]), each of which declined by 20% after 3 weeks of no therapy. These values returned to their prior levels shortly after resumption of physical therapy.[93]

Forced Expiratory Technique

A number of studies compared FET to conventional therapy. The authors of the studies postulated that if FET and conventional therapy were similar in effect, then FET should be recommended because of its easier use by the patient with no requirement for a second individual. Several studies were performed by the group at Brompton Hospital in London who first described and strongly advocated FET. Although those studies support the use of FET, the weak or absent statistical analyses and potential for bias among the therapists who collected the data raise questions about their validity.[94-97] Verboon and associates found no difference in pulmonary function in eight subjects treated with either FET and postural drainage or FET alone. When the results of one subject who produced little sputum were deleted, 24-hour sputum collection showed a significant difference supporting the conventional technique of postural drainage.[98] Although FET appears promising, a well-controlled study with appropriate subjects, design, and statistical analysis must be published in a refereed journal for true acceptance of this technique.

Positive Expiratory Pressure Mask

The PEP mask, described earlier in the chapter, may hold the greatest promise in terms of independent removal of excess secretions in children with CF. Several studies have found that the efficacy of the PEP mask, when used in conjunction with FET, was superior to, or at least equal to, that of conventional bronchial hygiene measures, including positioning, manual techniques, and coughing.[99-102] One study found conventional treatment to be superior, but that study used statistical analysis only for within-group changes, rather than between-group changes.[103] Only one study claimed to have found FET superior to PEP and conventional treatment. Not surprisingly, that study was reported by the Brompton group, whose possible bias for the FET has already been noted.[23]

Directed Coughing

At least three studies have examined the efficacy of directed coughing for secretion removal in CF. Each study compared coughing alone with conventional therapy and found that the benefits derived did not differ among the approaches.[104-106] The study by DeBoeck and Zinman, however, found that flows at low lung volume, which are usually indicative of small airway function, were significantly improved with conventional physical therapy.[104]

Modifications of usual treatment procedures are often necessary for acutely ill children or for those with certain complications. In a patient with major hemoptysis, chest percussion and vibration should be discontinued temporarily because the physical maneuvers may dislodge a blood clot and prolong the bleeding. FET and PEP may be useful. If the area of hemoptysis can be identified, the child should be positioned to drain the accumulated blood. Percussion and vibration may be reinstituted gradually within 24 to 48 hours if the bleeding abates.

Pneumothorax is often a complication of CF and is commonly treated with an intrapleural chest tube with suction. Gravity drainage is appropriate, although percussion and vibration at the site of tube insertion are contraindicated. FET, PEP, and directed coughing may enable the continued treatment of excessive secretion. Bronchial hygiene treatment for the noninvolved thorax should be continued.[107]

With far advanced destruction of the lung, the child at the final stage of disease will not tolerate drainage positions. These patients may be treated in any position of comfort, with vibration for all areas of the lungs, and this can then be followed by FET or PEP. Vibration during coughing and manual support of the chest will enhance the expulsive coughing effort in the terminal stage of CF. Improvement of diaphragmatic excursion, decreased use of accessory muscles, and relaxation are often advocated for children with CF. The rationale for using these measures in patients with CF is similar to that for those with asthma: decreased work of breathing, decreased dead space ventilation, and reduced anxiety. The efficacy of these treatments has not, however, been tested by appropriate clinical trials.

Keens and associates attempted to improve ventilatory muscle endurance, as measured by the maximal sustainable ventilatory capacity (MSVC).[27] This study documented an improvement of more than 50% in MSVC after specific ventilatory muscle training in children with CF. Additionally, a group of seven children at a summer camp who underwent a general physical activity program also showed more than a 50% improvement in MSVC. Once the ventilatory exercise or physical activity ceased, a decrease in MSVC was noted. Physical conditioning and training programs will, therefore, affect specific ventilatory muscle endurance.[27]

Formal and informal methods of physical conditioning are used for patients with CF. Cropp and associates showed that, in children with CF (except for those with severe lung disease), the cardiovascular response was normal during incremental exercise testing on a cycle ergometer.[108] The ventilatory response to exercise was abnormal because patients with CF and decreased pulmonary function

Display 8-1.
Case Study

H.E., a 14-year-old white boy with a history of Duchenne's muscular dystrophy diagnosed at 4 years of age, was referred for pulmonary physical therapy evaluation. At the time of his referral, a functional evaluation revealed that H.E. could ambulate 25 feet in 20 seconds, could roll from a prone to a supine position and back to a prone position, and had adequate sitting balance. He was unable to run, ascend or descend stairs, rise from the floor or from a chair, sit up from a supine position, or assume a posture on all fours. A modified manual muscle examination indicated strength that was graded from "poor" to "absent" for all isolated muscle groups with the exception of wrist extensors, which were graded as "fair" to "good." H.E. could function from an electric wheelchair, and he could ambulate slowly using a walker with supervision.

Pulmonary physical therapy evaluation included an assessment of H.E.'s breathing pattern, respiratory muscle strength, chest wall mobility, coughing ability, and oral motor functions. The results of these assessments are presented in Table 8-2.

In addition to the therapeutic regimen outlined in Table 8-2, H.E.'s parents were instructed in the techniques of bronchial drainage, chest percussion, vibration, and shaking. Although retention of secretions had not been a problem, the potentially severe effects of a respiratory tract infection were explained. The parents were instructed to begin bronchial hygiene procedures at the first sign of an infection of the respiratory tract.

increased their ventilation more than did normal controls at all levels of stress. This relative increase in minute ventilation was necessary to overcome

Table 8-2. *Physical Therapy Plan for H. E.*

Problem	Initial Evaluation	Treatment Plan

Breathing pattern
  Resting
  Exertion
	Diaphragmatic and intercostal (R > L)
	diaphragmatic, intercostal, accessory (R > L)
		Instruction in diaphragmatic breathing and lateral costal expansion with emphasis on unilateral increased expansion for (L) hemithorax

Respiratory muscle strength
  Inspiratory
  Expiratory
	Inspiratory capacity = 45% of predicted
	maximum inspiratory pressure = 60% of predicted
	vital capacity = 49% of predicted
	maximum expiratory pressure = 35% of predicted
		Instruction in the use of two incentive spirometers: one flow calibrated to be used in conjunction with diaphragmatic and lateral costal breathing. Blow bottle instruction for use as an expiratory exerciser

Chest wall mobility	1 inch expansion on inspiration (32–33 inches); full passive motion at glenohumeral joint	Maintain ROM through continued exercise program managed by parents

Coughing
  Inspiration
  Glottic closure
  Expiratory force
	Shallow
	Adequate
	Weak
		Functional–weak
		Incentive spirometry (noted above)
		Blow bottles and practice at forced expiratory maneuvers

Swallowing
  Solids
  Semisolids
	Adequate
	Adequate	

the airway obstructive element of the disease. Children with severe disease had increased arterial levels of carbon dioxide, indicating an inability to increase ventilation sufficiently. These severely involved children also experienced desaturation of arterial oxygen during exercise.[108]

The relevance of these findings is that physical training and reconditioning, in a formal or informal program, is safe and beneficial in all patients except those with severe lung disease. Even those with severe disease have been shown to benefit from an exercise program if supplemental oxygen is provided. Marcus and colleagues demonstrated that patients with advanced CF who exercised with an FIO_2 of 30% worked longer, had higher maximal oxygen consumption, and experienced less oxygen desaturation than while exercising at room air.[109] Treadmill walking or running, cycle ergometer training, free running or walking, and strengthening exercises are useful methods of increasing cardiovascular fitness, endurance, and general muscular strength. Although several investigators have ex-

amined the immediate effects of exercise on children with CF, the effects of a long-term training program have yet to be evaluated.

Summary

This chapter has attempted to provide a summary of unique characteristics of lung disease in children, growth and development of the respiratory system, and the reasons why children and infants are predisposed to acute respiratory failure. Assessment of the child with pulmonary disease and treatments aimed at reducing the severity of pulmonary disease in infants and children have been reviewed. Four major respiratory disorders have been described, along with a discussion of appropriate physical therapy assessment and management. Published evidence for the physical therapy methods has been reviewed. Physical therapy for children with lung disease has been shown to be efficacious depending upon the treatment employed and the problems addressed.

References

1. Lemen RJ, Parcel GS, Loughlin G, et al. Pediatric lung diseases. *Chest.* 1992;102(suppl):232S–242S.
2. Taylor WP, Newacheck PW. Impact of childhood asthma on health. *Pediatrics.* 1992;90:657–662.
3. *Vital Statistics of the United States, 1970.* Vol 2. Mortality, Part A. Rockville, MD: National Center for Health Statistics; 1974.
4. Waring WW. Respiratory diseases in children: An overview. *Respir Care.* 1978;20:1138–1145.
5. Avery ME: Normal and abnormal respiration in children. Presented at the 37th Ross Conference on Pediatric Research; 1961.
6. Dunhill MS. Quantitative observations on the anatomy of chronic non-specific lung disease. *Med Thorac.* 1965;22:261.
7. Holsclaw DS. Pediatric pulmonary disease: An overview. *Pediatr Ann.* 1977;6:438–443.
8. Woolcock AJ. Asthma—What are the important experiments? *Am Rev Respir Dis.* 1988;138:730–744.
9. Charnock EL, Doershuk CF. Developmental aspects of the human lung. *Pediatr Clin North Am.* 1973;20:275–292.
10. Avery ME. Hyaline membrane disease. *Am Rev Respir Dis.* 1975;111:657–688.
11. Polgar G, Weng TR. The functional development of the respiratory system. *Am Rev Respir Dis.* 1979; 120:625–695.
12. Downes JJ, Fulgencio T, Raphaely RC. Acute respiratory failure in infants and children. *Pediatr Clin North Am.* 1972;19:423–445.
13. Holsclaw DS. Early recognition of acute respiratory failure in children. *Pediatr Ann.* 1977; 6:467–475.
14. Haskins R, Lotch J. Day care and illness: Evidence, costs, and public policy. *Pediatrics.* 1986;77 (suppl):951–956.
15. Keens TG, Ianuzzo CO. Development of fatigue-resistant muscle fibers in human ventilatory muscles. *Am Rev Respir Dis.* 1979;119:139–141.
16. Pagliara AS, Karl IE, Haymond M, Kipnis DM. Hypoglycemia in infancy and childhood. *J Pediatr.* 1973;82:365–379.
17. Crane L. Physical therapy for the neonate with respiratory disease. In: Irwin S, Tecklin JS, eds. *Cardiopulmonary Physical Therapy.* St. Louis: CV Mosby; 1985.
18. DeCesare J. Physical therapy for the child with respiratory dysfunction. In: Irwin S, Tecklin JS, eds. *Cardiopulmonary Physical Therapy.* St. Louis: CV Mosby; 1985.
19. Dab I, Alexander F. Evaluation of a particular bronchial drainage procedure called autogenic drainage. In: Baran D, Van Bogaert E, eds. *Chest Physical Therapy in Cystic Fibrosis and Chronic Obstructive Pulmonary Disease.* Ghent, Belgium: European Press; 1977;185–187.
20. Dab I, Alexander F. The mechanism of autogenic drainage studied with flow volume curves. *Monogr Paediat.* 1979;10:50–53.
21. Pryor JA, Webber BA, Hodson ME, Batten JC. Evaluation of the forced expiratory technique as an adjunct to postural drainage in treatment of cystic fibrosis. *Br Med J.* 1979;2:417–418.
22. Partridge C, Pryor J, Webber B. Characteristics of the forced expiratory technique. *Physiotherapy.* 1989;75:193–194.
23. Hofmyer JL, Webber BA, Hodson ME. Evaluation of positive expiratory pressure as an adjunct to chest physiotherapy in the treatment of cystic fibrosis. *Thorax* 1986;41:951–954.
24. Shearer MO, Banks JM, Silva G, Sackner MA. Lung ventilation during diaphragmatic breathing. *Phys Ther* 1972;52:139–147.
25. Wetzel J, Lunsford BR, Peterson MJ, Alvarez SE. Respiratory rehabilitation of the patient with spinal cord injury. In: Irwin S, Tecklin JS, eds. *Cardiopulmonary Physical Therapy,* St Louis: CV Mosby; 1985:406–407.
26. Darbee J, Cerny F. Exercise testing and exercise conditioning for children with lung dysfunction. In: Irwin S, Tecklin JS, eds. *Cardiopulmonary Physical Therapy,* 2nd ed. St. Louis: CV Mosby; 1990:468.
27. Keens TG, Krastins IRB, Wannamaker EM, et al. Ventilatory muscle endurance training in normal subjects and patients with cystic fibrosis. *Am Rev Respir Dis.* 1977;116:853–860.
28. Orenstein D, Franklin BA, Doershuk CF, et al. Ex-

ercise conditioning and cardiopulmonary fitness in cystic fibrosis. *Chest.* 1981; 80:392.

29. Laennec RTH; Forbes J, trans. *Diseases of the Chest.* 4th ed. London: 1819.

30. Atelectasis. In: Schaffer AT, Avery ME, eds. *Diseases of the Newborn.* 4th ed. Philadelphia: WB Saunders; 1977:122–126.

31. Nemir RL. Atelectasis. In: Kendig EL, Chernick V, eds. *Disorders of the Respiratory Tract in Children.* 3rd ed. Philadelphia: WB Saunders; 1977.

32. Thoren L. Postoperative pulmonary complications: Observations on their prevention by means of physiotherapy. *Acta Chir Scand.* 1954;107:193–205.

33. Stein M, Cassara EL. Preoperative pulmonary evaluation and therapy for surgery patients. *J Am Med Assoc.* 1970;211:787–790.

34. Bartlett RH, Gazzinga AB, Graghty JR. Respiratory maneuvers to prevent postoperative complications. *J Am Med Assoc.* 1973;224:1017–1021.

35. Hymes AC, Yonehiro EG, Raab DE, et al. Electrical surface stimulation for treatment and prevention of ileus and atelectasis. *Surg Forum.* 1974;25:222–224.

36. Finer MN, Moriartey RR, Boyd J, et al. Postextubation atelectasis. A retrospective review and a prospective controlled study. *J Pediatr.* 1979;94:110–113.

37. Burrington JD, Cotton EK. Removal of foreign bodies from the tracheobronchial tree. *J Pediatr Surg.* 1972;7:119–122.

38. Tecklin JS, Holsclaw DS. Bronchial drainage with aerosol medication in cystic fibrosis. *Phys Ther* 1976;56:999–1003.

39. Mallory GB, Stillwell PC. The ventilator-dependent child: Issues in diagnosis and management. *Arch Phys Med Rehabil* 1991;72:43–55.

40. Polgar G, Promadhat V. *Pulmonary Function Testing in Children.* Philadelphia: WB Saunders; 1971.

41. Dereene JP, Macklem PT, Roussos CH. The respiratory muscles: Mechanics, control, and pathophysiology. Part III. *Am Rev Respir Dis.* 1978;118:581–601.

42. Black LF, Hyatt RE. Maximal respiratory pressures: Normal values and relationship to age and sex. *Am Rev Respir Dis.* 1969;99:696–702.

43. Braun NMT, Rochester DF. Muscular weakness and respiratory failure. *Am Rev Respir Dis.* 1979; 119:123–125.

44. Williams HE. Inhalation pneumonia. *Aust Paediatr J.* 1973;9:279–285.

45. Farber S. *Neurorehabilitation: A Multisensory Approach.* Philadelphia: WB Saunders; 1982.

46. Merrick J, Axen K. Inspiratory muscle function following abdominal weight exercises in healthy subject. *Phys Ther.* 1981;61:651–656.

47. Gross D, Riley E, Grassino A, et al. Influence of resistive training on respiratory muscle strength and endurance in quadriplegia (abstract). *Am Rev Respir Dis.* 1978;117(4):343.

48. Pontoppidan H. Mechanical aids to lung expansion in non-intubated surgical patients. *Am Rev Respir Dis.* 1980;122(5):109–119.

49. Leith DL, Bradley M. Ventilatory muscle strength and endurance training. *J Appl Physiol.* 1976; 41:508–516.

50. Siegel IM. Pulmonary problems in Duchenne muscular dystrophy: Diagnosis, prophylaxis, and treatment. *Phys Ther.* 1975;55:160.

51. Roth FG. Effects of respiratory exercises on the vital capacity and forced expiratory volume in children with cerebral palsy. *Phys Ther.* 1978;58:421–425.

52. Watts N. Improvement of breathing patterns. *Phys Ther.* 1968;48:563–576.

53. Adkins H. Improvement of breathing ability in children with respiratory muscle paralysis. *Phys Ther.* 1968;48:577–581.

54. Warren A. Mobilization of the chest wall. *Phys Ther.* 1968;48:582–585.

55. Bergofsky EH. Respiratory failure in disorders of the thoracic cage. *Am Rev Respir Dis.* 1979; 119:643–669.

56. National Heart, Lung and Blood Institute National Asthma Education Program Expert Panel Report. *Guidelines for the Diagnosis and Management of Asthma.* Bethesda: NHLBI; 1991.

57. Reed CE. Basic mechanism of asthma: Role of inflammation. *Chest.* 1988;94:175–177.

58. *National Center for Health Statistics Annual Summary of Vital Statistics.* Hyattsville, MD: US Dept of Health and Human Services; 1970–1986.

59. Prograis LJ, Zunich KM. NIAID Programs for Asthma Research, Education, and Outreach. *Chest.* 1992;101(suppl):357S.

60. Godfrey S. Childhood asthma. In: Clark TJH, Godfrey S, eds: *Asthma.* Philadelphia: WB Saunders; 1979.

61. Weiss KB, Gergen PJ, Crain EF. Inner-city asthma: The epidemiology of an emerging US public health concern. *Chest.* 1992;101(suppl):362S–367S.

62. Emergency room treatment of asthma. *Pediatr Ann.* 1977;6:490–492.

63. Middleton E. The biochemical basis for the modulation of allergic reactions by drugs. *Pediatr Clin North Am.* 1975;22:111–119.

64. Wood DW, Downes JJ, Lecks HI. A clinical scoring system for the diagnosis of respiratory failure in childhood status asthmaticus. *Am J Dis Child.* 1972; 123:227–228.

65. Lunsford BR. Clinical indicators of endurance. *Phys Ther.* 1978;58:704–709.

66. Kendall HO, Boynton DA. *Posture and pain.* Baltimore: Williams and Wilkins, 1952.

67. Huber AL, Eggleston PA, Morgan J. Effect of chest physiotherapy on asthmatic children (abstract). *J Allergy Clin Immunol.* 1974;53:2.

68. Rathbone JL. *Relaxation.* Philadelphia: Lea & Febiger; 1969.

69. Gayrard P, Orehek J, Grimand C, Charpin J. Bronchoconstrictor effects of a deep inspiration in patients with asthma. *Am Rev Respir Dis.* 1975; 111:433–439.

70. Shturman-Ellison R, Zeballos RJ, Buckley JM, Sourada JF. The beneficial effect of nasal breathing on exercise-induced bronchoconstriction. *Am Rev Respir Dis.* 1978;118:65–73.

71. Deal EC, McFadden ER, Ingram RH, et al. Role of respiratory heat exchange in production of exercise-induced asthma. *J Appl Physiol.* 1979;46:467–475.

72. Cropp GJA. Exercise-induced asthma. In: Middleton E, ed. *Allergy: Principles and Practice.* St Louis: CV Mosby; 1978.

73. Sly RM, Harper RT, Rosselot I. The effect of physical conditioning upon asthmatic children. *Ann Allerg.* 1972;30:86–94.

74. Fitch KD, Morton AR, Blanksby BA. Effects of swimming training on children with asthma. *Arch Dis Child.* 1976;51:190–194.

75. Cochrane LM, Clarke CJ. Benefits and problems of a physical training programme for asthmatic patients. *Thorax.* 1990;45:345–351.

76. Weiner P, Azgad Y, Ganam R, et al. Inspiratory muscle training in patients with bronchial asthma. *Chest.* 1992;102:1357–1361.

77. Rommens JM, Iannuzzi MC, Kerem B, et al. Identification of the cystic fibrosis gene: Chromosome walking and jumping. *Science.* 1989;245:1059–1065.

78. Riordan JR, Rommens JM, Kerem B, et al. Identifi-cation of the cystic fibrosis gene: Cloning and characterization of complementary DNA. *Science.* 1989;245:1066–1073.

79. Kerem B, Rommens JM, Buchanan J, et al. Identification of the cystic fibrosis gene: Genetic analysis. *Science.* 1989;245:1073–1080.

80. Shwachman H, Kowalski M, Khaw KT. Cystic fibrosis: A new outlook. *Medicine* 1977;56:129–149.

81. Holsclaw DS, Kovatch A. A clinical profile of adults with cystic fibrosis. *CF Club Abstr* 1977; 18:53.

82. diSant'Agnese PA, Davis PB. Cystic fibrosis in adults. *Am J Med.* 1979;66:121–132.

83. Holsclaw DS. Common pulmonary complications of cystic fibrosis. *Clin Pediatr.* 1970;9:346–355.

84. Goldring RM, Fishman AP, Turino GM, et al. Pulmonary hypertension and cor pulmonale in cystic fibrosis of the pancreas. *J Pediatr.* 1964;65:501–524.

85. Holsclaw DS, Grand RJ, Shwachman H. Massive hemoptysis in cystic fibrosis. *J Pediatr.* 1973; 76:829–838.

86. Gayton WF, Friedman SB. Psychosocial aspects of cystic fibrosis: A review of the literature. *Am J Dis Child.* 1973;126:856–859.

87. McCollum AT, Gibson LE. Family adaptation to the child with cystic fibrosis. *J Pediatr.* 1970; 77:571–578.

88. Lorin MI, Denning CR. Evaluation of postural drainage by measurement of sputum volume and consistency. *Am J Phys Med.* 1971;50:215–219.

89. Tecklin JS, Holsclaw DS. Evaluation of bronchial drainage in patients with cystic fibrosis. *Phys Ther.* 1975;55:1081–1084.

90. Weller PH, Bush E, Preece MA, et al. The short-term effects of chest physiotherapy on lung function tests in children with cystic fibrosis. *Monogr Paediatr.* 1979;10:58–59.

91. Feldman J, Traver GA, Taussig LM. Maximal expiratory flows after postural drainage. *Am Rev Respir Dis.* 1979;119:239–245.

92. Motoyama EK. Lower airway obstruction. In: Mangos JA, Talamo RD, ed: *Fundamental Problems of Cystic Fibrosis and Related Diseases.* New York: Intercontinental Medical Book Corp; 1973.

93. Desmond KF, Schwenk F, Thomas E, et al. Immediate and long-term effects of chest physiotherapy in patients with cystic fibrosis. *J Pediatr.* 1983; 103:538–542.

94. Pryor JA, Webber BA. An evaluation of the forced

expiratory technique as an adjunct to postural drainage. *Physiotherapy.* 1979;65:304–307.

95. Sutton PP, Parker RA, Webber BA, et al. Assessment of the forced expiratory technique, postural drainage, and directed coughing in chest physiotherapy. *Eur J Respir Dis.* 1983;64:62–68.

96. Webber BA, Hofmyer JR, Morgan MDL, et al. Effects of postural drainage incorporating the FET on pulmonary function in cystic fibrosis. *Br J Dis Chest.* 1986;80:353–359.

97. Partridge C, Pryor J, Webber B. Characteristics of the forced expiration technique. *Physiotherapy.* 1989;75:193–194.

98. Verboon JML, Bakker W, Sterk PJ. The value of forced expiration technique with and without postural drainage in adults with cystic fibrosis. *Eur J Respir Dis.* 1986;69:169–174.

99. Falk M, Kelstrup M, Andersen JB, et al. Improvement in the ketchup bottle method with positive expiratory pressure, PEP, in cystic fibrosis. *Eur J Respir Dis.* 1984;65:424–432.

100. Tyrell JC, Hiller EJ, Martin J. Face mask physiotherapy in cystic fibrosis. *Arch Dis Child.* 1986;61:598–600.

101. Tonnesen P, Stovring S. Positive expiratory pressure (PEP) as lung physiotherapy in cystic fibrosis: A pilot study. *Eur J Respir Dis.* 1984;65:419–422.

102. Oberwaldner B, Evans JC, Zach MS. Forced expirations against a variable resistance: A new chest physiotherapy method in cystic fibrosis. *Pediatr Pulmon.* 1986;2:358–367.

103. Van Asperen PP, Jackson L, Hennessey P, et al. Comparison of a positive expiratory pressure (PEP) mask with postural drainage in patients with cystic fibrosis. *Aust Paediatr J.* 1987;23:283–284.

104. DeBoeck C, Zinman R. Cough versus chest physiotherapy: A comparison of the acute effects on pulmonary function in patients with cystic fibrosis. *Am Rev Respir Dis.* 1984;129:182–184.

105. Rossman CM, Waldes R, Sampson D, et al. Effect of chest physiotherapy on the removal of mucus in patients with cystic fibrosis. *Am Rev Respir Dis.* 1982;126:131–135.

106. Bain J, Bishop J, Olinsky A. Evaluation of directed coughing in cystic fibrosis. *Br J Dis Chest.* 1988;82:138–148.

107. Tecklin JS, Holsclaw DS. Cystic fibrosis and the role of the physical therapist in its management. *Phys Ther.* 1973;53:386–393.

108. Cropp GJA, Pullano TP, Cerny FJ, Nathanson IT. Adaptation to exercise in cystic fibrosis. *CF Club Abstr.* 1979;20:32.

109. Marcus CL, Bader D, Stabile MW, et al. Supplemental oxygen and exercise performance in patients with cystic fibrosis with severe pulmonary disease. *Chest.* 1992;101:52–57.

Pediatric Physical Therapy,
second edition, edited by Jan
Stephen Tecklin. J. B. Lippincott
Company, Philadelphia © 1994.

9

Jan Stephen Tecklin

Orthopedic Disorders in Children and Their Physical Therapy Management

I would like to recognize that Donna DeMarco and Laura Boyle were authors of the chapter in the first edition of the text. I would also like to acknowledge the valuable assistance of Elizabeth Graber, M.S.P.T., in the research for this chapter revision.

Orthopedics is a challenging specialty area within pediatric rehabilitation. The term *orthopedia (orthos,* meaning straight; *paidos,* meaning child) was first used in the title of a book about childhood deformities by Nicholas Audrey in 1741.[1] This medical and surgical specialty area has grown to include infants, children, and adults with acute and chronic musculoskeletal derangements. Skeletal disorders can be traced to the earliest humans, but knowledge and treatment of orthopedic disorders is always changing and growing. Those people who work with pediatric orthopedic disorders find the challenge particularly great because they are working with a rapidly changing and growing system. Just as the physician's role in orthopedic care has increased, so too has the importance of the role of the physical therapist. Successful rehabilitation of children with orthopedic disorders requires a good working relationship among the physician, physical therapist, and other health care professionals.

Orthopedic disorders in children may occur prenatally or during the birth process, childhood, or adolescence. These problems may be congenital, acquired, acute, or chronic, and the presenting problem may not be the same as the underlying pathology.

Some common orthopedic anomalies in children are discussed in this chapter. Congenital hip dislocation, scoliosis, slipped capital femoral epiphysis, Legg-Calvé-Perthes disease, arthrogryposis multiplex congenita, osteogenesis imperfecta, tibia vara, fractures, and limb length discrepancy are discussed. Guidelines for physical therapy treatment are presented, but the specific components of treatment often vary among hospitals and referring physicians.

Physical Therapy Evaluation

When a child with a particular orthopedic disorder is referred for physical therapy, a thorough physical therapy evaluation is necessary to ensure appropriate treatment. This evaluation should include some, if not all, of the following: history, observation, range of motion (ROM) testing, manual muscle testing, sensory testing, skin evaluation, assessment of pain, general musculoskeletal assessment, orthotic examination, and analysis of gait. The specific tests and measurements depend on the disorder. The evaluation often requires two or more sessions, depending on the age of the child. Younger children have limited attention spans, and play must be included in the evaluation. One session may be needed in order to gain the child's trust. As the presence of parents or guardians may help or hinder the evaluation, therapists must use their judgment as to whether to include them. If parents are not present, they must be informed about the findings and recommendations.

History

The therapist must thoroughly review the child's medical and surgical history before initiating the physical examination. Old photographs may be useful in determining the course of a deformity. Previous surgical and medical records will help the therapist understand certain limitations in performance that may exist. An interview with the patient or parent is important, and emphasis should be placed on previous physical therapy and results, the emotional stability of the child, family interaction with the child, school performance, daily routine and schedule, and current treatment goals.

Range of Motion

Testing active and passive ROM of all extremities and the trunk is an important part of the initial evaluation. Joint ROM provides an objective method for documenting a child's progress or regression. Preoperative values for ROM are essential in order to determine postoperative treatment goals and to ascertain the effectiveness of surgery. Preoperative values are important when the surgery is done in an attempt to maintain range and prevent loss of range, rather than to increase range. Because changes in motion may be small, observation is inadequate, and classical goniometry must be done.

In similar fashion to an adult, the child, particularly one with a chronic disability, will use subtle compensatory movements at neighboring joints to the joint that is limited. Compensatory movements are often noted at the cervical spine, shoulder girdle, and pelvic girdle. The therapist must place the child carefully and properly in position and should stabilize proximally when doing goniometry in order to guard against these motions.

ROM must be frequently reevaluated because goniometric values can be affected by the child's fear, pain, spasm, or level of cooperation. Two or more sessions may be needed to complete the goniometric evaluation. In some instances, the orthopedic surgeon may believe that general anesthesia is necessary in order to accurately measure the ROM. It is very useful for the therapist to be present during this procedure in order to appreciate the difference in the passive movement of the particular joint and to do the measurement.

Manual Muscle Testing

Manual muscle testing in children can be a unique experience. Standard manual muscle testing is impossible on a young or uncooperative child. The physical therapist may need to rely solely on observational skills when the child cannot or will not cooperate. The therapist must fully understand the specific muscle activity required for specific postures and movement patterns in order to use observational skills effectively.

Accurate testing is difficult in smaller children and grading becomes subjective. Assessment of strength requires that the therapist be aware of the testing position used, proper stabilization, and substitution patterns of muscle function. The therapist must consider the child's weight and body size when considering the level of resistance. Strength can be estimated by observing muscle activity in antigravity positions and by examining the arc of motion against gravity. Movement against gravity through the full range of a particular muscle can be rated as "fair" or 3 on a scale of 1 to 5. A grade of "fair" is often considered to be a functional level as well as the antigravity level.

Careful and precise manual muscle testing can help the surgeon who is trying to decide on a particular procedure. Some surgical procedures require "good" strength of a particular muscle, rated 4 on a scale of 1 to 5. (Strength, more than a functional "fair" level, is necessary because one grade will be lost as a result of the surgery.) An example of this situation is an out-of-phase muscle transfer in which an agonist muscle becomes an antagonist muscle. A transfer from the hamstrings to the quadriceps muscles is an example in which the original knee flexor is expected to serve as knee extensor. The muscle, as such, loses some of its previous level of function.

The therapist should look for a symmetric pattern of strength and function of the extremities. When a young child has a clearly dominant side, the nondominant side should be evaluated carefully for weakness, abnormal tone, and deformity.

The child with spasticity should not be subjected to a standard muscle test. Offering resistance to a muscle with abnormally high tone often results in even greater tone that may be mistaken for increased strength and a falsely high grade. For muscles with increased tone, the therapist must examine the ability of the muscle to function in an antigravity posture and to take part in voluntary or involuntary patterns of movement.

Determination of the presence of muscle spasm is related to manual muscle testing. *Spasms,* or sudden, involuntary contractions of a muscle accompanied by pain, limited ROM, and reduced function are common in children. Spasms occur after injury or surgery, when a cast is removed, and with many diseases. When the therapist feels resistance when attempting to move the segment through its normal range, this resistance often indicates muscle spasms.

Sensory Testing

A thorough sensory evaluation may be done quickly and accurately. Any child with an orthopedic disease in which sensation might be affected should have a sensory test. Important testing is done before and after surgery and, if possible, before application of a cast when a fracture occurs.

The methods of sensory testing are identical in the child and adult. The pediatric therapist, however, must be more inventive in how to elicit a response from the child. Testing might incorporate various games or riddles presented at a level appropriate for the child.

Damage to sensory nerves may have differing mechanisms, including contusion, compression, traction, surgery, and laceration. The degree of injury may range from complete transection to minor compression with no anatomic derangement. When sensory impairment is noted, the therapist must document the type of sensation lost and the dermatomes in which the loss exists. This careful documentation provides baseline data against which regeneration or the efficacy of therapeutic intervention can be assessed.

Gait Assessment

Children begin to ambulate at between 9 and 18 months of age. The early gait pattern includes a wide base of support, externally rotated lower extremities, hip and knee flexion, pronated feet, anterior pelvic tilt with trunk leaning slightly forward, and upper extremities in a high-guard position. Stride lengths are short, and balance is precarious owing to the center of gravity being anterior to the body. The pelvis becomes more upright and the gait velocity decreases as the child matures. As equilib-

rium reactions mature, a rotational component to gait begins and a more mature pattern of gait emerges. By 3 years of age, all components of the adult gait cycle are present, although these components are not well integrated into the mature pattern until 7 to 9 years of age.[2]

The therapist must consider neuromuscular and musculoskeletal aspects of movement when analyzing gait. An abnormal gait can be caused by musculoskeletal, neuromuscular, or biomechanical disorders. Unlike gait assessment of an adult, the child's gait pattern depends on the developmental sequence and the child's level within that sequence. A normal gait pattern for an 18-month-old child, therefore, will differ from that of a 9-year-old child. The child should be observed ambulating while wearing shoes and also after taking them off. Shoes should be examined for signs of wear that may suggest deviations in gait. The child should be examined in an organized fashion. It is suggested that the therapist start with the head, then proceed to the shoulder girdle, upper extremity, trunk, pelvic girdle, and lower extremity. Specific components of the gait cycle include stance phase, propulsion (swing) phase, stride length, stride width, walking velocity, cadence, and reciprocal upper extremity motion. Most gait assessment is by observation, although more objective methods are available for little cost.[3] Some therapists will use the services of a fully instrumented gait laboratory at their institutions. These laboratories may include two- or three-dimensional motion analysis systems, force plates by which to measure ground reaction forces during gait, electromyographic systems, and a newly developed "gait measurement mat"* by which to easily measure time/distance/width parameters of gait.

Examples of deviations commonly seen in children's gait include gluteus medius and gluteus maximus lurches secondary to weakness. The gluteus medius lurch, or Trendelenburg gait, occurs when, during stance on one side, the opposite pelvis drops. The gluteus maximus lurch occurs when the child's trunk leans backward over the weight-

*EQ, Inc., Plymouth Meeting, PA.

bearing extremity. Children with quadriceps weakness, as occurs in myopathy, often place a hand on the knee to help with extension of the knee during early stance. Children with a slipped capital femoral epiphysis often have a Trendelenburg gait with the limb held in external rotation. Children with weakness in the dorsiflexors often show a drop-foot deviation in gait in which they compensate for the weak dorsiflexors by flexing the hip more than normal. This excessive hip flexion raises the lower part of the limb and enables the foot to clear the floor during swing phase. Each particular lower extremity or trunk disorder is likely to have a specific deviation in gait.

When assessing gait patterns in children, the therapist must, as with adult gait assessment, be knowledgeable about development, biomechanics, kinesiology, anatomy, and energy expenditure. Muscle function studies, assessment of kinematics and kinetics, and energy expenditure studies provide objective data regarding gait. These data provide a group of tools with which the therapist can determine the effectiveness and efficiency of surgical and nonsurgical procedures used to improve gait patterns.

Measurement of Leg Length

Leg length is important to document because numerous orthopedic disorders cause leg length inequality. One of three techniques is generally used when measuring leg length. Using two bony landmarks to ascertain limb length is a quick and reliable method to determine leg length, provided there are no significant bony or muscular disorders that might confound the measurement. Another method of measurement relies on placing lifts of various heights under the shoe of the shorter leg while the child is standing. The point at which the pelvis (anterior superior iliac spines [ASIS]) is level determines the appropriate size of lift and the approximate discrepancy in leg length. The third commonly used method requires a physician's referral for roentgenographic measurement. The measurement is done directly from the roentgenogram.

When using the bony landmark method for measurement of leg length, the therapist measures from the ASIS to the medial malleolus. An accurate comparison of limbs is achieved only when both extremities are placed in identical hip abduction and extension. Contractures at the hip and knee, particularly flexion contractures, will produce inaccurate measurements. Another related method, although less accurate, is used occasionally as a screening technique for leg length. The child lies in a supine position with a level pelvis, with hips and knees flexed, and with feet flat on the surface. When the knees are seen in an anteroposterior direction, a higher knee suggests a longer tibia on that side. When seen laterally, asymmetric knees suggest unequal femur lengths.

Numerous hip disorders in children are treated using surgical reconstructions that result in fixed pelvic obliquity and asymmetry of the ASIS. In these instances, measurements from the ASIS will provide inaccurate data. The umbilicus may be used as a substitute for the ASIS. Fixed adduction contractures of more than 30 degrees can also cause a functional pelvic obliquity. In order to uncross the legs, the child will raise the pelvis on the side of the contracture, thus causing a functional shortening of the limb. Although the limb appears shortened, a measurement from the ASIS to the medial malleolus should be accurate. Excessive valgus and varus, knee instability, other malalignments, and asymmetry in muscle mass should be noted when assessing limb length.

A lift for the shoe is required only when the leg length discrepancy is more than 1/2 inch. An adequate correction is achieved when the discrepancy is within 1/4 inch. Before and after the lift is used, a temporary one should be inserted first and gait analysis performed. The child with muscle weakness sometimes ambulates more efficiently and effectively when the discrepancy remains. A patient with hip or knee flexion contractures may require a larger lift than suggested by the measurement. The therapist must be aware that many factors in addition to the specific amount of discrepancy play a role in such assessments.

Developmental and Functional Assessment

A developmental or functional assessment should be included as part of the initial physical therapy evaluation. Orthopedic problems that occur congenitally or during early life often cause delayed acquisition of developmental skills. Numerous guidelines, tests, and scoring systems exist to determine the level at which the child is functioning based on gross motor, fine motor, social, emotional, and cognitive levels. Several of these tests of development are discussed in Chapter 2.

Children with significant orthopedic disorders often have delays in gross motor development secondary to limited ROM, inadequate strength, surgery, and long periods of immobilization with casting or bracing. Parents should be instructed in appropriate methods for enhancing motor development through exercise programs, handling techniques, and positioning. Because mobility and exploration are critical to the development of cognitive skills, older children who are restricted by casts or braces should use adapted equipment, such as prone scooters and wheelchairs, to allow safe exploration of their environment.

Functional evaluation and functional training are often necessary for the older child with impaired mobility. The therapist should teach transfers, ambulation, and wheelchair management skills as early as possible to promote independence. The physical therapist must be creative when attempting to teach functional skills to children with significant congenital anomalies, and typical methods of instruction are often inappropriate. Children are often the best teachers and devise ingenious means for efficiently accomplishing functional tasks. Communication with the family regarding the functional goals for the child and the expected support of the family is essential for the successes of any training program.

Congenital Hip Dislocation

Congenital hip dislocation (CHD) occurs in approximately 2 to 3 children per 1000 live births.

There is a female-to-male ratio of approximately 5:1. A higher incidence of CHD is found after breech delivery, in the firstborn child, and in the left hip. White infants are more susceptible to CHD than are black children.[4] Two prime etiologic factors in the development of CHD appear to be a familial mesenchymal tissue disorder resulting in ligamentous laxity around the hip, and mechanical stress on the joint related to the leg-folding mechanism.[5]

Standard nomenclature exists for describing CHD. A *subluxed hip* is one in which the femoral head lies partially beneath the acetabular roof. A *dislocatable hip* is one that can be dislocated and relocated by way of manipulation and positioning. The dislocated hip exists when the femoral head lies completely out of the acetabular confines. The *teratologic hip* is one that has dislocated at an early stage during embryonic or fetal development. The teratologic hip has structural changes in the joint present at birth and will require surgery (Fig. 9-1).[4]

The femoral head, hip joint capsule, and acetabulum are normally well developed at approximately 10 weeks of embryonic life. A congruent relationship must exist between the acetabulum and femoral head for continued growth and development of a healthy hip joint. With CHD, the femoral head most often dislocates posteriorly and superiorly. The abnormal position within the ilium causes reshaping of the femoral head. The ilium gradually develops a "false" acetabulum to accommodate the femoral head. The acetabulum may retain its shape for a period, but ultimately becomes more vertically oriented with a loss of the acetabular roof. Changes in soft tissue include muscles and ligaments whose resting length is altered.[4]

Clinical Features

CHD is usually identified early because neonatal screening examinations usually include a clinical test for CHD. A continuing study that began in 1967 demonstrated that screening is effective, early treatment improves the outcome, and the economic savings exceed $15,000 per 1000 infants screened.[6]

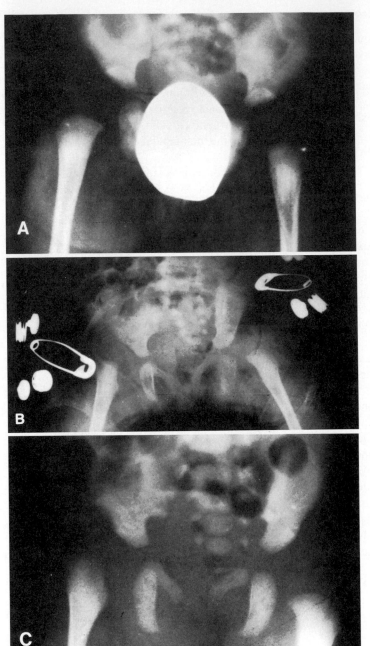

Figure 9-1. *Three types of dislocated hips recognized at birth. A. Lateral displacement occurring at birth reduces easily and responds well to simple treatment. There is only lateral displacement of the femur with no proximal displacement. B. Dislocation due to neuromuscular origin reduces easily but tends to redislocate owing to muscle imbalance. C. Teratologic dislocation occurs in utero. There is frank dislocation with lateral and proximal migration of the femur at birth, and the femoral head will not reduce into the acetabulum. A false acetabulum will have developed. (From Lovell WW, Winter RB, eds. Pediatric Orthopaedics. 2nd ed. Philadelphia. JB Lippincott; 1986:705.)*

The earlier treatment is initiated, the better the prognosis for correction of the deformity with a reduced risk for complications. Evidence of hip joint instability in the neonate is seen with provocative testing. Physical characteristics include asymmetric skin folds of the buttocks and adductor region; limitation of passive hip abduction; leg length inequality; and telescoping of the flexed and adducted thigh on the pelvis, a positive Ortolani sign (jerk or click), and a positive Barlow sign (Figs. 9-2 and 9-3). The older child who has begun to ambulate shows a positive Trendelenburg sign (associated with gluteus medius weakness) and limited hip extension. A child with bilateral CHD appears to have a waddling gait that is caused by bilateral positive Trendelenburg signs. This type of gait is easily dismissed as normal; therefore, when bilateral CHD is suspected, a careful observation of gait should be made. With a high degree of suspicion of CHD, the physician will order various imaging tests for a definitive diagnosis. In recent years, classical roentgenography has been replaced by real-time ultrasonography, with magnetic resonance imaging (MRI) still being evaluated for use in the diagnosis of CHD.[7,8]

Medical Management

Medical management depends on both the child's age and the degree of derangement of the hip. Nonoperative management often includes the Pavlik harness, which is used for the child with either dislocatable or dislocated hips during the first 9 months of life (Fig. 9-4). This harness provides gradual dynamic reduction, but requires a reliable, compliant parent and close supervision by the physician. A recent review of 74 affected hips treated with the Pavlik harness for an average of 12 years revealed that 17% of the hips had undesired changes in the acetabulum, and the authors stressed the importance of medical follow-up until skeletal maturity occurs.[9] Splints are used throughout the day in children of ages birth to 6 months and at night in older children to place the hips in a position of abduction and internal rotation. Hips that are either subluxed or dislocatable are commonly treated

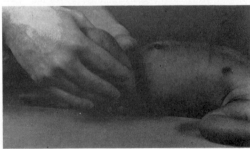
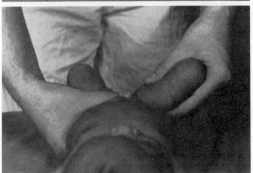

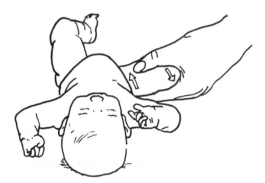

Figure 9-2. *The Ortolani maneuver. In this technique, the hip is gently abducted and the thigh is raised with the fingers to gently reduce the hip. When doing the test, one hand should always be used to stabilize the pelvis; therefore, only one hip at a time can be examined. (From Lovell WW, Winter RB, eds. Pediatric Orthopaedics. 2nd ed., Philadelphia: JB Lippincott; 1986:707.)*

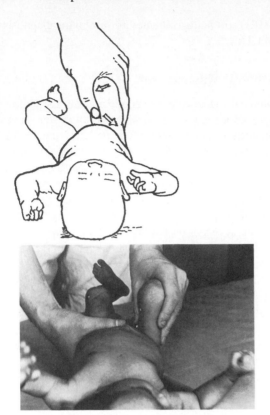

Figure 9-3. *The Barlow Test. The thumb is placed on the inner aspect of the thigh and the hip is abducted, with longitudinal pressure exerted on the thigh to push it toward the table. The examiner again uses one hand to stabilize the pelvis, testing one hip at a time. (From Lovell WW, Winter RB, eds.* Pediatric Orthopaedics. *2nd ed. Philadelphia: JB Lippincott; 1986: 707.)*

with splints. Low-temperature moldable material is used to customize these abduction splints.

Orthoses are often used with children who are active and ambulating. An A frame, a unilateral double upright long-leg brace with pelvic band, and the Scottish Rite brace are commonly used braces. The A frame has medial metal uprights connected by a horizontal bar under the groin and is used for children between 9 months and 4 years of age. The brace places the hips in position in abduction and internal rotation, the knees in extension with a me-

dial "cookie" to prevent valgus stress, and the feet in a neutral position with shoes wedged to accommodate the internal rotation at the hip (Fig. 9-5).

The unilateral metal double upright long-leg brace with pelvic band maintains the hip in abduction and internal rotation, and is commonly used for children over 4 years of age.

The Scottish Rite brace consists of a pelvic band with plastic thigh sockets. The brace places the hip in abduction, but does not control rotation. The Scottish Rite brace is most effective with children older than 4 years of age (Fig. 9-6).

Surgical Management

Surgical management depends on the child's age and the degree of hip pathology. Some type of skin traction may precede surgery. Buck traction and split Russell traction may be used to pull the hips into extension and abduction, and may be either unilateral or bilateral. Bryant traction is used in infants weighing less than 35 lb, and is applied bilaterally to place the hips in a position of flexion and abduction. Skeletal traction may be used when greater amounts of weight are required in an older child.

Closed and open reduction of the dislocation may be done with or without muscle tenotomies. The hips are placed in abduction with either flexion or extension. Immobilization in plaster, after reduction, may be maintained for as long as 9 months depending on the child's age at diagnosis and the particular type of surgery.

Pelvic osteotomy may be done when a child's hips are resistant to open reductions. A Salter innominate pelvic osteotomy is used for children between 18 months and 10 years of age. These children are immobilized in plaster hip spica casts for up to 8 weeks (Fig. 9-7). The Steel triple osteotomy is done on children 12 years of age and older and usually requires 12 weeks of immobilization in a hip spica (Fig. 9-8). Derotational femoral osteotomy or femoral shortening may be performed along with the pelvic osteotomy or with extra-articular shelf procedures. The Chiari procedure is an exam-

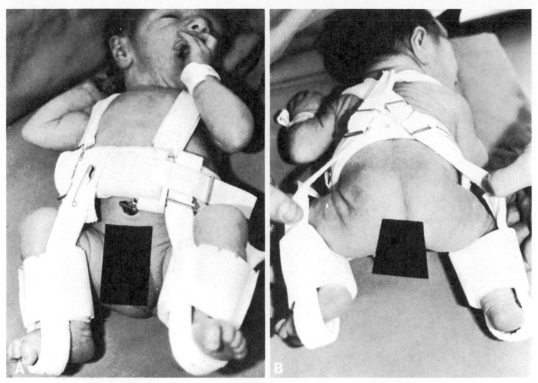

Figure 9-4. A. *The Pavlik Harness is applied so that the baby's hips are in flexion without force. The hips fall into abduction with 90 degrees of flexion. B. The prone position encourages gentle abduction. (From Lovell WW, Winter RB, eds. Pediatric Orthopaedics. 2nd ed. Philadelphia: JB Lippincott; 1986:712.)*

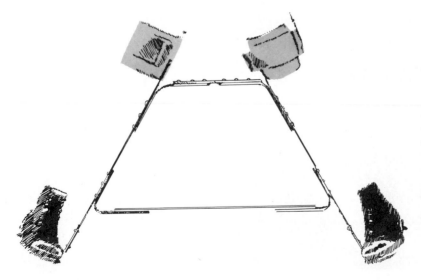

Figure 9-5. *Hip abduction orthosis (A frame). The frame is non-ambulatory and has metal or plastic bars that are adjustable for length and width. (Adapted from D'Astous J, ed. Orthotics and Prosthetics Digest: Reference Manual. Ottawa: Edahl Production; 1983; redrawn by Christopher Metzger, Beaver College, Glenside, PA.)*

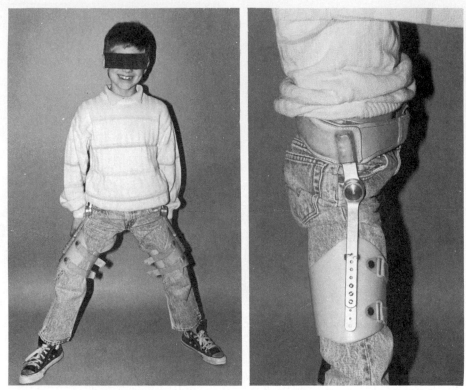

Figure 9-6. *The Scottish-rite Hospital Brace. (From Morrissy RT. Lovell and Winter's Pediatric Orthopaedics. 3rd ed. Philadelphia: JB Lippincott; 1990: 874.)*

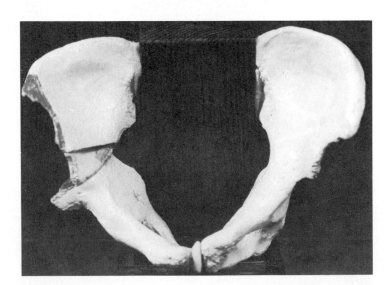

Figure 9-7. *A model of the Salter osteotomy. (From Lovell WW, Winter RB, eds. Pediatric Orthopaedics. 2nd ed. Philadelphia: JB Lippincott; 1986: 726.)*

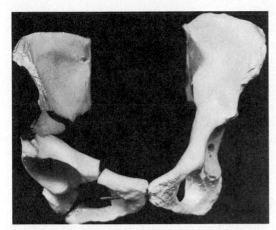

Figure 9-8. *A model of the Steele osteotomy shows a cut made on the innominate bone through the three appropriate areas. The pin is used only to stabilize the model and is not a part of the actual procedure. (From Lovell WW, Winter RB, eds. Pediatric Orthopaedics. 2nd ed. Philadelphia: JB Lippincott; 1986: 730.)*

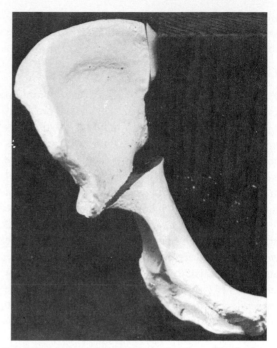

Figure 9-9. *A model of the Chiari procedure. The displacement should be at least 50% of the width of the pelvis. (From Lovell WW, Winter RB, eds. Pediatric Orthopaedics. 2nd ed. Philadelphia: JB Lippincott; 1986: 733.)*

ple of an extra-articular shelf procedure, and requires 6 weeks of immobilization (Fig. 9-9).

Salvage procedures are final attempts to relocate the hip and reduce pain. Capsular arthroplasty using a Vitallium cup are often used to reduce pain, as are hip joint fusions. Total hip joint replacement is seldom used in these children.

Physical Therapy Management

Physical therapy for the child with CHD should be individualized based on the findings of the evaluation. Children with CHD who have had surgery or immobilization will require intensive exercises to improve ROM. Hip flexion, abduction, and internal rotation are emphasized, whereas external rotation is allowed only to a neutral position. External rotation of greater magnitude will predispose to dislocation. Knee motion is often reduced when a child has spent time in a hip spica cast. When this occurs, it is important to regain complete motion of the knee. Younger children appear to regain lost motion more rapidly than do older children. Children treated with a Salter osteotomy or a Steele triple osteotomy are often limited in hip flexion, whereas

children who undergo a Chiari procedure usually lack hip abduction. The therapist must always measure ROM in the hip before surgery and should also determine range in the nonaffected extremity. The nonaffected extremity is often immobilized to ensure pelvic stability during healing, and that extremity often loses range despite being normal.

Muscle Strengthening

Muscle atrophy commonly results from surgery or immobilization. Strengthening exercises are needed to reverse the atrophy. Depending on the child's age, the therapist may need to be creative when designing a therapeutic exercise program. Both extremities should be exercised because the nonaffected extremity is often immobilized, too. Most children who have had hip surgery will need exercises to strengthen the gluteus maximus, iliopsoas, gluteus medius, quadriceps, and hamstrings. Active exercises usually precede resistive exercise.

Gait Training

Early weight bearing through standing or ambulation is encouraged to deepen the acetabulum. Gait training should not begin until the child has strength in the hip and knee musculature that is rated as "fair" or better and the ROM has reached a plateau. When assistive devices are used for gait training, children younger than 4 years of age are safer when using a walker as compared to crutches.

Children in an A frame can participate in gait training using either a walker or crutches. The walker is used in the usual manner. Crutches are usually used with one in front of and one behind the child. They are used in this manner owing to the wide stance caused by the position of extreme hip abduction instituted by the A frame. The child ambulates by lifting and advancing one foot, advancing the contralateral crutch, then advancing the opposite foot followed by the remaining crutch. This is similar to a four-point alternate gait pattern. If the child attempted any normal crutch pattern, there would be a severe mechanical disadvantage to effective and efficient ambulation.

Children with a unilateral metal double upright long-leg brace with a pelvic band may ambulate with crutches or unaided. Gait training is usually straightforward, uncomplicated, and easily learned by the child.

Children with the Scottish Rite orthosis will tend to ambulate with hips slightly abducted and externally rotated, with knees slightly flexed, and the feet in normal position. Older children do well with this orthosis, and often ambulate without assistive devices. Children younger than 4 years of age have a difficult time ambulating with the Scottish Rite orthosis and are often placed in an A frame.

Other Treatments

Physical methods, such as thermal and electrical agents, are not used with children as routinely as in adults. Hydrotherapy, however, is used to increase ROM, assist muscle strengthening, and for gait training. Children enjoy the water and often do exercises with less objection or concern than is shown outside the therapeutic pool. An increase over the past decade in the availability and use of therapeutic pools and self-contained aquatic systems has enhanced this approach to rehabilitation. Ice packs or cold hydrocollator packs are occasionally used to control pain, but heat is not commonly used with younger children who have CHD.

Arthrogryposis Multiplex Congenita

Arthrogryposis multiplex congenita (AMC) is a syndrome characterized by many nonprogressive, congenitally rigid joints. The syndrome was first described in 1841, but its pathogenesis has not been determined. Theories about the potential pathogeneses include nervous system disorders, muscle disorders, and joint abnormalities. A recent study of 21 infants with AMC who died shortly after birth showed that 11 had disease of myogenic origin, 5 had disease of neurogenic origin, and there was uncertain origin in the remaining 5 infants.[10] Restricted intrauterine movement resulting from an altered uterine environment may also be implicated as a cause.[11]

Clinical Features

The disease has a spectrum of severity ranging from mild to severe contractures with limited function of the extremities. Although the axial skeleton is not commonly involved, scoliosis may occur. Joint disorders are usually symmetric, and when only two extremities are affected, they are usually the lower extremities. Five clinical characteristics are common in children with AMC:

1. Extremities with little or no features and a shape that is cylindrical, absent skin creases, and thin subcutaneous tissue
2. Joint rigidity
3. Dislocated joints in the hips and, occasionally, in the knees

4. Muscle atrophy and absence of muscle groups
5. Intact sensation, but occasional loss of or decrease in deep tendon reflexes

Patients with classical deformities in the upper extremities usually have limited abduction and external rotation of the shoulder. Elbows may be either flexed or extended, with only a few degrees of motion available. Wrists are flexed and deviated toward the ulnar side. Fingers are slender, and polydactyly or syndactyly are common. The deltoids, biceps, and forearm muscles are often inactive (Fig. 9-10).

Lower extremity posture includes hips in abduction, flexion, and external rotation, with dislocation being common. Knees may be flexed or extended, but are usually rigid. The patellae may be dislocated or absent. Club feet are common. Muscle mass may be decreased or absent, with muscle replaced by adipose tissue. The severity of deformity is greater toward the distal extremity. These children have normal intelligence (Fig. 9-11).[12]

Robinson surveyed families of 87 individuals with AMC to determine their current health problems. More than one half of the individuals were affected by feeding disorders related to structural disorders of the jaw and tongue. The feeding difficulties were thought to have given rise to constipation, recurrent respiratory infections, and failure to thrive.[13]

Medical Management

The main goal of treatment is to provide maximum function. The goal for lower extremity position is to provide stable, well-aligned joints for weight bearing. The goal for the upper extremities is to provide for independence in activities of daily living. Nonoperative treatment includes manipulated casting, physical therapy, bracing, and splinting.

Surgical Management

The goal of lower extremity operative care is to correct, before 2 years of age, all lower extremity deformities that hinder walking. Upper extremity sur-

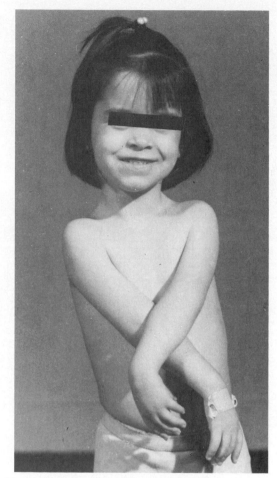

Figure 9-10. *Classical upper extremity deformity in arthrogryposis multiplex congenita. (From Morrissy RT. Lovell and Winter's Pediatric Orthopaedics. 3rd ed. Philadelphia: JB Lippincott; 1990: 445.)*

gery is often delayed for a few years until full function of the upper extremities can be determined.[14]

Because a unilateral hip dislocation can result in pelvic obliquity and scoliosis, the dislocation is usually surgically repaired. Bilateral hip dislocations are usually stable high on the pelvis, and symmetric, and the result is a balanced pelvis. For these reasons and because ambulation is not delayed, open reduction is not often done.

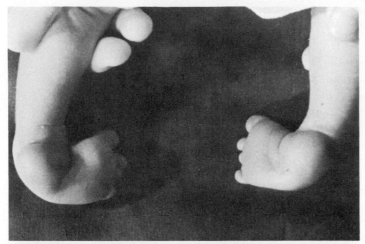

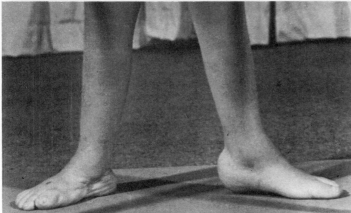

Figure 9-11. *Arthrogryposis multiplex congenita.* Top. *Talipes equinovarus.* Bottom. *Definitive correction is achieved with talectomy, after unnecessary posteromedial releases. (From Lovell WW, Winter RB, eds. Pediatric Orthopaedics. 2nd ed. Philadelphia: JB Lippincott; 1986: 323.)*

Surgery on the knee is usually aimed at correcting a flexion contracture and does not increase motion; rather, the surgery changes the arc of motion. The correction of flexion deformities at the knee is usually maintained with bracing.

Scoliosis resulting from arthrogryposis is treated by nonoperative methods if the deformity is identified when the child is young and before progression. A total contact thoracolumbosacral orthosis is recommended for curvatures between 20 and 40 degrees. Curvatures of greater than 50 degrees should be treated with surgery.[15]

Physical Therapy Management

A careful evaluation, as described previously, is essential. Goniometric assessment of joint motion throughout the body is important.

Exercise

Exercises to increase ROM are started during the neonatal period. Although the success of exercise in increasing motion is unpredictable, when improvement occurs, it usually happens before 3 years of age. Parents are instructed to do exercises for

ROM. They are instructed on hand placement and individual joint motion, rather than on motion of the entire limb, and they are encouraged to do the exercise regimen several times each day.

Passive ROM exercise is also important to maintain joint mobility in the older child with AMC. The exercise regimen is important immediately before and after surgery. Although the goal of improving motion is important and continuing, many operations are done to change the arc of motion in order to achieve better functional results. The physical therapist must be informed about the goal of surgery in order to provide appropriate and safe treatment.

Exercise to increase strength should follow manual muscle testing. The therapist must determine whether limitation in function is the result of muscle weakness or absence, or decreased joint mobility.

Splinting, Casting, and Bracing

Casts or splints are commonly used to maintain joint mobility. Parents are instructed in the application of devices and in how to check on the circulation and skin. The amount of time that they are worn will depend on the appliance and tolerance of the skin. Frequent modification of splints and casts is necessary as the child grows. Serial casting is often used to increase range in a specific plane of motion. Although the primary concern is on the joint being casted, the therapist and family must maintain range in the proximal and distal joints as well.

Orthotics are also used to maintain ROM, but, in addition, they provide support for the lower extremity during standing or gait training. The therapist must evaluate strength, ROM, and functional needs when deciding on the type of orthotic device needed. Braces should be checked periodically by parents and the therapist to ensure continued good fit and function. Moore et al. described an approach to orthotic management for a girl with AMC that included a plastic body section; thigh, calf, and foot sections; and articulating hips and knees and gas

springs to provide ". . . near-constant extending moments" in an attempt to gain motion at the hips and knees.[16]

Positioning

Recommendations for specific positioning will vary with the child's orthopedic deformities, ROM limitations, and tolerance. We encourage positions that will maintain or increase joint mobility, stimulate cognitive development, and enhance fine motor development. Specific suggestions about positioning are too numerous to identify because many joints may be involved. Two common examples of positioning include side-lying, which encourages upper extremity midline activity and lower extremity adduction, and the prone position, which encourages hip extension. A small towel roll placed under the axilla of a child in the prone position may encourage shoulder flexion and forearm weight bearing.

In addition to providing positioning that will help reduce or maintain the orthopedic deformities, therapists must also encourage normal motor development. Facilitation of normal developmental sequence and postural reactions should be a major concern. Parents should be instructed about the normal developmental sequence and should be shown basic handling techniques, especially as they apply to dressing, carrying, and positioning the child.

Functional Skills

After a functional assessment, the child may need to learn transfer techniques and mat mobility skills. These techniques are modified depending on the child's abilities. Because children with AMC usually have normal intelligence, they learn well and often function despite their disability.

Some children with more severe deformities will require adaptive seating and wheelchairs. Various commercial seating systems are available, or the therapist can make a seating system. The advantages and disadvantages of each method are given in Chapter 13. When a wheelchair is required, the therapist must work closely with the vendor to ensure proper fit, function, and control systems for the child.

Gait

Standing is encouraged as a preambulation skill as soon as lower extremity alignment permits. Prone or supine standers, or parapodiums, may be used to help promote early weight bearing.

The quality and quantity of gait, the age of onset of walking, and the assistive device used all vary with the degree of orthopedic deformity. Many children with AMC have the potential for ambulation without an assistive device, although most children begin gait training with some type of assistive device.

The therapist must be innovative and creative when an upper extremity deformity interferes with the use of a walker or crutch. A young child with limited hand function and elbow flexion may benefit from an infant walker with a sling seat. The seat provides support, while the upper bar of the walker is held against the child's trunk. This technique enables the child to direct the walker with the upper extremity while receiving support from the sling seat. When children with AMC have fixed elbow flexion contractures, platforms added to the walker or crutches can be used to assist weight bearing and support. A build-up of the handle on the walker or crutch can be helpful because most children have reduced grip strength and limited finger flexion. Two-point or four-point gaits are used most frequently for gait training. When limited hip flexion will not allow an adequate swing phase, forward progression is achieved by rotating the entire body to alternately place each foot forward.

Osteogenesis Imperfecta

Osteogenesis imperfecta (OI) is a common and serious abnormality resulting in weakness and fragility of the bones. This abnormality is transmitted genetically in an autosomal dominant pattern, although it also occurs occasionally in a recessive mode.[17] OI affects formation of collagen within developing bone, which impairs the development of normal Haversian systems.[18] The severity and type of disease is usually denoted by the age at which fractures first occur. The most severe form, a form which is often fatal, is characterized by many fractures during fetal life and at parturition. This fetal type is associated with a high mortality rate during infancy. The infantile form of OI is moderately severe, with many gross fractures occurring in the long bones during early childhood (Fig. 9-12). Children with the infantile form usually develop limb deformities, stunted growth, and a head size that, although normal for their age, appears large in relation to the body. The less severe juvenile type of OI is typified by fractures in later childhood.[19] A more contemporary, but less clinical, classification is based upon biochemical phenotypes of OI related to fibroblast secretion of abnormal collagen-related substances. Identification of these abnormal substances may help determine the mode of inheritance and the clinical severity of the disorder.[20] Classification of the disease by radiographic changes has also been proposed.[21]

Clinical Features

Common characteristics of children with OI include thin cortical bone that often fractures, shortness of stature, scoliosis, defective dentinogenesis of primary and secondary teeth, conductive hearing loss secondary to fractures of the ossicles, laxity of ligaments, blue sclera, an unusually shaped skull with wide intertemporal measurements and a small triangular face, thin skin, and narrow diaphyses in the long bones. The diagnostic triad of clinical signs include blue sclera, dentinogenesis imperfecta, and generalized osteoporosis in a child with many fractures and bowing of the long bones.[22]

Medical Management

Orthopedic management is concerned with bowing deformities of the long bones. These deformities have the potential of severely reducing the functional level of the child. Treatment of fractures is also a major focus of treatment.

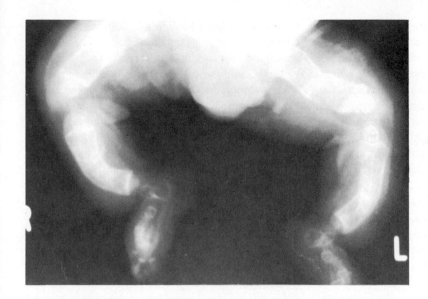

Figure 9-12. *Osteogenesis imperfecta. Note the multiple fractures in the femur and tibia. (From Lovell WW, Winter RB, eds. Pediatric Orthopaedics. 2nd ed. Philadelphia: JB Lippincott; 1986: 113.)*

The healing of a fracture is usually normal but, once healed, the bone may be as weak as it was before the fracture. In addition, nonunion of fractures and associated loss of functional ability is prevalent in children with OI.[23] After a fracture, the site is immobilized until bone healing has occurred. If the child is wearing an orthosis, the physician may elect not to use a cast, but may have the child continue with the orthosis and continue to bear weight or use the extremity. Because weight bearing and other stresses promote formation of osteoblasts, the activity may actually promote healing. Recent trials of calcitonin, delivered by nasal spray as opposed to injection, have resulted in a decrease in fractures.[24]

Surgical Management

A main form of treatment of OI involves the insertion of a Bailey-Dubow rod in the long bones. These intramedullary rods, which can elongate by telescoping, have a small hook fixed into cortical bone at each end. As the child grows, the rods can be lengthened, thus allowing several years of growth with the reinforcement offered by the rods.[25]

Scoliosis associated with OI is one of the most challenging orthopedic problems. Lateral curves in the child with OI progress rapidly after 5 years of age and reach a maximum at approximately 12 years of age.[26] Progression of the curvature should be prevented with either functional bracing or surgical fusion, with or without insertion of a Harrington rod or similar types of instrumentation.

Splinting and Orthotics

Splinting for the upper extremities is commonly used to decrease the bowing deformities associated with OI. Our facility uses low-temperature materials, such as Orthoplast and Aquaplast molds.

Bracing is used in the lower extremities to protect the long bones against additional fracture and deformity and to help with ambulation. Parapodiums or other long-leg braces may be used to promote weight bearing for the younger child. Older children with the moderate to severe type of OI will usually require bilateral knee-ankle-foot orthoses (KAFOs), with or without pelvic bands.

Physical Therapy Management

Exercise

Exercise to increase ROM is initiated after the fracture or surgical site has healed. Gentle passive exercise should be initiated because the areas of fracture or surgical repair are severely osteoporotic. More vigorous exercise can cause additional fractures. Full ROM for functional purposes is always the goal of these exercises; however, achieving this goal is often a slow, tedious process because of the fragile bones. The physical therapist must be aware of the signs of a fracture. Classical signs of inflammation, including warmth at the site, edema, pain, bruising, irritability, and deformity, suggest a fracture.

The therapist should immediately refer the child to the surgeon if a child with an intramedullary rod begins to suddenly lose ROM. This sudden loss of motion often indicates that the rod has moved from its original position. This complication requires immediate medical attention.

As with exercises for ROM, strengthening exercise should be initiated only after the fracture or surgical site is fully healed. Similar care should be taken with strengthening exercise to prevent fractures. We advocate using low weight with high repetitions for strengthening, and we often combine these exercises with those used for ROM.

Gait Training

Gait training is commonly initiated when the child has achieved strength with a rating of at least 3 of 5 ("fair") and when ROM has reached a plateau. Gait training is progressed in the usual fashion, beginning with the parallel bars and moving to various assistive devices. Children with OI frequently use braces during weight bearing and gait training. When children who use walkers bear a large percentage of body weight on the upper extremities, precautions against bowing deformities of the radius and ulna are often necessary. Splints may help protect against their further progression when these deformities begin.

Axillary and lofstrand crutches are commonly used for gait training. A four-point gait is the preferred pattern, although a swing-to or swing-through pattern may also be used.

Many children begin gait training with periods of weight-bearing because weight-bearing forces will promote bone healing and strengthening. Tilt tables, parapodiums, and prone and supine standers are all used for weight-bearing activity.

Gerber and associates presented their experience with a comprehensive rehabilitation program emphasizing ambulation for 12 children with OI. The program included strengthening exercises, aquatic exercise, molded seating, and gait training with long-leg braces. Of the 12 children, 9 were community ambulators, whereas 3 were home ambulators. The authors determined that the rehabilitation program resulted in a high level of function for the children, with an acceptable level of fractures that actually decreased in some children.[27]

Orthotics

Braces typically used for children with OI include either conventional metal bracing or plastic molded KAFOs. A pelvic band may be used, but is often unnecessary. When long-bone bowing is severe, a clamshell type of brace protects the extremities against a progression of the deformity.

Wheelchairs

Children who have moderate and severe types of OI often require wheelchairs for mobility. Because of the shortened extremities, the chairs are often specially ordered and may require adaptations. We recommend a lightweight chair because the wheelchair should be designed to provide for functional independence.

Therapeutic Methods

Thermal agents, including heat and cold, may be used to help achieve the therapeutic goals of increased motion and relief of pain and edema. Hydrotherapy and therapeutic pool activity can be used to increase ROM and strength and to promote gait training.

Family Education

The stigma associated with the "brittle bones" of OI causes fear in both parents and siblings. The physical therapist plays a major role in preventing fractures by teaching proper and safe methods of handling the child. Family members must be supported repeatedly in the belief that if a child suffers a fracture, no one is to blame. Parents often feel guilt or anger about their child's disease. The physical therapist who detects these feelings may choose to refer the family to a social service agency and may suggest the family contact the Brittle Bone Society.

Legg-Calvé-Perthes Disease

Legg-Calvé-Perthes disease (LCPD) is one of several osteochondroses typified by a self-limiting necrosis of the femoral head in otherwise normal children. The disease occurs in children between 2 and 12 years of age, although it is most prevalent between 4 and 8 years of age. The annual incidence is 1:1500 for children younger than 14 years of age, and boys are afflicted with LCPD five to six times as frequently as girls.[4]

The exact cause of LCPD is unknown, although both genetic and environmental etiologies have been suggested. Theories of pathogenesis include an interruption to the blood supply of the femoral head and increased intra-articular pressure secondary to disease or trauma resulting in ischemia to the femoral head. Strong experimental evidence supports the theory of interruption of blood supply to the femoral head.[28] A familial link occurs in 20% to 24% of patients. There is significant correlation between low birth weight and LCPD. Newborn children weighing less than $5\frac{1}{2}$ lb are five times as likely to develop LCPD as are those weighing $8\frac{1}{2}$ lb or more. Seventy-five percent of patients have a delay in skeletal maturity when compared to chronologic age.

Clinical Features

LCPD involves a process that begins with necrosis of the femoral head and may involve all or part of the capital femoral epiphysis. Progression occurs through four stages—condensation, fragmentation (lytic), reossification, and remodeling.[29] The necrosis may result in either collapse or flattening of the head. Resorption of necrotic bone occurs, with subsequent deposition of new bone that takes the smooth, regular shape of the normal epiphysis. The degree to which the newly deposited bone regains the normal characteristics of the femoral head relates to both the severity of the process and the age of onset.[30]

Catterall classified LCPD into four groups of severity. The first group (grade I) is characterized by no clear necrosis and involvement of only the anterior portion of the femoral head. Children with grade II disease have a greater portion of the anterior epiphysis involved, and necrosis and subsequent collapse occur. Grade III LCPD is characterized by necrosis and collapse of a major portion of the femoral head, but a normal medial and lateral border. Grade IV LCPD involves necrosis and destruction of the entire femoral head and neck. Lateral subluxation of the hip joint may occur with any grade, but is most commonly seen in Grades III and IV (Figs. 9-13 to 9-16). Subluxation places additional stress on the femoral head and greater deformity is likely.[31]

A painless limp that occurs intermittently is usually the first symptom, followed by a constant limp associated with pain in the hip, knee, or groin. The pain may be present for months before medical attention is sought. Some children report a recent injury associated with the initiation of limp and pain. Limitation is seen in hip internal rotation and abduction, and muscle spasms or shortening often cause limitation in hip flexion and extension. In more severe cases, the child may have a positive Trendelenburg sign, and a 1- to 2-cm leg length discrepancy when healing is finished. Approximately 10% of patients develop bilateral LCPD.

Prognosis is related to the extent of epiphyseal involvement, presence of subluxation, age of onset, and appropriate initiation of treatment. Children younger than 5 years of age at onset usually have a more favorable outcome than do older children.

Medical Management

Treatment of LCPD centers around providing the most beneficial environment in which the disease process can run its course. The specific goal of

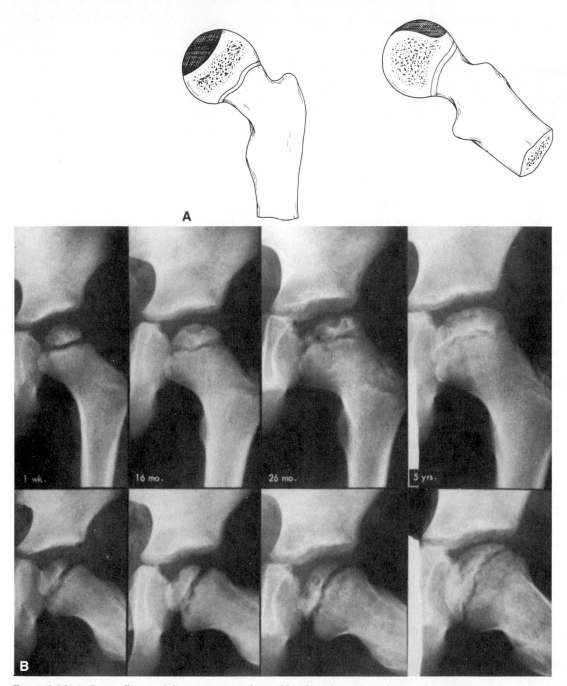

Figure 9-13. A. *Catterall group I disease: anterior femoral head involvement, with no evidence of sequestrum or of a subchondral fracture line or metaphyseal abnormalities. B. Catterall group I disease 1 week to 5 years after onset of symptoms. (From Morrissy RT. Lovell and Winter's Pediatric Orthopaedics. 3rd ed. Philadelphia: JB Lippincott; 1990: 863.)*

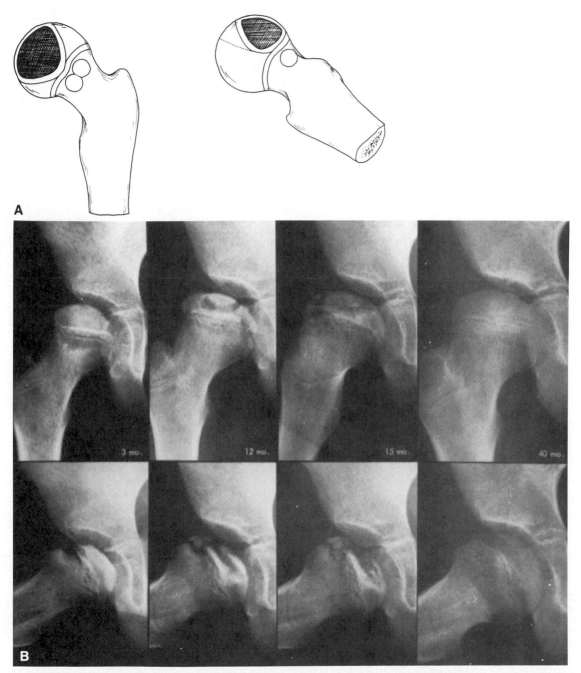

Figure 9-14. A. *Catterall group II disease: anterolateral involvement, sequestrum formation, and a clear junction between the involved and uninvolved areas. There are anterolateral metophyseal lesions, and the subchondral fracture line is in the anterior half of the femoral head. The lateral column is intact.* B. *Catterall group II disease 3 to 40 months after onset of symptoms. Note the intact lateral pillar. (From Morrissy RT. Lovell and Winter's Pediatric Orthopaedics. 3rd ed. Philadelphia: JB Lippincott; 1990: 864.)*

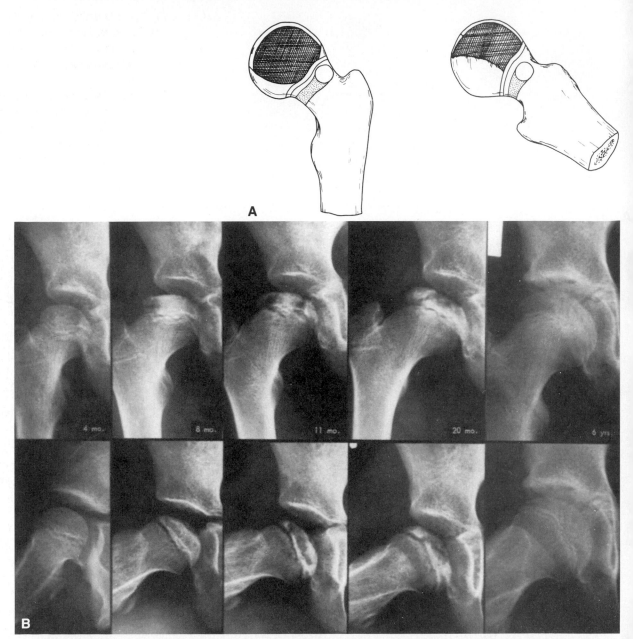

Figure 9-15. A. *Catterall group III disease: large sequestrum involving three quarters of the femoral head. The junction between the involved and uninvolved portions is sclerotic. Metaphyseal lesions are diffuse, particularly anterolaterally, and the subchondral fracture line extends to the posterior half of the epiphysis. The lateral column is involved. B. Catterall group III disease 4 months to 6 years after onset of symptoms. Note the involvement of the lateral pillar as well as the subchondral radiolucent zone on the radiograph taken 8 months after onset of symptoms. (From Morrissy RT. Lovell and Winter's Pediatric Orthopaedics. 3rd ed. Philadelphia: JB Lippincott; 1990: 865.)*

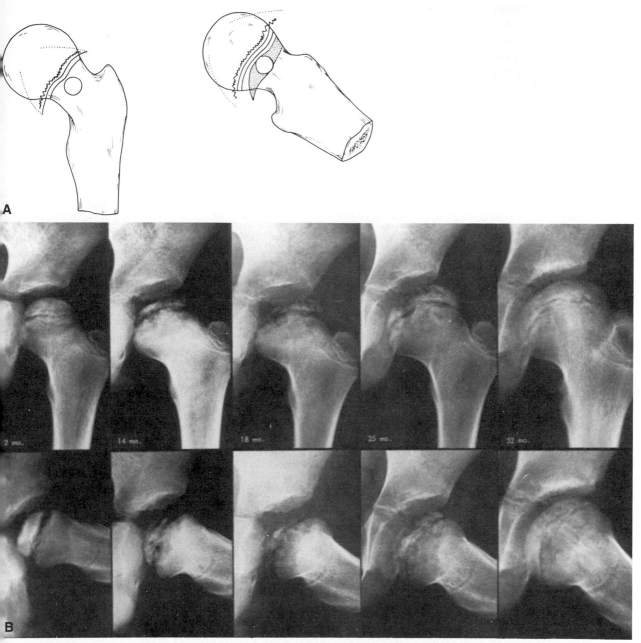

Figure 9-16. A. *Catterall group IV disease: whole femoral head involvement with either diffuse or central metaphyseal lesions and posterior remodeling of the epiphysis. B. Catterall group IV disease 2 to 52 months after onset of symptoms. Note the stages: 14 months—fragmentation; 18 months—early reossification; 25 months—late reossification; 52 months—healed. Note also the growth arrest line and evidence of reactivation of the growth plate along the femoral neck. (From Morrissy RT. Lovell and Winter's Pediatric Orthopaedics. 3rd ed. Philadelphia: JB Lippincott; 1990: 866.)*

treatment is to "contain" the femoral head in the acetabulum in order to keep full ROM and allow reformation of the femoral head. This containment can best be achieved with a position of hip abduction. Both conservative and surgical treatments are available, and the choice depends on the symptoms, roentgenographic findings, and the needs and attitudes of the parent and child.

If a child has pain or spasms, rest in bed and skin traction are initiated in the hospital or at home. This regimen continues until spasms have decreased and ROM has returned to normal.

A child with grade I involvement, or a child younger than 2 years of age with grade II involvement, should be monitored regularly with roentgenograms and goniometry. Such children can be treated with an abduction cast or orthosis provided there is no deterioration in status. Specific orthoses include the A frame, Toronto brace, Petrie cast, and Atlanta or Newington brace (Fig. 9-17). Physician preference and brace availability often dictate the choice of brace. The brace should provide sufficient abduction to keep the femoral head in the acetabulum, and it should also provide slight internal rotation. This position helps mold and stabilize the femoral head and places the hip abductor muscles at mechanical disadvantage, thus limiting the forces that place stress on the joint.[32]

Surgical Management

Surgery is usually recommended only for grades III and IV LCPD if the femoral head cannot be kept in place with an orthosis or if the child refuses to wear the device. Varus derotational osteotomy and innominate osteotomy are the two procedures used most commonly for LCPD. The femoral neck-to-shaft angle is decreased to approximately 115 degrees in a varus osteotomy. The patient is placed in a postoperative cast for up to 6 weeks. The pelvic osteotomy changes the position of the hip joint by altering the shape of the pelvis on the side involved. This procedure is usually followed by a hip spica cast for 6 to 8 weeks.[33] Regardless of medical or surgical management, the orthopedic surgeon must periodically monitor the child until bone growth is complete.

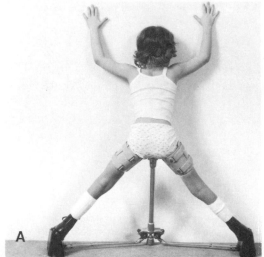

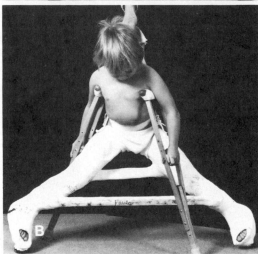

Figure 9-17. A. *The Toronto brace, an abduction containment orthosis. B. The Petrie cast, which achieves abduction with mild internal rotation. (From Lovell WW, Winter RB, eds.* Pediatric Orthopaedics. *2nd ed. Philadelphia: JB Lippincott; 1986. 765.)*

Physical Therapy Management

A thorough physical therapy evaluation is done on each child. Emphasis is on passive ROM of the hip in all planes. The range of the hip joint must be evaluated carefully and repeatedly. Internal rotation and abduction are motions that are commonly decreased.

A full orthotic examination should be done if the child is fitted with an orthosis. The physical therapist must instruct the child and parents in the proper donning and doffing of the device.

Gait training may be initiated with the orthosis. The specific gait pattern and assistive devices depend on the type of orthosis. A walker is recommended for younger children, and crutches may be used for older children. A modified gait pattern with one crutch in front of the child and one crutch behind, as was described for CHD, is often necessary for those with LCPD.

After surgery and removal of the cast, passive ROM exercise is initiated, along with muscle strengthening. Full weight-bearing gait training is allowed when the child shows adequate ROM and strength.

A comparison was made of the behavioral sequelae of children who received surgery versus those who were braced. A significant difference in three areas was noted between the two groups. Children who were braced were likely to have deficits in social, academic, and sexual behavior when compared to the surgery group. This issue must be considered by professionals and the family when working with children who are braced.[34]

Slipped Capital Femoral Epiphysis

Slipped capital femoral epiphysis (SCFE) is an uncommon orthopedic disorder of childhood. The disorder is characterized by a disturbance in the growth plate of the capital epiphysis, an associated weakening of the structure, and subsequent displacement of the femoral head on the femoral neck.[4] The femoral head usually shifts in an inferior and posterior direction in relationship to the femoral neck. The femoral head usually stays within the acetabulum, but the limb becomes externally rotated as a result of the slip. SCFE can occur only before growth plate closure. It occurs between one and three times per 100,000 children. Black boys are most susceptible to SCFE, and the incidence in that group is approximately 8:100,000. SCFE is twice as common in boys as in girls, and most patients are obese, with weights exceeding the 95th percentile, and have delayed skeletal and sexual maturity. The age range for onset in boys is 12 to 16 years of age, whereas the range is from 10 to 13 years of age in girls. Girls are rarely affected after menarche.[35] Slipping of the epiphysis is often seen during a growth spurt.[36]

The cause of the condition is unknown, but probably relates to both growth and mechanical factors. One theory suggests an inherent weakness of the epiphysis during adolescent growth spurts. Shear stress through the hip joint crack the cartilaginous growth plate and displacement occurs. Because of the large number of obese and sexually immature patients, some authorities believe that an imbalance between sex and growth hormones may be the cause, but all laboratory values are normal for these children. Infection, trauma, and genetic predisposition are other possible causes.

Clinical Features

SCFE is classified by clinical findings and roentgenographic results. Symptoms vary according to the degree of deformity and the time of onset. The severity is determined by measuring the percentage of slipping, as analyzed from the roentgenogram. A child with a "pre-slip" shows changes in the epiphyseal plate but has no displacement. A grade I slip is a deformity in which the femoral head is displaced less than one third of the width of the neck. A grade II slip occurs when the displacement is between one third and one half of the width of the femoral neck. A slip of more than one half of the width of the femoral neck is a grade III slip (Figs. 9-18 and 9-19).[4]

A patient who develops an acute and sudden displacement (less than 3 weeks of onset) has an abrupt onset of pain and develops a limp. These symptoms may be associated with an injury or fall. The child with a more insidious or chronic slip will complain of intermittent and gradually increasing pain in the hip, knee, buttock, or groin. It is important to note that hip pain is not a universal finding, and pain referred to other areas often results in the diagnosis of SCFE being missed.[37] The child with SCFE will have pain on motion, muscle spasms,

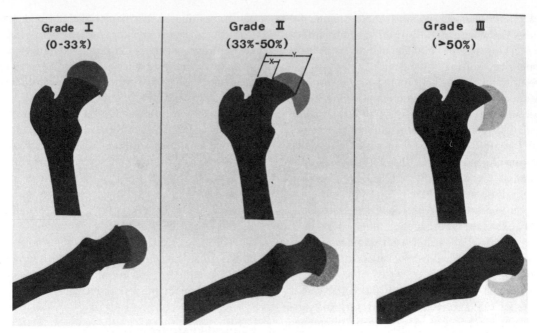

Figure 9-18. *Classification of the three grades of slipped capital femoral epiphysis. (From Lovell WW, Winter RB, eds.* Pediatric Orthopaedics. *2nd ed. Philadelphia: JB Lippincott; 1986: 746.)*

and be unable to bear weight on the affected hip. Internal rotation, abduction, and occasionally, hip flexion are limited. When the hip is flexed passively, the motion is accompanied by external rotation and abduction (Fig. 9-20). A small leg length discrepancy may exist. With a chronic slip, there may be a reactive bone formation seen on the roentgenogram. Most children have unilateral involvement, but approximately 20% have bilateral slips. Two thirds of those with bilateral involvement will have the two slips simultaneously, whereas the remaining third have the slip several months later.[38]

Medical Management

Several types of therapy may be used, depending on the severity of the slip and on physician's preference. Weight loss is strongly encouraged as an adjunct to treatment for all children with excess weight.

Nonoperative management of the child with the "pre-slip" condition usually consists of non–weight-bearing ambulation and restricted physical activity. The child is closely monitored at 1- to 3-month intervals.

Conservative treatment of adolescents with grades I, II, or III slips consists of initial rest in bed and traction. Bucks or split Russell traction is applied with the limb in slight internal rotation and abduction. A hip spica cast is applied once muscle spasms have decreased and the slip is reduced. The child will wear the cast for 12 to 14 weeks. Physical therapy begins after the cast is removed.[39]

Bed rest and traction precede most operations, and the length of time in traction depends on the grade of slip and the severity of symptoms. Operative techniques are varied for SCFE, but Canale states that most agree that in situ pinning of the epiphysis is done on patients with mild, moderate, and some severe slips.[40] This type of internal fixation will not restore normal alignment in children with moderate to severe deformity. However, a long-term follow-up of 124 patients at the University of Iowa with 155 involved hips found that in situ pinning provided the best long-term function

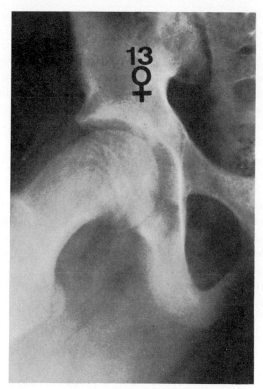

Figure 9-19. *Example of a moderately slipped epiphysis. (From Lovell WW, Winter RB, eds.* Pediatric Orthopaedics. *2nd ed. Philadelphia: JB Lippincott; 1986: 745.)*

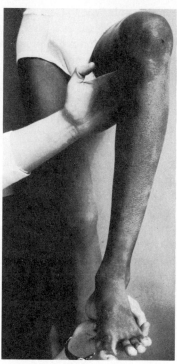

Figure 9-20. *As the thigh is flexed, it tends to roll into external rotation and abduction. (From Lovell WW, Winter RB, eds.* Pediatric Orthopaedics. *2nd ed. Philadelphia: JB Lippincott; 1986: 743.)*

and delay of degenerative joint disease.[41] An osteotomy may help correct alignment and compensate for the varus and retroversion deformity caused by the slip. A hip spica cast is applied for approximately 6 weeks after the osteotomy. Epiphysiodesis (epiphyseal fusion) may be performed in a child with a chronic slip. A hip spica may also be used after this operation.[42]

Physical Therapy Management

Exercise

Treatment should begin with a careful, thorough evaluation of the motion of the hip joint. Measurements of hip motion should be done regularly because the degree of spasm and pain may change the range at any time. After every operation and removal of a cast, a regimen of full ROM exercises, both active and passive, should be begun. Exercises should be done in all planes, with particular emphasis on hip flexion, internal rotation, and abduction. Knee flexion is also stressed when the knee has been immobilized in a cast for a long time. Patients respond in various ways, and those with a severe slip may not regain full motion.

Patients who have been immobilized in a cast will usually have strengthening exercises recommended immediately after removal of the cast. When the SCFE has been repaired surgically, the physician will indicate when strengthening exercises should begin.

Gait Training

Gait training is started once lower extremity strength and ROM is adequate for ambulation skills. When the child is treated without surgery, weight-bearing ambulation is usually tolerated when strength and range are adequate. Partial weight-bearing ambulation is begun approximately 14 days after epiphyseal pinning. When the child is treated with epiphysiodesis, full weight-bearing status is permitted when the growth plate has fused (within approximately 3 to 4 months).

Prognosis

Prognosis depends on the severity of the slip and the occurrence of complications. Complications commonly associated with SCFE include avascular femoral head necrosis, migration or penetration of a pin, chondrolysis, and, in later years, degenerative joint disease. Patients with grade I slips have a favorable prognosis when treated early. The prognosis becomes less favorable as the grade of slip becomes more severe. The goal for treatment is to provide a hip joint that functions as well as possible and is unlikely to undergo early degenerative changes.

Limb Length Discrepancy

Limb length discrepancy (LLD) is a common disorder in children and may result in marked impairment in posture and function. Causes of LLD are numerous. Congenital LLD may occur as a result of many deformities, including proximal focal femoral deficiency, hemiatrophy, and CHD. Abnormal shortening may be associated with trauma and with infections of the epiphyseal growth plate. Bony overgrowth may be a late complication of fracture or hemihypertrophy. The femur contributes 54% of length to the lower extremity, whereas the tibia accounts for 46%. The distal femoral and proximal tibial epiphyses account for the greatest increments of length in each bone. Injury to either of these areas will have an increased effect on bone growth.[43] The degree of LLD and the treatment depends on the cause and location of the altered growth, and the skeletal age of the child at the time of insult. Minor LLDs of less than 1 cm are often ignored. A lift in the shoe of the shorter leg may be adequate for an LLD of 1 to 2 cm. Surgery is often necessary when the LLD is 2 cm or more.[44] An LLD of greater than 18 cm cannot be corrected successfully by equalization methods of surgery, and a prosthesis or orthosis may be required, with or without amputation. Correction of LLD is important because the result of the asymmetry is abnormal stress on joints in the periphery, at the pelvis, and in the spine. An abnormal gait pattern may result from LLD.

Medical Management

The first step for the physician is to measure precisely the amount of shortening. Three techniques are commonly used. At least two of the three techniques are done on each child. Measurement of limb length using two bony prominences gives an accurate assessment, provided there are no other significant skeletal or muscular deformities. By placing a variable-sized lift under the short leg of the child who is standing, the physician can determine the functional degree of correction of the LLD. An orthoroentgenogram accurately determines the degree of discrepancy. After these measurements, the skeletal age of the child is determined from roentgenograms of the wrists and hands. When the skeletal age is known, the physician can determine the amount of growth still to occur in the bones. Unfortunately, it is difficult to make such a determination in an abnormal limb. Parental height and the degree of the child's sexual maturity can also be used as predictive factors. Using these several predictive measures, the orthopedic surgeon can ascertain the amount of correction required in order to regain symmetry.

For an LLD of less than 2 cm, a shoe lift is an effective means of correction. Larger discrepancies require larger and unattractive shoes that the child often refuses to wear. When a femoral discrepancy occurs, a heel lift, although useful, causes a cosmetic problem as a result of the knees being at different heights. Children with extreme or severe LLD will not be safe with a shoe lift because of a lack of balance. These children often benefit from a foot-in-foot prosthesis or an orthosis (Fig. 9-21).

Surgical Management

Epiphysiodesis

The goal of epiphysiodesis is to achieve growth arrest in the proximal tibial and fibular epiphyses or in the distal femoral epiphysis. The surgery involves creating a bony bridge across the epiphysis to the metaphysis.[44]

Bone Shortening

Bone shortening is recommended for children with excessive inequality who are too mature for epiphysiodesis and who are not candidates for lengthening procedures. Loss of height is a significant drawback of this surgery.

Limb Lengthening

The Wagner femoral lengthening procedure is complicated and prolonged and requires extensive hospitalization. The operation includes an osteotomy followed by gradual distraction to either the tibia or femur using a series of screws inserted into the bone. A special device provides a distractive force against the screws, thus increasing the length of the bone (Figs. 9-22 and 9-23). Once the desired lengthening is achieved, bone grafting and internal fixation of the bone are done to stabilize the limb segment. Complications with this surgery include pin track infection, bony angulation, delayed union or nonunion, knee and ankle contractures, subluxation, paresthesias, and circulatory disturbances.[45]

The Ilizarov limb lengthening procedures (Fig. 9-24) involves a series of metal rings and threaded rods that provide a distractive force while the bone is maintained by wires. A corticotomy is performed in an attempt to leave intact the blood supply of the periosteum and endosteum. The distraction provides a gap in the bone, which is ultimately filled via osteogenesis. The process provides lengthening of approximately 1 cm per month.[46]

Physical Therapy Management

The physical therapist may do many of the early and preoperative measurements and treatments (e.g., the shoe lift) for the child with LLD.

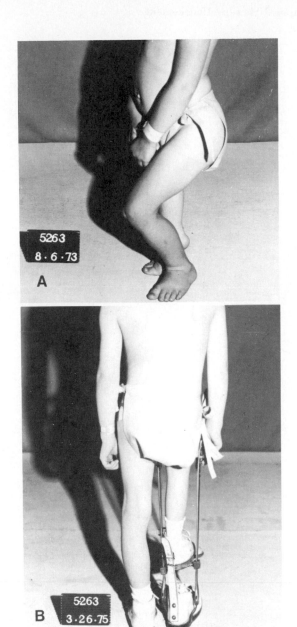

Figure 9-21. A. *A child with extensive shortening of the lower right limb. In order for her to stand on tiptoes on the right, she must bend the left knee to a right angle. B. This condition requires that she wear a large built-up caliper orthosis to allow more effective ambulation. (From Lovell WW, Winter RB eds. Pediatric Orthopaedics. 2nd ed., Philadelphia: JB Lippincott; 1986: 787.)*

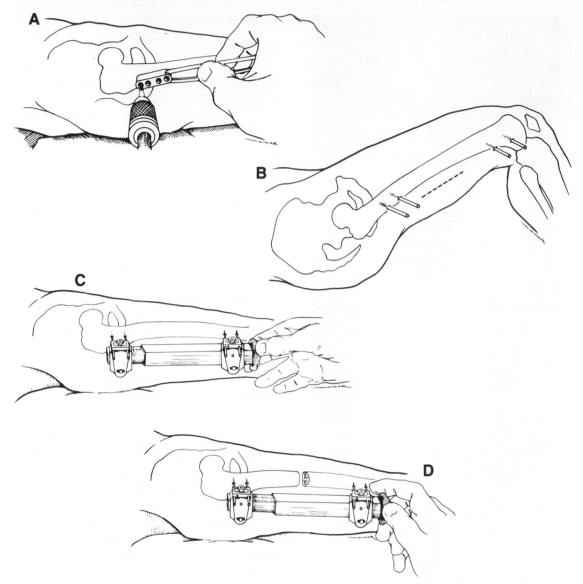

Figure 9-22. *The Wagner method of femoral lengthening consists of placing two 6-mm Schanz pins in the distal fragment. A. A template is used, and with the patient supine, a 3.2-mm drill hole is made at the level of the lesser trochanter. B. The Schanz screws are placed in the femur, well anterior to the incision for osteotomy. C. The lengthening device is applied, but the device should be reversed to that shown. D. The fragments are distracted at least 1 cm and the wound is closed. (From Lovell WW, Winter RB, eds.* Pediatric Orthopaedics. *2nd ed. Philadelphia: JB Lippincott; 1986: 834.)*

Figure 9-23. *Technique of Wagner femoral lengthening demonstrated on a 13-year-old boy with a congenital shortening of the right lower limb who had previously undergone tibial lengthening for a shortening of 8 cm. A. The orthoroentgenogram shows that the lower limb is still 4 cm short. B. 10 weeks after Wagner femoral lengthening, the amount of bone bridging the distracted fragment is obviously inadequate; therefore, an autogenous bone grafting and plating of the femur were accomplished. C. The results of the plating and grafting procedure. (From Morrissy RT.* Lovell and Winter's *Pediatric Orthopaedics. 3rd ed. Philadelphia: JB Lippincott; 1990: 804.)*

▶

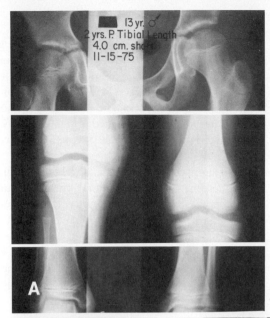

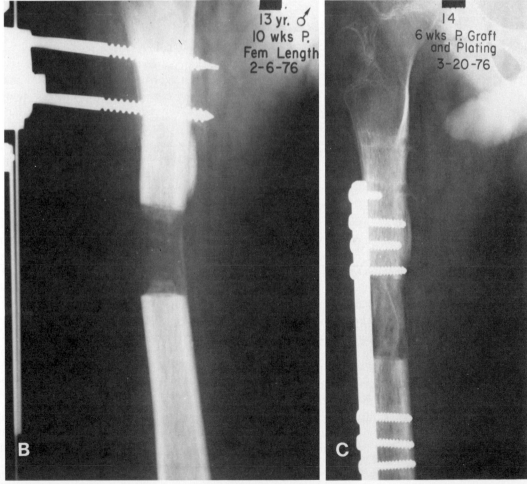

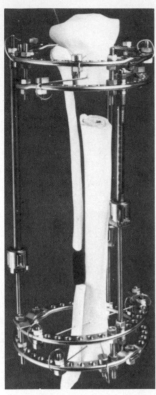

Figure 9-24. *Ilizarov lengthening device. External fixation is accomplished by tensioned wires affixed to circumferential rings. (From* The Ilizarov External Fixator (General Surgical Technique Brochure). *Richards Medical Company, 1988.)*

Orthopedic Assessment

Spinal alignment should be evaluated, with particular emphasis on scoliosis. Any curves should be identified as structural or functional, and compensatory curves should be identified. Pelvic obliquity is noted, as is hip subluxation or dislocation. Stability and alignment of the knee and ankle should be assessed. Lower extremity alignment and stability are important because surgery places extra stress on all joints, and may predispose the patient to varus/valgus or ligamentous laxity and instability.

Limb lengths should be measured with the child in a supine position. The pelvis must be level and the hips and knees in a neutral position with a symmetric degree of abduction at the hip. Limb length is measured from the anterosuperior iliac spine to the medial malleolus. The length measurements may be inaccurate if pelvic obliquity or asymmetry of the anterosuperior iliac spine exists. A second method of measurement can be used. This method uses the umbilicus and the medial malleolus. The therapist should document the sites used for measuring.

A postural evaluation with the child standing should be done by using a plumb line or posture grid. Abnormalities should be noted. The posture evaluation may be used to identify the proper lift to be used in a patient's shoe. A level pelvis is seen when the proper lift is used. The pelvis cannot be used to determine the fit of a lift when a fixed pelvic obliquity exists. The shoulders can be used as a point of reference in this instance (Figs. 9-25 to 9-27).

Range of Motion

Because contractures often alter limb measurements and gait patterns, careful goniometric assessment is important. Existing knee and ankle contractures are often exacerbated by tibial and femoral lengthening. Contracture of the Achilles tendon often follows years of compensation for the LLD. An active program of stretching, as necessary, will provide for a more normal gait pattern after equalization of the limb by surgery.

Strength

Careful and specific manual muscle testing will document weakness. The shorter limb, which is often preferred for function, commonly has reduced strength. Muscle absence or weakness are often concomitant findings if the LLD results from congenital anomalies. Because the surgical procedures can change bone length and muscle mechanics, weakness that is present before surgery is often more noticeable after surgery. The importance of strengthening exercises cannot be overstated.

Gait Analysis

Complete gait analysis should be done at the initial evaluation and after the insertion of a lift. Because shoe lifts will affect posture and function in differ-

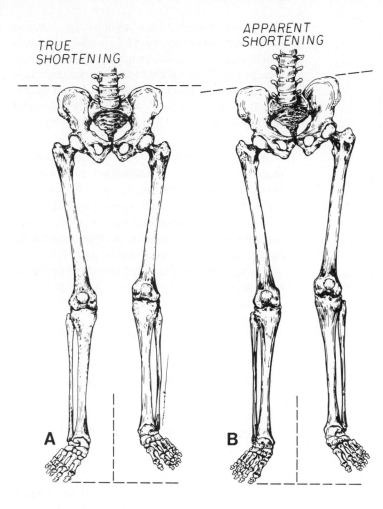

TRUE SHORTENING

APPARENT SHORTENING

A

B

Figure 9-25. *The difference between true shortening (A) and apparent shortening (B). A. In the case of true shortening, the limb from the hip joint to the ankle is short by actual measurement. B. As a result of pelvic obliquity, abduction contracture of the apparent short side or abduction contracture of the apparent long side (the side on which the pelvis is elevated) appears shorter than its opposite member. The limb lengths, however, are actually the same. (From Lovell WW, Winter RB, eds. Pediatric Orthopaedics. 2nd ed. Philadelphia: JB Lippincott; 1986: 799.)*

ent ways, the therapist must evaluate both before determining the proper lift height.

Prosthetic and Orthotic Evaluation

A complete evaluation of orthoses or prostheses is done when appropriate.

Skin

Integrity of the skin is evaluated, with particular emphasis before surgery and when orthoses or prostheses are used.

Sensation

A complete sensory evaluation should be done when surgery is planned. This is particularly impor-

tant to be able to compare postoperative sensation with the preoperative level.

Assessment of Functional Skills

The child's ability to ambulate; ascend and descend stairs, ramps, and curbs; and instruction in the use of crutches or other assistive devices should be part of this preoperative evaluation.

Physical Therapy for Specific Surgeries

EPIPHYSIODESIS. Physical therapy is minimal after epiphysiodesis. After the surgery, the child is placed in some type of soft dressing or a knee immobilizer. Physical therapy is directed toward gait training several days after surgery. Gait activities

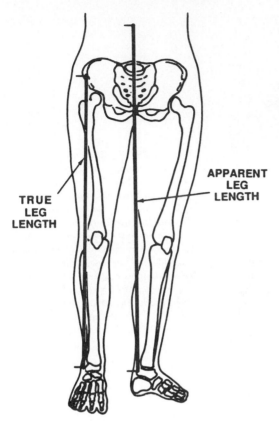

Figure 9-26. *Measurement of real and apparent lengths. The measurement of real length is relatively immune error because of pelvic obliquity, whereas measurement of apparent length is susceptible to such error. (From Morrissy RT. Lovell and Winter's Pediatric Orthopaedics. 3rd ed. Philadelphia: JB Lippincott; 1990: 781.)*

are done with either partial weight bearing or with weight bearing to tolerance. Strength and ROM are evaluated and treatment is provided as necessary. Fusion of the epiphysis occurs in approximately 3 months.

BONE SHORTENING. Children with weakness should be involved in preoperative strengthening exercises. In addition to exercises, non–weight-bearing crutch walking can be taught before surgery. A soft dressing is usually applied after surgery. Isometric exercise for the quadriceps and

gluteus maximus, and use of ankle pumps, is begun immediately after surgery. The exercise regimen is progressed to a complete program as pain and tolerance permit. Non–weight-bearing crutch training is begun when the patient has recovered from the initial effects of surgery and anesthesia. Partial weight bearing begins around 3 months after surgery.

BONE LENGTHENING. The Wagner procedure requires prolonged hospitalization and intensive physical therapy. Preoperative family education about the surgery and subsequent rehabilitation is essential. The preoperative program begins with assessment of lower extremity ROM and strength. Gait training and transfer techniques to be used after surgery are taught and practiced before the operation.

Quadricep-setting exercises are begun on the first day after surgery and the patient attempts to sit over the edge of the bed with the knee flexed to 90 degrees. Exercise sessions are scheduled twice a day as the patient progresses. Active-assisted knee flexion and extension is stressed, and hip and ankle exercise is done to increase motion and strength. Ice, heat, and gentle massage or vibration can help to control pain and facilitate ROM. Knee flexion or extension splints and a positioning schedule can help in regaining joint mobility. Partial weight-bearing ambulation may begin as early as the third day after surgery, but many orthopedic surgeons differ in this early approach. The therapist must be aware of subluxation of the patella or of the tibia resulting from the pull of the quadriceps and hamstrings. Sensation must be evaluated daily to identify any signs of nerve injury as soon as possible.

Physical therapy is similar to that following the Ilizarov procedure, which approach was recently reviewed.[46]

Scoliosis

Scoliosis is defined as a lateral curvature of the spine with a rotatory component. Scoliosis may develop in a localized area, or it may involve the entire vertebral column. The curve may vary in sever-

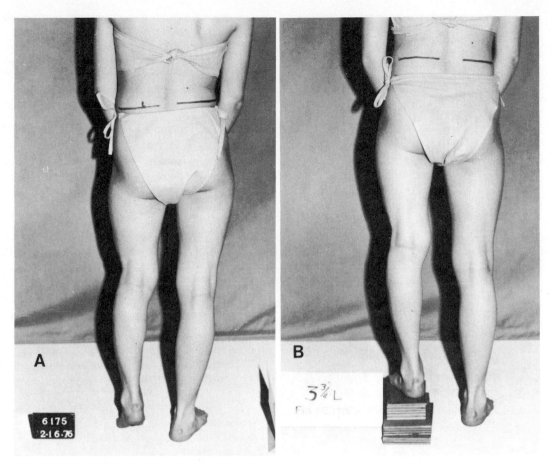

Figure 9-27. A. *A child with almost 4 inches of shortening as a result of traumatic distal femoral and proximal tibial epiphyseal arrests. B. The amount of lift needed under the heel to achieve a level pelvis. The exact height of the blocks necessary to achieve equalization is included. (From Lovell WW, Winter RB, eds. Pediatric Orthopaedics. 2nd ed. Philadelphia: JB Lippincott; 1986: 800.)*

ity from mild to severe. The incidence in young children is distributed equally between the sexes, but there is a female predominance of 90% beyond 10 years of age. Scoliosis may be idiopathic, neuromuscular, or congenital, based on its cause. This section discusses adolescent idiopathic scoliosis—the most common form of the disorder. Idiopathic scoliosis involves a lateral curvature of the spine of unknown cause. The four curve patterns seen include thoracic; thoracolumbar, with the apex at the T-12 or L-1 vertebral body; lumbar; or double

major curve. The right thoracic curve is the most common in the adolescent group (Fig. 9-28).

Idiopathic scoliosis is either structural or nonstructural. A *nonstructural scoliosis* may be defined as a lateral curve with no structural alterations in the vertebral column. The nonstructural curve disappears with forward trunk flexion, recumbency, suspension, and volitional correction. The nonstructural curve has no rotary component or compensatory curve and is nonprogressive. A discrepancy in leg length is the most common reason

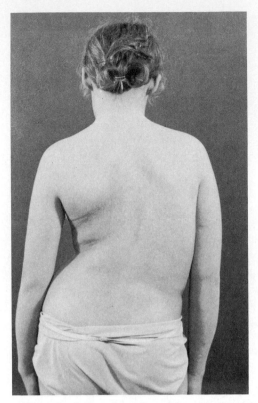

Figure 9-28. *Back view of a patient with a right thoracic curve. (From Morrissy RT. Lovell and Winter's Pediatric Orthopaedics. 3rd ed. Philadelphia: JB Lippincott; 1990: 627.)*

for nonstructural scoliosis. Other causes include postural abnormalities, muscle spasm, and spinal neoplasm. By contrast, structural scoliosis is characterized by distinct alterations in the vertebral column. There is no volitional correction, flexibility of the back varies, and structural changes depend on the degree of severity and progression of the curve. These curves frequently have compensatory curvature, and the vertebral bodies are rotated toward the convex side.

Some terminology used when identifying curvatures include the following:

• *Primary or major curve:* the largest lateral curve with structural changes and the greatest degree of vertebral body rotation

• *Double major curve:* two primary curves of equal or almost equal degree

• *Minor or compensatory curves:* curves that develop above and below the primary curve and in the opposite direction to the primary curve

• *Decompensation:* the degree to which the child's posture is out of balance or alignment

The minor or compensatory curves maintain the head vertically over the pelvis in accordance with the horizontal ocular righting reaction. Minor curves have a smaller rotational component at an early stage, but may develop structural changes.

Clinical Features

Signs and symptoms of scoliosis are straightforward. Because many otherwise obvious signs are hidden by clothing, diagnosis and treatment are often delayed, especially in the adolescent population. With the advent of school screening programs in the 1940s, which are currently mandated by school health codes or state law in many states, scoliosis is being detected and treated at an earlier stage. Clinical signs commonly seen with scoliosis include the following:

Shoulders that are not level
Prominent and slightly elevated scapula
Prominent breast
Pelvis that is not level
Asymmetric waist curves
Deformity of the back
Poor posture
Trunk rotation with rib prominence
Leg length discrepancy
Mild back pain (which should be completely evaluated)

The precise cause of idiopathic scoliosis is still unknown. Current theories include muscle weakness; disturbances in growth plates; and metabolic, hormonal, or genetic disturbances. Many support the idea that scoliosis is inherited as a multifactorial genetic disorder.[47] Pathologists have described scoliosis as distorted vertebrae with the vertebral body shifted toward the convex side. Because the ribs attach to the rotated vertebral bodies, the ribs themselves "project" or "hump." The greater the rotational component of the scoliosis, the greater is the clinical deformity (Fig. 9-29).[48]

In addition to musculoskeletal changes, restrictive pulmonary changes may occur as rib cage distortion compresses the lungs. Lung volumes become reduced, although at insignificant levels, in the patient with a 60-degree curve. The pulmonary component becomes significant and threatening when the curve reaches 90 degrees. Studies on pulmonary function should be done routinely for patients with severe curves.

Prognosis

Factors of prognostic significance include sex, curve pattern and severity, and growth potential. Girls whose scoliosis is detected before menarche have the greatest chance for progression of the condition (66%), whereas those whose curves are detected after menarche have a less severe progression (33%). Most girls reach skeletal maturity 2 years after menarche.[49]

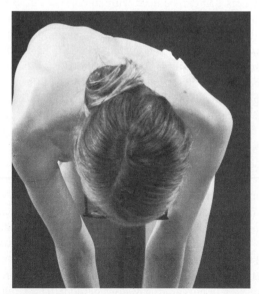

Figure 9-29. *Forward bending to show rib hump associated with thoracic rotation. (Lovell WW, Winter RB, eds. Pediatric Orthopaedics. 2nd ed. Philadelphia: JB Lippincott; 1986: 547.)*

Differing rates of progression are associated with different curves. Thoracic curves show the greatest progression in skeletally immature adolescents. The double major curve and thoracic lordosis concurrent with scoliosis are the next most rapidly progressive curves. The greater the initial degree of curvature, the greater is the potential for progression. Lumbar curves have the least risk for progression.[50]

Another predictor of progression is the Risser grade. The Risser sign indicates capping of the iliac apophysis and is graded from 1 to 4. The lower the grade, the further from skeletal maturity is the patient and the greater is the likelihood of progression.[51]

Despite several predictive techniques, it is impossible to accurately predict which curves will develop and which ones will not. Speculation about progression after an initial evaluation can be made only in general terms. Progression after skeletal maturity is seen in curves greater than 30 degrees and particularly in thoracic curves. Pregnancy does not appear to influence the progression of a curve.

Medical Management

When scoliosis is suspected, the child should be referred to an orthopedic surgeon who will do a complete evaluation. A roentgenographic series for scoliosis will enable the physician to calculate the degree of curvature and differentiate between primary and compensatory curves (Fig. 9-30). Two recent nonroentgenographic techniques for assessing curve progression are moiré shadow pattern topography and the Integrated Shape Investigation System.[52] The physician will decide on a type of treatment based on both the physical examination and the roentgenographic series. Most curves of 20 degrees or less are routinely seen on periodic roentgenograms, or using one of the nonroentgenographic techniques at 3- to 6-month intervals. In addition to the roentgenographic determination of the angle of curvature, one of various methods may be used to quantify the degree of rotation. These methods may include a Scoliometer (Orthopedic

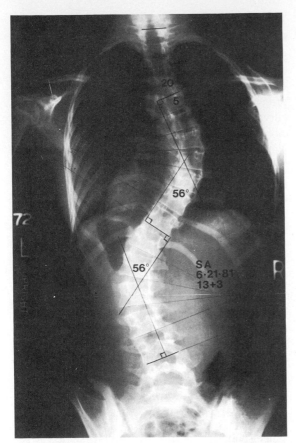

Figure 9-30. *A typical scoliosis with a line drawn along the lower endplate of each vertebra. Note that the lines converge to the left for the right thoracic curve and to the right for the left lumbar curve. The most tilted vertebrae are the end vertebrae of the curve. At the junction of the two curves, one vertebra is the end vertebra of both curves (the "transitional" vertebra). After selection of the lower end vertebra of the curve (the vertebra most tilted from the horizontal), a line is placed along the endplate of this vertebra, and a perpendicular is erected from that. Similarly, the upper end vertebra is selected, a line is drawn along its upper endplate, and a perpendicular is erected that crosses the first one drawn. The angle of intersection is the angle of the curvature (Cobb-Lippman technique of scoliosis measurement). The proper measurement of the double major curve pattern is shown here. One line on the transitional vertebra serves for measurement of both upper and lower curves. (From Morrissy RT. Lovell and Winter's Pediatric Orthopaedics. 3rd ed. Philadelphia: JB Lippincott; 1990: 628.)*

System Inc, Hayward, CA 94545), a type of inclinometer; the moiré topographic technique; and the back contour device. Pearsall, Read, and Hedden recently compared three methods for measuring scoliosis and found improved validity of measurement within the thoracic region as compared to the lumbar region.[53]

Bracing for children with progressive curves of 25 degrees or more has been used for more than 40 years. The goal of orthotic management is to maintain, rather than correct, the curve by using the three-point principle of fixation. This principle uses force directly at the apex of the curve in conjunction with two points of counterforce. Bracing is commonly initiated in a child whose curve is more than 30 degrees at the initial visit, or when a curve progresses by 5 degrees in 6 months. Although traditional treatment is based on the child wearing the brace for 23 hours a day, recent studies have suggested that 12-hour use is as effective.[54]

The Milwaukee brace, developed by Blount and Schmidt in 1946, is a cervicothoracolumbosacral orthosis that can be used with all curves. The Boston Bracing System employs a thoracolumbosacral orthosis (TLSO) used for low thoracic and lumbar curves. The TLSO is a custom-molded jacket with the same indications for use as the Boston jacket. The Boston System eliminates some of the unsightly metal portions of the Milwaukee Brace, thereby providing better cosmesis.

Lateral electrical surface stimulation is a nonoperative approach to treatment that was thought to hold great promise in the early 1980s.[55,56] This approach involved the application of stimulation via surface electrodes on the convex side of the curve using a portable single- or dual-channel electrical stimulator while the child was asleep. Sullivan and co-workers reported the results of a study in which 114 of 142 subjects were compliant in using electrical stimulation until skeletal maturity. A 10% progression in curvature was considered to be a failure of treatment. When subjects who were noncompliant were added to the failures, there was a total failure rate of 56%. Based on the results, the authors recommended that electrical stimulation not be considered an alternative to orthotic management. (Figs. 9-31 and 9-32).[57]

Surgical Management

Surgical management consists of spinal fusion and is considered when the curve develops to more than 40 degrees. The specific type of surgery depends on the severity and pattern of the curve and the personal preference of the surgeon. Cassella and Hall state that the traditional aims of surgery are to safely straighten the spine, balance the trunk on the pelvis, and stabilize the spine by arthrodesis or fusion.[52] Fusions can be done either anteriorly or posteriorly, and some curves may require both ap-

proaches. Rib resection is occasionally done for cosmetic purposes when the rib hump is severe and disfiguring. Common posterior fusions use the Harrington rod, which requires either bracing or casting for immobilization after surgery and results in restricted activity (Fig. 9-33). A newer procedure—the Cotrel-Dubousset procedure—requires no bracing or casting after surgery. The Cotrel-Duboussett apparatus includes cross-links that attach vertical rods, thereby providing good stability in most planes. Luque sublamina wiring with rods requires no immobilization, but restricted activity is suggested, with no exertion greater than walking for 1 year. Because of the specifics of the Luque procedure, there is increased risk of injury to the spinal cord. As a result of this risk, the Luque procedure is

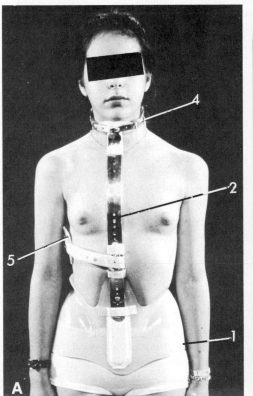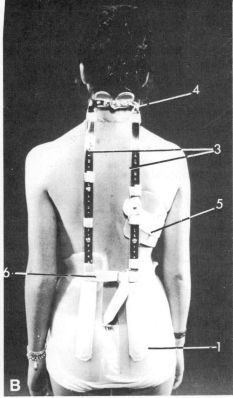

Figure 9-31. A *and* B. *Milwaukee brace. (From Morrissy RT.* Lovell and Winter's Pediatric Orthopaedics. *3rd ed. Philadelphia: JB Lippincott; 1990: 644.)*

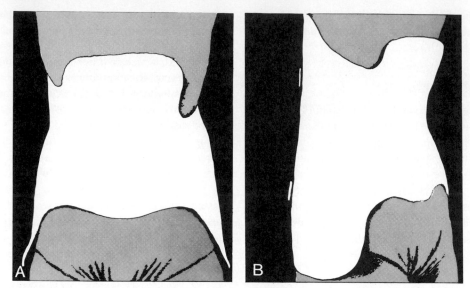

Figure 9-32. A and B. *The Boston Jacket, a thoracolumbosacral orthosis used for low thoracic and lumbar curves. (Adapted from Redford JWB:* Orthotics, Etcetera. *2nd ed. Baltimore: Williams and Wilkins; 1980; redrawn by Christopher Metzger, Beaver College, Glenside, PA)*

not the one preferred for idiopathic adolescent scoliosis, but is more commonly used in the child who is not neurologically intact.[58] Anterior fusions, including the Dwyer and Zielke procedures, are seldom used for idiopathic adolescent scoliosis.

Physical Therapy Management

Exercise

Exercise has no effect on either reducing the curve or on preventing its progression. The primary benefit of exercise, therefore, is to help with the bracing program, to help reduce back pain, and to maintain or improve ROM. Cassella and Hall identified five outcomes for an exercise program used during bracing:[52]

1. Maintain corrected alignment during and after bracing program
2. Maintain proper respiration and chest mobility
3. Maintain muscle strength, particularly in abdominals
4. Maintain ROM and spinal flexibility
5. Resume pre-bracing functional skills

Despite the importance the physical therapy and rehabilitation literature places upon exercise for children with scoliosis, particularly those treated with orthotics, others are not as optimistic about the efficacy of exercise. Carman et al. reported no attributable effects of exercise, either in decreasing curve progression or increasing curve correction, in a group of 24 females using the Milwaukee Brace.[59] Moreover, Kehl and Morrissy state that the efficacy of exercise in the orthotic management of scoliosis is questionable.[60]

Lateral Electrical Surface Stimulation

The physical therapist has a great deal of responsibility for the patient with scoliosis who is being treated by electrical stimulation. The physician and the therapist will usually work together in evaluating potential candidates for stimulation. The therapist is responsible for proper placement of electrodes, as identified by strong contraction of muscles. The therapist also teaches the patient and family about the stimulator, its use, associated skin

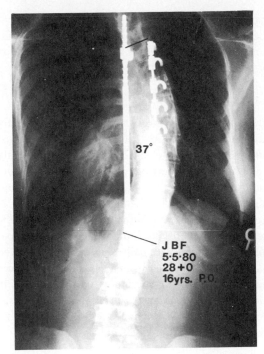

Figure 9-33. *A Harrington rod is used to correct to 37 degrees a scoliosis that had been 102 degrees. (From Lovell WW, Winter RB, eds.* Pediatric Orthopaedics. *2nd ed. Philadelphia: JB Lippincott; 1986: 597.)*

problems, and proper exercises for spinal movement. The therapist must be able to interpret from roentgenograms the proper placement of electrodes and make changes when necessary. The physical therapist assumes major daily responsibility, under the direction of the physician, for coordinating, implementing, and modifying the treatment of patients with electrical stimulation.[56]

Operative Concerns

The patient who undergoes surgery for scoliosis should benefit from preoperative respiratory instruction in deep diaphragmatic breathing, coughing, and other techniques of bronchial hygiene that will prevent postoperative pulmonary complications. In addition to the obvious pulmonary concerns, early mobilization and prevention of venous thrombosis are other major postoperative goals for physical therapy.

Fractures in Childhood

Fractures that occur during childhood are treated differently than those that occur during adulthood. Children's fractures may be classified into four types (Fig. 9-34). A buckle fracture, commonly

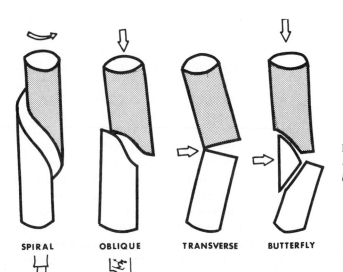

SPIRAL   OBLIQUE   TRANSVERSE   BUTTERFLY

Figure 9-34. *Fracture types in children. (From Rang M.* Children's Fractures. *2nd ed. Philadelphia: JB Lippincott; 1983: 5.)*

seen around the metaphysis of a young child, is a compression fracture that causes a crimping of the bone (Fig. 9-35). Bending or bowing fractures, usually seen in the ulna and fibula, are not true fractures, and the bone will straighten itself, but will do so incompletely (Fig. 9-36). A greenstick fracture occurs when the side of the shaft under greatest tension breaks, while the side being compressed suffers a bowing defect (Fig. 9-37). Complete fractures occur when the entire shaft of the bone loses its continuity; these may be classified as transverse, spiral, oblique, butterfly, or other (Fig. 9-38).[61]

Fractures in children usually heal quickly; therefore, reduction should be done promptly. When there is significant damage to the epiphyseal

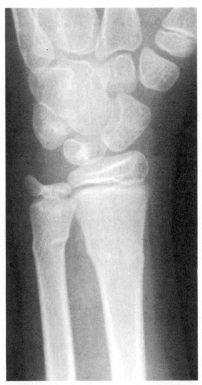

Figure 9-35. *Buckle fracture in a 10-year-old child. The compressed bone has erupted on the surface in the same way mountain ranges were pushed up on the earth. (From Rang M.* Children's Fractures. *2nd ed. Philadelphia: JB Lippincott; 1983: 2.)*

growth plate, children are at risk for the development of bony deformities. When the epiphysis is injured, slight overgrowth is the rule, and retardation of growth is the exception.

Clavicle

The clavicle is one of the bones most frequently fractured, and the mid-shaft is the area that is most often fractured. The clavicle, which is the only bony connection between the shoulder girdle and the trunk, is at risk for fracture when force is applied to an outstretched hand, elbow, or shoulder. A fractured clavicle is a common birth injury to the neonate. Symptoms are characterized by pseudoparalysis of the arm with pain when the arm is moved passively. Rest is usually an adequate and effective treatment. Greenstick fractures of the clavicle in older children are treated with a figure-of-eight harness for 4 weeks. Reduction may be necessary for a displaced or overriding clavicular fracture.

Femoral Shaft

Approximately 70% of femoral shaft fractures in childhood occur in the middle third of the shaft, 18% in the proximal third, and the remaining 12% in the distal third. Closed fractures of the shaft are treated conservatively with immobilization in a cast for 6 to 8 weeks, depending on the age of the child. Rotation of and angulation of the distal fragment must be prevented if the fracture is displaced. Prevention is accomplished by way of either Buck's or Bryant's skin traction, which holds the legs in a symmetric position while the distractive force is applied. Sloughing of skin and ischemic necrosis caused by circulatory compromise are two well-established complications of skin traction in children, and everyone working with the child must be aware of the early signs of these complications.

Open reduction is rarely necessary in children. When surgery is needed to reduce a fractured femoral shaft, complications may include osteomyelitis, gross deformity, nonunion, numerous fractures, and even death.

Recent studies have examined approaches with

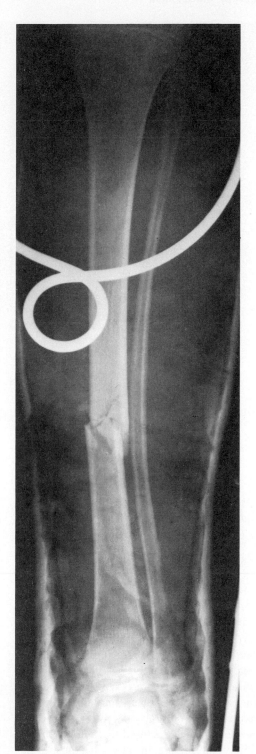

Figure 9-36. *Bending of the fibula in a 12-year-old child. The position remained unchanged, and no new bone formed around the fibula. Remodeling did not occur, even after 4 years. (From Rang M. Children's Fractures. 2nd ed. Philadelphia: JB Lippincott; 1983: 3.)*

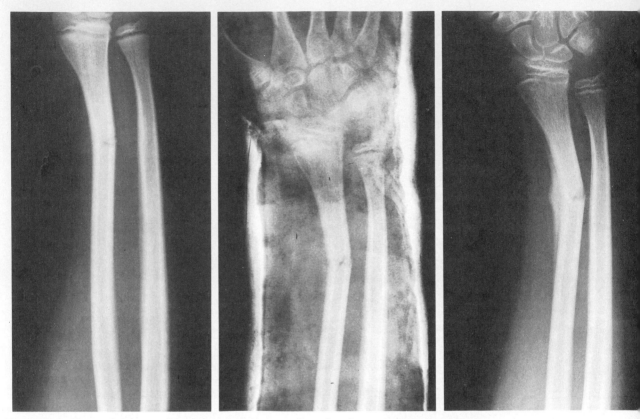

Figure 9-37. *Greenstick fracture of the radius. One cortex was bent, the other gaping. The initial angulation is acceptable, but it has increased and should have been corrected. (From Rang M. Children's Fractures. 2nd ed. Philadelphia: JB Lippincott; 1983: 4.)*

casting and bracing to provide for fracture stabilization while enabling the child to ambulate.[62,63]

Shaft of the Tibia and Fibula

The degree of injury to bones of the leg varies, depending on the age of the child. In infants and in children younger than 6 years of age, torsion of the foot produces a spiral fracture of the tibia with no break in the fibula. In the older child (5 to 10 years of age), direct trauma may produce a transverse fracture of both bones without displacement. These types represent the most common mechanisms for fractures of the leg.

Spiral fractures of the tibia require immobilization with a plaster long-leg cast for 3 weeks in the infant and for 4 to 5 weeks in the older child. When both the tibia and fibula are fractured and displaced, manipulation after administration of a general anesthetic is often necessary to provide satisfactory reduction.

Ankle

In the infant, a transverse greenstick fracture caused by trauma just proximal to the distal epiphysés may involve the tibia alone or both the tibia and fibula. Treatment usually consists of immobilization in a long-leg cast for 3 weeks. In children between 3 and 12 years of age, an ankle fracture often involves the epiphyses directly. The distal tibial epiphysis is often fractured in an ankle injury. After epiphyseal fracture, the physician must ascer-

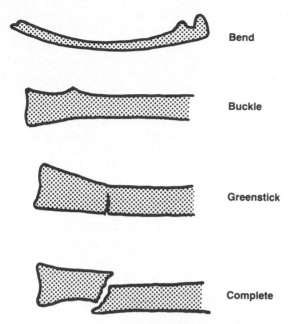

Figure 9-38. *The shape of the fracture indicates how it was produced. Spiral fractures are shaped like a pen nib, whereas oblique fractures are shaped like a ski jump. (From Rang M. Children's Fractures. 2nd ed. Philadelphia: JB Lippincott; 1983: 2.)*

Bend

Buckle

Greenstick

Complete

tain by review of roentgenograms that growth has not been disturbed.

Epiphysis

Epiphyseal fractures are generally treated like other fractures, but they always have the potential for growth disturbance. Crush injuries to the epiphyseal plate can result in either growth retardation of the segment or angular deformity as one portion of the epiphysis continues to grow. Although Salter and Harris have described five specific types of epiphyseal fracture, a discussion of each type is beyond the scope of this chapter.[64]

Physical Therapy Management

The physical therapist has a minimal role in treating fractures in children. The child may occasionally need instruction in gait training, self-help activity, or daily activities. When exercises are suggested,

they are usually intended to increase ROM and strength of the limb in which the fracture occurred. The therapist must be gentle in order to obtain the child's cooperation and to prevent displacement of healing fragments. Strong, aggressive exercise is not indicated for children with fractures.

Tibia Vara (Blount's Disease)

Tibia vara is a disorder caused by a growth disturbance of unknown etiology in the medial portion of the proximal tibial epiphysis. Because most children with tibia vara are overweight, abnormal stress on the epiphysis has been suggested as a possible cause. Neither trauma nor infection can be implicated as causes. Tibia vara occurs most commonly during the first 3 years of life, although a second type is seen after 9 years of age. A recent histopathologic evaluation of the physeal zones in children with late-onset tibia vara showed abnormalities that were very similar to early-onset disease, and to slipped capital femoral epiphysis. The authors of this study suggested that asymmetric compressive and shear forces acting across the physis were common to all three disorders.[65] The more common infantile disorder occurs in obese children who walk at an early age. The course of tibia vara is generally progressive.[66]

Clinical Features

The diagnosis of tibia vara is based on both clinical and roentgenographic findings, with the differential diagnosis including physiologic bowlegs, trauma, and rickets. The disease may be bilateral or unilateral, and is classified into six different stages based on the child's age and on the bony changes.[67] Bowing of the tibia is the only specific finding on physical examination. The varus deformity may increase during the stance phase of gait, and the child often walks with knee flexion. Knee instability is often a problem for the child with tibia vara (Fig. 9-39).

Medical Management

Treatment may be unnecessary for the young child with minimal deformity or roentgenographic

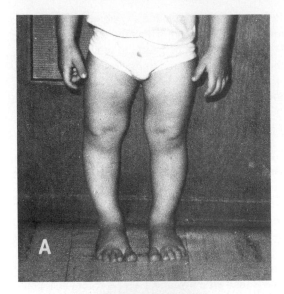

Figure 9-39. A. *A 2-year-old child with varus on weight bearing.* B. *A roentgenogram of the same patient at 2 years of age, showing early Blount's disease.* C. *At 2½ years of age, the changes of Blount's disease have progressed.*

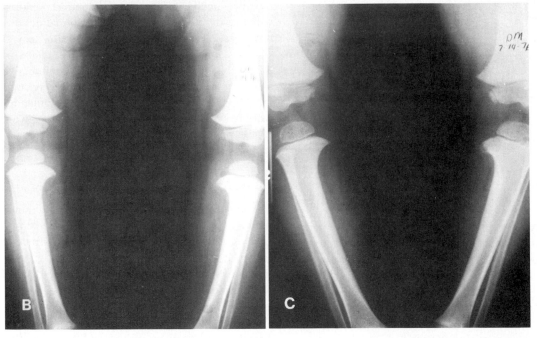

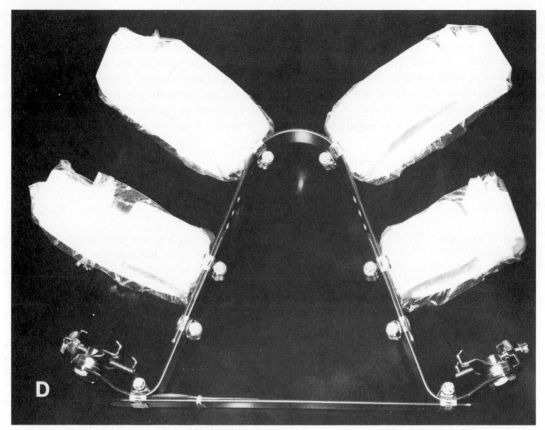

Figure 9-39. *(continued)* D. *The patient now wears this orthosis at night. (From Lovell WW, Winter RB, eds. Pediatric Orthopaedics. 2nd ed. Philadelphia: JB Lippincott; 1983: 872.)*

changes, as the deformity may resolve spontaneously. The preferred approach for the minimally involved child consists of periodic monitoring or use of a correct orthosis. It should be noted that these orthoses are difficult to fit and are often disliked by the children because of difficulty turning in bed. An osteotomy is often performed for an older child with more advanced bony changes, but is also indicated for a younger child with an obviously progressive deformity.[68] The initial osteotomy is usually totally corrective for the child 8 years of age or younger, but for the older child, a second operation is often necessary.[69]

Physical Therapy Management

The physical therapy evaluation should include lower extremity goniometry, manual muscle testing, gait analysis, sensory evaluation, and an orthotic evaluation, if appropriate. A recent study of goniometric reliability and effect of lower extremity position was reported by Lohmann and Rayhel. They determined that tibia vara measurements were reliable both within and between examiners within 2 to 3 degrees. They further determined that a significant difference in values existed among three different lower extremity positions.[70]

Parental instruction in proper donning and doffing of the orthosis is the major aspect of physical therapy for the young child. A younger child fitted with an orthosis may require gait training and an assistive device, often a walker, for a brief period. The type of orthosis depends on whether it is intended for gait or for use at night only.

The child who is treated with tibial osteotomy will usually be placed in a cast for up to 8 weeks. After removal of the cast, physical therapy takes the form of therapeutic exercise to gradually increase ROM and strength to the lower extremity. Gait training is begun when adequate knee motion and appropriate strength is achieved. Some physicians may choose to use an orthosis during ambulation for several weeks after surgery.

References

1. Audrey N. *Orthopedia.* Vols. 1 and 2. Philadelphia: JB Lippincott; 1961.
2. Tylkowski CM. Assessment of gait in children and adolescents. In: Lovell WW, Winter RB, eds. *Pediatric Orthopedics.* 2nd ed. Philadelphia: JB Lippincott; 1986:1076–77.
3. Shores M. Footprint analysis in gait documentation. *Phys Ther.* 1980; 60:1163–1167.
4. MacEwen GD, Bunnell WP, Ramsey PR. The hip. In: Lovell WW, Winter RB, eds. *Pediatric Orthopedics.* 2nd ed. Philadelphia: JB Lippincott; 1986.
5. Wilkinson JA. Etiologic factors in congenital displacement of the hip and myelodysplasia. *Clin Orthop.* 1992;281:75–83.
6. Tredwell SJ. Neonatal screening for hip joint instability. Its clinical and economic relevance. *Clin Orthop.* 1992;281:63–68.
7. Millis MB, Share JC. Use of ultrasonography in dysplasia of the immature hip. *Clin Orthop.* 1992; 274:160–171.
8. Harcke HT. Imaging in congenital dislocation and dysplasia of the hip. *Clin Orthop.* 1992;281:22–28.
9. Tucci JJ, Kumar SJ, Guille JT, Rubbo ER. Late acetabular dysplasia following early successful Pavlik harness treatment of congenital dislocation of the hip. *J Pediatr Orthop.* 1991;11:502–505.
10. Quinn CM, Wigglesworth JS, Heckmatt J. Lethal arthrogryposis multiplex congenita: A pathological study of 21 cases. *Histopathology.* 1991;19:155–162.
11. Stern WG. Arthrogryposis multiplex congenita. *J Am Med Assoc.* 1923;81:1507.
12. Drennan JC. Neuromuscular disorders. In: Lovell WW, Winter RB, eds. *Pediatric Orthopedics.* 2nd ed. Philadelphia: JB Lippincott; 1986: 320–321.
13. Robinson RO. Arthrogryposis multiplex congenita: Feeding, language, and other health problems. *Neuropediatrics.* 1990;21:177–178.
14. Thompson G, Bilenher R. Comprehensive management of arthrogryposis multiplex congenita. *Clin Orthop Rel Res.* 1985;194:7.
15. Saarwak JF, MacEwen GD, Scott CI. Amyoplasia (a common form of arthrogryposis). *J Bone Joint Surg.* 1990;72A:465–469.
16. Moore P, Major R, Stallard J, Butler P. Contracture correction device for arthrogryposis. *Physiotherapy.* 1990;76:303–305.
17. Sillence DO, Senn A, Danks DM. Genetic heterogeneity in osteogenesis imperfecta. *J Med Genet.* 1979; 16:101.
18. Zaleske DJ, Doppert SH, Mankin HJ. Metabolic and endocrine abnormalities in the immature skeleton. In: Lovell WW, Winter RB, eds. *Pediatric Orthopedics.* 2nd ed. Philadelphia: JB Lippincott; 1986:113–114.
19. Salter RB. *Textbook of Diseases and Injuries of the Musculoskeletal System.* Baltimore: Williams & Wilkins; 1983:138–139.
20. Wenstrup RJ, Willing MC, Starman BJ, Byers PH. Distinct biochemical phenotypes predict clinical severity in nonlethal variants of osteogenesis imperfecta. *Am J Hum Genet.* 1990;46:975–982.
21. Hanscome DA, Winter RB, Lutter L, et al. Osteogenesis imperfecta. Radiographic classification, natural history, and treatment of spinal deformities. *J Bone Joint Surg.* 1992;74A:598–616.
22. King JD, Bobechko WP. Osteogenesis imperfecta:

An orthopedic description and surgical review. *J Bone Joint Surg.* 1971;53B:72.

23. Gamble JG, Rinsky LA, Strudwick J, Bleck EE. Non-union of fractures in children who have osteogenesis imperfecta. *J Bone Joint Surg.* 1988; 70A:439–443.

24. Nishi Y, Hamamoto K, Kajiyama M, et al. Effect of long-term calcitonin therapy by injection and nasal spray on the incidence of fractures in osteogenesis imperfecta. *J Pediatr.* 1992;121:477–480.

25. Bailey RW, Dubow HI. Experimental and clinical studies of longitudinal bone growth: Utilizing a new method of internal fixation crossing the epiphyseal plate. *J Bone Joint Surg.* 1965;47A:1669.

26. Gitelis S, Whiffen J, DeWald RL. Treatment of severe scoliosis in osteogenesis imperfecta. *Clin Orthop.* 1983;175:56.

27. Gerber LH, Binder H, Weintrob J, et al. Rehabilitation of children and infants with osteogenesis imperfecta: A program for ambulation. *Clin Orthop.* 1990;251:254–262.

28. Freeman MAR, England JPS. Experimental infarction of the immature canine femoral head. *Proc R Soc Med.* 1969;62:431.

29. Canale ST. Osteochondroses. In: Canale ST, Beaty JH, eds. *Operative Pediatric Orthopedics,* St. Louis: Mosby-Yearbook; 1991:743.

30. Jonsater S. Coxa plana: A histopathologic and arthrographic study. *Acta Orthop Scand* 12 (suppl): 1953.

31. Catterall A. The natural history of Perthés disease. *J Bone Joint Surg.* 1971;53B:37.

32. Petrie JG, Bitenc I. The abduction weight-bearing treatment in Legg-Perthés disease. *J Bone Joint Surg.* 1971;53B:54.

33. Salter RB. Legg-Perthés disease: The scientific basis for the methods of treatment and their indications. *Clin Orthop.* 1980;150:49.

34. Price CT, Day DD, Flynn JC. Behavioral sequelae of bracing versus surgery for Legg-Calve-Perthés disease. *J Pediatr Orthop.* 1988;8:285–287.

35. Burrows HJ. Slipped upper femoral epiphysis: Characteristics of one hundred cases. *J Bone Joint Surg.* 1957;39B:641.

36. Chung SM, ed. *Hip Disorders in Infants and Children.* Philadelphia: Lea & Febiger; 1981.

37. Ledwith CA, Fleisher GR. Slipped capital femoral epiphysis without hip pain leads to missed diagnosis. *Pediatrics* 1992;89:660–662.

38. Boyer DW, et al. Slipped capital femoral epiphysis: Long-term follow-up study of 121 patients. *J Bone Joint Surg.* 1981;63A:85.

39. Brashear HR, Raney RB. *Shands Handbook of Orthopedic Surgery.* St. Louis: CV Mosby; 1978:373–374.

40. Canale ST. Fractures and dislocations. In: Canale ST, Beaty SJ, eds. *Operative Pediatric Orthopedics.* St. Louis: Mosby-Yearbook; 1991;902–903.

41. Carney BT, Weinstein SL, Noble J. Long-term follow-up of slipped capital femoral epiphysis. *J Bone Joint Surg.* 1991;73A:667–674.

42. Canale ST. Fractures and dislocations in children. In: Crenshaw AH, ed. *Campbell's Operative Orthopedics.* 8th ed. St. Louis: Mosby-Yearbook, 1992:1163.

43. Coleman SS. Lower limb length discrepancy. In: Lovell WW, Winter RB, eds. *Pediatric Orthopedics.* 2nd ed. Philadelphia: JB Lippincott; 1986: 782.

44. Phemister DB. Operative arrestment of longitudinal growth of bones in the treatment of deformities. *J Bone Joint Surg.* 1933;15:1.

45. Wagner H. Operative beinverlangerung. *Der Chirurg.* 1970;42:260.

46. Simard S, Marchant M, Mencio G. The Ilizarov procedure: Limb lengthening and its implications. *Phys Ther.* 1992;72:25–34.

47. Filho NA, Thompson MW. Genetic studies in scoliosis. *J Bone Joint Surg.* 1971;53A:199.

48. Nash CL, Moe JH. A study of vertebral rotation. *J Bone Joint Surg.* 1969;51A:223.

49. Lonstein JE. Prediction of curve progression in untreated idiopathic scoliosis during growth. *J Bone Joint Surg.* 1984;66A:1070.

50. Bunnell W. A study of the natural history of idiopathic scoliosis. *Orthop Trans.* 1983;7:6.

51. Risser JC. The iliac apophysis: An invaluable sign in the management of scoliosis. *Clin Orthop.* 1958;11:111.

52. Cassella MC, Hall JE. Current treatment approaches in the nonoperative and operative management of adolescent idiopathic scoliosis. *Phys Ther.* 1991;71: 897–909.

53. Pearsall DJ, Reid JG, Hedden DM. Comparison of three noninvasive methods for measuring scoliosis. *Phys Ther.* 1992;72:648–657.

54. DiRamando CV, Green NE, MacLean WE. Brace compliance in adolescent idiopathic scoliosis. Presented at a meeting of the Scoliosis Research Society; September 19–22, 1984; Orlando, FL.

55. Faraday JA: Current principles in the non-operative

management of structural idiopathic adolescent scoliosis. *Phys Ther.* 1983;63:512–513.

56. Eckerson LF, Axelgaard J. Lateral electrical surface stimulation as an alternative to bracing in the treatment of idiopathic scoliosis: Treatment protocol and patient acceptance. *Phys Ther.* 1984;64:483–490.

57. Sullivan JA, Davidson R, Renshaw TS, et al. Further evaluation of the Scolitron treatment of idiopathic adolescent scoliosis. *Spine.* 1986;11:903–906.

58. Donaldson WF. Scoliosis. In: Ferguson AB, ed. *Orthopedic Surgery in Infancy and Childhood.* 5th ed. Baltimore: Williams & Wilkins; 1981: 855–927.

59. Carman D, Roach J, Speck G, et al. Role of exercises in the Milwaukee brace treatment of scoliosis. *J Pediatr Orthop.* 1985; 5:65.

60. Kehl DK, Morrissy RT. Brace treatment in adolescent idiopathic scoliosis. *Clin Orthop.* 1988;229:34–43.

61. Rang M. *Children's Fractures.* 2nd ed. Philadelphia: JB Lippincott; 1983: 3–6.

62. Guttmann GG, Simon R. Three-point fixation walking spica cast: An alternative to early or immediate casting of femoral shaft fractures in children. *J Pediatr Orthop.* 1988;8:699–703.

63. Cheng JC, Cheung SS. Modified functional bracing in the ambulatory treatment of femoral shaft fractures in children. *J Pediatr Orthop.* 1989;9:457–462.

64. Salter RB, Harris WR. Injuries involving the epiphyseal plate. *J Bone Joint Surg.* 1963;45A:587.

65. Carter JR, Leeson MC, Thompson GH, et al. Late-onset tibia vara: A histopathologic analysis. *J Pediatr Orthop.* 1988;8:187–195.

66. Blount WP. Tibia vara: Osteochondrosis deformans tibiae. *J Bone Joint Surg* 1937;19A:1.

67. Langenskiold A, Riska EB. Tibia vara: A survey of seventy-one cases. *J Bone Joint Surg.* 1964;46A: 1405.

68. Canale ST. Osteochondroses. In: Canale ST, Beaty JH, eds. *Operative Pediatric Orthopedics.* St. Louis: Mosby-Yearbook; 1991. 768–769.

69. Tachdjian MO. *Pediatric Orthopedics.* Philadelphia: WB Saunders, 1972.

70. Lohmann KN, Rayhel HE, Schneiderwind WP, Danoff JV. Static measurement of tibia variability and effect of lower extremity position. *Phys Ther.* 1987;67:196–202.

Pediatric Physical Therapy,
second edition, edited by Jan
Stephen Tecklin. J. B. Lippincott
Company, Philadelphia © 1994.

10

Shirley A. Scull

Juvenile Rheumatoid Arthritis

- **Types of Juvenile Rheumatoid Arthritis**
- **Medical Management**
- **Management with Medications**
- **Musculoskeletal Problems**
- **Assessment**
  History
  Observation and Inspection
  Range of Motion
  Strength Testing
  Posture
  Gait
  Activities of Daily Living
  Special Tests
  Summary of Evaluation
- **Treatment**
  Therapeutic Exercise
  Recreation
  Activities of Daily Living
  Pain Management
  Splints and Orthotics
  Gait Training
  Surgery
- **Management Strategies**
- **Other Rheumatic Disorders of Childhood**
  Dermatomyositis
  Ankylosing Spondylitis
  Scleroderma
- **Summary**

Rheumatic diseases are characterized by inflammation of connective tissue. A frequent manifestation of this inflammation is *arthritis,* or inflammation of a joint. According to estimates from the American Rheumatoid Association, more than 250,000 children in the United States may have some type of rheumatoid arthritis. Juvenile rheumatoid arthritis (JRA) is the most common type of chronic arthritis in children. Other rheumatic diseases that occur in pediatrics include systemic lupus erythematosus, dermatomyositis, scleroderma, and juvenile ankylosing spondylitis.

In a child younger than 16 years of age, persistent arthritis that lasts for more than 6 weeks can be diagnosed as JRA if other causes of joint pathology have been ruled out. Some of those other causes of joint pathology may include trauma, infection, or, less commonly, malignant disease. Joint symptoms may include swelling, heat, loss of motion, and pain when motion is attempted. Joint pain (*arthralgia*) when found alone, is not sufficient for a diagnosis of arthritis.

JRA is called by other names, including the British term juvenile chronic arthritis, or the historical term Still's disease. The term JRA is misleading because it implies that the disease is a childhood version of the adult type of rheumatoid arthritis. Most children with JRA have a negative blood test for rheumatoid factor (RF−) and may not have the systemic manifestations found commonly in the adult type of the disease. Nonetheless, the term JRA is the accepted nomenclature in medical literature in the United States.

The cause of JRA is unknown. Several possible factors have been implicated in its pathogenesis, including infection, autoimmunity, trauma, stress, and a genetic predisposition.[1] The chronic joint inflammation that we call JRA may actually be many factors grouped together under the one diagnosis; alternatively, a single pathogenic vector may manifest itself differently, depending on the specific reaction of each host.

A history of recent systemic infection or trauma is commonly found in many cases of JRA. One theory suggests that the genetically predisposed host is subjected to a foreign agent, such as an infection, or to trauma and then undergoes immunologic changes that result in inflammation of the joint. The body's normal formation of antibodies becomes altered so that it no longer recognizes certain antibodies as "self." This altered immune function triggers a chain of events that propagates the inflammatory reaction.[1]

The child usually has no family history of rheumatoid arthritis. Some studies however, show an association between histocompatibility of antigens and JRA. For example, children with JRA who have ankylosing spondylitis often have human leukocyte antigen HLA-B27 in their blood. Children with impaired defense mechanisms or overt forms of immunodeficiency may also develop arthritis.

Types of Juvenile Rheumatoid Arthritis

Juvenile rheumatoid arthritis is not a single disease, but rather a group of diseases. The disease has at least three different subtypes. The subtypes differ in clinical symptoms, epidemiology, immunologic features, and prognosis. The major differences among the various types of JRA are summarized in Table 10-1.[2]

Systemic JRA occurs in approximately 10% of patients, affecting boys and girls equally.[1] The child presents to the physician with a high, spiking fever of up to 39°C that returns to normal a short time later. This cycle of fever occurs once or twice each day. An evanescent salmon-colored rash accompanies the fever and usually appears on the trunk and proximal portions of the limbs. Extra-articular findings may include hepatosplenomegaly, lymphadenopathy, pleuritis, pericarditis, and myocarditis. Joint disease may appear later than involvement of other organs. Approximately 25% of those with systemic JRA will develop an arthritis that is severe and unremitting and that has a poor prognosis.[2]

Polyarticular JRA occurs in approximately 40%

Table 10-1. *Subtypes of Juvenile Rheumatoid Arthritis*

Subtype	Joints	Age	Female:Male	Clinical Findings	Prognosis for Severe Arthritis
Systemic	Multiple	Any age	1:1	Fever; rash; organomegaly	25%
Polyarticular	5 or more; symmetric	RF+ in teenager	3:1	Erosive joint changes	RF+ :50%
		RF− at any age	3:1		RF− :10%–15%
Pauciarticular	4 or less; unilateral	1–4 yrs.	5:1	ANA+; iridocyclitis	10%–20% ocular damage; severe arthritis rare
	4 or less; unilateral	>10 yrs.	Male	HLA-B27; hip and sacroiliac joints	Some have ankylosing spondylosis

RF, *rheumatoid factor;* **ANA,** *antinuclear antibody;* **HLA**, *human leukocyte antigen.*

of patients, with a preponderance for females. Five or more joints are involved, usually in a symmetric distribution. Knees and ankles are frequently affected, as are elbows, wrists, and the small joints of the hands. The temporomandibular joint and the cervical spine may also be involved with polyarticular JRA. The average age of onset for polyarticular JRA is 8 years, which is older than the onset for other types.[3] Some children with polyarticular disease show a positive rheumatoid factor. Of children with the RF+, 50% develop severe arthritis with erosive joint changes. These children are usually teenagers, and the disease in this group is more analogous to adult rheumatoid arthritis.[2]

Pauciarticular JRA is the most common type, occurring in 50% of children with JRA. Pauciarticular, by definition, involves four joints or less. The joint disease often presents itself asymmetrically and often involves larger joints, such as the knees. Involvement of only one joint is sometimes seen. The physician must be particularly careful to rule out infection or trauma in these cases.

Two subtypes of pauciarticular JRA exist. One subtype is found in girls of 1 to 4 years of age. These children are at risk for chronic inflammation of the iris, a condition which, if not diagnosed and treated at an early stage, can lead to blindness. Patients with this subtype are monitored with slit lamp ophthalmology examinations biannually, even if the joint disease resolves. A laboratory test for antinuclear antibodies (ANA) is often positive in patients with this subtype. Severe arthritis is uncommon with this subtype, but 10% to 20% of children have ocular damage from iridocyclitis.[2]

The second subtype of pauciarticular JRA occurs in children older than 10 years of age and has a male predilection. These children frequently develop arthritis of the hips and sacroiliac joints, which may progress to ankylosing spondylitis.

The diagnosis of JRA is established by exclusion of other diseases. More than 50 other conditions can imitate JRA. No single laboratory test is diagnostic. The time required to rule out other diseases and to make a diagnosis of JRA is often frustrating to the parent and child who do not understand the process of diagnosis by exclusion.

Medical Management

Most children with JRA can lead active lives with proper medical management. The goals of medical treatment should be to provide a program of medication that is less dangerous than the disease; to preserve joint function; and to educate the child and family so that the child may lead a life that is as normal as possible.[4] Most professionals who treat children with JRA believe that a team of professionals provides optimal management for the child. A pediatric rheumatologist, nurse, social worker, and physical and occupational therapists should be included in that team, and consultation should be obtained as needed from orthopedic surgeons, ophthalmologists, nutritionists, and orthotists.

The role of the physical therapist in the treatment of the child with JRA may vary depending on the setting. The physical therapist may treat the child on a daily basis in the acute care or rehabilitation hospital—for example, after reconstruction of a joint by surgery. The therapist may play a more limited treatment role in an outpatient setting or in the school, and may function more as a consultant. This consultative role may include designing a home treatment program, with subsequent teaching of the family who will be expected to participate in the program; or it may include making referrals to a community-based therapist; or it may include making splints and ordering adaptive equipment.

Management with Medications

Although JRA cannot be cured, the disease can usually be controlled with various medications. Four major groups of medications are used in the management of children with JRA. These are nonsteroidal anti-inflammatory drugs (NSAIDs), slow-acting antirheumatoid drugs (SAARDs), corticosteroids, and immunosuppressive and cytotoxic agents.[5]

NSAIDs are the traditional approach to controlling joint inflammation, and appear to be sufficient in 50% of patients when combined with physical therapy, psychosocial support, and attention to the educational plan.[5] Only tolmetin and naproxen are approved by the FDA for use by the young child. However, other NSAIDs may be prescribed, such as ibuprofen or indomethacin. Salicylates, or aspirin, can be used in high doses for an anti-inflammatory effect, but have become less popular because of the dangers of Reye's syndrome.

SAARDs are so called because their effects are not evident for 2 to 4 months. They are also called disease-modifying antirheumatic drugs (DMARDs). They include antimalarials, gold salts, penicillamine, and sulfasalazine. They are usually prescribed in addition to one of the NSAIDs for disease that is insufficiently controlled by the latter. Children are carefully monitored for the side effects of toxicity.

Systemic corticosteroids are usually reserved for severe cases of JRA because of their potential side effects. Corticosteroids, when taken daily, will suppress the hypothalamic–pituitary–adrenal axis. An alternate-day schedule, therefore, is preferred for corticosteroids. The child often reports an increase in "stiffness" during the day on which the medication is not taken. Side effects of systemic corticosteroids include growth retardation, severe osteoporosis, infections, hypertension, and features similar to Cushing's disease.

Immunosuppressive agents are reserved for severe polyarticular or systemic disease that is potentially life-threatening secondary to pericarditis, rapidly progressive disease, or amyloidosis. The potential for future oncogenic or teratogenic side effects is cause for concern. An exception is methotrexate, which is now used in early disease management and is thought to be safe except for the possible risk of fibrosis of the liver.

Experimental therapy involves the use of cytotoxic agents, such as cyclosporine A, and forms of immune modulation, such as intravenous human immunoglobulin (IVIG). These drugs are being studied for use in children with intractable disease that cannot be managed by more conservative drugs.

The physical therapist must understand the medication regimen because intervention by physical therapy can be enhanced when used at appropriate times within the course of the medication program. The acutely ill child whose disease is not being adequately controlled by medication may not tolerate a therapeutic exercise program initially. Resting in therapeutic or functional positions, use of various therapeutic modalities, and encouragement of activities of daily living (ADLs) may be the only realistic treatment until the disease is under good medical control. The child whose acute illness is controlled by medication can begin an active exercise program that also emphasizes conservation of the joints. The child whose disease is in remission, but who has contractures, can be treated more aggressively with passive stretching of muscles and joints. These guidelines are aimed at ensuring that exercise does not exacerbate inflammation of the joints.[6]

Musculoskeletal Problems

The physical therapist is concerned primarily with the child's musculoskeletal problems. In order to appreciate the pathophysiology of JRA, the following discussion is divided into the effects of the disease on the joints, muscles, the skeletal system, and functional abilities.

Inflammation of the joints with loss of motion is characteristic of all types of arthritis. A palpable proliferation of synovial tissue is often present. The joint appears grossly edematous and is warm when touched. Pain may be present with joint motion, but pain is usually not as pronounced as in adult arthritis. Stiffness may preclude ambulation for several hours in the morning when the patient arises from bed. The joint tends to "gel" during periods of inactivity, such as sleep. Changes in the joint seen later in the course of the disease include destruction of the articular cartilage, loss of joint surface congruity, adhesions, and osteophytes, or bone spurs.[7]

Many of these advanced changes can be appreciated from a roentgenogram.

Muscles that surround the affected joint may suffer from disuse atrophy. This atrophy leaves the joints less protected from external forces, such as weight bearing. Muscle tightness can also contribute to joint contracture. In addition to assessing joint range of motion (ROM) in a standard fashion, certain muscles should be examined closely. These muscles include the tensor fasciae latae, the hamstrings, and the gastrocnemius muscle. Tendon sheaths that are lined with synovium may also become inflamed, and the result may be tenosynovitis. Tenosynovitis of the extrinsic muscles of the fingers often occurs in the wrist.

The immature skeletal system can be permanently disfigured from abnormal weight-bearing forces. Postural deformities, such as scoliosis or genu valgum, may develop from muscle imbalance or with abnormal weight bearing. Chronically increased blood flow near the knee joint can cause an overgrowth of the femur or the tibia, with resultant discrepancy in leg length.[7] Limb shortening can also occur when the joint destruction causes closure of an adjacent epiphysis. Systemic JRA can also produce growth retardation, as can the effects of treatment with systemic corticosteroids.

Musculoskeletal problems cause various functional difficulties. Deviations in gait or an inability to ambulate occurs in severe cases. The child may have difficulty dressing, toileting, bathing, or with other ADLs. Decreased cardiovascular endurance and also muscular endurance may require frequent rest periods during the child's functional activities or recreation. The American College of Rheumatology has defined four categories that describe the various degrees to which musculoskeletal difficulty may interfere with functional activities. These categories are shown in Table 10-2.

Assessment

Assessment of the musculoskeletal problems of each patient is an important part of physical ther-

Table 10-2. *The American College of Rheumatology Categories of Disabilities based on Functional Deficits*

Class I	Completely able to perform usual activities of daily living (self-care, vocational, and avocational)
Class II	Able to perform usual self-care and vocational activities, but limited in avocational activities
Class III	Able to perform usual self-care activities, but limited in vocational and avocational activities
Class IV	Limited in ability to perform usual self-care, vocational, and avocational activities

(Source: Hochberg MC, Chang RW, Dwoshi F, Lindsey S, Pincus T, Wolfe F. The American College of Rheumatology 1991 revised criteria for the classification of global functional status in rheumatoid arthritis. Arthritis & Rheumatism *1992;35:498–502.*

apy. A comprehensive assessment has several benefits, including facilitating establishment of a differential diagnosis for a new patient, especially if there may be trauma to the joint. Assessment is used to identify the patient's problems and to establish the treatment goals and plans. As treatment progresses, reassessment allows an evaluation of progress toward the previously identified goals. Assessment data may be grouped to begin to answer questions about program effectiveness in a formal research format.

The physical therapy clinician should approach the assessment with an organized outline in mind. Flow sheets may simplify and organize the recording of data, thus facilitating the assessment and providing for easy recall of data (Display 10-1). Areas that should be covered in a physical therapy assessment for the child with JRA include:

1. Patient history
2. Observation and inspection
3. Range of motion
4. Strength
5. Posture
6. Evaluation of gait
7. Activities of daily living
8. Special tests

The results of the assessment are analyzed to identify major problems, and findings are correlated to

Display 10-1.
Children's Seashore House Physical Therapy Department Evaluation
for Juvenile Rheumatoid Arthritis

Date: _____

Problem list: _____

_____

_____

Subjective: _____

_____

_____

_____

Objective: _____

_____

_____

_____

Range of Motion	**Right**	**Left**		**Right**	**Left**
Hip flexion	_____	_____	Shoulder flexion	_____	_____
Hip extension	_____	_____	Shoulder abduction	_____	_____
Hip abduction	_____	_____	Shoulder internal rotation	_____	_____
Hip internal rotation	_____	_____	Shoulder external rotation	_____	_____
Hip external rotation	_____	_____	Elbow flexion	_____	_____
Knee flexion	_____	_____	Elbow extension	_____	_____
Knee extension	_____	_____	Forearm pronation	_____	_____
Ankle dorsiflexion	_____	_____	Forearm supination	_____	_____
Ankle plantar flexion	_____	_____	Wrist flexion	_____	_____
Ankle inversion	_____	_____	Wrist extension	_____	_____
Ankle eversion	_____	_____	Cervical flexion	_____	_____
			Cervical extension	_____	_____
			Cervical rotation	_____	_____
			Cervical lateral bending	_____	_____
			Comments: _____		

_____

(continued)

Display 10-1.
Evaluation for Juvenile Rheumatoid Arthritis (continued)

Leg length: Right _____   Left _____

Posture: _____

_____

_____

_____   Back view   Lateral View

Quick Manual Muscle Test	Right	Left	Comments
Hip flexion	_____	_____	_____
Hip extension	_____	_____	_____
Hip abduction	_____	_____	_____
Knee flexion	_____	_____	_____
Knee extension	_____	_____	_____
Ankle plantar flexion	_____	_____	_____
Ankle dorsiflexion	_____	_____	_____
Shoulder abduction	_____	_____	_____
Elbow flexion	_____	_____	_____
Elbow extension	_____	_____	_____

Joint Circumference (Cm)	Right	Left
Knee		
Ankle		

Gait pattern: _____

_____

_____

_____

Activities of Daily Living: _____

_____

_____

_____

(continued)

Display 10-1.
Evaluation for Juvenile Rheumatoid Arthritis (continued)

Assessment: _____

_____

_____

Goals: Short-Term _____

_____

Goals: Long-Term _____

_____

Plan: _____

_____

Therapist's signature _____

_____

Pain: | Red | | Yellow | | Green | | Blue |

Front   Back

detect relationships between cause and effect. For example, a lordotic posture may be the result of a bilateral hip flexion contracture. The treatment plan evolves easily once the comprehensive assessment is completed.

History

The history is usually taken from the parent, but an older child may provide useful information. Questions should be asked in a neutral manner, thus eliciting responses that describe the problem. Leading questions with an obvious "yes" or "no" response should be avoided. The initial question should focus on a description of the chief complaint, which may include identifying the joints involved and how joint involvement has affected the overall functional ability of the child. The therapist should also explore the history of the present illness. If a home remedy has been tried, its effect on the particular symptom should be ascertained.

A useful interview technique involves asking the parent to describe a typical day in the life of the child. This description will provide information about the degree of pain and the child's functional limitations. The therapist may also learn about coping strategies used by the family and the description will help predict the family's ability to start a home care program. If other caretakers are routinely involved with the child, this information will also emerge during the interview.

The physical therapist may also wish to determine how well the parents understand the diagnosis. A question, such as "Tell me what the doctor has said about Susie," is one method of asking the parents to describe their knowledge and understanding of the disease. This type of question should be asked even when the source of referral indicates that the diagnosis was explained to the family. There is frequently a difference between what the parents were told by the physician and what they understand about the disease.

Observation and Inspection

While the therapist is taking a history from the parents, the child has an opportunity to become accustomed to the environment. The therapist may choose to offer the child a toy in order to begin to develop a rapport with him or her. The therapist should casually observe the child's movement patterns. The parents and child should now be oriented to the examination and the child should be undressed.

The child's limbs are observed for gross abnormalities, such as muscle atrophy, joint swelling, or joint malalignments. Palpation for heat around the joint is done using the dorsum of the hand. Gentle palpation can be done at the joint line to determine whether proliferation of synovial tissue has occurred. Girth measurements, using standard bony landmarks, allow objective documentation of the degree of edema. A figure-of-eight wrap with a tape measure provides an indication of swelling of the ankle.

Range of Motion

Goniometry is used to determine if restricted joint motion exists. Before doing a formal goniometric test, a screening examination for active ROM may help identify joints that are grossly restricted. A screening of the upper extremities includes asking the child to complete the following motions:

1. Arms above the head
2. Hands behind the head (external rotation)
3. Hands behind the back (internal rotation)
4. Palms up
5. Palms down
6. Hands in a position of prayer
7. Opening and closing the hands

The game "Simon Says" is a useful method for having the child participate more enthusiastically.

Restricted joints should be measured with standard goniometric technique. When a child has polyarticular disease, restriction often occurs in flexion and external rotation of the shoulder, extension of the elbow, supination of the forearm, and extension of the wrist and fingers.

Lower extremity ROM can also be screened actively by observing the child's gait and by asking the child to bend down to pick up a toy. Assessment of passive ROM at the hip should include a Thomas test to identify hip flexion contractures. Abduction and rotations of the hip are also frequently restricted. The knee is examined for full extension and for available flexion. An active ROM for the knee of 0 to 100 degrees of flexion is optimal for functional activities.

The ankle is a joint complex and should be examined accordingly. Dorsiflexion and plantar flexion occur between the ankle mortise and the talus. Dorsiflexion to at least a neutral position is necessary for functional gait. Subtalar motion of the hindfoot is examined by rocking the calcaneus on the talus, with the foot dorsiflexed. Supination and pronation of the forefoot are examined with the hindfoot stabilized. The toes must also be examined to assess the available motion and to identify the presence of deformities. Seventy degrees of metatarsophalangeal extension of the great toe is necessary for toe-off during the gait cycle.

The cervical spine is examined using active motion only. The therapist should stabilize the shoulder girdle, then instruct the child to do the six cardinal motions of the cervical spine. Children with polyarticular disease may have ankylosis of the cervical spine with limitation of extension, rotation, and lateral flexion.[8] Forward flexion is not commonly restricted. The temporomandibular joint is assessed by asking the child to open the mouth and insert three fingers held vertically. Underdevelopment of the mandible (*micrognathia*) may cause malocclusion of the upper and lower teeth.

Strength Testing

Manual muscle testing may be modified to avoid undue stress on an inflamed joint. Resistance is used judiciously, and only when pain allows. Break testing of the muscle using isometric contraction is preferred to offering resistance through the range. In the early stages of inflammatory disease, girth measurement of the quadriceps and gastrocnemius muscles may be substituted for manual muscle testing.

Because a goal of the assessment is to identify general patterns of disuse atrophy, muscles may be tested in functional groups, rather than in isolation. Special attention is paid to antigravity muscles. In the lower extremities, these muscles include hip extensors, hip abductors, knee extensors, and ankle plantar flexors. Major groups examined in the upper extremities include the deltoids, biceps, triceps, wrist extensors, and finger flexors and extensors.

Posture

Assessment of sitting and standing posture is important. The child should be viewed from the front and the side and should be compared to an optimal alignment. The "bend over" test is used to detect early signs of scoliosis. Postural deformities found in children with JRA frequently include forward head, kyphosis, lordosis, scoliosis, hip and knee flexion contractures, genu valgus, and a variety of deformities of the foot and ankle. Problems with alignment in the lower extremities rarely occur at a single joint because of the "kinetic chain," and joints above and below a deformity should be inspected for compensatory deformities.

Gait

Gait evaluation is commonly done by visual inspection. The child should be observed from both anteroposterior views, and from left and right lateral views. The trained therapist's eye watches each joint as the joint progresses through the various phases of gait. Linear assessments, including stride length, step length, and width of base of support, help to document abnormalities. Typical gait deviations include decreased velocity, cadence, and stride length. Anterior pelvic tilt is increased, with lack of hip extension and plantar flexion at toe-off.[9]

Activities of Daily Living

ADLs may be assessed by directly watching the child or by conducting an interview. Self-care and mobility in the child's natural environment, including both home and school, should be examined in the assessment. In the child younger than 6 years of age, the normal developmental sequence of ADLs will serve as a basis for interpretation of assessment results. Age-appropriate activities should be explored for feeding, toileting, dressing, grooming, and mobility. An occupational therapist may share the responsibility of assessing for ADLs.

Newly developed pediatric tests of function include the Functional Independence Measure for Children (WeeFIM)[10] and the Pediatric Evaluation of Disabilities Inventory (PEDI).[11] Functional tools specific to children with JRA include the Juvenile Arthritis Functional Assessment Scale (JAFAS)[12] and the Health Assessment Questionnaire (HAQ)[13] (see Display 10-2).

Special Tests

Special tests are added to the evaluation procedures when appropriate. Tests for joint play are frequently done. Valgus and varus stress at the knee will detect collateral ligament laxity. Anterior and posterior drawer signs are used to test the cruciate ligaments of the knee. The therapist can use the Ober test on the hip to assess tightness of the iliotibial band, which, when tight, contributes to genu valgum. The child is placed in a side-lying position for the Ober Test, and the iliotibial band is placed on a stretch by extending and adducting the hip.

A review of available roentgenograms may help to delineate destruction of the joint. Discrepancy in leg length should always be determined in pediatric patients because of the potential for a compensatory scoliosis. Leg length is measured from the anterior superior iliac spine to the medial malleolus. When there is a knee flexion contracture, femoral length and tibial length should be measured separately to determine leg length.

Summary of Evaluation

After gathering all the data, the therapist analyzes the major problems and tries to identify items from the assessment that may correlate. A list of the patient's problems is developed and short-term and long-term goals are established. The goals of treatment often fall into the following general categories:

1. Maintain or increase joint ROM.
2. Maintain or increase strength.
3. Independent ADLs or ambulation
4. Control of pain
5. Prevention of deformity

Treatment

Therapeutic Exercise

Exercise is the most important part of the treatment regimen for children with arthritis. Exercise should be designed to be appropriate for the child's developmental age and to accomplish the goals of (1) improving ROM, (2) increasing strength, and (3) improving endurance.

Improving or maintaining joint ROM can be achieved with active and passive exercise or with a positioning program. All joints should be moved through their available range at least once each day. Specific joints are also targeted for increased ROM when limitations interfere with function. When the child's disease is under medical control, a stretching exercise regimen may be started. The contract–relax technique, advocated by proponents of proprioceptive neuromuscular facilitation, may be used for muscle elongation. Muscles antagonistic to those shortened by contracture should be exercised to increase strength.

Prevention of flexion contractures in the lower extremities is the best method of treatment. A daily program that will maintain extension in most cases consists of the child lying in a prone position for 20 minutes with hips and knees fully extended with the feet over the edge of the mattress. If a knee flexion contracture exists, this position will take advantage

Display 10-2.
Health Assessment Questionnaire*

In this section, we are interested in learning how your child's illness affects his/her ability to function in daily life. Please feel free to add any comments on the back of this page. In the following questions, please check the one response which best describes your child's usual activities (averaged over an entire day) OVER THE PAST WEEK. If your child has difficulty in doing a certain activity or is unable to do it because he/she is too young but NOT because he/she is RESTRICTED BY ARTHRITIS, please mark it as "Not Applicable." ONLY NOTE THOSE DIFFICULTIES OR LIMITATIONS WHICH ARE DUE TO ARTHRITIS.

	Without Any Difficulty	With Some Difficulty	With Much Difficulty	Unable To Do	Not Applicable
Dressing & Grooming					
Is your child able to:					
• Dress, including tying shoelaces and doing buttons?	_____	_____	_____	_____	_____
• Shampoo his/her hair?	_____	_____	_____	_____	_____
• Remove socks?	_____	_____	_____	_____	_____
• Cut fingernails/toenails?	_____	_____	_____	_____	_____
Arising					
Is your child able to:					
• Stand up from a low chair or floor?	_____	_____	_____	_____	_____
• Get in and out of bed or stand up in crib?	_____	_____	_____	_____	_____
Eating					
Is your child able to:					
• Cut his/her own meat?	_____	_____	_____	_____	_____
• Lift a cup or glass to mouth?	_____	_____	_____	_____	_____
• Open a new cereal box?	_____	_____	_____	_____	_____
Walking					
Is your child able to:					
• Walk outdoors on flat ground?	_____	_____	_____	_____	_____
• Climb up five steps?	_____	_____	_____	_____	_____

(continued)

Display 10-2.
Health Assessment Questionnaire* (continued)

*Please check any AIDS or DEVICES that your child usually uses for any of the above activities:

_____ Cane

_____ Walker

_____ Crutches

_____ Wheelchair

_____ Devices used for dressing (button hook, zipper pull, long-handled shoe horn, etc.)

_____ Built-up pencil or special utensils

_____ Special or Built-up chair

_____ Other (Specify: _____)

*Please check any categories for which your child usually needs help from another person BECAUSE OF ARTHRITIS:

_____ Dressing and grooming

_____ Arising

_____ Eating

_____ Walking

	Without Any Difficulty	With Some Difficulty	With Much Difficulty	Unable To Do	Not Applicable
Hygiene					
Is your child able to:					
• Wash and dry entire body?	_____	_____	_____	_____	_____
• Take a tub bath (get in & out of tub)?	_____	_____	_____	_____	_____
• Get on and off the toilet or potty chair?	_____	_____	_____	_____	_____
• Brush teeth?	_____	_____	_____	_____	_____
• Comb/brush hair?	_____	_____	_____	_____	_____
Reach					
Is your child able to:					
• Reach and get down a heavy object, such as a large game or books, from just above his/her head?	_____	_____	_____	_____	_____
• Bend down to pick up clothing or a piece of paper from the floor?	_____	_____	_____	_____	_____
• Pull on a sweater over his/her head?	_____	_____	_____	_____	_____
• Turn neck to look back over shoulder?	_____	_____	_____	_____	_____

(continued)

Display 10-2.
Health Assessment Questionnaire (continued)*

	Without Any Difficulty	With Some Difficulty	With Much Difficulty	Unable To Do	Not Applicable
Grip					
Is your child able to:					
• Write or scribble with a pen or pencil?	_____	_____	_____	_____	_____
• Open car doors?	_____	_____	_____	_____	_____
• Open jars which have been previously opened?	_____	_____	_____	_____	_____
• Turn faucets on and off?	_____	_____	_____	_____	_____
• Push open a door when he/she has to turn a door knob?	_____	_____	_____	_____	_____
Activities					
Is your child able to:					
• Run errands and shop?	_____	_____	_____	_____	_____
• Get in and out of car or toy car or school bus?	_____	_____	_____	_____	_____
• Ride bike or tricycle?	_____	_____	_____	_____	_____
• Do household chores (e.g., wash dishes, take out trash, vacuum, do yardwork, make bed, clean room)?	_____	_____	_____	_____	_____
• Run and play?					

*Please check any AIDS or DEVICES that your child usually uses for any of the above activities:

_____ Raised toilet seat   _____ Bathtub bar

_____ Bathtub seat   _____ Long-handled appliances for reach

_____ Jar opener (for jars previously opened)   _____ Long-handled appliances in bathroom

*Please check any categories for which your child usually needs help from another person BECAUSE OF ARTHRITIS:

_____ Hygiene   _____ Gripping and opening things

_____ Reaching   _____ Errands and chores

(continued)

Display 10-2.
Health Assessment Questionnaire* (continued)

Pain

We are also interested in learning whether or not your child has been affected by pain because of his or her illness.

• How much pain do you think your child has had because of his or her illness IN THE PAST WEEK?

Place a mark on the line below to indicate the severity of the pain.

No Pain   Very Severe Pain

├───┤
0   100

Health Status

1. Considering all the ways that arthritis affects your child, rate how your child is doing on the following scale by placing a mark on the line.

├───┤
0   100
very   very
well   poorly

2. Is your child stiff in the morning?   _____ Yes _____ No

   If YES, about how long does the stiffness usually last (in the past week)?   Hours/Minutes _____

*Adapted from Singh G, Athreya B, et al. Measurement of functional status. Arthritis Rheum. In press.

---

of the forces of gravity to help reduce the contracture (Fig. 10-1).

A badly damaged joint, such as an ankle or wrist, may occasionally be allowed to fuse in a functional position rather than making continual attempts to improve ROM. If movement of the joint causes significant pain, improved function may be achieved with a stable, immobile joint. Generally this approach of allowing natural joint fusion is best used for distal joints.

The position of the various joints should be varied throughout the day to avoid development of contractures. Exercise to increase ROM seems pointless when the joint is rested in a position of deformity for the rest of the day.

Optimal sitting alignment should be monitored closely. The feet should be supported with the ankles in a neutral position, and the child's desk or table should be high enough to encourage trunk extension. An easel, desk or book holder that raises the work toward a vertical position can help with extension of the trunk and can prevent flexion of the cervical spine.

It is difficult to control the posture of the sleeping child. When the child's cervical spine is involved, either a thin flat pillow or no pillow should

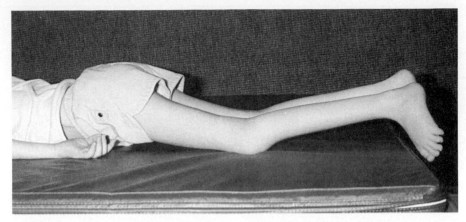

Figure 10-1. *Child with bilateral knee flexion contractures lying in a prone position.*

be used when sleeping in the supine position. The tendency for flexion contractures of the neck can be reduced by avoiding using a pillow. Resting splints may be used during the night to obtain optimal alignment of the knees or wrists and to decrease morning stiffness.

Exercises to improve muscle strength should focus on antigravity muscles, particularly those lower extremity stabilizers that function during gait. Isometrics, which minimize pain by avoiding joint motion during contraction, should be begun at an early stage. Gluteal sets and quadriceps sets can be done while lying in a prone position. Isotonic exercises are also useful for lower extremity extensors and abductors. Although resistive exercise improves strength, damage to a joint can occur when a strong contraction is interrupted suddenly by pain. Resistance, when used, should be light in order to prevent an exacerbation of inflammation of the joint.

Elastic bands, such as Theraband, can be used effectively for strengthening lower extremity extensors and abductors. The band can be placed just above the knees or above the ankles, depending on the child's strength. The child contracts hip and knee extensors and hip abductors while trying to stretch the band by pushing the legs apart.

Improving endurance is another goal of therapeutic exercise. The child should be encouraged to increase either the number of repetitions of an exercise or the time of the exercise session to improve endurance. A child with arthritis whose natural activity level is decreased will suffer from reduced cardiovascular capacity. A 20-minute session of exercise three times per week that elevates the heart rate to 65% to 85% of predicted maximum capacity will improve aerobic conditioning.[14] A program of cycling or swimming will improve the child's cardiovascular status without exacerbating the inflammation of the joint.

Various adjuncts to the exercise program may be used to help in the achievement of goals. Biofeedback with surface electrodes may reinforce muscle reeducation or may teach muscle relaxation. Functional electrical stimulation may be considered to help improve ROM or strength. Continuous passive motion devices may be used to gradually improve ROM.

Recreation

Play and recreation are used routinely to help achieve exercise goals. The therapist's advice regarding recreational activities should be based on the child's developmental level, the child's interests, and the severity of the disease.

Toddlers enjoy gross motor activity involving balls, swings, and toys that can be ridden. A tricycle provides exercise for the lower extremities, but avoids weight bearing. The therapist should adjust the seat to an appropriate height to provide almost full knee extension with each revolution of the tricycle pedal, and foot straps may need to be applied. Some children may choose to enroll in dance class. Positions used in classical ballet should be modified as necessary to avoid undue stress on the joints. Upper extremities, particularly hands and wrists, can be exercised during play involving modelling clay. As previously noted, the game "Simon Says" is an excellent method of making ROM exercises more fun. The pediatric physical therapist must be creative in order to analyze play options and select those actions that will reinforce the desired goals of exercise.

School-aged children should be encouraged to participate in a physical education class whenever feasible. However, to avoid potentially harmful activity, these classes should be adapted with guidance from the therapist. For example, activities such as somersaults and headstands may be harmful to the child with cervical spine disease. Likewise, contact sports and activities requiring weight bearing of the upper extremities should be avoided.

Swimming and cycling are excellent methods of exercising the large joints of the body for children of all ages. Both sports provide for vigorous exercise, but minimize weight bearing and stress on the joints. Swimming in a heated pool is recommended throughout the year. The buoyancy of the water reduces the weight of the limbs to make exercising easier. The use of flotation devices may give the nonswimmer enough confidence to participate in the sport; these devices facilitate movement, as well.[15]

Activities of Daily Living

A primary goal for the child with JRA is to achieve independence in age-appropriate ADLs. For the child with minimal involvement, training in ADLs may involve advice on the most efficient method of doing an activity. For the more severely disabled, training in ADLs may take the form of instruction in the use of assistive devices, or environmental modification to achieve functional independence.

Principles of protection of the joints are taught to the patient and family and must be integrated into all daily tasks.[16] Protection of the joints preserves the integrity of the joint during an activity by reducing physical and mechanical stresses. Because large joints of the body tolerate stress better than small joints, large joints should be used whenever feasible. For example, rather than carrying school books by hand and placing stress on the wrists and hands, the child should use a backpack. The child should be issued two sets of books (one set for school and one set for home) whenever possible to completely eliminate the task of carrying books.

Dressing is complicated in the morning by stiffness that usually results in the morning being the worst time of the day for the child with JRA. If limited ROM makes reaching for the feet impractical, a dressing stick may help a child to don garments on the lower extremities. A hoop made from a wire coat hanger can help with donning shirts (Fig. 10-2). Velcro can simplify the manipulation of fasteners, such as zippers or buttons.

Custom-designed feeding utensils may be required to help with grasping of the utensil and to allow a normal hand-to-mouth pattern of motion. Maintenance of ROM at the elbow is important for eating. When extension of the cervical spine is limited, a glass with a straw may be used to help drink without tilting back the head.

Architectural modification of the bathroom is often necessary, particularly for the child who depends on a wheelchair. The child should have access to the bathtub, toilet, and sink with adequate support to provide safety and privacy. Items that may help promote independence include special tub seats, hand-held shower hoses, longhandled sponges, and grab bars.

Handwriting may be a tedious task for the school-aged child with JRA. A cock-up splint may be used to support the wrist during writing tasks. A pencil with a large circumference will provide for easier grasp. Alternatives to writing, such as the use of typewriters, tape recorders, and computers, may

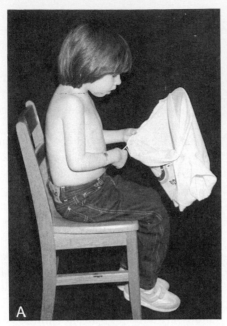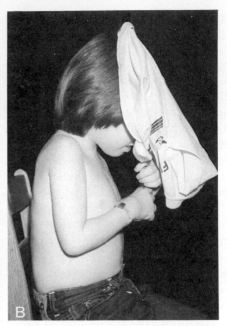

Figure 10-2. A and B. *A wire hanger may be used to facilitate donning a shirt by a child with limited motion at the shoulder.*

be appropriate for the child with an impairment of the upper extremities.

Children with JRA may reach a point at which functional mobility requires either partial or complete use of a wheelchair. This point is commonly reached when the energy costs of ambulation become excessive. A lightweight sports wheelchair is recommended in such cases. The reduced weight of the chair is important for conservation of the joints and should improve endurance for self-propulsion. A stroller-type transporter is sometimes prescribed for the young child who needs help during outings. Parents should be advised, however, to restrict the use of these strollers because the sling-backs do not provide for good posture. When feasible, a tricycle is probably a better means of mobility for a younger child or toddler. Powered wheelchairs may sometimes be required in order for the most severely involved youngsters to achieve independent mobility. An accessible home, school, and transportation system is mandatory when considering powered mobility for the child.

Pain Management

Heat can be used to decrease pain or control stiffness in the morning. Applications of superficial heat are easily done at home and may provide pain relief. A warm tub bath or shower on arising in the morning will help to alleviate stiffness and can be recommended for all children with JRA. Exercises and toys that float are used to encourage movement. a sleeping bag or blanket-sleeper pajamas may be useful in maintaining the body's natural heat to reduce stiffness.[17] A paraffin bath is used occasionally for the small joints of the wrist and hand. Hydrocollator packs may be used for the cervical or lumbar spine. Exercise should follow any heat treatment. Therapeutic methods, such as heat, are adjuncts to the exercise program but, when used alone, are not sufficient to achieve therapeutic goals.[18]

Application of deep heat, such as by ultrasound or diathermy, is contraindicated in pediatric patients with JRA. Its potential for increasing inflammation and accelerating the bioenzymatic chain of events resulting in destruction to cartilage has caused deep heat to come under careful scrutiny even for adults with rheumatoid arthritis.[19,20] In addition to these changes with deep heat, its effect on the growing epiphyseal plate is not fully understood and is a cause for concern in the child.[21]

Although cold also provides relief from pain, many children find cold uncomfortable. In our clinic, cold treatment is reserved for acute injuries and is used along with elevation and partial weight bearing. With the exception of acute injuries, cold is not routinely used to treat pain in the joints in children with JRA, although patient preferences should be considered as a guide.

Transcutaneous electrical nerve stimulation (TENS) may be useful in alleviating localized, severe pain. Most complaints of pain in patients with JRA, however, do not follow this pattern. Moreover, there is always the concern that, by disguising or reducing pain, we are eliminating a protective signal suggesting further damage to the joint. Most patients can control pain adequately with medication, a tub bath in the morning, and rest during the day when pain interrupts activity.

Splints and Orthotics

Splints and orthotics are important adjuncts to treatment for many children with JRA. The type of splint selected for a particular purpose may depend on the therapeutic goal. There are three categories of splints, as follows:

1. Resting splint
2. Corrective splint
3. Functional splint[22]

The resting splint is used to place an inflamed joint at rest. The joint is placed in a functional position rather than a position of potential deformity. The splint must be removed for daily exercises. For most patients, resting splints are worn only during sleep or when needed during an acute exacerbation. The wrist and fingers are often placed in a resting splint (Fig. 10-3). The knee may also be splinted using a posterior shell when the patient is asleep.

The concept of position of function or most useful position is important when splinting arthritic joints. For example, 20 degrees of wrist extension is commonly considered an optimal position for hand function.

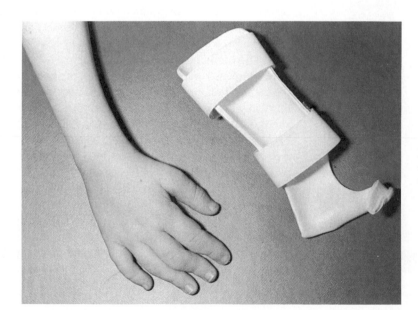

Figure 10-3. *A resting splint that was customized for the child with rheumatoid arthritis.*

Corrective splints may include serial splinting and dynamic splinting. Corrective splints are used to improve joint ROM. With this concept in mind, the joint is usually splinted by placing it at its maximum range and by holding it in that position. The splint is adjusted accordingly as the range increases. A dial-lock joint on an orthosis allows the therapist to adjust the brace as ROM increases. Dial-lock joints are used most commonly at the knee (Fig. 10-4).

Dynamic splints use springs or rubber bands to provide a constant stretching force to the contracture. The forces applied must be monitored in order to assure proper alignment of segments. Improper alignment and stretching at the knee could cause

posterior subluxation of the tibia on the femur. Commercially available dynamic splints can be ordered and fitted to specific joints. The splinting program should be reevaluated if gradual improvement in motion is not seen.

Functional splints or orthoses are used to support the joint during ADLs. A lower extremity orthosis may be used if pain or weakness occurs during the stance phase of gait. In the upper extremity, a small wrist splint may be used to help with hand activities at school.

Gait Training

Crutches or a rolling walker may be needed for the child who experiences pain on full weight bearing. The use of an assistive device for gait is complicated by the fact that this device merely shifts weight bearing to the upper extremity. In order to protect the hands and wrists from the forces of weight bearing, forearm platform devices are usually added to the crutches or walker to shift weight bearing to the elbows and shoulders, which are usually less involved (Fig 10-5).

Soft, comfortable footwear is usually recommended for children with JRA. Sneakers with a flexible sole and a longitudinal arch are usually a good choice. When fitting the child for shoes, leg length discrepancy should be corrected to within $\frac{1}{4}$ inch. This correction of leg length will prevent postural compensations, such as flexion of the knee in the longer limb, or scoliosis. Children with pain in the feet may ask for sandals and refuse to wear shoes. Unfortunately, sandals should be avoided because they provide inadequate support during weight bearing. Lining the shoe with a foam insole will cushion the force of impact at heel strike.

Orthoses may be used to achieve functional gait. A heel cup or custom orthotic insert may decrease pain in the feet and may correct alignment during weight bearing. A molded ankle foot orthosis can be used to stabilize the ankle during stance. Bracing above the knee may be indicated for quadriceps weakness, significant flexion contracture at the

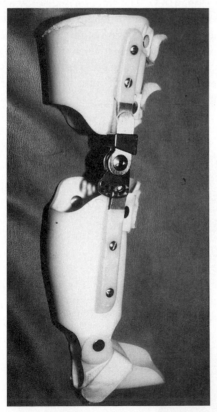

Figure 10-4. *Example of a dial-lock knee joint.*

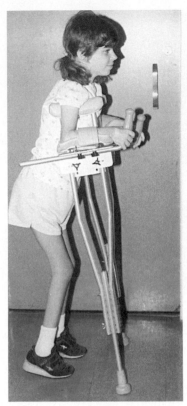

Figure 10-5. *Platform crutches facilitate ambulation by shifting weight bearing of the upper extremities from the hands and wrists to the larger, more proximal joints.*

knee, and for genu valgum. All orthotics should be made of lightweight polypropylene to avoid further stress while a person is walking.

Surgery

Children with JRA may require orthopedic surgery when contractures interfere with function.[23] Surgery should be considered only after a trial of medication and exercise. Contractures are managed orthopedically by manipulation of the joint with the child under general anesthesia, or by soft tissue releases, such as tenotomy or capsular release. A

bony procedure, such as an osteotomy or a joint fusion, may occasionally be necessary. Synovectomy is done less commonly.[24] Some children will require arthroplasty, usually of the hips and knees.[23] Because a joint prosthesis has a finite life span, arthroplasty is usually deferred as long as possible to prevent the need for a second joint replacement. Arthroplasty has the potential to damage the epiphysis and to interfere with growth.

The physical therapist plays a major role both in preoperative planning and in postoperative rehabilitation. Selection of patients for surgery requires a thorough interdisciplinary assessment. The parents and child must understand the goals of surgery and must commit themselves to intensive postoperative rehabilitation.[23]

Postoperative immobilization is kept to a minimum in order to avoid further loss of motion. A continuous passive motion machine may be used as an alternative choice rather than immobilization.[25]

Splinting and positioning are important considerations after soft tissue surgery. The newly acquired ROM should be maintained by splinting during the hours of sleep. The exercise program, too, should emphasize the postoperative ROM.

Rehabilitation is extensive after total joint replacement. A continuous passive motion machine is used immediately after surgery for most of the day (Fig. 10-6). The therapist tries to achieve a functional range in the early rehabilitation phase. At the hip, a functional range includes 0 to 90 degrees of flexion, 0 to 40 degrees of abduction, and 0 to 30 degrees of external rotation. Movements that should be avoided after hip arthroplasty include flexion of more than 90 degrees, adduction past the neutral position (across midline), and all internal rotation. A reclining wheelchair that can be gradually adjusted toward 90 degrees at the hip is useful when alternated with continuous passive motion and prone positioning for extension. An abduction pommel reminds the child to keep his or her legs uncrossed. At the knee, functional ROM includes 0 to 90 degrees of flexion. After knee arthroplasty,

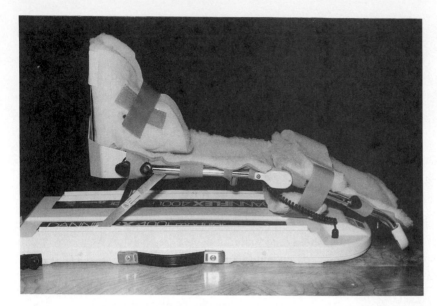

Figure 10-6. *A continuous passive motion machine for use at the knee.*

prone positioning is used to achieve extension and gravity-assisted flexion is attained with sitting.

Strengthening exercises are crucial for the lower extremity musculature after arthroplasty. Because many children who have orthopedic surgery have not been walking for a long time before surgery, disuse atrophy and osteoporosis in the lower extremities are major concerns. A program of standing on a tilt table at angles that move toward a vertical position may promote calcium deposition.

Hydrotherapy is a useful adjunct to rehabilitation. Exercise and ambulation in water may be begun as soon as wound healing allows the use of a community pool. The child is only partially weight bearing by ambulating in water. The child can be gradually moved to more shallow parts of the pool as the tolerance to weight bearing improves.

Gait training after orthopedic surgery may involve using a sequence of assistive devices, including a rolling walker, platform crutches, and canes. Not all patients achieve independent ambulation without assistive devices. Patient endurance and the need for joint conservation should be considered when deciding on the type of assistive device for gait training.

Management Strategies

The need for daily therapeutic management of children with rheumatic disease requires that parents be instructed in correct administration of a home therapy program. When appropriate, the child must assume some responsibility for treatment and for learning about the disease. The home program should be designed for each child and should be expressed in simple terms and described with stick figures as necessary. The therapist should first show each exercise to the child, then allow the parent to practice the exercise with the child under the therapist's supervision. The successful home program will be appropriate for the child's developmental age and should be limited to five or six important exercises. It is probably unrealistic to expect any family to spend more than 30 minutes each day working on the exercise program. The therapist must be certain that the program fits the daily schedule of the family.

Knowledge and understanding of the exercise program can be assessed at the time of the family's next visit to the clinic. The therapist should request that the family demonstrate the exercise program. The family that has been practicing the home program will do the exercises with little or no difficulty. Alternatives must be considered when the family does not comply with the program. Outpatient treatment with a therapist in the community or in a school are possible alternatives.

Patient and parent education is also the responsibility of the therapist. Many good pamphlets and other resources are available from the Arthritis Foundation and from regional pediatric rheumatology centers.[26] Parents can reinforce information received at the rheumatology clinic by reading about the disease and principles of its treatment.

The physical therapist may also play the role of advocate to maintain the child within the school system and to obtain necessary related services. The Education for All Handicapped Children Act (Public Law 94-142) mandates for handicapped children a free and appropriate public education in the least restrictive environment. If related services, such as physical or occupational therapy, or specialized transportation is necessary to allow the child to benefit from the educational program, these services must be stated in the child's individualized educational plan. School personnel should be educated about rheumatic diseases. Architectural barriers must be removed or avoided. An optimal education for the child with rheumatic disease can be achieved and the physical therapist may play an important role as child advocate to help achieve that education.

Other Rheumatic Disorders of Childhood

Dermatomyositis

Dermatomyositis is a rare disease affecting skin and muscle. Muscles, especially proximal muscles, become inflamed and weak. This weakness results in difficulty climbing stairs and problems in rising from the floor. The skin is red and shiny, with dry scaly areas over the elbows, knuckles, fingertips, and knees. A heliotrope rash may be present on the eyelids. Edema of the hands, feet, and eyelids may occur. Gastrointestinal hemorrhage or perforation can occur and is often life-threatening. Aspiration pneumonia is also possible when the muscles of the upper airway are involved. The disease is called *polymyositis* if the myopathy occurs in the absence of the rash.

Most children with dermatomyositis respond to treatment with corticosteroids, and the muscle and skin disease usually stabilizes within 2 years. In disease that is not well controlled by medication, scarring of muscle tissue may occur, causing contractures and stiffness. Soft tissue calcification—*calcinosis universalis*—occurs in approximately one third of patients. Calcium may extrude through the skin to produce painful sores that are predisposed to infection. Scarring of the skin may also contribute to immobility.

Muscles are tender and painful during the active stage of this disease. Exercise should not be instituted until the pain and tenderness have subsided. Deep breathing exercises aimed at increased thoracic expansion may be started at an early stage if intercostal muscles are involved. Loss of motion caused by calcium deposits is managed with exercise and splinting. Aggressive stretching is avoided because it may cause an acceleration of calcium deposits. A whirlpool may be needed for infected sores.

Ankylosing Spondylitis

Ankylosing spondylitis is one of the spondyloarthropathies that may have onset in childhood.[27] Ankylosis of the spine accompanied by a dorsal kyphosis are common findings of the disease. Sternal and costovertebral joints may be affected, as may large joints in the extremities. Inflammation of tendons where they insert into bones is commonly found, as is heel pain. Ankylosing spondylitis has the strongest genetic etiology of any of the rheumatic diseases and is associated with the blood marker HLA-B27.

Patients with ankylosing spondylitis should have their posture monitored closely. The height of the chair or the work surface should be adjusted to promote extension of the trunk during periods of sitting. Breathing exercises that emphasize expansion of the chest should be taught to the patient. Stiffness secondary to inactivity is a common problem in patients with ankylosing spondylitis, and this stiffness should be managed similarly to the stiffness seen with JRA.

Scleroderma

Scleroderma, or systemic sclerosis, is a disorder of the small blood vessels and connective tissue. Induration and thickening of the skin, as well as inflammatory changes in numerous body tissues, characterize scleroderma. Muscles, joints, heart, lungs, gastrointestinal tract, and kidneys can all be affected by the inflammatory changes. Early edema and stiffness of the hands and face are typical signs of the disease. Arthritis or arthralgia and muscle weakness are common symptoms.[28]

Patients with scleroderma commonly develop Raynaud's phenomenon. Wearing protective clothing and minimizing exposure to cold may control the tendency for vasospasm. Prevention of contractures is difficult, especially within the fingers and hands. A claw hand is typically seen. This deformity is caused by extension contractures at the metacarpophalangeal joints and flexion contractures of the interphalangeal joints. Aggressive stretching exercises and splinting are used to prevent or treat the contractures. Tightness of the soft tissue of the face leads to a classical mask-like face. This tightness causes difficulty in opening the mouth and restricts the use of facial expressions as a means of communication. Facial exercises are taught to maintain facial muscle strength and mobility.

Summary

The purpose of this chapter is to introduce the beginning physical therapist to principles and methods of assessing and treating children with JRA. An interdisciplinary team is an essential feature to meet the complex needs of the child with arthritis. A total program of care should include medical and surgical management, patient and family education, and psychosocial support, in addition to the program of physical rehabilitation presented in this chapter. The ultimate goal is for each child is to lead as normal a life as possible. This goal can be achieved only if the care delivery team is also invested in teaching the child, the family, and school personnel how best to manage the child's disease on a daily basis.

References

1. Cassidy JT, Petty RE. *Textbook of Pediatric Rheumatology.* 2nd ed. New York: Churchill Livingstone; 1990.
2. Schaller JG. Chronic arthritis in children. *Clin Orthop.* 1983;182:79–89.
3. Brewer EJ, Giannini EH, Pearson DA. *Juvenile Rheumatoid Arthritis.* Philadelphia: WB Saunders; 1982.
4. Athreya BH. Juvenile rheumatoid arthritis. In: Rose LF, Kaye D, eds. *Internal Medicine for Dentistry.* St. Louis: CV Mosby; 1983.
5. Athreya BH, Cassidy JT. Current status of the medical treatment of children with juvenile rheumatoid arthritis. *Rheum Dis Clin North Am.* 1991;17:871–889.
6. Wilson CH. Exercise for arthritis. In: Basmajian J,

ed. *Therapeutic Exercise.* Baltimore: Williams & Wilkins; 1984:529–545.

7. Ansell BM, Swann M. The management of chronic arthritis of children. *J Bone Joint Surg.* 1983;65B:536–543.

8. Fried JA, Athreya BH, Gregg JR, et al. The cervical spine in juvenile rheumatoid arthritis. *Clin Orthop Rel Res.* 1982;79:102–107.

9. Lechner DE, McCarthy CF, Holden MK. Gait deviations in patients with juvenile rheumatoid arthritis. *Phys Ther.* 1987;67:1335–1341.

10. SUNY at Buffalo Center for Functional Assessment Research, Department of Rehabilitative Medicine. *Guide for the Use of the Uniform Data Set for Medical Rehabilitation Including the Functional Independence Measure for Children (WeeFIM).* Research Foundation SUNY, 1991.

11. Hayley SM, Coster WJ, Faas RM. A content validity study of the Pediatric Evaluation of Disability Inventory. *Pediatr Phys Ther.* 1991;3:177–189.

12. Lovell DJ, et al. Development of a disability measurement tool for juvenile rheumatoid arthritis. The Juvenile Arthritis Functional Assessment Scale. *Arthritis Rheum.* 1989;32(11):1390–1395.

13. Singh G, Athreya B, Fries JF, Goldsmith DP. Measurement of functional status in JRA. *Arthritis & Rheumatism.* In press.

14. Giannini MJ, Protas EJ. Exercise response in children with and without juvenile rheumatoid arthritis: A case comparison study. *Phys Ther.* 1992;72:365–372.

15. Baldwin J. Pool therapy compared with individual home exercise therapy for juvenile rheumatoid arthritic patients. *Physiotherapy.* 1972;58:230–231.

16. Cordery J. Joint protection. *Am J Occup Ther.* 1965;19:285–294.

17. Brewer EJ. Reduction of morning stiffness and/or morning pain using a sleeping bag. *Pediatrics.* 1975;56:621.

18. Michlovitz S. The use of heat and cold in the management of rheumatic diseases. In: Michlovitz S, ed. *Thermal Agents in Rehabilitation.* Philadelphia: FA Davis; 1986.

19. Feibel A, Fast A. Deep heating of joints: A reconsideration. *Arch Phys Med Rehabil.* 1976;57:513–514.

20. Harris ED, McCroskery PA. The influence of temperature and fibril stability on degeneration of cartilage collagen by rheumatoid synovial collagenase. *N Engl J Med.* 1974;290:1–6.

21. Lehmann JD, ed. *Therapeutic Heat and Cold.* Baltimore: Williams & Wilkins; 1985.

22. Donovan WH: Physical measures in the treatment of juvenile rheumatoid arthritis. *Arthritis Rheum.* 1977;20:553–557.

23. Hyman BS, Gregg JR. Arthroplasty of the hip and knee in juvenile rheumatoid arthritis. *Rheum Dis Clin North Am.* 1991;17:971–983.

24. Jacobson ST, Levinson JE, Crawford AH. Late results of synovectomy in juvenile rheumatoid arthritis. *J Bone Joint Surg.* 1985;85:8–15.

25. Salter RB. The biologic concept of continuous passive motion of synovial joints; the first 18 years of basic research and its clinical application. *Clin Orthop* 1989;242:21–25.

26. Arthritis Foundation: *We Can: A Guide for Parents of Children with Arthritis.* Atlanta: Arthritis Foundation; 1985.

27. Schaller JG. Ankylosing spondylitis of childhood onset. *Arthritis Rheum.* 1977;20:398–401.

28. Melvin JL, Brannan KL, Leroy EC. Comprehensive care for the patient with systemic sclerosis (scleroderma). *Clin Rheumatol Pract.* May/June 1984;112–130.

Bibliography

Ansell BM. Rehabilitation in juvenile chronic arthritis. *Clin Rheum Dis.* 1981;7:469–484.

Emery HM, Bowyer SL. Physical modalities of therapy in pediatric rheumatic diseases. *Rheum Dis Clin North Am.* 1991;17:1001–1014.

Koch B. Rehabilitation of the child with joint disease. In:

Molnar GE, ed. *Pediatric Rehabilitation*. Baltimore: Williams & Wilkins; 1982.

Rhodes VJ. Physical therapy management of patients with juvenile rheumatoid arthritis. *Phys Ther*. 1991;71:910–919.

Scull SA, Dow MB, Athreya BH. Physical and occupational therapy for children with rheumatic diseases. *Pediatr Clin North Am*. 1986;33:1053–1077.

Pediatric Physical Therapy,
second edition, edited by Jan
Stephen Tecklin. J. B. Lippincott
Company, Philadelphia © 1994.

11

Dolores B. Bertoti

Physical Therapy for the Child with Mental Retardation

I was full of anticipation and bravado that first day of my student affiliation. The classroom days were behind me and in my mind's eye, all that I had learned academically about mental retardation was crystal clear. As I followed the supervising therapist into the special education classroom, my footsteps slowed. A sea of faces turned towards us with eagerness to both greet and investigate the newcomers. I was panic stricken. Where do I start? How will I know what to do? Help!!

That was many years ago, and I am still eager with anticipation each time I meet new children. My footsteps are more self-assured and firm with the understanding and knowledge which only experience provides. Each evaluation is a new challenge and the innovative programming necessary for the population of mentally retarded children is the biggest challenge. There are parents to interview and teach. There are teachers and classroom aides to instruct and train. There is equipment which needs adaptation and modification.

And there are the children to learn about, to teach, to listen to, so that I can continue to learn from them. With experience, this is the single most important thing which I have learned.

REFLECTIONS OF A PHYSICAL THERAPIST

The physical therapist plays a challenging and important multifaceted role in the management of mentally retarded children. The challenge lies in the fact that mentally retarded children often have various developmental problems, such as difficulty in sensory processing and maturation of reflexes. There may be deficits in attaining gross and fine motor skills.[1] The physical therapist must be able not only to assess the weaknesses of the child, but must also innovatively develop, implement, and modify treatment. These activities and related suggestions must then be shared effectively with the various people involved with the care of the mentally retarded child, including family members, teachers, classroom aides, and other professionals. In this chapter, an approach is offered to the physical therapist for developing a strategy for dealing with the numerous needs of the mentally retarded child.

Historical Review

Society and the mentally retarded population have had many interactions. In the earliest of recorded interactions between the two groups, mentally retarded people were ignored, received little or no care, or were actually left to die.[2] Spartan society believed in survival of only the fittest, and many people, including the physically and mentally handicapped, were left to die.

Conversely, during the Middle Ages and in ancient Rome, it was not uncommon for wealthy people to help a "fool" or "court jester" in response for the amusement these people provided for the household and its guests.[2] Artistic work of the Middle Ages shows people who have the physical attributes of Down's syndrome serving as jesters.[3] In the later Middle Ages, particularly in Europe, superstitious religious beliefs led to the execution of many people who were considered "witches and warlocks." Mentally retarded people were undoubtedly included in these groups.[2] This idea that mentally retarded people were social menaces and outcasts persisted throughout the 19th century with the trend away from execution but toward punishment, imprisonment, and isolation.[4]

In the early 20th century, there was a publicly perceived need to shelter and protect mentally retarded people from the misunderstanding, abuses, and wrath of society. As a result, they were socially isolated in asylums, shelters, and farm communities. These communities rapidly became overcrowded. The goal of this public effort was clearly housing, and not provision of other services.

Interest in providing services to help mentally retarded people had a difficult beginning. In the early 1800s, Jean Marc Itard, a French physician, became intrigued with a mentally retarded youngster whom the physician had captured in the forests of Aveyron in France. Acting on the premise that intellectual performance could be affected by environmental stimulation, Itard succeeded in teaching this "Wild Boy of Aveyron." Although Itard's work helped the boy improve over a 5-year period, the gains were not sufficient for acceptance of the boy into the Parisian society at that time. Society frowned on the child and Itard believed he had failed.[5]

Johann Jacob Guggenbuhl, in 1840, established a center in Switzerland for group teaching for mentally retarded children. His work received worldwide acclaim as a major reform. This reform influenced the work in France and in the United States of Edouard Seguin, who was a leader in the development of educational and residential services for mentally retarded people. In 1876, Seguin was made president of the newly formed Association of Medical Officers of American Institutions for Idiotic and Feeble-Minded Persons. This Association later became the American Association of Mental Deficiency (AAMD),[5] currently called the American Association on Mental Retardation (AAMR).

In the United States, the social organization accompanying the Industrial Revolution reinforced the concept of group care of children, as well as stimulating a sense of social responsibility.[2] Throughout the 1800s, small gains fluctuated with a sense of frustration and futility, and there was a movement to house the "incurables" in large, overcrowded facilities in isolated areas.[3]

By the end of World War II, emphasis for care of mentally retarded people changed to include "programming." This shift to a plan of activity was mainly the result of efforts by the National Association for Retarded Citizens (NARC) and other parent or professional advocacy groups.[3] A growing awareness of the negative effects of residential segregation and the limitations of existing programs led to a critical reappraisal of existing care for mentally retarded people. Influenced by the civil rights movement, the 1960s represented a time of expansion in program legislation and funding allocations for all handicapped people. Discrimination against and segregation of mentally retarded people were recognized as negative and undesirable.[3]

In the early 1970s, American visitors to Scandinavian countries encountered the concept of "normalization," which is defined as the principle of educating handicapped people in and for the "normal" environment of the nonhandicapped to the maximum extent feasible.[6] This process obviously requires major development and use of community-based support systems. The era was one of "deinstitutionalization" for mentally retarded people. Living arrangements in the community have now become the norm for long-term care for retarded citizens.[6] Many community-based services, often created and operated by parent associations, are appearing.

The most current approach to programming in the field of mental retardation can be described as a functional, integrated approach. The focus of this approach, which involves use of integrated program models, is to help make the mentally retarded person more functional within the world.

Mental retardation is now seen as a functional and social problem, the consequences of which can be alleviated by social acceptance, training, and a wide range of educational, medical, and socially supportive services. The main idea is to humanize and normalize the lives of all mentally retarded people.[4]

This rapid expansion of services and the trend toward normalization through use of community resources have major implications for physical therapists. As services for mentally retarded people expand, service models and roles of the physical therapist also expand. The physical therapist has been involved traditionally with evaluation and treatment. With the recent expansion of roles, the physical therapist now serves as consultant, educator, researcher, and planner. The physical therapist is in the forefront of this expansion and can improve various aspects of the entire life span of the mentally retarded person.

Definition and Description

The terms used to define mental retardation previously came from observations and descriptions of typical types of behavior.[2] Retarded people were described as "simple," "stupid," and "feeble." Terminology and definitions of mental retardation reflected the prevailing views of society. It was not until 1961 that an official definition of mental retardation was developed by the AAMD. The original definition was revised in 1973 and states:

> Mental retardation refers to significantly subaverage general intellectual functioning existing concurrently with deficits in adaptive behavior, and manifested during the developmental period.[7]

It is obvious from this definition that deficits in two dimensions—measured intelligence and adaptive behavior—are characteristics of mentally retarded people. Subaverage intellectual functioning means earning a score that is two or more standard deviations below the mean on an intelligence quotient (IQ) test. Adaptive behavior refers to such skills as communication, sensorimotor function, social skill, and vocational ability.[8] It is also apparent from the definition that the deficit of mental retardation is multidimensional and has interactive effects on social, psychological, cultural, and physical factors.

Incidence

Approximately 2% of any population is composed of mentally retarded people.[7] The largest percentage of these people are those who are only mildly retarded. The AAMR estimates that there are currently between 4 and 6 million citizens with mental retardation in the United States.

Classification

Systems used to classify mentally retarded people have changed greatly over the years and are still being modified. Although used with varying frequency, the most common systems are based on measured intelligence or severity of symptoms; medical causes; adaptive behavior; educational expectations; and function.[3]

Measured Intelligence

Classification by measured intelligence requires grouping people according to IQ test scores. For many years, this was the only classification system used, and it is still common. The AAMD IQ classification is shown in Table 11-1. These scores are derived from a standardized intelligence test that is given by a psychologist. Psychologists may use various testing instruments. The more commonly used tests are described as follows.

Stanford Binet Intelligence Scale

The Stanford Binet Intelligence Scale, which has been revised, is considered to be a strong, sensitive tool for assessing intelligence in mentally retarded people and in children younger than 8 years of age.[9] One drawback is that this tool relies heavily on verbal ability.[3]

Wechsler Intelligence Test for Children

The Wechsler test is both effective and quick to administer. It is used to assess intelligence in children older than 5 years of age.[3]

McCarthy Scales of Children's Abilities

The McCarthy scale provides a general cognitive index and is a valuable tool for testing young children.[9]

Briggance Diagnostic Assessment of Basic Skills

The Briggance test is a compilation of criterion-referenced tests appropriate for individuals up to 21 years of age. The test has many subtests that are excellent for testing specific skill areas and is particularly suited for physically handicapped people.

Bayley Scales of Infant Development

The Bayley developmental scales were developed for infants and young children from 2 to 30 months of age. The test identifies a developmental level based on mental, motor, and behavioral limits, and is both standardized and reliable.[3]

Peabody Picture Vocabulary Test

The Peabody test, which has been revised, is a good tool for assessing receptive language in nonverbal people. Physically handicapped children can be tested by using the large, widely spread pictures.[3]

Although most states require a numerical IQ score, that score is only part of a composite classification that describes the child. A descriptive clarifying statement usually accompanies the numerical IQ score. Using an IQ test in an isolated manner can give an unjust assessment of the child's abilities, which is true particularly for the multiply handi-

Table 11-1. *Intelligence and Educational Classification of the Mentally Retarded*

Descriptive Terminology	Intelligence Quotient	Educational Classification	Mental Age	Possible Placement Using Functional Curriculum Model
Profound	<20	Dependent; needs life support	0–2 yrs	Multiple disabilities support
Severe	20–35	Dependent; trainable	0–2 yrs	Life support
Moderate	36–51	Trainable	3–7 yrs ⎫	Life support or learning support
Mild	52–67	Educable	8–12 yrs ⎭	

capped child. Children with motor, language, or emotional disabilities are unlikely to do well on the standardized IQ test. The IQ test should never be the sole measure for the handicapped child.

Classification of Medical Causes

In the United States, the International Classification of Disease is used in an effort to classify mental retardation according to its medical cause.[7,10] This classification and the classification presented by the AAMR describe 10 categories of causes:

1. Infections and intoxications (e.g., rubella, congenital syphilis, and encephalitis)
2. Traumatic injury or a physical agent (e.g., mechanical injury at birth, head trauma)
3. Disorders of metabolism or nutrition (e.g., hypothyroidism, Tay-Sachs disease)
4. Postnatal gross brain disease (e.g., intracranial neoplasm, neurofibromatosis)
5. Unknown prenatal influences (e.g., hydrocephalus, microcephaly)
6. Chromosomal abnormalities (e.g., Down's syndrome, Klinefelter's syndrome)
7. Disorders of gestation (e.g., prematurity, low birth weight)
8. Secondary to a major psychiatric disorder
9. Environmental deprivation (cultural or familial retardation)
10. Associated with other conditions or influences

Adaptive Behavior

The definition from the AAMR states that mentally retarded people manifest deficits in adaptive behavior.[7] *Adaptive behavior* can be defined as appropriate social performance in daily living as expected of a person of a particular age by the community, or culture, of which that person is part.[11] An important aspect of using adaptive behavior as a type of classification is that it attends rather specifically to human development. An assessment of adaptive behavior indicates at what level on the developmental continuum the person is functioning. Deficits in adaptive behavior vary at different ages and may be reflected in many areas. They may be seen during infancy and early childhood in sensorimotor

skill and development; communication skill; self-help skill; and socialization. Deficits during childhood and early adolescence may be reflected in application of basic academic skills, in activities of daily living (ADLs), in the use of appropriate reasoning and judgment, and in social interpersonal skills.[10]

The adaptive behavior classification system, as updated by the AAMD, delineates age-level skills in several areas, including physical, social, occupational, communication, and ADLs.[1] Tests commonly used to assess adaptive behavior are given by psychologists. Two such tests are described in the following sections.

American Association of Mental Retardation Adaptive Behavior Scale

The AAMR Adaptive Behavior Scale is preferred for evaluating adaptive behavior. This test is easily administered and presents a broad, global view of the child's ability to function.[3]

Vineland Social Maturity Scale: Scales of Independent Behavior

The Vineland Social Maturity Scale is a new and promising means of assessing adaptive behavior in people up to 40 years of age. Table 11-2 shows adaptive behavior levels according to age.[6] The Vineland focuses on testing adaptive and social behavior.

Educational Classification

The educational classification system, first defined by Scheerenberger in 1964,[10] is rarely used as a sole classification system. This system is shown in Table 11-1. Terms such as "educable" (IQ of 50 to 75), "trainable" (IQ of 20 to 49), dependent (IQ of less than 20), and life support are designated.[12] This terminology is now considered to be out-of-date.

Functional Curriculum Programming

Most recently, programming for children with mental retardation has followed a functional, commu-

Table 11-2. *Adaptive Behavior in the Mentally Retarded*

| | Age of the Mentally Retarded Person | | |
Category	*Preschool*	*School-aged*	*Adult*
Mild	Often appears normal; develops social and communication skill	Academic skills of 6th grade are possible; special education needs for secondary school	Can learn social and vocational skills
Moderate	Poor social skills; can communicate; may need supervision	Can develop up to 4th grade skills with special training	Unskilled or semiskilled vocation
Severe	Lacks communication; poor motor skills	May learn to communicate; basic personal health habits; no academic skills	Needs complete supervision for any self-support activity
Profound	Dependent for care; poor sensorimotor development	Some motor development; continues to be dependent for care; limited success with training	Limited motor ability and communication; continued dependency for care

(Adapted from Sloan W, Birch JW. A rationale for degrees of retardation. Am J Mental Defic. 1955;60:262.

nity-based model. The basic assumptions underlying this functional approach are as follows:

- Students with developmental disabilities should be provided age-appropriate and application-oriented skills.
- Students with developmental disabilities should be prepared to participate more independently in less restrictive settings (community-based curriculum).
- The curriculum should include procedures for maintenance of skills that generalize to the environments in which the skills will ultimately be performed.
- Students with developmental disabilities should participate, at least partially, in community activities.[13]

This functional, or community-based, approach uses the following descriptive terminology in determining program placement for the mentally retarded:

- Academic support class or gifted support
- Learning support
- Life skills support
- Emotional support
- Sensory and communication support class (services for the deaf and hearing-impaired)
- Blind and visually-impaired support
- Speech and language support
- Physical support

- Autistic support
- Multiple disabilities support

It is important to note that the terminology cited refers to the programming, not necessarily to the mentally retarded student. The intent is to describe a child's needs and, based upon those needs, to place the child in appropriate programming.

Composite Classification

Each of the systems of classification has strengths and weaknesses. Composite descriptions are commonly being used. These descriptions often include IQ score, medical diagnosis, and functional level. These composites are more appropriate than single tests, and facilitate programming designed for the specific and individual needs of each child.

Physical Therapy Assessment

Important Elements

A successful and effective physical therapy assessment of the child with mental retardation depends largely on the therapist's approach to the child. Four important elements should facilitate the process of assessment.

Throughout the assessment, the therapist must analyze not only what the child can do, but also the *processes underlying the observed skills and behaviors.*[1] Thus, the therapist must determine not only what tasks the child can do, but also why the child can do those specific tasks and not others. Movements must be broken down into components, and basic mental, physiological, and physical processes must be analyzed in relation to those tasks.

Evaluative procedures used for children, particularly mentally retarded children, often differ from the more rigid clinical procedures used for adults. As in all of pediatrics, much information can be gathered by interacting with the child through observation and during play. Standard evaluative tests and procedures may be used as rapport is established, depending on the functional level of the child. Owing to the attention deficits and associated problems of the mentally retarded child, the evaluation should be done serially, and should be ongoing. With the new functional approach to curriculum planning, the physical therapist should perform an evaluation with as many *functional aspects,* using age-appropriate materials, as is reasonable.

The third important element necessary for a good evaluation is related to the basic orientation of the therapist. As with other areas of physical therapy, but more importantly with the multiply handicapped child, the therapist must be able to identify not only the disability, but also the child's abilities, however minimal. The skilled therapist will identify even the smallest of abilities and effectively communicate the importance of those abilities to the child, parents, and other professionals working with the child. A major focus of treatment involves attempts to increase those abilities. This *"positive" orientation and approach* will have a beneficial effect on the child's self-image and on those people working with the child.[14] If our actions suggest a true concern and expectation for progress, however limited that progress may be, the effect of this attitude should encourage the child, the teachers, and the family to strive toward goals that have been identified.[14]

The fourth important element in evaluation is that the therapist must always first assess *sensory processes and attention.* Children experience their world through sensory (afferent) pathways. They assimilate the information; then they take action. Because the sensory or receptive abilities must be intact for normal movement to occur, the therapist must include assessment of the sensory systems as a major component in the overall evaluation of the child.[1] The therapist must understand by what means—or even whether—the child is perceiving the world before continuing with the evaluation.

Sensory Assessment and Treatment

The therapist must determine the basic responsiveness of the child before deciding on an appropriate interaction strategy for the rest of the evaluation. Kinnealy distinguished two broad categories of mentally retarded children on the basis of their reactions to various sensory stimuli.[15] She described one group as having difficulty monitoring the intensity of sensory input and, therefore difficulty in modulating the response. The other group was described as having reduced perception of the incoming stimuli. This group required more intense input for arousal or elicitation of a response. This initial difference in perception of sensory stimulus is a critical point of departure that the therapist must ascertain during the first attempt at interaction with the child.

Visual

When assessing the child's visual sense, the therapist should note the ability of the child to orient to, focus on, and track a visual stimulus. A flashlight, or a brightly colored, patterned toy should be placed approximately 7 to 15 inches from the child's face for this assessment (Fig. 11-1). This range of distance affords optimal visual clarity in early development.[16] Getman and associates have suggested that horizontal tracking is easier than vertical tracking, and that diagonal tracking is the most difficult.[17] Notable responses include difficulty in tracking across the midline and resting eye movements (nystagmus). The term *cortical blind-*

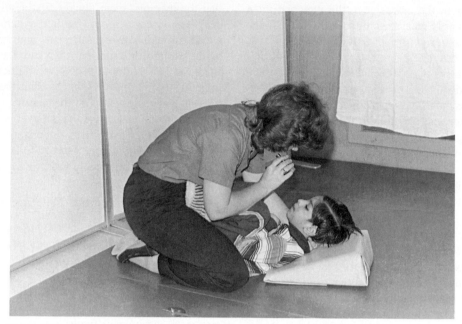

Figure 11-1. *A physical therapist uses a small flashlight to assess visual sense.*

ness describes an inability to interpret visual information owing to severe brain damage or occipital lobe atrophy.

During treatment, visual stimulation activities can be used to provide practice in both focusing and tracking (Fig. 11-2). Children who have poor head control may have an inadequate base of support for eye movements. Treatment aimed at improving postural mechanisms may improve visual skill.[1] Adaptive aids to ensure proper body positioning should be used at all times. Vestibular input may also improve visual focusing and processing because vestibular reflexes, in combination with optic and tonic neck reflexes, maintain a stable image on the retina while the head and body are in motion.[1] The vestibulo-oculomotor pathways contribute to skilled movements of the eyes that can be used for educational skills, including reading and writing.[18]

Auditory

The child's response to auditory stimuli may range from an absence of response, to simple orientation to and movement toward the stimulus, to a startle response[1] (Fig. 11-3). Although it is difficult to assess hearing loss in a retarded or multiply handicapped child, referral for a complete audiologic evaluation is indicated whenever there is a possibility of a hearing loss. Audiologic testing can be used to identify a hearing loss, to differentiate between conductive and sensorineural loss, and to quantify the degree of loss. Tympanometry (an objective measure of eardrum function) helps identify a conductive loss when behavioral testing is unreliable. Testing for brain-stem–evoked response traces the passage of an auditory stimulus from the ear to the brain stem. Central or cortical deafness describes a lack of interpretation of auditory information owing to brain damage.

Vestibular stimulation is a component of treatment aimed at enhancing auditory integration. Although the vestibulocochlear nerve (cranial nerve VIII) has been described as comprising two separate entities (vestibular and auditory), it developed phylogenetically as a unit, and its portions appear to

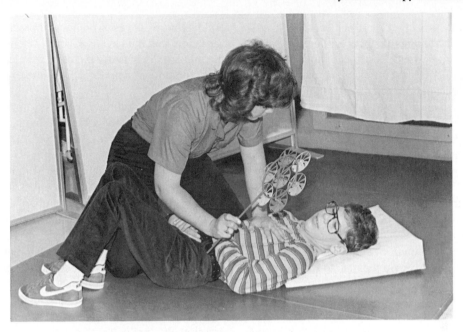

Figure 11-2. *A physical therapist uses a brightly colored toy to work with older child on visual tracking skill.*

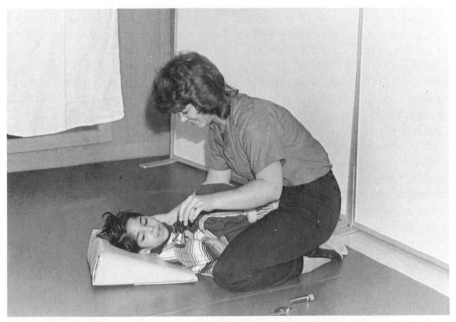

Figure 11-3. *A physical therapist uses a small bell to assess gross response to sound. Proper positioning to reduce tone and isolation of the auditory stimulus are important aspects of this procedure.*

be related functionally.[1] There is clear clinical evidence that difficulties in hearing interfere with equilibrium responses. Vestibular input may not only improve equilibrium reactions, but may also sometimes enhance auditory attention and integration.[19]

Tactile

The tactile system is the largest sensory system, and it plays a major role in both physical and emotional behavior.[20] The tactile system develops earliest in utero, and the ability to process tactile input is important for neural organization.

As early as 1920, Head described two cutaneous systems: the "protopathic" and the "epicritic" systems.[21] The primitive protopathic system was described as protective, causing a person to react to tactile stimuli with increased affect and alertness.[21] The protopathic system may be synonymous with the spinothalamic system described by Poggin and Mountcastle.[22] The epicritic system was described as having a more discriminative function, and is synonymous with the described lemniscal system.[22] This epicritic system allows a person to respond to light touch with a well-localized sensation. The dualism of these systems may actually be more of an intermingling of the two, or portions of a continuum, rather than a strict dichotomy. Normal neural organization is likely characterized by a continuous gradient of functional organization of the two paths.[23] The systems are normally in balance. When threatened, there is a predominant response of increased alertness and increased affect. When not challenged, however, the person is free to explore and manipulate the environment.[24]

Many children with brain damage show an imbalance between the two pathways. With neurologic impairment, many children show an aversive response to some types of tactile stimulation. This aversion to tactile stimuli, called *tactile defensiveness,* is often manifested by such behavior as hyperactivity or distractibility.[23] Children who show tactile defensiveness may display avoidance reactions around the hands, feet, and face. This behavior has obvious implications for the manner in which a child explores the environment, appreciates tactile sensation, and thus learns. Tactile defensiveness in the oral area may cause the child to reject textured or flavored food in preference to smoother, blander foods.

Although no data are available to support the idea, some professionals suggest that tactile defensiveness is part of a generalized "set" of the nervous system by which the child interprets stimuli as "danger."[23] Tactile functions were among the first means by which the child received information about his or her environment in order to adapt appropriately. The result of neurodevelopmental disorders is often behavior that appears to be less completely evolved and less discriminatory than normal. Tactile defensiveness or overresponsiveness may be seen in this context as poorly developed mechanisms for the interpretation of information. Clinically, the child may appear anxious, emotionally labile, or threatened and unable to cope. Compensatory behavior may be characterized by withdrawal, irritability, or distractibility.[23]

Ayres has suggested various treatment regimens designed to alter the balance of the two systems in favor of increased discrimination. The postulate on which treatment is based is that certain types of sensory input will normalize the neural process and will elicit a protective response. This response will cause a balance between the protective and discriminative aspects of the total system. The sensory input that appears to be particularly effective in influencing the modulating mechanism operates through the tactile system. The proprioceptive system serves a cooperative role in this functional scheme.[23]

The physical therapist can easily incorporate into treatment appropriate activities for both the tactile and proprioceptive systems. Heavy touch and pressure or weight bearing are excellent activities for decreasing tactile hypersensitivity and promoting proximal joint stability. Light touch or stimuli that tickle or irritate the child should be avoided in favor of activities that offer deep pressure.

The response of the mentally retarded child to tactile input must be observed and monitored during evaluation and treatment. The therapist must note whether the child responds to the stimulus (i.e., the touch of the therapist's hand) and, if a response is noted, the therapist must identify the type of response. If the input is noxious, does the child respond with a grimace, or does the child move actively to avoid the stimulus? One might surmise that the child who actively removes or withdraws from the noxious stimulus is not only aware of the stimulus but also has some proprioceptive sense by which to locate and remove the stimulus. Conversely, the therapist must be aware of the child who is so totally unaware of sensory input that the therapist is unable to penetrate and reach the child by any means. Clearly, knowing the level of awareness of the child will direct the therapist through subsequent stages of the evaluation process.[1]

Vestibular

Along with the tactile system, the vestibular system is one of the earliest developing sensory systems in the human being. The tracts within the vestibular system are fully myelinated by 20 weeks of gestation.[23] Information from the vestibular system tells us our position exactly in relation to gravity, whether or not we are moving, and our speed and direction of movement.[20] Semicircular canals within the inner ear are the vestibular receptors that provide dynamic information regarding angular acceleration around the body's axis. The utricles are receptors that provide static information concerning the position of the body in relation to gravity.[25] The vestibular system is so sensitive that changes in position and movement have a powerful effect on the brain, and this effect changes with even the most subtle adjustments of movement or posture.[23]

Vestibular sensations are produced mainly within the vestibular nuclei and the cerebellum.[23] Stimuli are sent caudally in the spinal cord and into the brain stem where they serve a powerful integrative function. Some stimuli are also sent rostrally from the brain stem to the cerebral hemispheres.[20]

The vestibular system has a strong effect on muscle tone and movement. This influence is mediated through the lateral and medial vestibular nuclei and affects efferent transmission down the spinal cord. Vestibular influence usually exerts a facilitatory effect on the gamma motoneuron to the muscle spindle and may influence the alpha motoneurons supplying skeletal muscle. By activating the gamma efferent to the muscle spindle, the afferent flow from the spindle is maintained and regulated for assistance with motor function. This basic role in muscle function and mobility gives the vestibular system an important role in the development and maintenance of body scheme that depends on interpretation of movement.[23] Impulses ascending to higher brain stem and cortical levels synapse with tactile, proprioceptive, visual, and auditory impulses to provide both perception of space and orientation of the body within that space.[20] Vestibular input seldom enters conscious thought or awareness except when the stimulus is so intense that we are rendered dizzy.

Vestibular function can be assessed clinically by noting the presence of and duration of nystagmus after vestibular stimulation, such as spinning. Nystagmus is a slow movement of the eyes in one direction followed by a rapid movement in the opposite direction.[1] Ayres has developed a procedure for testing postrotatory nystagmus. Her procedure has been standardized on children between 5 and 9 years of age.[26] If there is no nystagmus, or if nystagmus lasts only for a short time, the child's vestibular nuclei are either not receiving the correct amount of vestibular input or processing of the input is inadequate. If nystagmus is hyperactive, Ayres suggests that the vestibular system is overresponding, possibly as a result of a lack of inhibitory forces.[20] As part of the evaluative process, the therapist, or someone trained in giving the postrotatory nystagmus test, assesses the response of the child to the movement. It is important to know whether the child overreacts to or is threatened by movement, or has difficulty in attending to and assimilating movement experiences.

The physical therapist may choose to include various movement or vestibular activities in a child's program with the hope of achieving several goals. With a knowledge of the child's response to vestibular stimulation, activities can be chosen to improve balance, simulate experience of movement, influence muscle tone (specifically, antigravity extensors), promote awareness and eye contact, and increase spatial awareness and perception. Examples of equipment used in these movement activities include swings, barrels, and scooter boards. A type of swing being used to assess postrotatory nystagmus is shown in Figure 11-4.

Self-Stimulation

Self-stimulation in some mentally retarded children is an area of concern. This type of behavior can take many forms, including self-abuse. Examples of self-stimulation include constant mouthing of objects or the hand, spinning, head banging, hand or arm flapping, teeth grinding, rocking, and self-biting. Evaluation of the sensory status of the child may identify the reason for self-stimulation. The child may be performing self-stimulation to fulfill a basic sensory need, or he or she may be overstimulated and may be reacting out of frustration or an inability to cope with sensory overload.[1]

In educational programs, the tendency is to discourage self-stimulation, especially when the stimulation is abusive or socially unacceptable. When stimulation is restricted, an appropriate sensory input must be substituted or the child may substitute another form of self-stimulation. For example, a child whose elbows are restricted to extension in an effort to prevent hand biting may respond with head banging. A child who cannot cope with the sensory stimuli in the environment and is being overstimulated needs to have sensory input graded to tolerance.[1] As in all other areas of evaluation and treatment, the therapist must look beyond the behavior to the processes that are initiating it. Underlying sensory abnormalities or deficiencies must be recognized and treated before a change in behavior can be expected.[27]

The manner in which the child provides self-stimulation can suggest strategies that may be effective in improving or eliminating the behavior. Slow, rhythmical rocking may be the distractible child's method of calming himself or herself, whereas violent, irregular rocking may be the hypo-

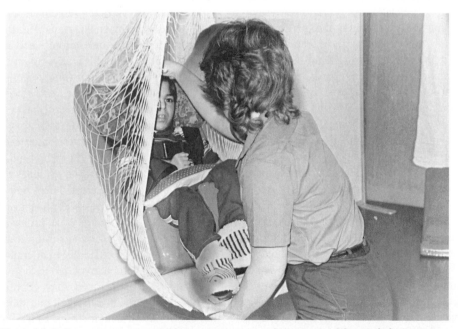

Figure 11-4. *Preparing to spin a child in a swing to assess the response of the vestibular system.*

tonic child's method of providing sensory input that will increase muscle tone and alertness. The type of behavior must also be considered in light of the developmental age of the child. Constant mouthing of objects and hands is socially unacceptable for a school-aged child. If, however, that child is functioning at a lower developmental and functional level than age would dictate, oral exploration is a primary component of the learning process.[1] Rather than restricting such oral exploration and stimulation, the child must be provided means of oral stimulation, such as gum rubbing, tooth brushing, and foods of various textures, in order to help facilitate progression to the next developmental and functional level.

Assessment of Motor and Developmental Skills

A knowledge of the numerous comprehensive tests of motor development is important when assessing the motor abilities and developmental level of a mentally retarded child. The therapist must be able to draw from a knowledge of many tests to conduct a smooth and efficient evaluation session. Much useful information can be gathered by watching the child during play and other activities. This ability to gather information by observation is important when working with a child whose comprehension, attention span, and level of cooperation may be limited. This section of the chapter discusses motor evaluation as it is accomplished with a mentally retarded child. A more thorough review of tests of development and information regarding musculoskeletal assessment can be found in Chapters 2 and 7.

Reflexes

Reflexes are the substrate of human movement; they are the raw material on which the central nervous system builds volitional movement.[28] An evaluation of reflex integration is essential in determining a basic level of neuromotor development.[1] Tests of motor function that include an assessment of the effects on motor skill development of reflexes are valuable tools for the therapist. Although not yet standardized, the Early Intervention Developmental Profile offers a simple but comprehensive means of assessing development and skill quality in children up to 5 years of age.[29] Classic reflex testing is used universally as an assessment tool in pediatrics, and can be used for mentally retarded children. In addition to classical testing, or when classical testing is not feasible, reflex abnormalities can be observed during motor activities. An analysis of postural responses can be done while the child is rolling, crawling, creeping, standing, and walking. For example, several areas of inadequate reflex integration can be identified by watching the child while rolling. An overly flexed position with the child prone, or an extended position with the child supine suggests poor integration of tonic labyrinthine responses. "Log rolling" or rolling without segmental rotation may indicate that the righting reflexes are not incorporated into functional activities.[1]

Muscle Tone and Strength

Muscle tone may range from extreme hypotonia to extreme hypertonia and, in many children with cerebral palsy, to spasticity.[1] As abnormalities in muscle tone are commonly seen in mentally retarded children, a review of this topic seems appropriate.

When hypotonia occurs in combination with mental retardation, the cause is thought to be general integrative deficits within the central nervous system (CNS) and, possibly, a lack of "gamma" efferent biasing of the muscle spindle.[1] Activity of the gamma efferent system has been linked to general levels of activity within the CNS.[30] Children with mental retardation and subsequent limited movement or limited movement experience may display hypotonia as a result of inadequate sensorimotor experience.

During treatment, sensory stimuli that are effective in increasing arousal and alertness may also be used to elicit an increase in muscle tone. Children with hypotonia should be encouraged to engage in activities that enhance muscle co-contraction and proximal stability. Resistance activities, such as pushing weighted carts or toys, using push-pull scooter board games against resistive tubing strips, and scooting or creeping using weights and dowels, may be effective in increasing muscle tone, providing opportunities for joint approximation and weight bearing, and facilitating proximal stability. Some possibilities for treatment are shown in Figure 11-5.

Hypertonia must be distinguished from a pathologic increase in muscle tone (i.e., spasticity). Increased muscle tone may be seen in some mentally retarded children in the absence of neurobiologic signs of spasticity. These children may be described as being unusually tense; they may have tactile defensiveness and may be distractible. Sensory input for the child with hypertonia or with spasticity should be geared toward decreasing or normalizing muscle tone.[1] In the absence of cerebral palsy, hypertonia is seen less often than hypotonia in mentally retarded children.

Strength testing and goniometry for children with mental impairment must be as innovative as other aspects of the physical therapy evaluation. Many children, especially those with cognitive deficits, are unable to follow directions and have difficulty understanding the concept of resistance and range of motion (ROM). It is usually necessary to structure a play situation in which general observation regarding strength can be made. The child may need to imitate the postures made by the therapist. Activities to assess strength can be improvised. These improvisations may include manually resisting a pull-toy, providing resistance against creeping, or observing the child's ability to lift and carry a weighted toy.[1] Goniometric assessment of the mentally retarded child may require a two-person team. Proper positioning to decrease the effects of abnormal tone will facilitate the accuracy of measurement of joint ROM (Fig. 11-6).

Developmental Testing

Assessment of motor function and developmental skill level can be accomplished using various tests. The most commonly used tests of motor development are reviewed in Chapter 2. In clinical situations, the Early Intervention Developmental Profile, although not standardized, is an excellent tool for assessing development in the young child.[29] This test measures five areas of development: gross motor, perceptual-fine motor, language, social-emotional, and self-help. Test items are fun for the child and are easily given by the therapist. The assessment test also includes a program component, translating developmental skills into goals and objectives for easy incorporation into an Individualized Educational Program. Therapists are reminded that all developmental testing must be clarified and supplemented with observations regarding the quality of movement, skill attainment, and functional abilities of the child.

Summary

To summarize, the physical therapist assessing the mentally retarded child must have various skills and must approach the evaluation with a flexible but organized strategy. Assessment must include not only developmental testing, functional assessment, goniometrics, posture, and strength, but also a complete evaluation of the sensory systems. Because the main goal of treatment is to enhance basic developmental processes and to improve function, there must be a thorough examination of all sensory and motor components of development. It is challenging and rewarding to evaluate such a complex group of skill areas and still have a concise picture of the whole child.

Physical Therapy Treatment Strategies

General Principles

Treatment and management of the mentally retarded child must be directed toward the development of the child's full potential in all areas of learning: motor, cognitive, and affective. The child's ability to respond appropriately and effectively in terms of movement, intellectual function, and attitudes and feelings serves as the major long-range goal of treatment. This concept of treatment

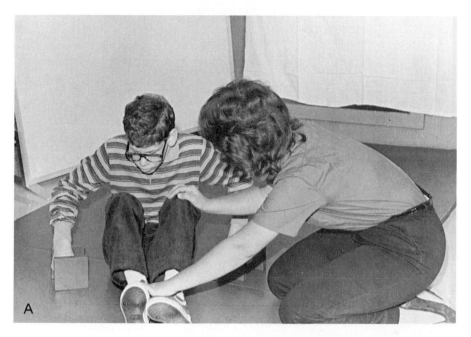

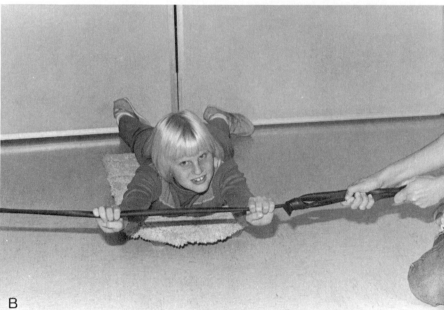

Figure 11-5. A *and* B. *Children perform resistance activities as a means of improving proximal joint stability.*

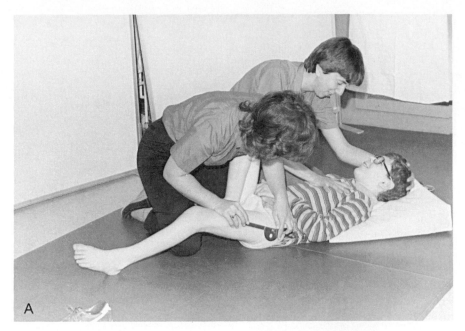

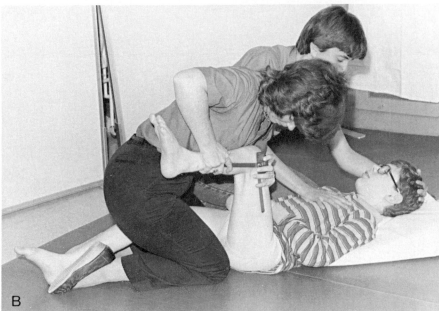

Figure 11-6. A *and* B. *Two therapists perform goniometric measurements on a mentally retarded child.*

applies to the total function of the child. A deficit in one type of behavior may influence all other types. The child who needs motor stability may also benefit from psychological stability. Influences used to change the former may also have an effect on the latter and vice versa.[14] Although the physical therapy setting is structured to provide mainly for the acquisition of motor skills, the environment should facilitate development in all areas of behavior.

There are several important elements to remember when designing effective treatment programs for mentally retarded children. The therapist must recognize the importance of choosing activities that accommodate the mental age of the child, but that are also as age-appropriate as possible. Table 11-3 offers several examples of how purely developmental activities can be translated into functional activities.

Activities in the treatment program should be interesting, fun, and meaningful. Because children with mental retardation often have a poor attention span, therapeutic activities should be chosen that most effectively and efficiently meet the identified goal. Rather than asking a child to do a standard exercise regimen for strengthening, the necessary therapeutic activities can be translated into a functional task or social game (Fig. 11-7). This approach not only sustains interest, cooperation, and enthusiasm, but it emphasizes carryover into ADLs. It may also promote achievement of goals in other areas, such as social, emotional, self-help, and cognitive skills. The therapist must be imaginative and should integrate many different approaches in order to develop an effective treatment approach for a particular child in a particular situation.

Repetition and consistency are crucial aspects of any treatment plan in which learning is expected to occur. Because repetition is important for learning any task, the therapist must design several activities that teach the same component task, but do so in different ways. For example, if the treatment goal is to improve extension of the trunk, the therapist may use activities such as a basketball drop or scooterboard games (Fig. 11-8). These activities are varied but enjoyable methods of attaining the same

Table 11-3. *Examples of Functional Activities That Incorporate Developmental Skills*

Assessment Item	Underlying Skill	Examples of Alternative Materials/Activities
Walks on balance beam	Balance	Walking on bleachers, walking between rows of chairs
Holds rattle for 5–10 seconds	Can hold an object for 5–10 seconds	Cup, spoon, book, hairbrush, coin, pencil and ball
Stacks 3 wooden blocks	Perceptual-motor coordination of stacking	Glasses, bowls, dishes, trays, records, and cassette tapes
Strings 3 1-inch beads	Perceptual-motor coordination of inserting and pushing/pulling through	Lace shoes
Places peg in pegboard	Eye-hand (or hand-hand) coordination of placing an object in another object	Straw in milk carton, sock in shoe, toast in toaster, coin in vending machine slot, key in lock, pencil in sharpener
Picks up raisin with pincer grasp	Uses pincer grasp to pick up items	Food, table game pieces, coins, pages of book, vocational items (nails, hooks)
Anticipates being picked up	Anticipates routine event	Being fed, bathed, tickled, greeted, and being put to bed

Downing J, Bailey B. Presented at the TASH Annual Conference; December 9, 1988; Washington, DC.

goal. This approach to treatment planning ensures not only the necessary repetition of activities, but also offers the dimensions of interest and fun for a child with limited comprehension or attention.

One of the most important yet most difficult skills for the therapist to master is the ability to delineate priorities for treatment and to establish effective and appropriate long-term plans. When the therapist is faced with the challenge of a child with numerous deficits in many areas of development, it is easy for the therapist to become overwhelmed.

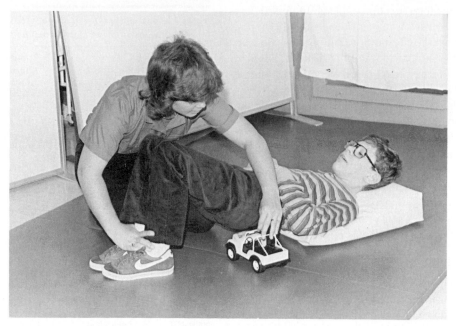

Figure 11-7. *Strengthening exercises for the hips and trunk can be done as part of a game.*

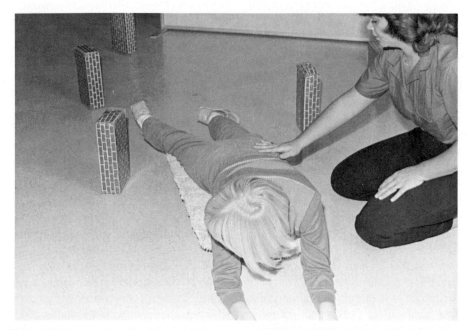

Figure 11-8. *A physical therapist supervises a scooter board activity that has been set up as an obstacle course.*

When developing treatment plans, it is important to consider the child as a whole person. All pieces of the evaluation puzzle should merge to provide the therapist with a composite picture of how the child is or is not functioning within the child's world. The priorities for treatment should become clear by looking at the child's overall development in this functional sense.

Learning Characteristics

An overview of cognitive development is necessary in order to understand the cognitive limitation of the mentally retarded child and to design effective treatment programs to overcome those cognitive limitations.

Piaget's Theory of Intellectual Development

Jean Piaget, in order to explain normal and abnormal intellectual development, divided the developmental process into four stages: the sensorimotor period (0–18 months); the preoperational stage (2–7 years); the stage of concrete operations (7–12 years); and the period of formal operations (12 years and older).[31] The delineations offered by Piaget's stages provide a basis for understanding the sequence of normal development and the limitations at various levels of mental retardation.

Children learn mainly through exploration of the senses and through movement during the sensorimotor stage. The ability to coordinate sensorimotor activity to reach certain goals is apparent in primitive forms of intelligence. During this early stage, exploration of the environment includes much experimentation. Learning cannot be generalized to new situations during this period, and most discoveries are made by trial and error. A child who is severely retarded may never progress beyond this stage of intellectual development.[31]

The preoperational stage is characterized by the development of language and the beginnings of abstract thought. Children at this stage can use symbols to represent objects that are not present, and may be able to classify and group objects, although not proficiently. A child with moderate retardation may not develop beyond this stage.[31]

During the concrete operations stage, the ability to order, classify, and relate experience to an organized whole begins to develop.[11] The child can solve some mathematical problems and can read well. The child can generalize learning to new situations and can begin to recognize another person's point of view. There is still an inability to deal with hypothetical problems. Persons with mild retardation often remain at this level of cognitive development.[31] Piaget's final stage—formal operations—normally begins at 12 years of age and continues throughout life. The abilities to reason and hypothesize are characteristic of this stage. The mentally retarded child seldom reaches this level of development.[31]

Concrete Concepts Compared with Abstract Concepts

Mentally retarded people are less able to grasp abstract concepts than concrete concepts.[32] When working with mentally retarded people, the therapist must present treatment concepts using meaningful, concrete directions. Activities are best understood when demonstrated, done passively first, or translated into familiar activities pertaining to daily life.

Memory

The literature regarding the mentally retarded person's ability to remember shows that that ability is related to the type of retention task involved.[11] Use of short-term memory is consistently difficult for the mentally retarded person.[33–35] Smith indicates that a high level of distractibility by external, irrelevant stimuli is associated with these short-term memory deficits. With this knowledge in mind, some of the following strategies can be used during physical therapy sessions.

1. Remove irrelevant, distracting material from the treatment area. Do not work with the child in distracting surroundings, even if room dividers or cur-

tains must be used to separate a small space from a larger, busy area (Fig. 11-9).

2. Present each component of the task clearly and separately.
3. Begin with simple tasks and then progress to more difficult tasks.
4. Explain your expectations of the child at each stage.
5. Give immediate and consistent positive reinforcement.
6. Repeat directions as often as necessary.
7. Check the accuracy of performance frequently.
8. Keep the child informed of progress and give the child an opportunity to demonstrate or practice the new skill independently.

Most researchers agree that practice, review, and overlearning help the mentally retarded child with long-term retention of skills. The therapist can promote learning and retention by providing ample opportunity to use the newly learned material. Physical therapists inform parents and teachers of a child's progress and should encourage practice of the newly learned task at home or in the classroom

(Fig. 11-10). Learning cannot occur or be retained when the physical therapy sessions are an isolated segment of the child's day. Extended practice and communication are both vital.

Transfer of Learning

Transfer of learning is regarded as the ability to apply newly learned material to new situations having components that are similar to those of the material that was newly learned.[34] The literature on transfer of learning suggests that two factors, in particular, be considered when formulating a plan for treatment.

Meaningfulness is an important element in transfer of learning for the retarded child. A meaningful task is both easier to learn at the outset and easier to transfer to a second setting than one that has no meaning for the learner. This concept strongly supports the use of functional activities during physical therapy as opposed to meaningless "splinter skills."

Moreover, learning can be transferred best when

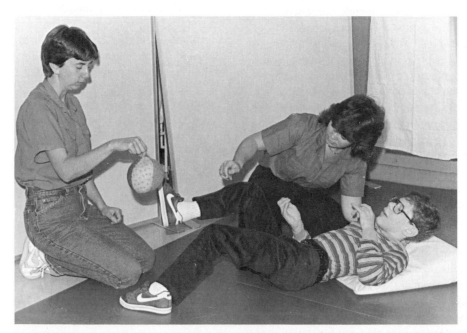

Figure 11-9. *Vertical room dividers and towels are used to reduce environmental distraction during therapeutic play.*

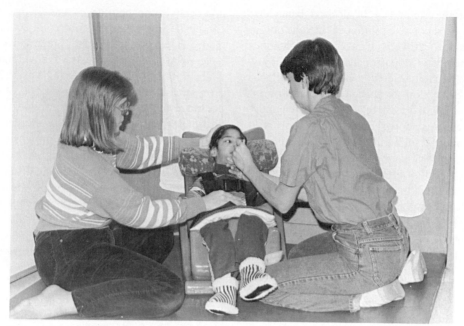

Figure 11-10. *A physical therapist demonstrates proper feeding technique.*

both the initial task and the transfer task are *similar.* If, for example, the therapist is working on the ability to push rather than to pull on crutches, all of the therapy tasks, such as pushing in a prone position, sitting push-ups, and other tasks, can be transferred more readily to the task of pushing on crutches. *Consistency* also helps the child see the connection between therapy tools and their function.

Knowledge of basic learning concepts and an understanding of cognitive development are crucial for the physical therapist working with an intellectually impaired child. Physical therapy is a learning situation, and some modifications in approach will be necessary to accommodate the differences in performance seen in the mentally retarded child.

Behavior Modification

Behavior modification is a technique that is often used in the education and training of the mentally retarded child. Behavior modification, sometimes called behavioral therapy, is classically defined as a systematic application to the area of human behavior of scientifically established principles of learning. It assumes that behavior can be modified to some degree. It further assumes that significant variables can be found within the person's environment, and that these variables control behavior and can be altered to make a change in response.[2]

The foundations of this approach were established by Pavlov and Thorndike at the turn of the century. The first use of the applied science of behavior modification in humans is mainly accredited to Watson, Wolpe, and Skinner.[36] The techniques are based on concepts derived from various learning theories and on behavioral principles concerning stimulus–response relationships.[2] The focus of behavior modification is generally either to increase or strengthen the frequency of desired behaviors or to decrease the frequency of or eliminate undesired behaviors.[37] Conditioning procedures, such as positive reinforcement, shaping of behavior, stimulus control, and conditioned reinforcement, are some of the approaches used to establish or increase the frequency of desired behaviors. Commonly used positive reinforcers include praise, food, attention, or tokens. Conversely, techniques that are designed to stop or reduce the frequency of undesirable behaviors include extinction and punishment.[36] Extinction involves a privilege or reinforcer that is immediately taken away when undesirable behavior is shown. Punishment involves an aversive stimulus, such as "restraint" (isolating the child). The use of punishment has come under scrutiny and is used less often than in the past. When punishment is used, the undesirable behavior is examined by a psychologist and a specific program is designed. The preferred approach is to use positive reinforcement to encourage even minimal lessening of the frequency of maladaptive behavior. For example, to stop head banging, a positive reinforcer could be used to reward increasing periods of time during which the child refrains from head banging, rather than punishing the child for head banging.

Physical therapists working with mentally retarded children can use methods of behavior modification to change behavior related to physical therapy goals. In addition to using behavioral modification to help attain goals, the therapist must also be aware of any overall behavioral programs for the child. For example, if a school psychologist has recommended specific, consistent methods to stop tantrums in a child, the therapist must be aware of these methods should the tantrums occur during a physical therapy session. Consistency of approach for all professionals is essential for learning, especially for the mentally retarded child.[38]

The Team Concept

When working with the mentally retarded or multiply handicapped child, physical therapists must view themselves and their treatment goals as part of a total management plan. Use of an interdisciplinary team of professionals is the standard approach for children with special needs. Comprehensive delivery of services for the mentally retarded child is beyond the scope of any one professional discipline. One of the main values of an interdisciplinary

approach is the pooling of knowledge so that a composite and relevant course of action can be made. Because the mentally retarded child will have delays in many areas of development, the skills of many professionals can be used. No single professional has the necessary scope of expertise nor the resources to effectively provide care and education throughout the life of the retarded child.[10]

In order to be effective, each professional on the team must understand the periodic shift of authority and emphasis at different times and different stages of development. Input from the physical therapist will sometimes be of paramount importance, whereas at other times, the priorities will lie in other areas of care. During these latter periods, the physical therapist may play a consultative or advisory role. Success of the team in its primary purpose of helping the child achieve his or her maximum potential will depend on each professional considering the whole child, while offering the needed expertise to alleviate specific problems or handicaps.[14] Communication among team members and respect for one another's unique knowledge and skills are keys to making the team process work.

Effective use of all team members will ensure that consistency and reinforcement are present throughout the child's total program. For example, if certain sounds are being taught in speech therapy, the learning of these sounds can be reinforced by using them during physical therapy sessions. The physical therapist and special education teacher must work as partners in caring for the child. The teacher must be taught handling techniques, positioning, and simple techniques of stimulation. The therapist is uniquely qualified to assist the teacher in understanding the impact of abnormal sensorimotor function on the achievement of cognitive milestones. For example, consider the child with extensor hypertonus, average head control, and obvious interference from tonic neck reflexes. In such a case, knowledge of the basics of muscle tone management could be invaluable to the teacher when working on a cognitive skill with the child, such as performing a simple cause-and-effect activity (e.g., manipulating a "busy-box"). A simple

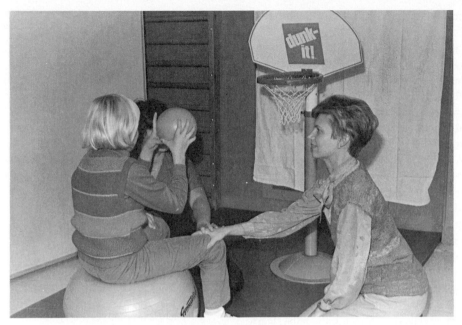

Figure 11-11. *Adapted physical education activity used for therapeutic endeavors in a recreational mode. It is important for the adapted physical education teacher to have a thorough understanding of the sensory and motor skills being developed.*

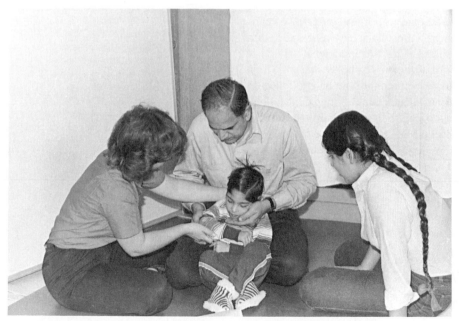

Figure 11-12. *A physical therapist teaches proper handling techniques and proper positioning skills.*

suggestion from the therapist that the child be side-lying rather than supine could reduce the extensor tone and enable the child to reach for and manipulate the "busy box." Such a cooperative approach both facilitates the child's accomplishment of the educational goal and reduces the frustration of the teacher. In addition, were the teacher unaware of the physical therapy goal to reduce extensor tone and the influence of the tonic neck reflex, postures that would be inconsistent with physical therapy goals might be used unknowingly.[39] The physical therapist must communicate and work with all members of the team, including the nurse, occupational therapist, psychologist, physician, teacher, physical education teacher, speech therapist, and parent (Fig. 11-11).

Whenever they work with children, physical therapists must recognize the importance of the parents as part of the therapeutic team. Program carryover into the home is important for maximum treatment effectiveness. The parents must learn how to handle the child and must be able to help achieve the goals of the program (Fig. 11-12). This concept is true not only for physical therapy, but for all areas of treatment and education. When asking parents to participate in a home program of care, physical therapists must be able to assess the abilities of the parent. The therapist must recognize problems or conditions in the home that may limit the successful participation of the parents.[39] Referral to appropriate agencies may help parents alleviate or resolve those problems or conditions. Several books that discuss the special needs of families of retarded children may be useful for physical therapists.[40–43] The long-term nature of problems associated with mental retardation and management of those problems usually requires a major commitment from the family.

Overall Role of the Physical Therapist

Role Expansion

The evaluation, treatment, and management of the mentally retarded child presents an intriguing chal-

Table 11-4. *Types of Delivery for Physical Therapy Services for the Mentally Retarded Child*

I.   Direct Services
  A. Evaluation
  B. Treatment
  C. Establishment of goals and program plans—active participation in Individual Education Plan (IEP) development (see chapter)
  D. Family education
  E. Communication with members of service delivery team
  F. Record-keeping and dissemination of information to a referring physician

II. Indirect Services
  A. Administrative
    1. Budget planning
    2. Personnel recruitment
    3. Equipment recommendations
    4. Architectural consultations
    5. Development of policies and procedures
  B. Program planning and development
    1. IEP committees
    2. Various decision-making groups
  C. Screening
    1. Surveying large groups of students to identify problem areas and to determine program needs
    2. Developmental
    3. Postural
    4. Classroom observations
    5. Chart reviews and adults
  D. Consultation to various groups
    1. Teachers
    2. Parents
    3. School administration
    4. Other educational or medical personnel
  E. In-service education—formal or informal sessions to explain physical therapy strategies and treatment
    1. Treatment plans
    2. Treatment rationale
    3. Lifting techniques
    4. Body mechanics

(Adapted from Pennsylvania Physical Therapy Association: Guidelines for Delivery of Physical Therapy Services in Educational Settings in the Commonwealth of Pennsylvania. *Harrisburg, Pennsylvania Physical Therapy Association; 1977.)*

lenge for the physical therapist. The therapist must function not only as an effective, contributing member of an interdisciplinary team, but must be aware of various roles that must be assumed in the care of the mentally retarded child. Physical therapy services for the mentally retarded child can be divided into two broad categories—direct services and indirect services. The available models of service delivery are shown in Table 11-4.[44] All services can be provided either as a direct employee of a school or agency or on a private, contractual basis. The diversity of choices offers a stimulating challenge.

Role Release

To contribute effectively to the management of children with many complex and changing needs, the physical therapist must first understand the concept of being unable to be individually responsible for the overall management of the child's physical needs. If consistency and carryover of intervention techniques are the most effective means of promot-

ing the development of the child, the logical next step is to recognize that this effort must be a cooperative venture by parents, teachers, and health professionals. The physical therapist must accept the concept that other professionals can be taught certain therapeutic techniques. This "release of role" carries with it many responsibilities. First, the physical therapist must be able to communicate and teach the skill effectively. The therapist must, therefore, have a thorough understanding of both the developmental or functional skill to be taught and the purpose of the intervention. The skill and activity can each be broken down into understandable components and translated into a language appropriate for the parent or other professional. Clinical experience has shown that the accuracy of carryover depends directly on the learner's grasp of what must be done and the rationale for doing it. An understanding of this rationale gives meaning and importance to the task. The therapist must ensure that the parent or professional receives not only ad-

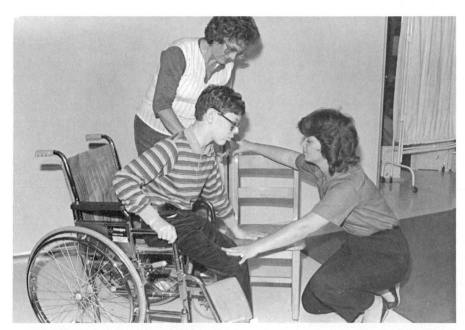

Figure 11-13. *A physical therapist teaches proper transfer techniques to parents of a mentally retarded child.*

equate, but continuing instruction and supervision, with periodic observation of performance (Fig. 11-13). Finally, the physical therapist must develop sensitive listening skills. This last skill will establish the therapist as a welcome adjunct to care and as someone who is attentive to the changing needs of the caregiver and the child.

Summary

In the management of the child with mental retardation, the physical therapist is challenged to use various skills. The many complex and persistent difficulties encountered by retarded children often require innovative methods of physical therapy evaluation and treatment. These methods must incorporate not only the basic principles of physical therapy, but also an understanding of the principles of teaching and learning as they relate to the mentally retarded person.

Communication of program needs to parents and other professionals requires not only technical expertise on the part of the therapist, but also psychosocial skills and the ability to be a sensitive listener and teacher. Through an effective interdisciplinary approach to the child and family, we can help the mentally retarded child strive to attain goals in life.

References

1. Montgomery PC. Assessment and treatment of the child with mental retardation. *Phys Ther.* 1981;61:1265–1272.
2. Nichtern S. *Helping the Retarded Child.* Grosset and Dunlap; 1974.
3. Sebelist RM. Mental retardation. In: Hopkins HL, Smith HD, eds. *Willard and Spackman's Occupational Therapy.* 5th ed. Philadelphia: JB Lippincott; 1978.
4. National Institute on Mental Retardation: *Orientation Manual on Mental Retardation.* Ontario, Canada: York University, 1981.
5. Itard J. *The Wild Boy of Aveyron.* Englewood Cliffs, NJ: Prentice-Hall; 1962.
6. Reynolds MC, Birch JW. *Teaching Exceptional Children in All America's Schools.* Reston, VA: The Council for Exceptional Children; 1977.
7. Luckasson RA, Coulter DL, Palloway EA, et al. *Mental Retardation: Definition, Classification, and Systems of Support.* 9th ed. Washington, DC: American Association of Mental Retardation; 1992.
8. Reference deleted.
9. Mitchell JV, ed. *The Ninth Mental Measurement Yearbook.* Lincoln, NE: University of Nebraska Press; 1985.
10. Scheerenberger RC. Mental retardation: Definition, classification, and prevalence. *Ment Retard Abstr.* 1964;1:432–441.
11. Hardy RD, Cull JB. *Mental Retardation and Physical Disability.* Springfield, IL: Charles C Thomas; 1974.
12. Chinn PC, Drew CJ, Logan DR. *Mental Retardation: A Life Cycle Approach.* St Louis: CV Mosby; 1979.
13. Downing J, Bailey B. Presented at the TASH (The Association for Persons with Severe Handicaps) Annual Conference; December 9, 1988; Washington, DC.
14. Pearson PH, Williams CE, eds. *Physical Therapy Services in the Developmental Disabilities.* Springfield, IL: Charles C Thomas; 1972.
15. Kinnealy M. Aversive and nonaversive responses to sensory stimuli in mentally retarded children. *Am J Occup Ther.* 1973;27:464–472.
16. McCall RB. *Infants.* New York: Vintage Books; 1979.
17. Getman GN, Kone ER, et al. *Developing Learning Readiness.* St Louis: McGraw-Hill; 1966.
18. DeQuiros JB. Diagnosis of vestibular disorders in the learning disabled. *J Learn Disabil.* 1976;9:50–58.
19. Moore J. Cranial nerves and their importance in current rehabilitation techniques. In: Henderson A, Coryell J, eds. *The Body Senses and Perceptual Deficit.* Boston: Boston University; 1973:102–120.

20. Ayres AJ. *Sensory Integration and the Child.* Los Angeles: Western Psychological Services; 1979: 34–35.

21. Head H. *Studies in Neurology.* Vol. 2. London: Oxford University Press; 1920:396–397.

22. Poggin GF, Mountcastle VB. A study of the functional contributions of the lemniscal and spinothalamic systems to somatic sensibility. *Johns Hopkins Med J.* 1960;106:266–316.

23. Ayres AJ. *Sensory Integration and Learning Disorders.* Los Angeles: Western Psychological Services; 1972.

24. Ayres AJ. Tactile functions: Their relation to hyperactive and perceptive motor behavior. *Am J Occup Ther.* 1964;18:6–11.

25. Clark RG. *Essentials of Clinical Neuroanatomy and Neurophysiology.* 5th ed. Philadelphia: FA Davis; 1975.

26. Ayres AJ. *Southern California Postrotary Nystagmus Test.* Los Angeles: Western Psychological Services; 1975:1–9.

27. Lemke H. Self-abusive behavior. *Am J Occup Ther.* 1974;28:94–98.

28. Easton TA. On the normal use of reflexes. *Am Sci* 1972;60:591–599.

29. Rogers SJ, Donovan CM, D'Eugenia DB, et al. Early Intervention Developmental Profile. Vol 2. In: Schafer DS, Maersch MS, eds. *Developmental Programming for Infants and Young Children.* Ann Arbor: University of Michigan Press; 1981.

30. Buchwald JS, Eldred E. Relation between gamma efferent discharge and cortical activity. *Electroencephalogr Clin Neurophysiol.* 1961;13:243–247.

31. Batshaw NL, Perret YM. *Children with Handicaps: A Medical Primer.* 2nd ed. Baltimore: Paul H. Brookes; 1986.

32. Weiner H. *Comparative Psychology of Mental Development.* New York: International University Press; 1948.

33. Hermelin B, O'Connor N. Short-term memory in normal and sub-normal children. *Am J Ment Defic.* 1964;69:121–125.

34. Smith R. *Clinical Teaching: Methods of Instruction for the Retarded.* New York: McGraw-Hill; 1968.

35. Ellis NR. Memory processes in retardates and normals. In: Ellis NR, ed. *International Review of Research in Mental Retardation.* Vol 4. New York: Academic Press; 1970:1–32.

36. Martin G, Pear M. *Behavior Modification: What It Is and How to Do It.* Princeton, NJ: Prentice-Hall; 1978.

37. Nawas MM, Braun SH. The use of operant techniques for modifying the behavior of the severely and profoundly retarded. Part II. In: Anderson RM, Greer JS, eds. *Educating the Severely and Profoundly Retarded.* Baltimore: University Park Press; 1976:81–96.

38. Tymchuk AJ. *Behavior Modification with Children.* Springfield, IL: Charles C Thomas; 1974.

39. Connolly BH, Anderson RM. Severely handicapped children in the public schools—A new frontier for the physical therapist. *Phys Ther.* 1978;58:433–438.

40. Odel SJ, Greer JG, Anderson RM. The family of the severely retarded individual. In: Anderson RM, Greer JG, eds. *Educating the Severely and Profoundly Retarded.* Baltimore: University Park Press; 1976:251–261.

41. Barsch RH. *The Parent of the Handicapped Child.* Springfield, IL: Charles C Thomas; 1968.

42. Roos P. Parents and families of the mentally retarded. In: Kauffman JM, Payne JS, eds. *Mental Retardation: An Introduction and Personal Perspectives.* Columbus, OH; Charles E. Merrill; 1975.

43. Farber B. Family organization and crisis: Maintenance of integration in families with a severely retarded child. Lafayette, IN: Child Development Publication, Society Research Child Development, 1960.

44. Pennsylvania Physical Therapy Association: *Guidelines for Delivery of Physical Therapy Services in Educational Settings in the Commonwealth of Pennsylvania.* Harrisburg: Pennsylvania Physical Therapy Association; 1977, updated 1993 (soon to be released).

Pediatric Physical Therapy,
second edition, edited by Jan
Stephen Tecklin. J. B. Lippincott
Company, Philadelphia © 1994.

12

Julaine M. Florence

Neuromuscular Disorders in Childhood and Physical Therapy Intervention

- **Duchenne Muscular Dystrophy**
  Clinical Presentation and Progression
  Treatment
  Physical Therapy Evaluation
  Physical Therapy Intervention
- **Other Related Disorders**
  Myotonic Dystrophy
  Facioscapulohumeral Dystrophy
  Spinal Muscular Atrophy
- **Summary**

Children with neuromuscular disorders have a life-long challenge to maintain function. That challenge can be met with the help of a knowledgeable physical therapist. In this chapter, the term *neuromuscular disease* refers to disorders whose primary pathology affects any part of the motor unit from the anterior horn cell out to the muscle itself. Common to all of these disorders is muscle weakness, which may be produced by pathology at any part of the motor unit. When characterizing neuromuscular disorders and their pathology, it is convenient to consider the various anatomic divisions of this motor unit: the anterior horn cell, peripheral nerve, neuromuscular junction, and the muscle.

Neuromuscular diseases may be either hereditary or acquired and are variously classified as myopathies, in which the cause of the muscle weakness is attributable to pathology confined to the muscle itself, or neuropathies, in which the muscle weakness is secondary to an abnormality of either the anterior horn cell or peripheral nerve. Further characterization is based on a particular disorder's characteristic pattern of presentation.

The term *muscular dystrophy* describes a group of myopathies that are genetically determined and have a steadily progressive degenerative course. Further classification of the muscular dystrophies is based on their clinical presentation, including the distribution of weakness and mode of inheritance.

The terms *spinal muscular atrophy* and *motor neuropathy* refer to neurogenic disorders whose underlying pathology affects the anterior horn cell or the peripheral nerve. Further classification is based on clinical presentation and mode of inheritance.

The neuromuscular disorders vary significantly in their presentation, pathology, and progression, but are linked with regard to physical therapy intervention by their common characteristic of muscle weakness leading to loss of function and physical deformity. A physical therapist with an understanding of these disorders can help identify, predict, intervene, and possibly prevent unnecessary complications throughout the course of each disorder. The purpose of this chapter is to provide an overview of select neuromuscular diseases, including clinical presentation, pathology, diagnosis, disease progression, medical treatment, and physical therapy intervention.

Because Duchenne's muscular dystrophy (DMD) is one of the most common myopathies and best known of the dystrophies affecting children, much of this chapter is devoted to a discussion of this disorder. Physical therapy interventions and principles that apply to the management of weakness and deformity in patients with DMD are also applicable to other neuromuscular diseases that present with similar symptoms and complications. Knowledge of the various disorders will allow appropriate decisions to be made about the suitability and timing of various physical therapy interventions. Other neuromuscular diseases that are reviewed in this chapter include myotonic and fasioscapulohumeral dystrophy and the spinal muscular atrophies.

Duchenne Muscular Dystrophy

Duchenne muscular dystrophy, also known as pseudohypertrophic muscular dystrophy or progressive muscular dystrophy, is one of the most prevalent and severely disabling of the childhood myopathies.

DMD is among the most severely disabling of all childhood disorders. Unlike disorders such as cerebral palsy or poliomyelitis, DMD represents a progressive disease in which the child becomes weaker and usually dies of a respiratory infection or cardiorespiratory insufficiency in the late teens or early 20s. Estimates of DMD's incidence vary between 13 and 33 patients per 100,000 live male births.[1] There is an X-linked inheritance pattern to DMD whereby male offspring inherit the disease from their mothers, who are most often asymptomatic. Advances in molecular biology have shown the defect to be a mutation at XP21 in the gene coding for the protein, dystrophin.[2]

Clinical Presentation and Progression

The onset of the disorder is insidious, usually resulting in symptoms before 3 years of age; however, symptoms may not be noticed for months or years, and the disease may be misdiagnosed for years.[3]

Earliest symptoms may include a reluctance to walk or run at appropriate ages, falling, toe walking, clumsiness, and an increase in size of several groups of muscles. The gastrocnemius is the most notable muscle that commonly shows this "pseudohypertrophy," but the infraspinatus and deltoid muscles are also commonly enlarged (Fig. 12-1). These pseudohypertrophic muscles have a firm consistency when palpated. Histologic examination of muscle shows degeneration of muscle fibers with increased connective tissue and adipose cells (Figs. 12-2 and 12-3). Motor and sensory neurons are undamaged, and there is no significant change in either the central nervous system (CNS) or in the vascular system.[4] A high rate of intellectual impairment and emotional disturbance has been associated with DMD.[5]

The clinical presentation gives the first clues to the diagnosis, which is confirmed by the results of laboratory studies. Laboratory findings include an abnormally high serum creatinine kinase level, myopathic electromyogram (EMG), and abnormal muscle biopsy results (see Fig. 12–3)[4] or characteristic deletion on genetic analysis.[2] With the availability of genetic analysis, all male family members may be screened for the disorder and all female family members may be screened for their carrier status.

The weakness is steadily progressive with the boys losing strength at 0.322 units per year (SD = 0.318) on a 10 point scale (Fig. 12-4). This average muscle score represents the sum score of 34 mus-

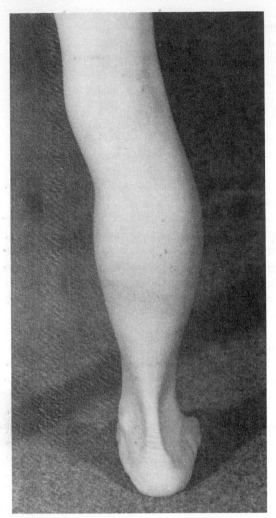

Figure 12-1. *Duchenne dystrophy. Pseudohypertrophy of the calf. (From Lovell WW, Winter RB, eds.* Pediatric Orthopaedics. *2nd ed. Philadelphia: JB Lippincott; 1986:264.)*

cles graded using the Medical Research Council Scale[6] for manual muscle testing, converted to a 10 point scale.[7] This slope of decline associated with the increasing age of the child was documented by following 378 boys, 6–18 years of age with the diagnosis of DMD, for a mean of 2.7 years (SD = 3.1, maximum = 10.7 years). This natural history study[8] of DMD was conducted by the Collaborative Investigation of Duchenne Dystrophy (CIDD) group. This natural history data has been re-analyzed with

the inclusion of 95 new cases for presentation in this chapter (Figs. 12-4, 12-5, and 12-7). Although the overall decline in strength is 0.3 units per year, different muscles decline at varying rates (Fig. 12-5), with proximal muscles tending to be weaker earlier in the course of the illness and progress faster.

Early weakness of the hip and knee extensors often results in an exaggerated lumbar lordosis that is characteristic of the early stages of disease. The lordosis occurs in response to the attempt to align the center of gravity anterior to the fulcrum of the knee joint and posterior to the fulcrum of the hip joint. This realignment gives maximum stability at both joints. The child attempts to broaden the base of support during walking and thus develops a gait that resembles waddling. The child may develop iliotibial band contractures made worse by this wide-based stance. As the weakness progresses, the child rises from the floor by "climbing up the legs." This maneuver, known as Gower's sign, is indicative of proximal muscle weakness (Fig. 12-6.)

As the weakness progresses, there is a tendency to develop contractures. These contractures typically result in plantar flexion at the ankle with inversion of the foot and flexion at both the hips and knees.

This early loss of range of motion (ROM), noted in the hip flexors, iliotibial bands, and heel cords, limits stance and ambulation in that patients find it difficult to achieve the mechanical alignment necessary to hold themselves in an upright posture using their weak musculature. As these boys spend more time sitting, an increasing degree of contracture is seen at the hips, knees, and elbows.

Functional activities may be performed more slowly by children with DMD than by normal children, but most of those affected are able to walk, climb stairs, and stand up from the floor without too much difficulty until 6 or 7 years of age. At this time, a relatively rapid decline in function has been documented, which generally results in a loss of unassisted ambulation at 9 to 10 years of age and loss of ambulation, even in long-leg braces, at 12 to 13 years of age.[8] A graphic representation of the ages at which the children have increasing difficulty

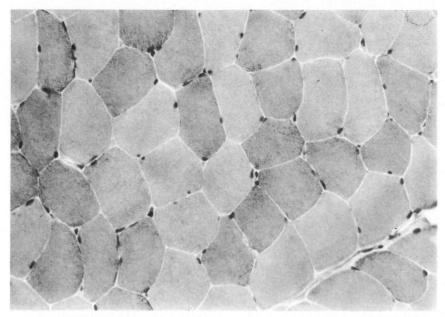

Figure 12-2. *Normal adult muscle. Muscle fibers are cut in a plane transverse to their long axis and appear to have round, oval, or slightly irregular profiles. One or more darkly stained nuclei are seen at the edge of most fibers. (Trichrome, × 300) (From Maloney, Burks, Ringel, eds.* Interdisciplinary Rehabilitation of Multiple Sclerosis and Neuromuscular Disorders. *Philadelphia: JB Lippincott; 1984:202.)*

with various functional activities is presented in Figure 12-7. These functional activities are considered to be "milestones," and represent significant points in disease progression. The arm grades awarded were developed by Brooke and associates[8] (Table 12-1), whereas the leg grades are based on a scale proposed by Vignos (Table 12-2).[9]

As is demonstrated, by the range and distribution of percentiles in Figures 12-4 and 12-7, the clinical course of disease progression in individual children is not homogeneous. The mildest of the X-linked progressive dystrophies has been termed Becker's muscular dystrophy. This classification applies to individuals who maintain independent ambulation until after the age of 15 years. Brooke and colleagues have coined the term "outliers"[8] to describe a population of boys who fulfill the diagnostic criteria for DMD but who, when compared to the DMD population's usual pattern of disease progression, fall outside the usual limits. Investigators

are studying genetic heterogeneity with regard to DNA mutations and resulting dystrophin expression in an attempt to explain the varying levels of clinical severity associated with DMD.

Scoliosis develops as the age of the child with DMD increases; significant curves are generally not noticed until after the age of 11 years.[10] This scoliosis tends to progress as the back muscles become weaker and as the child spends less time standing and more time sitting, resulting in a positional scoliosis (Fig. 12-8) which, over time, becomes fixed.

In addition to the voluntary muscles, DMD affects other organs. As the respiratory musculature atrophies, coughing becomes ineffective and pulmonary infections become more frequent, often leading to the patient's early death. Dystrophic cardiomyopathy is common and often contributes to death.[11] Although intelligence may be reduced among children with DMD, this deficit is not pro-

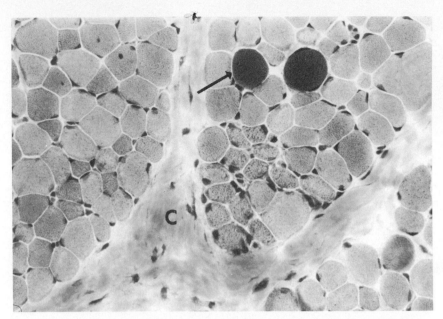

Figure 12-3. *Duchenne dystrophy. Compare these fibers to those of normal muscle in Figure 12-2. Dystrophic changes include a marked variability in fiber size; dark, "opaque" fibers (arrow); and abnormal quantities of fibrous connective tissue (C). (Trichrome, × 300) (From Maloney, Burks, Ringel, eds.* Interdisciplinary Rehabilitation of Muscular Dystrophy and Neuromuscular Disorders. *Philadelphia: JB Lippincott; 1984:203.)*

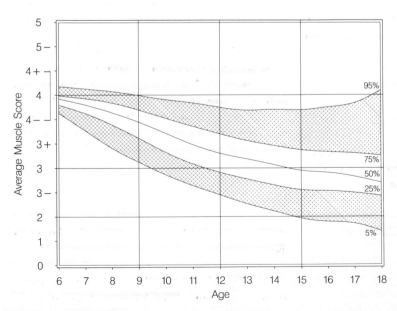

Figure 12-4. *Average muscle scores plotted as percentiles of the population. The center line represents the 50th percentile. The shaded areas span the 5th to the 25th and the 75th to the 95th percentile. (Courtesy of the Collaborative Investigation of Duchenne Dystrophy [CIDD] Group)*

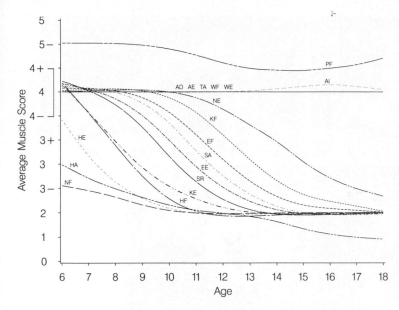

Figure 12-5. *The lines represent the 50th percentiles for the strength of individual muscles plotted against age.* PF, *plantar flexor;* AI, *ankle invertor;* AD, *ankle dorsiflexor;* AE, *ankle invertor;* TA, *thumb abductor;* WF, *wrist flexor;* WE, *wrist extensor;* NE, *neck extensor;* KF, *knee flexor;* EF, *elbow flexor;* HE, *hip extensor;* SA, *shoulder abductor;* EE, *elbow extensor;* HA, *hip abductor;* SR, *shoulder external rotator;* KE, *knee extensor;* HF, *hip flexor;* NF, *neck flexor.* (*Courtesy of the Collaborative Investigation of Duchenne Dystrophy [CIDD] Group*)

gressive and is not related to the severity of disease.[12] Although not progressive, this intellectual deficit may hinder the child's development and may make a physical evaluation of the child difficult. Fortunately, children with DMD seldom lose bowel or bladder control, and other neurologic signs do not appear.

Treatment

Although definitive treatment is lacking, proper management, as outlined by Ziter and Allsop, can prolong the maximum functional ability of the child.[13] This program of management begins once the diagnosis is established, and it is initiated concurrently with parental counseling in an attempt to reduce the guilt, hostility, fear, depression, hopelessness, and numerous other emotions commonly experienced by the parents.

The clinician faced with this situation can propose a positive approach based on the following: 1) some of the complications which magnify the functional disability of DMD are predictable and preventable; 2) an active program of physical therapy and the timely application of braces can prolong ambulation and more closely approximate the normal independence of later childhood; and 3) if a specific treat-

ment ever becomes available, those in optimal physical condition are most apt to benefit.[13]

There is no pharmaceutical treatment that will cure DMD, but several studies[14,15] have confirmed an initial report that prednisone increases strength in patients with DMD.[16] Further investigation has shown that prednisone, despite its many side effects, keeps those affected by DMD "stronger for longer."[17,18]

Myoblast transplant has been proposed as a treatment for DMD with the aim of replacing the missing protein, dystrophin.[19] However, at present, this procedure is still being investigated. Various other strategies for replacing the defective gene and missing protein are under study, but currently, none are available for clinical use.

Physical Therapy Evaluation

Each child with DMD should undergo a physical therapy evaluation. Such an evaluation involves the gathering of information that contributes to the development of a plan of care. That care plan will be based largely on the functional significance of the therapist's findings.

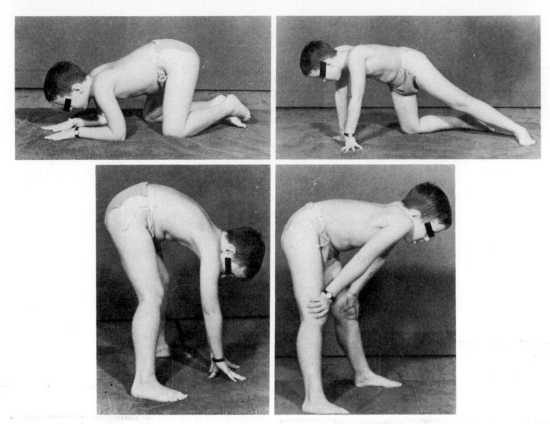

Figure 12-6. *Gower's sign. This series of maneuvers is necessary to achieve an upright posture, and it occurs with all types of pelvic and trunk weakness. The child "climbs up the legs" when rising from the floor. (From Lovell WW, Winter RB, eds.* Pediatric Orthopaedics. *2nd ed. Philadelphia: JB Lippincott, 1986:265.)*

Functional Ability

Systematic and serial recording of standard tasks shows that the child with DMD is in one of two general phases: stable performance or declining performance. During the stable phase, which may continue for several years, the child may demonstrate normal performance of various tasks during the serial evaluations, despite a continuing decline in strength. A discrepancy exists in the age at which the aforementioned tasks are failed, as illustrated in Figure 12-7.

Ziter and associates and Allsop and Ziter have demonstrated that, although functional ability appears to remain at a constant stage in many children

with DMD, actual muscle strength continues to decline insidiously.[20,21] These findings suggest that, although timed functional tests are useful in determining the patient's current status, they have limited value in monitoring the progressive loss of strength in DMD. As a result of these studies, Allsop believes that, when timed trials are used as dependent variables in drug trials, they may overestimate therapeutic efficacy. A patient who appears to be stable in a series of timed trials may actually be experiencing a continual decline in strength, in which case the drug has had no effect on the progression of the myopathy.

Brooke and co-workers[22] and Florence and associates[7] have presented a clinical evaluation protocol

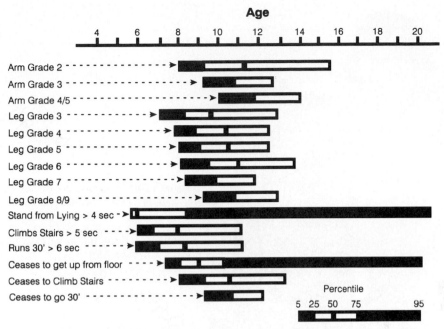

Figure 12-7. *Graphic representation of the ages (expressed as percentiles) at which children with Duchenne muscular dystrophy have increasing difficulty with functional tasks. (Courtesy of the Collaborative Investigation of Duchenne Dystrophy [CIDD] Group)*

Table 12-1. *Functional Grades: Arms and Shoulders*[8]

Grades	Functional Ability
1	Standing with arms at the sides, the patient can abduct the arms in a full circle until they touch above the head.
2	The patient can raise the arms above the head only by flexing the elbow (i.e., by shortening the circumference of the movement) or by using accessory muscles.
3	The patient cannot raise hands above the head, but can raise an 8-oz glass of water to the mouth (using both hands if necessary).
4	The patient can raise hands to the mouth, but cannot raise an 8-oz glass of water to the mouth.
5	The patient cannot raise hands to the mouth, but can use the hands to hold a pen or to pick up pennies from a table.
6	The patient cannot raise hands to the mouth and has no useful function of the hands.

Table 12-2. *Functional Grades: Hips and Legs*[9]

Grade	Functional Ability
1	Walks and climbs stairs without assistance
2	Walks and climbs stairs with the aid of a railing
3	Walks and climbs stairs slowly (elapsed time of more than 12 seconds for four standard stairs) with the aid of a railing
4	Walks unassisted and rises from a chair, but cannot climb stairs
5	Walks unassisted but cannot rise from a chair or climb stairs
6	Walks only with assistance or walks independently with long-leg braces
7	Walks in long-leg braces, but requires assistance for balance
8	Stands in long-leg braces, but is unable to walk even with assistance
9	Is in wheelchair
10	Is confined to bed

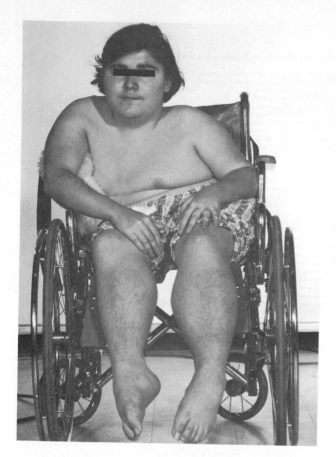

Figure 12-8. *Obesity with fixed equinocavovarus and scoliosis in a child with advanced Duchenne's muscular dystrophy. (From Maloney, Burks, Ringel, eds.* Interdisciplinary Rehabilitation of Muscular Dystrophy and Neuromuscular Disorders. *Philadelphia: JB Lippincott; 1984:290.)*

for DMD—assessing strength, pulmonary function, and functional tasks in combination—that has been demonstrated to be reliable in documenting disease course in patients with DMD.[8] In addition, the protocol is able to detect not only the therapeutic effect of pharmaceutical intervention, but the time course and differences in various dose levels of such intervention.[23]

Muscle Testing

Measurement of muscle strength by way of manual muscle testing (MMT) remains a valid approach to assessing the progression of disease in children with DMD.[8] MMT has been shown to be both reliable[24] and sensitive to changes in strength in patients with DMD.[23]

Because muscle weakness is characteristic of all myopathies, MMT must be a routine part of the physical therapy evaluation of the child with myopathy. Serial use of MMT provides data against which the efficacy of management can be monitored. The longitudinal results of MMT in children with DMD show a linearity in the decline of muscle strength. Although some authors describe an apparent stabilization of strength between 5 and 8 years of age, Allsop and Ziter,[21] Ziter and associates,[20] and Brooke et al.[8] have found neither plateaus nor accelerated periods of the disease process. Bracing does not slow down the deterioration, and use of a wheelchair does not increase the rate of decline.

By the time the child reaches 7 years of age, or with serial strength scores recorded for 1 year, it is possible to estimate the rate of progression as either rapid (> 10% deterioration per year), average (5% to 10% deterioration per year), or slow (< 5% deterioration per year). There is a variation in the rapidity of progression, and MMT, along with performance of functional tasks, helps to determine when bracing or wheelchairs will be needed.

The following muscles are routinely graded:

Upper trapezius	Rhomboids
Lower trapezius	Iliopsoas
Deltoid	Quadriceps
Serratus anterior	Gluteus maximus
Pectorals	Gluteus medius
Latissimus dorsi	Anterior tibialis
Triceps	Abdominals

Although this list of muscles may be useful for monitoring the child's status in the clinical setting, the only muscle groups in which reliability of testing has been documented are those graphed in Figure 12-5. It has been demonstrated that, although MMT is a reliable means of assessment in DMD when performed by the same examiner, the interrater reliability of MMT varies among individual muscles and grades.[7,24] It is apparent that one's purpose for performing MMT—whether it is to answer clinical questions or to serve as a research measurement tool—determines the vigor with which one approaches strength testing.

Because of the difficulty in testing the serratus anterior, a supplementary position may be used. The child holds both hands at eye level with arms horizontally abducted and elbows extended. The amount of scapular winging is noted and a subjective grade is given. The traditional testing position is then attempted in order to achieve a more refined and specific grade.

Although the iliopsoas muscle is tested in the standard position, its ability to generate force decreases at an early stage in the disease. Most of the hip flexion strength is generated by the long head of the rectus femoris and by the sartorius. No attempt is made to differentiate between the often nonexistent sternal head and the clavicular portion of the pectoralis major.

In the later stages of the disease, differentiation between the fair and fair–poor range of muscle strength becomes difficult to ascertain for the abdominal muscles. Weakened neck flexors provide additional resistance to the abdominal muscles. This resistance is caused by the head not being able to flex onto the thorax during abdominal contraction, thereby resulting in a longer lever arm for the abdominal muscles.

Range of Motion

Standard assessment of joint motion with goniometry should be done periodically. Pandya and associates studied the intratester and intertester reliability of goniometry for children with DMD.[25] They found high intratester values, but intertester values varied. As a result, they have recommended that serial goniometric evaluations be done by the same examiner.[25] Early loss of ambulation is more frequently caused by loss of motion and contracture than by weakness in specific muscle groups. Loss of full ankle dorsiflexion, knee extension, and hip extension, with resultant contractures, occurs commonly in patients with DMD. Measurement of ankle dorsiflexion, knee extension, hip extension, and iliotibial band (ITB) tightness are probably the most important aspects of goniometric testing.

Physical Therapy Intervention

We believe that physical therapists manage patients and their problems, not diseases. The primary problems encountered by children with DMD include the following:

1. Weakness
2. Decreased active and passive ROM
3. Loss of ambulation
4. Decreased functional ability
5. Decreased pulmonary function
6. Emotional trauma—individual and family
7. Progressive scoliosis

When physical therapy management has been appropriate, physical pain should not be a problem for the child. After a physical examination of the patient, the physical therapist can identify current problems and, based on a thorough understanding of the disease process, should be able to predict the next major difficulties to be encountered. Based on the specific areas of concern for each family, it is possible to identify four major goals of management common to all children with DMD.

1. Prevent deformity.
2. Prolong functional capacity.
3. Facilitate the development and assistance of family support and support of others.
4. Control pain, if necessary.

Home Program

Because much of the responsibility for daily treatment must be assumed by the family or friends of the patient with DMD, an effective program of care at home is essential. Although sustaining enthusiasm and compliance with the home program may be difficult, the likelihood of success can be improved by giving simple instructions, requesting a limited number of exercises and repetitions each day, and offering extensive feedback and positive reinforcement to people in the support system. By reducing the anxiety associated with noncompliance and outlining both short- and long-term goals for the family, compliance and rapport can be improved. In the case of a single-parent family, we suggest extra support from older siblings, clergy, social groups, neighbors, and schools. The home program is convenient and inexpensive. Professional physical therapy once or twice each week is probably neither necessary nor cost-effective, unless it is provided within the school setting. Periodic reevaluation, retraining, and motivation sessions for parents are mandatory.

Preventing Deformity

The tendency for development of plantar flexion contractures is usually the earliest problem. Daily stretching of the Achilles tendons should slow down the development of this deformity. The use of night splints in combination with heel cord stretching has been shown to play a significant role in preventing the often relentless equinovarus deformity associated with DMD.[10] No studies are available

upon which to base a passive stretching prescription, but the regimen often prescribed is between 10 and 30 repetitions, held for 5 to 10 seconds each, performed at least once, and preferably twice, daily.

As soon as the physical therapist sees any change in length of the hamstring muscles during a periodic evaluation, hamstring stretching is added to the home program. As with the Achilles tendon, hamstrings are stretched daily by performing ten repetitions of 10 seconds each. The ITB, hip flexors, and foot evertors are other structures that must be monitored carefully for loss of ROM, which usually occurs in all these structures as a result of either weakness or static position.

If plantar flexion contractures and the resultant knee, ITB, and hip flexion contractures are allowed to continue unchecked, the child will progress much sooner than necessary to the late ambulation stage, and will lose the ability to ambulate at an earlier age than with intervention.

Activity Level/Active Exercise

Normal activities for a young boy are stressed when possible, and active resistive exercise is not encouraged. There should be no concern about the level of activity causing undue fatigue unless fatigue is present after a full night's sleep.

Several studies have indicated that submaximal exercise has limited value in increasing strength or changing function in DMD.[26,27] At the same time, however, these studies have demonstrated no negative effects of exercise. Other have documented an increased metabolic stress associated with increased activity in boys with DMD[28] and with endurance exercise in individuals with other neuromuscular diseases.[29] This increased metabolic stress may be an indicator of muscle damage, although neither study documented a negative effect on muscle strength or function.

Scott et al. have suggested a possible beneficial effect of chronic low-frequency electrical stimulation in DMD. They demonstrated an increase in maximum voluntary strength of the tibialis anterior muscle of boys who were so stimulated for 6 weeks.[30] The effects of prolonged low-frequency stimulation are being investigated in other muscle groups. This finding is very interesting but, once again, such stimulation targets the strength of only one muscle group. With appropriate selection of muscles, this treatment may promote prolonged maintenance of function, but it does not address the systemic nature of the disorder.

Prolonging Ambulation

As patients with DMD become weaker, their gait pattern is altered in an attempt to improve stability during walking. Stride length decreases, and the width of the base of support increases to provide a more stable base. The ITB accommodates to the new, shortened position associated with the wider base of support. Weakness in the gluteus medius becomes more pronounced, and the child assumes the typical waddling gait.

The lordotic curve increases with progressive weakness of the gluteus maximus. As that muscle weakens, the child attempts to increase stability, moving the center of gravity posterior to the fulcrum of the hip joint by pulling the arms back and by exaggerating the lordosis. Stability at the hip joint during standing is now provided passively by structures anterior to the hip joint, primarily the iliofemoral ligament. Even a mild knee flexion contracture would make ambulation difficult or impossible with the child in this position.

Treatment programs combining passive stretching and lower extremity bracing have demonstrated a reduction in the rate of progression of lower extremity contractures and have prolonged ambulation.[31,32] Various surgical interventions—including Achilles tendon lengthening and Yount fasciotomies,[33] tibialis posterior transpositions,[34] and percutaneous tenotomies[35,36]—in combination with vigorous physical therapy and orthotic intervention, have been reported to improve and prolong ambulation.[37–39] However, there is a paucity of prospective studies that statistically substantiate which type of intervention is appropriate during what time period, and whether the patient and/or family was satisfied with such intervention. A recent prospective study has demonstrated "that a comprehensive program of single early surgical intervention followed by a definite course of rehabilitation can significantly stabilize and possibly prolong ambulation without resorting to long leg braces."[40]

Whatever the surgical methods, a vigorous postoperative physical therapy program should aim to get the patient up and standing and walking as soon as possible. Active joint stretching will help maintain, and may even increase, ROM at those joints that have been percutaneously released; this is because with release of the superficial layers, there is improved access to the deeper structures that may be shortened. The goal of the postoperative physical therapy program is independent ambulation with a minimum of 3 to 5 hours per day of standing and/or walking. Even when no steps are possible, the child is asked to stand at least 1 hour a day (in a standing table if necessary). Optimal stance is with the back in extension so that the center of gravity falls behind the hip joint. Some have proposed that this extension promotes a straight spine, as it keeps the facets locked in extension, thereby prohibiting side-bending.

Wheelchair Use

The decision to buy a wheelchair should be delayed until all other means of ambulation have been exhausted. However, use of a wheelchair or "buggy" strictly for long-distance transport may be most helpful for the child and family.

Only when a family is adamant in its opposition to bracing, or if braced ambulation is no longer possible, should a wheelchair be considered for the primary means of mobility. In many cases, efforts aimed at prolonging ambulation will cease when the child sees the improved independence, increased comfort, convenience, reduced fatigue, and peer attention afforded by wheelchair use. Deformities, particularly hip, knee, and ankle flexion contractures and scoliosis, will often increase when the child uses a wheelchair. Even when ambulation is not possible, use of a standing table of some type helps to postpone these deformities and may reduce the risk of early pulmonary complications.

Because the wheelchair is a personal piece of equipment for the child, he or she should be involved in decisions regarding its design, and color.

The therapist and the child should discuss the following wheelchair options.

1. Wrap-around, removable adjustable-height desk arms
2. Swing-away, elevating, detachable leg rests with heel loops. Elevation can be done periodically during the day to help maintain knee extension and prevent ankle edema.
3. Solid seat to maintain the pelvis in a horizontally aligned position that may help to postpone the development of scoliosis
4. Lateral trunk supports for thoracic positioning (Fig. 12-9)
5. Appropriate width—it is best to select a chair that is too narrow rather than one that is too wide.
6. Reclining back—may be useful in the later stages of disease when the upright posture is not tolerated; may promote spinal extension
7. Seat cushion to provide comfort and prevent decubiti
8. Headrest
9. Molded seat or back insert

During the later stages of the disease, if it is financially feasible, a powered wheelchair will provide for continued independent mobility. A proportional drive will make it both easier and safer for the child to manipulate the powered wheelchair, and should be considered along with the previously mentioned items.

Weight Control

The need to guard against obesity is as important for the child who is limited to a wheelchair as for the ambulatory child. Despite good use of transfer techniques and proper body mechanics by others, excessive weight gain can reduce the child's transfers and may restrict both mobility and social activity. Moreover, excessive weight gain in the child with neuromuscular disease may not only reduce mobility but may also have a deleterious effect on self-esteem, posture, and respiratory function.

Edwards and associates have demonstrated that controlled weight reduction in obese children with DMD is a safe and practical way to improve mobility and self-esteem.[41] However, it is probably easier to prevent excessive weight gain in the young, ambulatory child than to initiate severe dietary restriction in an obese, seated adolescent. It has been proposed that this philosophy of weight control be promoted early for children with neuromuscular disease (taking into account the need for fat intake in early development). Normal growth charts make no allowance for the progressive loss of muscle in

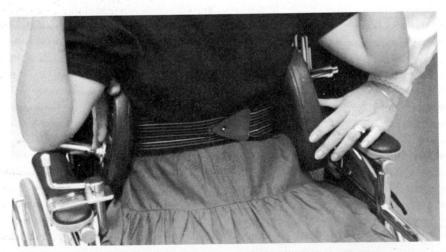

Figure 12-9. *Adjustable scoliosis pads fitted on a wheelchair facilitate trunk positioning. (From Maloney, Burks, Ringel, eds.* Interdisciplinary Rehabilitation of Muscular Dystrophy and Neuromuscular Disorders. *Philadelphia: JB Lippincott; 1984:275.)*

DMD, so if the child continues to gain weight according to normal standards, accumulation of fat tissue may occur as, at this stage, there is muscle wasting in DMD. Griffiths and Edwards studied the relationships between body composition and breakdown products of muscle.[42] They developed a chart, based on their research, which gives ideal weight guidelines for weight control in boys with DMD.[42] The physical therapist can play a major role in promoting this weight control philosophy with the child and family. When weight control is not effective, use of a hydraulic lift becomes important. One or more family members must be trained in the safe and proper use of such a lift.

Minimizing Spinal Deformity

As the child's sitting time increases, so does kyphoscoliosis. Previous clinical observations have documented that the convexity will likely be toward the dominant extremity.[43] Because of this relationship, we recommend that the child with adequate bilateral manual skills have the wheelchair drive moved from side to side every 6 months in order to prevent the scoliosis from becoming structural.

Various pads fitted onto wheelchairs, or custom molded backs and seats fitted into wheelchairs, have been used in an attempt to provide appropriate hip and spinal positioning while seated in the wheelchair, but no studies are available to prove their clinical efficacy. A light plastic body jacket extending from the pelvis to under the armpits has been used by some in an attempt to slow down or maintain the position of the spine, but again there are no studies to confirm its effectiveness. For this type of spinal orthosis to be effective, it must be worn the entire time the child is out of bed, which may be both impractical and uncomfortable. Moreover, such an orthosis does not work well on an obese individual, and it may reduce a child's ability to take a deep breath.[44]

The increasing sophistication of spinal instrumentation within the field of orthopedics has made spinal fixation an option for children with DMD. Previously, the amount of "down time" following surgery precluded these children from choosing this option, both because of the muscle weakness and

the risk of respiratory complications. Currently, physical therapy plays an important role in getting these children "up and moving" within days to a week after surgery, depending on their medical status. Any child with a thoracolumbar curve that has progressed past 30 degrees should be considered for spinal fixation, taking into consideration the child's functional level and cardiac and respiratory status. Initially, referrals for spinal stabilization were attempts on our part to improve or stabilize our patients' respiratory function, as we were concerned about the mechanical disadvantage the kyphoscoliosis placed upon the already weak respiratory muscles, as well as the potentially deleterious effect of this scoliosis on respiratory function. Recent studies have demonstrated no salutary effect of segmental spinal stabilization on respiratory function based on either short- or long-term follow-up, but all studies have documented improved sitting comfort, appearance, and stabilization, or improvement of kyphoscoliosis.[45–47]

Facilitating Sleep

Air mattresses or commercial flotation pads often improve sleeping comfort for children with advanced deterioration who have difficulty positioning themselves or changing position at night. These devices also provide relief for family members who might otherwise be up 3 to 5 times per night to turn the patient. A hospital bed may be useful in the later stages of disease to assist with positioning and transfers, as well as to elevate the head of the bed in an attempt to ease the respiratory distress that can occur during sleep as the contents of the abdominal cavity push against the diaphragm, increasing the effort required in taking a deep breath.

Respiratory Considerations

The major cause of respiratory complications in DMD is the progressive weakness of the muscles of respiration. This weakness may or may not be exacerbated by the mechanical disadvantages associated with kyphoscoliosis. The signs and symptoms of respiratory insufficiency include excessive fatigue and daytime sleepiness, headaches upon awakening (secondary to increased carbon dioxide levels that may accompany decreased respiratory efficacy while supine), sleep disturbances (nightmares), or feeling the need to strain to "gulp for air."

A good history and periodic pulmonary function testing with the child in both the seated and supine positions are the most effective means of monitoring respiratory insufficiency. In addition, family members should be trained in the techniques of bronchial drainage, chest percussion, and assisted coughing. One study demonstrated improved pulmonary function after performance of breathing exercises, but this effect was not sustained.[48]

If the history and pulmonary function test results suggest that the lungs are not being adequately ventilated, the child should be referred to a pulmonologist for further testing and discussion of options for assisted ventilation. A relatively new method of ventilatory assistance—nasal positive pressure ventilation—may be used at night to assist breathing and to provide a rest for overworked respiratory muscles.[49] An adjustment period is often necessary when this type of ventilation is used, but after a period of time the patient often derives the benefits of improved sleep and increased energy and alertness in the daytime. Ventilatory assistance might be required both day and night for children with advanced respiratory failure. Thanks to modern technology, this is a feasible option.[50] Technology has provided advances so that speech and eating are not severely affected by a tracheostomy, and ventilators are compact, battery-driven devices that can be attached to an appropriately modified wheelchair. The physical therapist may play a major role in positioning and adapting wheelchairs for individuals requiring assisted ventilation. This type of multidisciplinary program can optimize function and prolong life. Not all individuals choose these options, and some do not have the resources to pursue them, but those who have the means generally report a very satisfying life, including higher education and gainful employment.[51]

Activities of Daily Living

The physical therapist should routinely assess the child's ability to perform activities of daily living (ADLs). The patient's ability to feed himself, turn

pages in a book, and do necessary personal hygiene tasks must all be assessed periodically. The physical therapist may choose to request an occupational therapy consultation. A home visit is most helpful in assessing adaptive equipment needs.

Facilitating Family Support

The physical therapist plays an important role in providing support, motivation, and training of the patient with DMD and his family members. Successful family support depends on the early involvement of the physical therapist and the ability of the therapist to have the family comply with a home program that is monitored and adapted appropriately. Assessment of the social situation of the family should be part of each visit.

The mild to moderate intellectual impairment in these young boys often imposes both educational and emotional handicaps, in addition to the obvious physical changes accompanying DMD. The child learns that the disease will continuously erode the quality and quantity of his existence, and the resultant reliance and dependence on others frequently gives rise to stress within the family. Although not a psychotherapist, the physical therapist must be aware of the emotional factors involved with the illness and must provide strong emotional support, as well as help in reinforcing and attaining goals and preventing conflicts. A healthy emotional environment for the family and the child with DMD is at least as important to the child as the prevention of contractures.

Management of Pain

If the aforementioned goals are achieved, management of pain should be unnecessary. Pain occurs at the limits of ROM in all joints, and because contractures reduce the ROM, they also increase the opportunity for the development of pain. If pain becomes a problem, routine methods of treatment and appropriate positioning techniques should help to minimize the discomfort.

Summary

A successful treatment program should result in several additional years of independent ambulation, improved self-sufficiency, substantial postponement of the restrictions imposed by a wheelchair, and the maintenance of the maximal functional independence allowed by the child's level of strength.

Other Related Disorders

Although the neuromuscular disorders have varying etiologies and lack a cure, these disorders result in similar physical problems that can be managed by applying similar principles. As previously presented for DMD, the major physical therapy goals include preventing deformity, prolonging functional capacity, facilitating family knowledge and involvement through education and counseling, and helping in the management of pain, if necessary.

For each disorder, treatment should help to prevent complications. None of the habilitative approaches used can alter the underlying neuromuscular destruction. Prevention should serve as the focus of our efforts. The basic tenets of treatment should ensure that a carefully planned home program is carried out and appropriately monitored. In addition to these tenets, weight control is important. Caloric intake and physical activity level must be considered, and the family must be educated about the secondary complications associated with obesity.

Myotonic Dystrophy

Myotonic dystrophy (MTD) is an autosomal dominant disorder whose location is on chromosome 19. In the most typical form of MTD, the symptoms are first noticed during adolescence and are characterized by myotonia, a delay in muscle relaxation time, and muscle weakness. As the weakness progresses, the myotonia often decreases. The individual will present to the clinic with complaints of weakness and stiffness. Stiffness, which is often the major complaint, is characteristic of the myotonia. Patients often have a characteristic physical appearance that includes a long, thin face with temporal and masseter muscle wasting; frontal balding; and weakness and wasting of the sternocleidomastoids. The pattern of weakness in MTD presents first with distal wasting and weakness, manifested by a foot drop and difficulty opening jars. Proximal muscle weakness occurs in the later stage of the disease. The most severe form of MTD is congenital and is associated with generalized muscular hypoplasia, mental retardation, and a high incidence of neonatal mortality. Children with congenital MTD are born to mothers afflicted with the disorder. Because MTD is inherited in an autosomal dominant pattern, an individual with the disease has a 50/50 chance of each offspring having the disease. The severe congenital form of MTD is characterized by maternal transmission only. The latter group is often plagued with severe mental retardation, speech disturbances, delayed motor milestones, distal weakness, and spinal deformities. With survival to adulthood, these individuals follow the pattern of the classical course of the disease, in which cataracts are common. There is involvement not only of skeletal muscle, but smooth muscle, too, and cardiac conduction defects are often seen, particularly first-degree heart block. There may be associated infertility, decreased respiratory drive, and numerous endocrine problems. Currently, there is no treatment for the disorder, and the etiology of the genetic defect is unknown, as is the gene that produces the deletion causing MTD. There is no curative pharmacologic treatment, although some medications may be used to ameliorate the symptoms of myotonia. The objectives of current therapeutic intervention are to reduce the distal wasting and weakness and control the spinal deformities.

Death in these individuals is usually caused by heart block or problems secondary to decreased respiratory drive. The respiratory complications may be severe and, when mechanically ventilated, these patients are very difficult to wean. The congenital forms of MTD may be accompanied by severe developmental delays, in which case intervention that employs various motor development approaches may be beneficial.

Facioscapulohumeral Dystrophy

Facioscapulohumeral dystrophy (FSH) can arise at any time from childhood until adult life. There is an

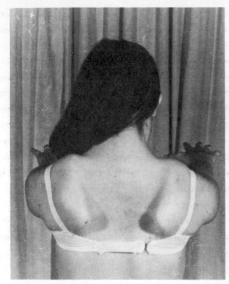

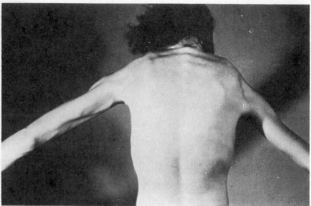

Figure 12-10. *Facioscapulohumeral dystrophy. Bilateral scapular winging and elevation are indicative of diffuse shoulder girdle involvmenet. (From Lovell WW, Winter RB, eds.* Pediatric Orthopaedics. *2nd ed. Philadelphia: JB Lippincott; 1986:268.*

autosomal dominant pattern of inheritance. The gene defect appears to be located on chromosome 4. Initial muscular involvement includes the face and shoulder girdle, but subsequent progression may include the pelvic girdle. Progression of the disease is usually insidious, with long periods of apparent arrest of the process. Some cases occur in which there is a rapid progression and disability, but most patients survive and are active throughout adulthood and do not die prematurely.[52] The disease commonly begins during childhood, but because of its wide variance, it may show up as late as the third or fourth decade. Therefore, a child at risk for inheritance of FSH should not be pronounced free of the disease just because no signs or symptoms occurred during childhood.

Although the progression of weakness in FSH proceeds proximal to distal, as in DMD, the pattern of muscle weakness is different. The lower trapezius and facial musculature in patients with FSH show weakness the earliest but, unlike DMD, the latissimus dorsi is seldom involved. During the early stages of the disease, a physical therapist with good muscle testing skills may be the person best qualified to identify or diagnose the muscle disease. A good test of facial weakness involves having the child blow air into the cheeks to cause them to bulge but not to let air escape through the lips. The therapist can then exert manual pressure on the cheeks to see the point at which the orbicularis oris muscle allows air to escape. The major problem for the physical therapist is to determine the difference between normal and reduced strength in the facial muscles. The brachioradialis is another characteristically weak muscle in children with FSH. However, because a strong biceps brachii confounds testing of the brachioradialis, palpation and observation are the main tools for identifying weakness in this muscle.

Allsop has conducted hand dynamometer grip strength tests on approximately 150 patients with FSH and has compared the results to similar results in approximately 50 physical therapy students. Most students had greater grip strength in the dominant hand or had similar strength bilaterally. The group with FSH showed a consistent reduction in grip strength in the dominant extremity when compared with the nondominant hand. These data raise the question of the advisability of strenuous exercise for weakened muscles in patients with FSH.[53]

The main problem caused by FSH early in the course of the child's life is pain in the upper thoracic region that results from lack of stability secondary to weakness of the trapezius, rhomboids, and other scapular musculature (Fig. 12-10). In severe cases, some recommend a modified Taylor brace to support the midthoracic region and to retract the scapulae (when properly fitted and stabilized at the pelvis). In those cases when the deltoid is preserved but scapular stabilization is absent, a scapulothoracic fusion may be helpful.[54,55]

Spinal Muscular Atrophy

Three categories of spinal muscular atrophy (SMA) occur in childhood:

1. Infantile SMA, or Werdnig-Hoffman disease
2. Intermediate SMA (type II muscular atrophy or chronic Werdnig-Hoffman disease)
3. Juvenile SMA (Kugelberg-Welander disease)

All are inherited as autosomal recessive disorders located on chromosome 5.[56,57] All three have pathology affecting the anterior horn cell and, although all are located in chromosome 5, there are primary differences in their clinical presentation. Diseases of the anterior horn cell (motor neurons) are associated with wasting and weakness of the muscles. Sensory changes are absent. In the childhood and juvenile forms, the lower motor neurons are chiefly affected and the diseases are often similar. This similarity is in contrast to amyotrophic lateral sclerosis, an adult form of motor neuron disease, which is less often inherited and more commonly associated with upper motor neuron involvement.

Infantile Spinal Muscular Atrophy

Infantile SMA is almost always noted within the first 3 months of life. The mother often complains of decreased fetal movement. At birth, the affected child is hypotonic, has difficulty feeding, commonly has respiratory distress, and may present with "failure to thrive." Muscle wasting is often severe, and spontaneous movements are few. The pattern of breathing is abnormal, with the abdominal muscles playing a greater role than the thoracic muscles (i.e., these children are "belly breathers"). The child may continue to have difficulty feeding and swallowing. On close inspection, the tongue may be atrophic, and when the child cries, one may see fasciculations or "jumping" of the tongue. Deep tendon reflexes are usually decreased or absent, and plantar responses are usually flexor or absent. No sensory abnormalities are noted. During the first several years of life, hospitalizations for pulmonary infections are common. These children do not achieve motor milestones at a normal rate, if at all. Most children with infantile SMA do not survive beyond 3 years of age, with respiratory failure being responsible for their death.[4]

Intermediate Spinal Muscular Atrophy

Intermediate SMA (or type II SMA) also affects infants, but is more benign than the acute or infantile (Werdnig-Hoffman) form. This form of SMA refers to a group of "floppy" children with lower motor neuron disease who are slow to attain motor milestones. Prior to differentiation between infantile SMA and intermediate SMA, it was noted that a group of children with SMA never walked, but did not die at an early age. These children are presumed to have had intermediate or type II SMA. Today, these children are usually involved in habilitative intervention, including physical therapy and orthotic training, to provide for early standing or ambulation. Type II SMA usually presents after 3 to 6 months of age when the children are noted to be slow in reaching their motor milestones. These children are characterized by weakness and wasting of the extremities and trunk musculature. Feeding and swallowing difficulties are seldom a problem. There is often a fine tremor when the child attempts to use the limbs. This is not a true intention tremor, but has been referred to as a mini-polymyoclonus.[4] These children may or may not learn to walk. Most will require orthotic intervention to ambulate, but often, the ambulation is not functional. Nonetheless, it is important in these patients to encourage stance, to maintain joint mobility, to prevent problems associated with long-term wheelchair sitting, and to attempt to keep the patient's back as straight as possible for as long as possible. These children often survive into adulthood, but are vulnerable to pulmonary infection at any point. Children with intermediate SMA are predisposed to the complications, such as joint contractures and kyphoscoliosis, that affect other children with neuromuscular weakness. Although respiratory insufficiency is a problem in both the infantile and intermediate forms of SMA, there is not the same cardiac involvement as is seen in Duchenne muscular dystrophy because the children with SMA appear to have normal cardiac tissue. In both forms of SMA, the diagnosis is made on the basis of the clinical presentation and laboratory tests, including electromyography, which will show denervation with fibrillations and a paucity of motor units. Nerve conduction velocity tests are usually normal for the child's age. Muscle biopsy helps to confirm the diagnosis by demonstrating a characteristic pattern of denervation. However, a muscle biopsy does not often differentiate between infantile and intermediate SMA. There is no diagnostic test available that can differentiate accurately between infantile and intermediate SMA; therefore, initial prognosis is often based on the clinical acumen of the physician and recommendations by other professionals. Most often, the prognosis is left for time to tell, and is dependent primarily upon the number of respiratory infections suffered each year.[4]

Both diseases have been located on chromosome number 5,[56] but no other etiology is apparent. Studies of anterior horn cell metabolism have not been helpful, and current treatment is primarily symptomatic. The treatment approach includes physical therapy, orthotics, spinal management, wheelchair seating, and appropriate treatment of respiratory distress.

Administration of neurotrophic factors—specifically, ciliary neurotrophic factor—is a pharmacologic treatment that has been newly proposed for individuals with anterior horn cell disease. Studies are presently underway on adult motor neuron disease syndromes.

Juvenile Spinal Muscular Atrophy (Kugelberg-Welander Disease)

Juvenile SMA is characterized by symptoms of progressive weakness, wasting, and fasciculations that are noted between the ages of 5 and 15 years. Proximal muscles are usually involved first and, because of the age of presentation, this disease may be confused with the muscular dystrophies. Deep tendon reflexes are decreased, but contractures are unusual, and progressive spinal deformities are uncommon. A mild, progressive weakness is common. Diagnosis is established on the basis of the clinical picture and the results of diagnostic laboratory studies, including an electromyogram and muscle biopsy, which show denervation. As with other forms of SMA, treatment is supportive in the hope of gaining time until a neurotrophic factor may become available to either cure or retard the progression of this disease.

Summary

The disorders discussed in this chapter are all characterized by weakness and wasting of the skeletal musculature, progressive deformity, and increasing disability. The physical therapist plays an important role as counselor, motivator, facilitator, and provider of emotional support for the affected child and family. These expanded roles may be as important as the actual physical assistance and training that physical therapists traditionally provide.

References

1. Dubowitz V. *Muscle Disorders in Childhood*. London: WB Saunders; 1978:22.
2. Koenig N, Hoffman EP, Bertelson CJ, et al. Complete cloning of the Duchenne muscular dystrophy (DMD) cDNA and preliminary genomic organization of the DMD gene in normal and affected individuals. *Cell*. 1987;50:509–517.
3. Crisp DE, Ziter FA, Bray PF. Diagnostic delay in Duchenne muscular dystrophy. *J Am Med Assoc*. 1982;247:478–480.
4. Brooke MH. *Clinicians' View of Neuromuscular Disease*. 2nd ed. Baltimore: Williams and Wilkins; 1986:117–159.
5. Leibowitz D, Dubowitz V. Intellect and behavior in Duchenne muscular dystrophy. *Dev Med Child Neurol*. 1981;23:577–590.
6. Medical Research Council of the United Kingdom. *Aids to Examination of the Peripheral Nervous System: Memorandum No. 45*. Palo Alto, CA: Pedragon House; 1978.
7. Florence JM, Pandya S, King W, et al. Clinical trials in Duchenne dystrophy. Standardization and Reliability of Evaluation Procedures. *Phys Ther* 64:41–45.
8. Brooke MH, Fenichel G, Griggs R, et al. Clinical investigations in Duchenne dystrophy. Part 2. Determination of the "power" of therapeutic trials based on the natural history. *Muscle Nerve*. 1983;6:91–103.
9. Vignos PJ, Spencer GE, Archibald KC: Management of progressive muscular dystrophy of childhood. *JAMA* 1963;184:89–96.
10. Brooke MH, Fenichel G, Griggs R, et al. Duchenne muscular dystrophy: Patterns of clinical progression and effects of supportive therapy. *Neurology*. 1989;39:475–481.
11. Griggs RC, Reeves W, Moxley RT. The heart in Duchenne dystrophy. In: Rowland LP, ed. *Pathogenesis of Human Muscular Dystrophies*. Amsterdam: Excerpta Medica; 1977:661–671.
12. Prosser JE. Intelligence and the gene for Duchenne muscular dystrophy. *Arch Dis Child*. 1969;44:221–230.
13. Ziter FA, Allsop K. The diagnosis and management of childhood muscular dystrophy. *Clin Pediatr* 1976;15(6):540–548.
14. Brooke MH, Fenichel G, Griggs R, et al. Clinical investigation of Duchenne muscular dystrophy. Interesting results in a trial of prednisone. *Arch Neurol*. 1987;44:812–817.
15. Mendell JR. Randomized, double-blind six-month trial of prednisone in Duchenne's muscular dystrophy. *N Engl J Med* 1989;320:1592–1597.
16. Drachman DB, Toyka RV, Meyer E. Prednisone in Duchenne muscular dystrophy. *Lancet*. 1974;2:1409–1412.
17. DeSilva S, Drachman D, Mellits D, Kunel R. Prednisone treatment in Duchenne muscular dystrophy. Long-term benefit. *Arch Neurol*. 1987;44:818–822.
18. Fenichel G, Florence J, Pestronk A, et al. Long-term benefit from prednisone therapy in Duchenne muscular dystrophy. *Neurology*. 1991;41:1874–1877.
19. Partridge TA. Myoblast transfer: Possible therapy for inherited myopathies? *Muscle Nerve*. 1991;14:197–212.
20. Ziter FA, Allsop KG, Tyler FH. Assessment of muscle strength in Duchenne muscular dystrophy. *Neurology*. 1977;27:981–984.
21. Allsop KG, Ziter FA. Loss of strength and functional decline in Duchenne dystrophy. *Arch Neurol*. 1981;38:406–411.
22. Brooke MH, Griggs R, Mendell J, et al. Clinical trial in Duchenne dystrophy. The design of the protocol. *Muscle Nerve*. 1981;4:186–197.
23. Griggs R, Moxley R, Mendell J, et al. Prednisone in Duchenne dystrophy. A randomized, controlled trial defining the time course and dose response. *Arch Neurol*. 1991;48:383–388.
24. Florence J, Pandya S, King W, et al. Intrarater reliability of manual muscle test (Medical Research Council Scale) grades in Duchenne muscular dystrophy. *Phys Ther*. 1992;72:115–126.
25. Pandya S, Florence JM, King W, et al. Reliability of goniometric measurements in patients with Duchenne muscular dystrophy. *Phys Ther*. 1985;65:1339–1342.
26. Vignos P, Watkins M. The effect of exercise in muscular dystrophy. *J Am Med Assoc*. 1966;197:121–126.
27. de Lateur B, Giaconi R. Effect on maximal strength

of submaximal exercise in Duchenne muscular dystrophy. *Am J Phys Med.* 1979;58:26–36.

28. Florence JM, Fox P, Planer J, Brooke MH. Activity, creatine kinase, and myoglobin in Duchenne muscular dystrophy: A clue to etiology? *Neurology* 1985;35:758–761.

29. Florence JM, Hagberg J. Effect of training on the exercise responses of neuromuscular disease patients. *Medicine and Science in Sports and Exercise* 1984;16:460–465.

30. Scott O, Vrbová S, Hyde S, Dubowitz V. Chronic electrical stimulation: Muscle function studies in children with neuromuscular disease. In: *Comprehensive Neurologic Rehabilitation.* Vol. 3. New York: Demos; 1989:307–313.

31. Harris SE, Cherry DB. Childhood progressive muscular dystrophy and the role of physical therapy. *Phys Ther.* 1974;54:4–12.

32. Scott OM, Hyde SA, Goddard C, Dubowitz V. Prevention of deformity in Duchenne muscular dystrophy. A prospective study of passive stretching and splintage. *Physiotherapy.* 1981;67:177–180.

33. Archibald DC, Vignos PJ Jr. A study of contractures in muscular dystrophy. *Arch Phys Med Rehabil.* 1959;40:150–157.

34. Spencer GE. Orthopaedic care of progressive muscular dystrophy. *J Bone Joint Surg (Am).* 1967;49:1201–1204.

35. Roy L, Gibson DA. Pseudohypertrophic muscular dystrophy and its surgical management: Review of 30 patients. *Can J Surg.* 1970;13:13–20.

36. Siegel IM. Management of musculoskeletal complications in neuromuscular disease. Enhancing mobility and the role of bracing and surgery. In: Fowler WM Jr, ed. *Advances in the Rehabilitation of Neuromuscular Diseases: State of the Art Reviews.* Vol. 4. Philadelphia: Hanley & Belfus; 1988;553–575.

37. Ziter FA, Allsop KG. The value of orthoses for patients with Duchenne muscular dystrophy. *Phys Ther.* 1979;59:1361–1365.

38. Heckmatt JZ, Dubowitz V, Hyde SA, et al. Prolongation of walking in Duchenne muscular dystrophy with lightweight orthoses. Review of 57 cases. *Dev Med Child Neurol.* 1985;27:149–154.

39. Vignos PJ. Management of musculoskeletal complications in neuromuscular disease: Limb contractures and the role of stretching, braces and surgery. In: Fowler WM Jr, ed. *Advances in the Rehabilitation of Neuromuscular Diseases: State of the Art Reviews.*

Vol. 4. Philadelphia: Hanley & Belfus; 1988:509–536.

40. Bach JR. Orthopedic surgery and rehabilitation for the prolongation of brace-free ambulation of patients with Duchenne muscular dystrophy. *Am J Phys Med Rehabil.* 1991;20:323–331.

41. Edwards RHT. Weight reduction in boys with muscular dystrophy. *Dev Med Child Neurol.* 1984;26:384–390.

42. Griffiths R, Edwards R. A new chart for weight control in Duchenne muscular dystrophy. *Arch Dis Child.* 1988;63:1256–1258.

43. Johnson E, Yarnell S. Hand dominance and scoliosis in Duchenne muscular dystrophy. *Arch Phys Med Rehab.* 1976;57:462–464.

44. Florence JM, Brooke MH, Carroll J. Evaluation of the child with muscular weakness. *Orthoped Clin North Am* 1978;9(2):421–422.

45. Miller F, Moseley C, Koreska J, Eng J, Levison H. Pulmonary function and scoliosis in Duchenne dystrophy. *J Pediatr Orthop.* 1988;8:133–137.

46. Miller R, Chalmers A, Dao H, et al. The effect of spine fusion on respiratory function in Duchenne muscular dystrophy. *Neurology* 1991;41:37–40.

47. Shapiro F, Sethna N, Colan S, Wohl M, Specht L. Spinal fusion in Duchenne muscular dystrophy: A multidisciplinary approach. *Muscle Nerve.* 1992;15:604–614.

48. Adams M, Chandler L. Effects of physical therapy program on vital capacity of patients with muscular dystrophy. *Phys Ther.* 1974;54:494–496.

49. Leger P, Jennequin J, Gerard M, Robert D. Home positive pressure ventilation via nasal mask for patients with neuromuscular weakness or restrictive lung or chest-wall disease. *Respir Care.* 1989;34:73–79.

50. Bach J, O'Brien J, Krotenberg R, Alba A. Management of end-stage respiratory failure in Duchenne muscular dystrophy. *Muscle Nerve.* 1987;10:177–182.

51. Bach JR, Campagnolo DI, Hoeman S. Life satisfaction of individuals with Duchenne muscular dystrophy using long-term mechanical ventilatory support. *Am J Phys Rehabil.* 1991;70:129–135.

52. Walton JN, Garder-Medwin D. Progressive muscular dystrophy and myotonic disorders. In: Walton JN, ed. *Disorders of Voluntary Muscle.* 3rd ed. London: Churchill Livingstone, 1974:561–613.

53. Allsop KG. Unpublished data.

54. Bunch WH. Scapulo-thoracic fusion for shoulder stabilization in muscular dystrophy. *Minn Med.* 1973;56:391–394.

55. Copeland SA, Howard RC. Thoracoscapular fusion for facioscapulohumeral dystrophy. *J Bone Joint Surg.* 1978;60B:547–551.

56. Guillian T, Brzustowicz L, Castilla L, et al. Genetic hemogeneity between acute and chronic forms of spinal muscular atrophy. *Nature* 1990;345:823–825.

57. Brzustowicz L, Lehner T, Castilla L, et al. Genetic mapping of chronic childhood-onset spinal muscular atrophy to chromosome 5q 11.2–13.3. *Nature* 1990; 344:540–541.

Pediatric Physical Therapy,
second edition, edited by Jan
Stephen Tecklin. J. B. Lippincott
Company, Philadelphia © 1994.

13

Jodi Barkin Oren

Adaptive Equipment for Handicapped Children

- **Role of Adaptive Equipment**
- **Precautions When Using Adaptive Equipment**
  - **Misuse**
  - **Poor Planning**
  - **Equipment Use Versus Facilitation**
- **Determining a Child's Equipment Needs**
  - **Initial Evaluation**
  - **Assessment of the Home and Family**
  - **School Assessment**
  - **Summary**
- **Equipment Selection**
  - **Purchasing Equipment**
  - **Making Equipment**

- **Selection of Materials**
- **Commonly Used Equipment for Various Positions**
  - **Sitting**
  - **Standing**
  - **Side-Lying**
  - **Overall Considerations**
- **Equipment for Infants and Toddlers**
  - **Hospitalized Children**
  - **Normal Infants and Toddlers**
- **Activities of Daily Living**
- **Conclusions**

Physical therapists have many products at their disposal to help provide the handicapped child with better means for positioning, achieving mobility, and performing activities of daily living (ADLs). New products are being developed every year in an attempt to satisfy the needs of children with disabilities. Products and materials are available in both standard, commercially produced forms and custom-fabricated forms to satisfy individualized specifications for each child.

The great variety of products and materials available and the constantly changing and expanding market present a formidable problem for the therapist who tries to give parents useful suggestions regarding equipment. How can students or recent graduates acquaint themselves with these products in order to feel confident in guiding families who need adaptive equipment for their child? What conditions should be evaluated before making decisions regarding adaptive equipment? What is the true role of adaptive equipment for children with handicapping conditions, and are there particular dangers or contraindications to adaptive equipment? These questions are addressed in this chapter, the main goal of which is to provide the student and the therapist who is inexperienced in pediatrics with a theoretical construct to facilitate decision making about adaptive equipment, regardless of familiarity with any particular piece of equipment. Commonly used equipment—prone standers, sidelyers, and wheelchairs—are evaluated, and case studies are used to further delineate approaches to practical decision making. There are few, if any, clear, scientific, objective guidelines on which to base a decision about adaptive equipment. The selection of adaptive equipment for children is still an art, rather than a science. As physical therapists, our goal is to try to meet the needs of handicapped children by using a critical approach to document our successes and failures in the hope of consequently transforming this "art" into a science.

Role of Adaptive Equipment

Adaptive equipment is becoming increasingly necessary as an adjunct to direct treatment. No child can realistically receive the constant handling needed throughout the day to prevent abnormal movement patterns. Although the physical therapist may teach families, day-care providers, and teachers about methods of handling the child to encourage optimal development, the child must be allowed time to move, explore, and relax without constant help. The increased cost of direct care and the crowded conditions often found in programs for the handicapped suggest a need for alternatives to direct patient handling.

One alternative is the judicious use of adaptive equipment to allow correct positioning during free, independent time for the child. Adaptive equipment can also provide for the reinforcement and use of positions and movements introduced to the child during treatment sessions. Similarly, abnormal or undesirable positions or movements can often be prevented by use of correct equipment.

Adaptive equipment may encourage functional

skills that the child may otherwise be unable to do. These uses of adaptive equipment not only promote motor and sensory development, but concurrently improve cognitive, perceptual, emotional, and social development.

Adaptive equipment, in addition to its direct therapeutic benefits, may serve an important role by assisting in the daily management of the handicapped child at home. Some indispensable items include bathtub seats, hydraulic lifts, and adapted high chairs. Adaptive items that facilitate safe and effective transportation may include many types of car seats, strollers, and wheelchairs.

Although adaptive equipment should be prescribed with the goal of achieving maximum benefits, this ideal approach may occasionally need to be compromised. For example, some families may be unwilling to adjust the routines of all family members to meet the needs of only one member. Ideal goals may also not be possible because of architectural barriers that prohibit the use of certain adaptive devices. When barriers (behavioral, architectural, or financial) exist, the therapist must analyze the short-term needs of the family and the long-term goals of the child before making a decision or recommendation. Whenever adaptive equipment is recommended, its use must be monitored to ensure that therapeutic goals and family needs are being met.

Precautions When Using Adaptive Equipment

Can adaptive equipment be dangerous? This is a difficult question to answer, especially because most equipment has a design that is inherently free of dangers. Problems may arise from the way in which equipment is used by various caretakers. Although a particular piece of equipment may have been prescribed, fitted, and properly explained, its overuse or misuse may cause difficulties.

Misuse

Adaptive equipment is often static and, although beneficial, may not provide a rich environment for learning new movements or transitions from one position to another, or for exploration. Gross motor development in normal children is known to require learning through doing, moving, and feeling. Sensory, vestibular, and tactile input are all required to produce varied and competent motor output. Static positioning, which occurs when some adaptive equipment is used excessively, can retard motor development. A carefully developed plan for therapeutic use of a piece of adaptive equipment must take into consideration not only the potential benefit, but also the potential deleterious effects. Normal motor development relies on coordination of both agonist and antagonist muscle groups to complete a pattern of movement. Adaptive equipment tends to "fix" a child into one pattern, albeit therapeutic, while denying the opportunity to experience the competing or antagonist pattern. For example, a side-lyer provides an opportunity for the child to play while placed in a neutral, midline orientation. Although a neutral, midline orientation may be an appropriate goal, it is important to note also that an asymmetric orientation is not inherently bad or undesirable. An asymmetric orientation is a normal precursor to weight shifting, lateral flexion, and lateral rotation. The pathologic or abnormal pattern or orientation may compete with the pattern facilitated by the equipment. Although the competing pattern may be abnormal, the therapist is responsible for teaching normal or "balanced" movement patterns. The person who places the child in a position must be aware of the benefits of various positions and must avoid constant and unchanging positioning habits. Inappropriate use of equipment, which places the child in static postures, can also lead to orthopedic complications, such as joint contracture, which may eventually require surgical repair. Anyone who has responsibility for the child must understand the therapeutic goals and must monitor equipment use to maximize the benefits and minimize the deleterious effects.

Poor Planning

Poor planning for growth can lead to misuse of equipment. With the current difficulty experienced in receiving authorization for third-party payment for expensive equipment for the handicapped child, the therapist must anticipate and plan carefully for both the physical and developmental growth of the child. The inexperienced therapist may overlook the changing needs of the child. A child who requires positioning in sitting during the early years may be given an expensive chair that will provide fine positioning and optimal use of the upper extremities for fine motor skills. However, despite the initial advantages of the chair, it may be inappropriate for future mobility and socialization needs. Predicting the child's needs in the areas of growth and development, education, and recreational alternatives (e.g., wheelchair sports) is a monumental task, but one in which physical therapists must often participate at the request of insurers and local and state funding agencies. Therapists must learn how various agencies and providers prefer to reconcile those requirements and reimbursement patterns with the patient's needs. Some providers prefer devices that, although more frequently replaced than costlier items, are more cost-effective at the outset. Other providers prefer an initial, larger expenditure for a device that will last for 3 to 5 years. These considerations must be addressed in order to meet the child's best interest. The consequences of miscalculations in these decisions will be a child who is poorly accommodated in an ill-fitting device that does not meet his or her current needs. In such instances, the therapist must then explore difficult alternatives, such as borrowing or adapting old equipment, until the patient is eligible for new equipment. The growth potential of various pieces of equipment is discussed later in this chapter. Clearly, growth and developmental considerations are a critical aspect when selecting adaptive equipment.

Equipment Use Versus Facilitation

The use of equipment in place of facilitation is the final danger or concern relating to adaptive equipment. We have already discussed how positioning devices may not allow for "balanced" development. Unfortunately, many therapists and parents are biased toward the idea that, because there are so many equipment options, equipment is equivalent to therapy. The child is thus "plugged into" many types of equipment (e.g., progressing from high chair to car seat to side-lyer to stander). Although each piece of equipment allows the child to challenge current patterns and to develop alternative patterns, the equipment is not a substitute for treatment. Equipment restricts the two types of experiences of learning—active motor transitions and movement for exploration—which are the ultimate goals of normal motor development. Some therapists believe that a child who is poorly fitted for adaptive equipment or a child who uses no adaptive equipment receives more treatment through oral feedback and handling (to reposition) than the child who is "well-equipped." That belief advocates neither malpositioning nor denial of needed equipment to maximize therapeutic input; rather, it suggests that, just as appropriate equipment can be useful for satisfying the overall needs of a child, overuse or misuse of equipment can also be equally detrimental.

Determining a Child's Equipment Needs

The therapist who provides routine, continuing care for the handicapped child is often not the same therapist responsible for purchasing adaptive equipment. Sometimes, because of the size or nature of the facility at which the child receives routine treatment, a referral to a larger, more well-equipped institution may be appropriate to determine equipment needs. Whether the child is referred to a children's hospital, to a wheelchair clinic in a major medical center, or directly to the vendor's establishment, the provision of appropriate apparatus depends mainly on detailed and accurate information about both the child and the child's environment. The primary therapist should be present during the evaluation of the equipment to give an accurate assessment of the child's needs. If the therapist is unable to attend, a report with an assessment of the child's needs and a recommendation for choices of equipment must be included in the referral. A stan-

dardized initial assessment is required whether a therapist is serving in a primary care or a consulting role. The therapist should assess the child in relation to a specific piece of apparatus. Because of time restrictions, the assessment may concentrate on one specific equipment or functional need (e.g., sitting), and additional assessments may be required for other equipment needs. Once a piece of equipment has been received, the therapist must examine the child to ensure that the apparatus suits the child, that it meets the identified goals, and that those people who will be using the equipment understand its correct use. Observing the child use the equipment after initial assessment and equipment selection also provides the new therapist with a measure of self-assessment for personal growth.

Initial Evaluation

The parameters to be considered when evaluating a child's need for adaptive equipment are similar to those of most other evaluations. The goal of such an evaluation, however, is to clarify and direct the therapist to the most appropriate equipment options available. The following specific items should be considered in the evaluation.

Range of Motion

Range of motion (ROM) is important in selecting almost all equipment because accommodating the patient in most apparatuses will depend on adequate ROM and joint mobility. The device being considered will dictate the motions that are critical to success. The ROM assessments that play an important role in various positioning devices are shown in Table 13-1.

Muscle Tone, Control, and Strength

Muscle tone, control, and strength deserve careful consideration when selecting equipment. The degree of strength or motor control needed for functional use of the device must be determined. For example, use of a manually controlled wheelchair requires strength and coordination of the upper extremities. If the child does not have adequate upper

Table 13-1. *Range of Motion Assessment*

	Side-Lying	Sitting	Standing
Head and Neck			
Rotation	When asymmetry exists, sidelying to only one side may be desirable to inhibit rotation, which may result in improved alignment.	Difficult to control neck rotation without maximal support	*
Extension	Inhibition or control of hyperextension of the neck is a major reason for using a side-lyer. The device may prevent contracture and reduce extensor tone.	May be inhibited or accommodated with a collar placed to avoid the occipital region, which is known to stimulate extension[†]	May result in choosing supine stander in an attempt to control extension
Flexion	With tracheostomy, avoid positions that will obstruct the airway.	Excessive flexion cannot be easily controlled and may require that a sitting device be reclined.	May use prone stander positioned only several degrees from neutral in an attempt to facilitate active extension
Trunk			
Scoliosis (see also pelvic obliquity)	May require positioning to only one side so that gravity or weight bearing can assist in stretching the concave side.	May be accommodated with lateral trunk support. In severe cases, custom molding to the patient may be needed. Sitting is not a method of remediating scoliosis, but may be designed to reduce progression.	If severe, may be uncomfortable and reduce breathing
Kyphosis (See also hip extension)	*	Excessive flexion cannot be easily controlled and may require that a sitting device be reclined. Kyphosis severely limits function.	If severe, the prone position may be tolerated poorly
Lordosis	Severe lordosis may negate the benefit of the device in controlling trunk and neck extension.	If severe, the lordosis may compromise stability and require added support or strapping. Custom molding may also be required when lordosis is severe.	May create compensatory lower extremity flexion
Pelvis			
Obliquity (See also hip abduction/adduction and scoliosis	*	Because the pelvis is the main base of support, obliquity may hamper proper alignment; this should be considered in design of a chair. If a discrepancy in leg length occurs, seat depth requires a change to avoid pressure on the popliteal fossa of the shorter leg. Obliquity may occur in the anterior/posterior (protraction/retraction plane, as well as the superior/inferior plane (hip hiked).	May cause a discrepancy in leg length that may be treated by lift under affected leg

Table 13-1. *Range of Motion Assessment (continued)*

	Lide-Lying	Sitting	Standing
Hip			
Flexion on extension	*	Hip flexion of 90 degrees is critical for a neutral sitting position. A lesser range requires posterior pelvic tilting with kyphosis or reclining the chair (greater than a 90-degree angle between seat and back).	Contracture of greater than 20 to 30 degrees compromises alignment and results in lordosis and knee and ankle flexion.
Abduction or adduction (see also pelvic obliquity)	If severe abduction contracture exists, side-lying to the side of the contracture may be impossible or may cause compensatory pelvic obliquity	Can usually be accommodated, although may be a problem when "windswept" (abduction of one lower extremity with adduction of opposite limb); this deformity results in a rotated base of support.	Abduction increses the base of support but if excessive, may encourage valgus feet; Adduction results in a decreased base of support, which may lead to instability.
Knee			
Flexion or extension	*	Limitation in flexion may require elevation and support in extension, but can usually be accommodated.	Flexion contractures compromise upright weight bearing. Kneel-standing may achieve weight bearing if hips are mobile; knees then will not become a limiting factor for good alignment.
Ankles			
Plantar flexion; inversion; eversion	*	A plantar grade foot is desirable but not critical for sitting. Avoid pressure over the bony prominences to reduce the risk of skin breakdown. Avoid pressure over the ball of the foot to reduce primitive extensor thrust.	A weight-bearing surface must be established for upright alignment and to avoid pressure and breakdown of skin.

*Indicates that position is rarely, if ever, a problem to accommodate within the apparatus, although the position may play an important role in "quality" of function.
†From Trefler E. Seating for Children with Cerebral Palsy—A Resource Manual. *University of Tennessee, 1984:62.*

extremity function, or if the child is functioning asymmetrically, a manually controlled wheelchair is an inappropriate choice. A motorized device that does not require the strength needed for a manually controlled chair may be more useful for the child. A motorized chair also has options for control that do not require upper extremity function. A specific, detailed assessment by an experienced technician can help the therapist identify alternative methods by which to attain optimal management of the equipment. In the exam-

ple of a motorized device, strength is only one determinant of success. One must also evaluate cognitive, visuomotor, perceptual, and social functions.

Positioning devices, such as standers, side-lyers, and seats, require little strength or motor control, but often have a modifying effect on muscle tone that must be examined. The child's orientation to gravity will have significant bearing on muscle tone when the child tries to assume an upright position. Therefore, in addition to active muscle control and strength, the therapist must assess patterns of involuntary movement and evaluate the child with regard to:

Spasticity
Athetosis
Flexor predominance
Extensor predominance

Is the movement pattern of mild, moderate, or severe magnitude? Does the patient have cortical control manifested by a voluntary ability to initiate and complete the pattern of motion? A child positioned in a prone stander and tilted slightly forward from a vertical position may show increased extensor tone in an attempt to achieve an upright position against the force of gravity. Increased scapular retraction and hyperextension of the neck may have detrimental side effects in the patient with hypertonus. The child who has a strong extension pattern may show reduced tone when sitting in a chair that is reclined 15 degrees from an upright position. Although the child may not demonstrate optimal upper extremity function when tipped back, this position may suit him or her better for transportation in a car or bus. Appreciation of particular short-term goals for such a child is important for proper selection of positioning. The tilted chair would be unacceptable for use in the classroom, but very useful for improving mobility.

Reflexes

A change of position with respect to gravity will also influence the child whose motor patterns are dominated by reflexes. The prone or supine position may improve the tonic labyrinthine reflex, whereas side-lying may facilitate the asymmetric tonic lumbar reflex. Because inadvertent facilitation of primitive reactions may create a block in the normal developmental pattern, each piece of equipment should be evaluated for its effect on reflexes. For example, some devices for mobility, such as bicycles, may aggravate a persistent asymmetric tonic neck reflex. As the child pushes the pedal with the right foot, the head is turned toward the right side to enhance the effectiveness of the push.

The child reverses this pattern when pushing with the left foot. Only in unusual circumstances would a therapist choose to use a technique that encourages using obligatory reflexes. The use of devices to restrict or inhibit primitive reflexes is more common, thus providing an opportunity for more normal and symmetric patterns of movement.

Sensation

Although it is unusual for a child with cerebral palsy to have a major sensory deficit, children with myelomeningocele offer tremendous challenges to the therapist attempting to develop a program that involves the use of adaptive equipment. Priorities for the child with myelomeningocele include providing safe, pressure-tolerant seating and upright positioning. The therapist must have a thorough knowledge of the patient's sensation in order to achieve these goals. The patient and family should be consulted with regard to sensation, as they usually have a keen awareness of the sensory loss, as well as potential danger zones. This situation is particularly true for the older child. Particular attention must be paid to bony prominences, including the ischial tuberosities, greater trochanters, sacrum, knees, and heels, as well as the skin over the spinal lesion.

Perception, Cognition, and Socioemotional Factors

Most physical therapists are not trained specifically to assess perception, cognition, or socioemotional development; as a result, these areas are often ignored. This is a serious omission for the pediatric patient whose prognosis for function with adaptive equipment often depends more on perception, cognitive function, and socioemotional skill than on physical abilities. Motivation, intelligence, and normal perception often overcome even severe physical handicaps. The opposite is also true. Limitations in perception, cognition, or social-emotional skills may result in function that is lower than would be predicted by physical findings alone. In order to develop realistic goals for a child, the therapist must know the "whole" child and must integrate information from the teacher, social worker, occupational therapist, and psychologist into the therapeutic plan.

Function

Functional skills are both important and difficult to assess because they require integration of all other information in an attempt to determine why a child behaves in a certain manner. The therapist must discover what the child does and how he or she achieves a goal, and why the child does not do more. If the therapist does not evaluate the child in this manner, it is probably impossible to develop appropriate goals for treatment and to select appropriate adaptive equipment. For example, some children tend to "bunny hop" rather than crawl. It is important to know if this tendency to "bunny hop" is secondary to a strong symmetric tonic neck reflex or because of weakness in the extensors of the hip and knee. Although each factor could cause the movement pattern observed, treatment, including the use of adaptive equipment, would be different for the two. A similar thought process should be used when deciding on adaptive equipment. For example, if a 2-year-old child is not rolling or exploring the environment, is a device aimed at improving mobility an appropriate goal? The therapist must first assess whether the child is mentally retarded and, therefore, disinterested in the environment; whether the child is afraid of mobility because of visual impairment; whether the child has a strong asymmetric tonic neck reflex or hypertonus that poses physical limitations; or whether the child has been placed in devices that limit the opportunity to develop independent mobility at home. If this information is not acquired and assimilated, realistic recommendations for equipment cannot be made. Only when working with a child who is severely limited by tone and reflexes would it be appropriate to turn immediately to adaptive devices for remediation. The severely retarded child may not gain from the use of equipment because the child will need to deal with both the device and the environment. In order to allow the visually impaired child to manipulate the environment, we need to improve

methods for exploration of that environment. Equipment may add another obstacle that the visually impaired child must overcome. When the child lacks experience in exploring the environment, the therapist must offer as much freedom of movement and equipment-free mobility as is possible. Although equipment may eventually play a role in each of these situations, adaptive equipment should not be the first type of treatment used. The child who is physically limited may show great improvement in cognitive ability, social interaction, and independence when mobility is improved. When adaptive equipment or devices are used judiciously, this improvement in mobility should occur without increases in abnormal reflexes or patterns of movement.

Evaluation of ROM, muscle tone, motor control, strength, reflexes, perception, cognition, and social-emotional status is an integral component of the assessment of the child. Only when these parameters are considered and we understand why a child is behaving in a particular manner can we treat the child effectively. Included in an overall treatment plan is the use of adaptive equipment that can provide a useful adjunct to treatment.

Once the type of device and the goals for the device are identified, the therapist should evaluate the family and school environments. Goals for the child must be compatible with the goals of the caregivers at home and at school. Because adaptive equipment is often used in several settings, there may be many conflicts and problems to solve while trying to achieve the short- and long-term goals for the child. Problems may arise for the child who is institutionalized or in a school placement. For example, the ability to teach the correct use of equipment to members of a changing or rotating staff is a major consideration. Ease of maintenance and minimizing the number of easily lost parts are additional considerations in institutional care.

Assessment of the Home and Family

Useful information can be obtained by asking the family about its expectations for the apparatus being considered. This opportunity for members of the family to express their opinions promotes a dialogue between family and therapist whereby the therapist can determine whether the family goals are realistic or whether compromises are necessary. Objective data about the family should encompass the following categories and questions:

1. *Physical layout of the dwelling.* The therapist should seek to answer the following questions:
   - Is the dwelling a house or apartment?
   - How many steps are found in the home?
   - Is there easy access to the home (i.e., no stairs, availability of an elevator, etc.)?
   - How large are the rooms?
   - Can equipment for mobility be used in the home?
   - Is there space for equipment use and storage?
   - How wide are the doorways?
   - Are the floors carpeted?
   - Are bathrooms, tubs, and toilets accessible?
2. *Community.* The therapist should determine whether the family lives in an urban, suburban, or rural community in order to assess the availability of and options for transportation and socialization. Families in the suburbs may use privately owned automobiles, whereas city dwelling families may rely on public transportation. This information is important when the therapist is considering mobility equipment. Also important are such issues as the weight of the device, its versatility on various surfaces, and its ease of transport, all of which must be tailored to the child's living conditions.
3. *Socioeconomic factors.* The cost of equipment may have a serious impact on the final decision made regarding apparatus for the handicapped child. When making a decision about buying adaptive equipment, the therapist, in conjunction with the social worker, must examine insurance coverage, other third-party payment systems, funding agencies within the community, and potential rental options. Size of the family, daily routine, and the time available for the handicapped child, as well as potential options for additional help, must be considered. Compliance with the suggested use of adaptive equipment may ultimately be the main issue to be considered in the decision to obtain the equipment. If there is little realistic expectation, based on many

of the aforementioned issues, that the child will benefit from having the equipment, there may be little justification for its purchase.

School Assessment

When assessing a child's need for equipment, the physical therapist must consider the school setting in which the child may spend a large portion of the day. It is important to determine whether the child is enrolled in a special school or mainstreamed into a regular classroom. In a special school, teachers and staff are usually very open to suggestions and are well-equipped to handle any devices being considered. It is often these teachers who initiate the purchase or procurement of the equipment, and they are eager to learn and work with the child.

When the child is mainstreamed—attending a regular school—teachers and other staff may be reluctant to accept adaptive equipment because of their limited experience with special apparatus. This reluctance of the staff may be related not only to the health and developmental needs of the child, but also to concerns about the time, space, liability for, and acceptability of these devices in a classroom of children without handicapping conditions. A thoughtful compromise is often necessary in order to meet the physical, educational, emotional, and social goals of the handicapped child.

Summary

Clearly, there are many aspects to consider in determining a child's need for adaptive equipment. The case study presented in Display 13-1 should clarify both the dynamics of the problems involved in selection of equipment and the thought processes and compromises involved in developing rational solutions to these problems.

Equipment Selection

When the evaluation of the child is completed and goals are established, the types of equipment available, or, alternatively, the practicality of making equipment, are determined.

Display 13-1.
Case Study

Ellen is a 5-year-old girl with a spastic diplegia pattern of motor function secondary to cerebral palsy. She was integrated into a normal elementary school. Ellen is intelligent and alert, and she enjoys all aspects of her school routine. Ellen's classroom teacher has two main concerns about Ellen. First, although Ellen is ambulatory, her gait is slow and labored, making it difficult for her to walk to classes in distant locations in the school building. Class trips have also been a problem for Ellen. The teacher's second major concern is Ellen's socialization during recess. Because mobility is a large part of the recess activity, Ellen's limited mobility makes socialization difficult. Ellen's mother was notified of the teacher's concerns and she sought help from Ellen's physical therapist. Ellen receives treatment twice a week from her therapist, who is aware of Ellen's strengths and limitations. Ellen's mother presented to the physical therapist the concerns of the teacher and her own personal concerns. These additional concerns included the fact that Ellen recently had a growth spurt and has become increasingly difficult to lift and carry. This new difficulty occurs mainly when the family goes on outings. It has also become difficult for Ellen to keep up with her active older brother and with her 3-year-old sister. Although mobility in the family's split level home in the suburbs has not been a problem, Ellen rarely plays outside because the children who live closest to her and who are the same age live several blocks away. Therefore, the family car is needed to transport Ellen almost everywhere she needs to go.

Ellen's therapist must satisfy the needs of the child, the family, and the school. Although the school's needs suggest that independent mobility is important and could be achieved with a properly fitted wheelchair, the family does not presently need this equipment. Because Ellen is ambulatory within the home and has help when she goes out with her family, a large, lightweight, easily folding umbrella stroller should be adequate. The difference in price between the two items is several hundred dollars, but each device has advantages and disadvantages. Ellen's therapist chose a systematic approach to the problem. She re-evaluated Ellen and added to her own list of goals those concerns expressed by the school and family. The list was as follows:

Problem

1. ROM—presently within normal limits. Tightness in hip and knee flexors is increasing as Ellen grows taller.

Solutions

a. Daily ROM exercises
b. Night splints to maintain ROM
c. Frequent positional changes; avoidance of long periods of sitting

Problems

2. Tone, control, and strength—inadequate antigravity back extensor and abdominal control for normal gait, causing trunk reversal. Poor endurance; moderate spastic extensor pattern in lower extremities; poor control when movement is isolated out of pattern; asymmetry of involvement, with right side more spastic and shortened.

Solutions

a. Weekly outpatient treatments
b. Training in upright and other positions to use more normal movement pattern
c. Positioning to avoid asymmetry
d. Avoidance of positions or activities that increase fixing and extensor pattern
e. Family education and home program

(continued)

Display 13-1.
Case Study (continued)

Problems

3. Social and emotional development—copes well with handicap; unable to participate in many group activities at home and school, especially those requiring mobility; encouragement and facilitation of progress in social and emotional development will be both the problem and the goal.

Solutions

a. Provide alternative means of mobility
b. Educate and support patient in developing strategies for coping with and compensating for handicap

Problems

4. Functional ability—able to ambulate functionally and independently but with poor endurance; poor reciprocal movement of the lower extremities secondary to abnormal extensor tone; poor weight shifting as a result of weak antigravity trunk muscles; independently makes transition from prone→supine→sitting→standing.

Solutions

a. Treatment to reduce extensor tone and maintain adequate ROM
b. Improve strength and control of trunk musculature
c. Gait training
d. Home training in proper movement pattern for gait
e. Avoidance of activities that will increase asymmetry and tone of extensor muscle groups

After the reevaluation and generation of this list of problems, Ellen's therapist was more confident about the decision to purchase the umbrella-type stroller with adequate support to achieve proper positioning and alignment.

1. With ROM a potential problem for Ellen, increased sitting time had to be discouraged and positional changes encouraged. Because the stroller does not offer independent mobility, Ellen would not enjoy sitting in the stroller for a long time.
2. Although a wheelchair provides more options for positioning in symmetric alignment using lateral pads, these attachments provide passive positioning and do not encourage active work on righting and equilibrium. Because Ellen was able to right herself with facilitation by verbal feedback or light tapping, Ellen's therapist believed that lateral supports were excessive and not indicated. The stroller must provide a firm seat and back support in order to allow Ellen to align herself properly.
3. When Ellen was tested for upper extremity function using a loaner wheelchair, the results suggested that a wheelchair would not be useful. The result of attempts at propulsion with the upper extremities was an overflow of tone into the lower extremities. This overflow increased extensor tone in the lower extremities and caused increased asymmetry in Ellen's trunk. This response was considered to be counterproductive to gait, and the possibility of propulsion in a wheelchair was ruled out for the present time.
4. Because Ellen has not complained of feeling left out or rejected in classroom activities and because she appears to be well adjusted to school without a wheelchair, independent mobility does not seem to be an important issue to her. Although the teacher has a valid concern about Ellen's mobility, the issue does not interfere with Ellen's social or emotional well-being. Periodic reevaluation, however, is necessary.
5. Because Ellen's family transports her in the

Display 13-1.
Case Study (continued)

family car where she is stable and comfortable wearing a standard seatbelt, a wheelchair is probably too heavy and cumbersome for their needs. The umbrella-type stroller is more practical for transporting Ellen. The stroller tends, however, to infantilize Ellen, who deserves to be treated as an increasingly mature and responsible person. Should Ellen's parents show signs of having difficulty accepting her disability or should they treat her as an infant or overprotect her unnecessarily, reconsideration of the stroller compared with the wheelchair might be appropriate. Ellen's family realizes that, although she is ambulatory and intelligent, she will continue to be restricted by her physical limitations and will require special consideration. They also realize that her emotional health and development

require that the family relate to Ellen as often as possible, and in the same manner as the other children. The umbrella-type stroller meets both Ellen's needs and the needs of the family without jeopardizing her normal social and emotional development.

6. Ellen's physical therapist had a final insight after reevaluating the child's equipment needs. The therapist realized that a possible third option—a three-wheeled motorized scooter (Fig. 13-1) might be most appropriate for Ellen's future mobility. The three-wheeled scooter is often used as an outdoor mobility device for ambulators with limited endurance or difficulty negotiating rough surfaces and terrain. This device is lighter in weight than standard motorized devices and is much more manageable

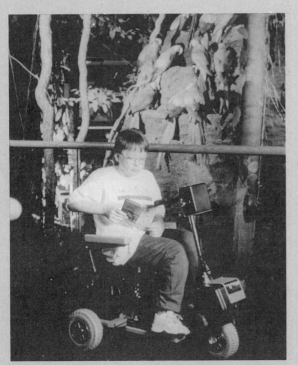

Figure 13-1. *The three-wheeled scooter.*

(continued)

Display 13-1.
Case Study (continued)

(i.e., it can be placed in a car). The physical effort required to use the scooter is less than the effort required to propel a manual wheelchair, and so the undesirable asymmetry and increased tone observed when Ellen propelled a standard wheelchair could be avoided. By introducing this device to Ellen and her family, the therapist could help clarify whether the scooter would be acceptable to all concerned. If the scooter was deemed acceptable, the umbrella-type stroller would still be a valuable addition for short excursions or as a back-up device should the scooter malfunction (as from a dead battery).

Ellen's therapist telephoned the classroom teacher to discuss the reasons for using an umbrella stroller both at school and at home. After an appropriate explanation, the teacher agreed with this solution on a temporary basis. The teacher reserved the right to present the issue again, if necessary. Constant reevaluation of all aspects of Ellen's physical, cognitive, psychological, and social development was agreed upon. Any significant changes would require a reassessment of the decision.

Purchasing Equipment

Selection of equipment is difficult because many companies make devices and equipment that are identical. Many criteria must be considered.

1. *Dimension of the apparatus.* The device should not only be adequate when purchased, but should also, if feasible, allow for some future growth. Some equipment has a built-in system for extending or enlarging the device. The therapist must determine which company makes the particular size best suited for each child.
2. *Availability of optional adaptations.* Are there parts that help improve the fit and specificity of the device? Are these options cost-effective, easily adjusted, and durable?
3. *Reputation of the manufacturer.* Is the product covered by a guarantee? Has the company previously provided support when problems with equipment have arisen? Is service readily available and is equipment for trial use available? Will a company representative train or instruct the staff in optimal use of the device?
4. *Promptness of delivery.* Is the product kept in stock by most local vendors or medical supply houses? Is there a backlog of orders that will delay the equipment's delivery? Is the product custom-made?
5. *Cost.* Is the price reasonable for the anticipated use of the product, or will less expensive alternatives provide the same benefits?
6. *Aesthetics.* Is the device cosmetically acceptable to the patient and family, or will it be rejected on this basis?
7. *Weight, size, and manageability.* Is the device easy to use and can it be stored? Can it be transported if necessary? (That is, does it fold or disassemble in some way?)

Brochures or catalogs available from the manufacturer or vendor will provide much of this information. Local vendors who may have extensive experience with the equipment can help in answering many of the questions. Physical therapists in local hospitals or in the community can recommend vendors or specific salespeople. The therapist should not feel obligated to order from any person in particular. Although one salesperson might be knowledgeable about wheelchairs, another person may have more experience with positioning devices or self-help equipment.

Anyone procuring or fabricating equipment on a regular basis should keep records on the various devices, manufacturers, and vendors they use. Records should indicate ease of fit, wear of the device (how well it holds up over time), acceptance or criticism from patients and family, and the efficiency of customer service, including the elapsed time from placement of an order to delivery of equipment. Records may be kept on computer or in card catalog form (or some similar system), and may be a useful resource for future recommendations and orders. In addition, the catalog file may provide the basis for quantitative data regarding benefits and deficits of various adaptive devices. Perhaps the compilation of these data can serve to help the profession evolve from an art to science.

Making Equipment

The decision to make equipment is based on many variables that must be considered carefully.

Personnel

Will physical therapists be building the equipment themselves, or will they be serving as consultants to other builders? If the therapists build the apparatus, how will their schedules allow for this time expenditure? Will patients be cancelled or will special time be allotted? Will overtime hours be needed? If the physical therapist is a consultant, how will this time be allocated and at what expense? If other people are building the equipment, will they be compensated, and if so, by whom? Will parents pay directly or will insurance companies pay the cost? Will the facility offering the services assume the cost? Will permission be given to build the equipment only after approval by third-party payers of the needed funding, or will the facility assume the cost in the hope that funds will be forthcoming? Who will bear the cost if funds are unavailable?

Space

Is adequate space available for building the apparatus on the premises? If space is available, will the safety and comfort of patients be compromised by this building site? Building is noisy, dirty, and potentially dangerous because of the tools and materials used. Ventilation must be provided if fumes from toxic paint or varnish are expected. This item may be a major problem when working with children with lung disease.

Cost

A decision must be made initially about the cost-effectiveness of making equipment. Items that must be accounted for include tools, space needs, building materials, time for planning and designing, time for measuring and building, and time away from patient care. In making a decision, the advantages of customized equipment must be weighed against the expense of designing, planning, and building the apparatus. Will adapting a commercially available device be the best compromise?

Failures

Can and will the facility absorb the loss in revenue that accrues from equipment that is inadvertently incorrectly fitted or that appears to be inappropriate when completed? This issue of equipment failure must be considered, because even the most experienced equipment technician will make mistakes.

Timing and Setting

An advantage of custom-made devices is evident when equipment is needed immediately. Therapist-fabricated equipment is usually available in days or weeks rather than the months often required for bureaucracies to approve, fund, order, and receive the equipment. Building the equipment might also be an attractive alternative when the device is required only for one specific setting, such as the classroom, but not for transport or home use.

Summary

Despite the potential drawbacks, many therapists still choose customized equipment. Customization may be particularly useful for the young child who is growing rapidly and for the child whose need is only temporary. In each of these situations, a sim-

Table 13–2. *Adaptive Equipment Comparison Chart: Adjustable Side-Lyer (Goal: Provide a durable adjustable side-lyer that is economical and may be obtained quickly)*

Base Material	Support Material	Cost	Fabrication Time	Skill Required	Tools	Durability	Level of Adjustability	Ease of Remodification	Ease of Cleaning	Weight	Special Considerations
Commercially Made											
Wood, custom-made	n.a.	$280–$600	Weeks	n.a.	n.a.	Average	Varies per item	Difficult and costly	Average	Heavy	Repairs or remodifications are usually costly and sometimes unavailable; vinyl padding may tear or may become detached from the wood base.
Prefabricated foam	n.a.	$190–$360	Varies depending on stock	n.a.	n.a.	Fair	Minimal	Impossible	Good	Medium	Only available in one basic size; may not be adjusted to fit a person's size; adjustability or accessories may be limited
Commercial; Adaptafoam	Adaptavinyl	$50–$80 for material, plus fabricator's hourly fee (usually $60–$80/hr).	1 hr	n.a.	n.a.	Excellent	Varies per side-lyer	Excellent	Excellent	Light	One piece of bonding and coating provide excellent serviceability; material's flexibility allows for dynamic positioning; no special personnel are required for adjustment or remodifications.
Self-made											
Adaptafoam	Adaptavinyl covering	$50–$80	1 hr	Minimal	Heat gun; electric knife	Excellent	Excellent	Excellent	Excellent	Light	

Material	Materials needed	Cost	Time		Tools					Weight	Comments
Wooden side-lyer	Hardware; dowels; glue; foam; vinyl; staples	$50–100	3–6 hrs	High	Saws; sanders; drills; hammer; stapler	Excellent	Average	Difficult	Average	Heavy	Repairs and modifications are time-consuming and usually require trained personnel
Cardboard (triwall); temporary	Hardware; glue; dowels; covering	$20–$30	1½–2½ hrs	Average	Saw; drill	Very poor	Average	Average	Very poor; temporary	Light	Only useful as a temporary measure; easily breaks down in time; the interior open walls trap food, bacteria, and insects unless they are completely covered.

(Adapted with permission from Modular Medical Corp., Bronx, NY 10461; prices reflect 100% mark-up from 1980 prices.)
n.a., not available.

ply made piece of equipment could satisfy the short-term needs of the patient. The child could use the fabricated equipment until he or she outgrows it, at which time another piece could be made, or, if growth has slowed, a commercially available piece could be substituted. One of the main reasons for building equipment is that commercially available equipment often does not satisfy the needs of a child with unique problems. Recently, however, manufacturers have shown an increased interest in handicapped children, which has resulted in a wider variety of and improvements in apparatuses.

Selection of Materials

Adaptive equipment can be built using various materials, each of which has unique qualities, advantages, and disadvantages. Personal preference often plays a major role in the decision to use a particular type of material. Although each material has its specific properties, most can be adapted to various uses. Some materials are lighter in weight, some are easier to use, some are easier to wash and keep clean, and some are more durable. Because none of the products is perfect, the therapist should have knowledge of several different materials. The therapist can try to match the material's advantages to the specific needs of the child. A comparison of wood, triwall, and Adaptafoam is made in Table 13-2. These materials are used commonly by pediatric therapists.

Wood

Wood is inexpensive, durable, and available, but requires a moderate measure of skill. Large work areas are required because wood has a "messy" quality and requires many different hand and power tools, some of which are expensive. Many therapists prefer to have professional carpenters construct adaptive devices from wood because of the level of skill required. Parents, however, are often familiar with woodworking, and a therapist may enlist the help of such a parent, providing plans and specifications for the equipment needed. Fabrication by family members can be a rewarding and sat-

isfying means of helping in the care of the handicapped child. Wooden equipment is often heavy, but it is also durable. Strength and durability are important qualities when material is to be used by a larger child. Wooden devices often need padding for comfort, and either painting, varnishing, or sealing for protection against liquids. Wood is often used for making inserts for seats, side-lyers, prone standers, and various ingenious mobility toys.

Triwall

Triwall consists of triple-thickness corrugated cardboard that is lightweight, firm, and inexpensive. Triwall is fast and easy to use, although its use requires an electric sabre saw (or other alternative saw), glue gun, and hand tools, such as a hammer, screwdriver, and utility knife. Although not waterproof, triwall can be treated with acrylic latex paint or fabric for sealing and preservation. Triwall is less durable than wood, which makes it most appropriate for temporary or trial pieces of equipment, or for children who are growing rapidly (Fig. 13-2). Like wood, triwall is a firm, solid medium and may require padding for comfort. Many therapists consider triwall useful for making customized chairs that must be measured precisely for the child. A "bolster-type" chair available commercially and a similar chair made from triwall are shown in Figures 13-3 and 13-4. Although selection of a design and measuring the child and the triwall are time-consuming chores, actual building with triwall is a fast process. Working with this material is noisy, messy, and potentially dangerous because of the tools. A separate workplace is recommended. As with wood, family members and volunteers can be recruited to make apparatuses from triwall. Special training is usually necessary, and many parents are reluctant to try because of fear of mistakes and failure. Some judicious support and praise for the family member can help overcome reluctance, and the parent may become an essential part of the team that is making the adaptive equipment for the child. A seating insert made from triwall is shown in Figure 13-5.

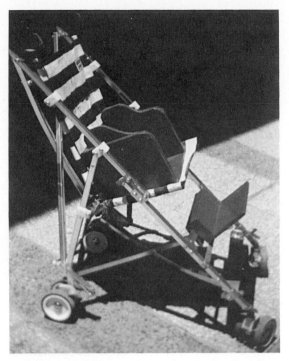

Figure 13-2. *Umbrella-type stroller with a triwall insert and foot support.*

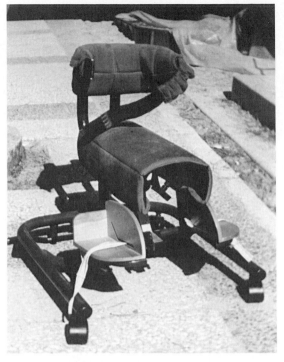

Figure 13-3. *Commercially made "bolster" chair.*

Adaptafoam

Adaptafoam is another commonly used medium for pediatric equipment because it is a dense, nonporous, nontoxic foam that is both fast and easy to use, but is more expensive than wood or triwall. The need for tools is minimal (e.g., heat gun, electric knife, and utility knife). Although a work area is useful, Adaptafoam is less messy than wood or triwall and poses less risk because of the limited use of tools. A special coating—Adaptavinyl—is the only paint that can be used, and its safe application requires excellent ventilation. However, because Adaptafoam is nonporous, it can be left unpainted and cleaned with soap and water when it becomes soiled. Covers can be made for the apparatus if the family prefers. Adaptafoam is available in several dimensions and different densities. With some experience, a physical therapist can determine the best use of the various types of Adaptafoam. Adaptafoam is easy to construct with because it bonds to itself when heated for a short time. Glue and nails are unnecessary. However, this self-bonding property loses some attractiveness when Adaptafoam is used with other material, such as wood, which Adaptafoam will not bond. Adaptafoam is commonly used to make prone-lyers, seats, inserts, small standers, and various components, including headrests and utensil handles for other apparatuses. Because many therapists work well with Adaptafoam, they must adjust their schedule if they choose to make equipment. Adaptafoam, unlike triwall, is easy to adjust for growth by inserting an additional piece of material when necessary. Like wood and triwall, Adaptafoam provides a firm surface and may need to be padded or covered to improve comfort.

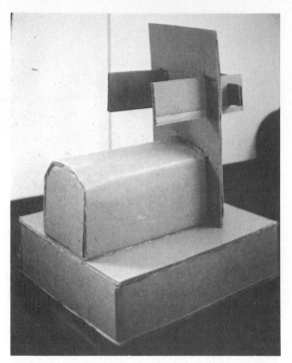

Figure 13-4. *Triwall alternative to the commercially made bolster chair shown in Figure 13–3.*

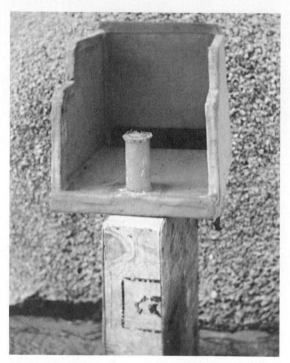

Figure 13-5. *Sideview of a triwall seat insert.*

Commonly Used Equipment for Various Positions

We have already discussed general uses for equipment as adjuncts to treatment. We have noted that physiological benefits will accrue when properly conceived and frequent changes of position are used. Among those benefits are inhibition of pathologic tone, reduction of abnormal reflexes, and prevention of soft tissue contractures. Let us now look more specifically at some of the issues involved in providing children with equipment to support various positions and activities—sitting, side-lying and standing.

Sitting

General Considerations

The sitting position is optimal for function and, therefore, is important for the older child and adult.

Although maintained sitting posture is a goal achieved by most normal infants before 1 year of age, sitting is used for prolonged function much later in life. By watching children in preschool and kindergarten, it is apparent that a goal of many teachers is maintenance of sitting for group activities. Children in the early school years who are younger than 7 years of age require frequent changes in position. They prefer to play and work in the prone position, standing by a table, and in other positions that easily allow for transitional movements and change. Sitting, as a position for optimal function, occurs only after the children "learn" to sit for prolonged periods of time. Sitting is defined as ". . . a position in which the weight of the trunk is transferred to the support area mainly by the ischial tuberosities and surrounding tissues."[1] Proper alignment in sitting is thought to improve patient function by providing an adequate and secure base, inhibiting abnormal tone, and improving perception of the environment. There are also significant social benefits to being upright and mobile.

Although there is a large body of literature devoted to seating for the pediatric age group, most of the material reports clinical experience and empirical data rather than controlled scientific data. The result of this lack of scientific documentation is poor standardization when evaluating and providing adaptive seating devices. Conflicts regarding the value of various positioning options could be more easily and completely resolved if a scientific basis existed for each option. Because the literature on pediatric seating is limited, we can, as an alternative, examine the adult literature and attempt to apply it to the pediatric age group. The factors that follow should be considered when evaluating a chair.

The first concern is the purpose of the chair. We know that chairs can be "function-specific." A lounge chair is uncomfortable when a person is eating a meal, yet a straight-backed chair with little padding is undesirable for relaxation. Similarly, a physical therapist must consider function when designing chairs for handicapped children. Many therapists believe that a custom-built chair is always preferable, but whether one is buying or making a chair, the following parameters, established for adults, should be considered.

Seat

HEIGHT. The height of the chair seat should allow the feet to be placed flat on the floor. Comfortable placement of the feet should prevent excessive pressure on the popliteal fossa caused by the front edge of the seat.[1,2]

DEPTH. The seat should be shallow enough to provide for flexion of the knee without pressure in the popliteal area without slouching. Slouching negates contact of the lumbar region with the backrest, thus nullifying any gain offered by backrest options. The seat should be deep enough to allow maximal distribution of weight.[2]

PADDING. Padding helps to distribute pressure away from the 6-mm^2 surface of each ischial tuberosity that normally bears weight in sitting. This allows for increased sitting tolerance.[3,4] However, surfaces that are too soft increase the difficulty with which postural changes are made during sitting, and this lack of postural change can lead to back strain. Akerblom judged movement while sitting to be the most important requirement of a comfortable chair.[3] He designed a chair that allowed for various conditions (i.e., the trunk off of the support surface, sitting with lumbar support, or reclining back with both lumbar and thoracic support). These options reduce muscle strain and increase tolerance.[3]

Back

Consideration must be given to trunk musculature and spinal ligaments in order to avoid back discomfort. The anterior and posterior longitudinal ligaments provide their best support with the back in neutral position. Increasing the normal lordosis may stretch the anterior longitudinal ligament, whereas exaggerated kyphosis will stretch the posterior longitudinal ligament and may cause posterior protrusion of degenerating intervertebral discs. These changes produce low back pain and cause difficulty in achieving the back extension needed to rise from sitting. In addition to the need for movement in the chair to prevent muscular fatigue, support for the weight of the trunk will reduce the muscular work of sitting. This support can be provided by a reclining backrest. Support for the lumbar curve and allowance for the posteriorly protruding sacrum and buttocks are also recommended. The height of the backrest need not extend above the shoulder. Freedom to change position and improved mobility are provided by limiting the height to this level.[5]

Armrests

Armrests should be positioned to bear approximately 50% of the weight of the patient's arms. Armrests are also used by a person to change from a sitting to a standing position.

Angle of the Back of the Seat

The angle formed between the seat and backrest is most comfortable between 95 and 110 degrees. This angle may cause the person to slide forward, particularly a problem with increased extensor tone in the hips and back musculature. The entire chair can be tilted back so that gravity pushes the patient back into the chair to avoid the problem of sliding. Attention to avoidance of pressure in the popliteal area is important when the chair is reclined.[1] Lumbar supports are also recommended for the reclined chair.

The same parameters addressed in an adult population are addressed in the pediatric population. However, working with children results in a greater number of variables to be assessed and fewer tools and guidelines to help in that assessment. Not only must the orthopedic and biomechanical needs of the child be considered, but the effects of those needs on muscle tone, reflexes, and function must also be considered. There is a lack of available information throughout the scientific literature regarding the effects on children of changing seating parameters. Most therapists use an empirical or trial-and-error approach to determine good positioning for a particular child. Because most therapists agree that the pelvis is important for correct stabilization, the pelvis serves as the keystone for seating. Once the pelvis is aligned properly, the trunk, head, and lower extremities will have a more stable base. The specific approaches, options, and adaptations are too numerous to review here. However, the objectives of providing seated weight bearing on the ischial tuberosities, as occurs with adults, and maintaining a slight lumbar lordosis, are reasonable expectations for the child. Ninety-degree angles at the hip and knee during seating have been advocated by many therapists as a correct method of positioning the child with cerebral palsy. This position seems to have developed as a reaction to the accentuated posterior pelvic tilt that commonly occurs when the child with spasticity is seated in a standard upholstered wheelchair. When the child is allowed to stay in the position that encourages posterior pelvic tilt, there is a likelihood of increased dorsal kyphosis, with protracted scapulae, and hyperextension of the neck. The 90-degree angle at the hips and knees will provide solid weight bearing and correct sensory input to aid stabilization. Bergan suggests that normal wheelchair seats provide sensory feedback and a spatial orientation that the child is "backward."[6] One of the problems associated with this unusual sensory feedback and orientation is an increase in extensor tone thought to accompany the "sling" effect of most wheelchair seats. A firm seat and back should reduce the unwanted feedback and orientation.

Despite the fact that many advocate using the 90-degree angle at hip and knee, I have found the position unsuccessful and can personally tolerate the position for only brief periods. The discomfort that occurs tends to stimulate an effort to escape the position by increasing the angle at the hip by posteriorly tilting the pelvis and sliding out of the chair, or by flexing the trunk forward and increasing the dorsal kyphosis. Although the 90-degree angle is suggested for children, studies in the adult population suggest that an angle of 95 to 110 degrees at the hip may be more advantageous for seating. In addition to altering the hip angle, the chair may be tilted, anteriorly or posteriorly, until the desired results of positioning are achieved. The issues of concern when making these adjustments continue to be pelvic alignment for stability while in a sitting position and the effects on tone of the various angles of the hip and of the seat itself. Nwaobi and colleagues, using electromyograms, found that orientation of the body and head in relation to gravity plays a significant role in controlling extensor activity.[7] Perception and hand function will also be altered as differing angles and positions are used. Therefore, an individualized approach, examining the effects of each change in position, will be necessary in determining optimal seating arrangements for children.

Once it appears that the various angles of hips, seat, and chair have been established and pelvic stability with minimal abnormal tone and reflexes has been achieved, the therapist must consider the trunk, head and neck, and the lower extremities of the child. Ninety degrees of knee flexion and good weight bearing on the foot should be encouraged to enhance stability. Too much weight bearing on the plantar surface can result in a primitive extensor thrust pattern that will significantly reduce stability. Alignment of the trunk should encourage maximal symmetry, yet provide for movement and active postural adjustment. A headrest or supports should be used if needed to improve positioning or to protect the child during mobility. The ultimate goal of the sitting position should be to align the child without restricting the movements and postural adjustments available to the child. Reassessment of the seating device is necessary when the patient's postural tone improves and skills are acquired.

Consideration of the Specific Disability

The criteria and limits described for seating are applicable to all types of seating systems and for all disabilities. The emphasis changes with the disability, but the concepts are constant. Appropriate seating for the child with cerebral palsy, for instance, must take into consideration the effects on tone and abnormal reflexes. Padding and pressure relief warrant increased attention in the child with myelodysplasia. Height of arm rests and enhancement of function are of great concern for the child with myopathy. The limitation of the seating devices and concerns regarding their use will be reasonably constant across disability groups. These limitations and precautions include limitation of joint motion secondary to static positioning; poor skin tolerance as a result of prolonged use of the seating device and a limited ability to change position; and reduced independent functional mobility resulting from abuse of seating devices.

Wheelchairs

Providing a wheelchair for a patient requires an understanding and application of all the criteria previously discussed about proper alignment and positioning. It is also beneficial to know about the options available in purchasing a wheelchair and the compromises involved when selecting certain options over others.

Before continuing, it is worth stating that the wheelchair industry is in constant flux. This is why a well-informed and capable vendor or manufacturer's representative is critical to the rehabilitation team. The representative can provide information about changes and innovations in durable medical equipment (DME), as well as about the comparative adaptability, durability, cost, and features of wheelchairs and other equipment supplied by competing manufacturers.

It may be easiest to discuss options by looking at a typical order form for a pediatric chair (see Display 13-2). These forms are traditionally completed by the vendor, patient, and physical therapist working together to meet the patient's needs.

The first consideration is chair design. For independent mobilizers, two basic options exist—a *rigid frame or folding* x-*frame wheelchair*. Most people are familiar with a cross-braced folding wheelchair and opt for this type as it is easiest to transport in cars and store in home closets. The rigid-frame chair does not fold, but the wheels are removable and the back drops down, leaving a small box type structure. The rigid-frame chair offers increased stability and ease of rolling, and it is always the chair of choice in sports and recreation. In many instances, once the child adjusts to it, families find the rigid chair to be as manageable as the folding chair. The disadvantage of the rigid-frame wheelchair is its limited growth adjustability resulting in it often being overlooked for the pediatric population. If properly fitted, however, in many instances it can provide years of use.[*] In patients who are not independently mobile owing to cognitive function, upper extremity involvement, asymmetry, or other problems, a standard wheelchair may not be the best option. The vendor should be consulted

---

[*]*Modified rigid wheelchairs have now been devised that combine rigidity but allow for some growth. Because they are still new to the market and uncommon, they are not be addressed in depth in this chapter. Additional information can obtained from an informed vendor.*

Display 13-2.

A sample order form for a pediatric wheelchair.

Effective July 5, 1993   **ORDER FORM**

Date: _____ P.O.#: _____
Buyer: _____ Customer#: _____

Bill To:
Name _____
Mailing Address _____
City _____ State _____ Zip _____
Phone (_____) _____

☐ **Drop Ship/Ship To:**
Name _____
Street Address _____
City _____ State _____ Zip _____
Phone (_____) _____ Marked For _____

QUICKIE 2   ☐ *Adult*   ☐ *Kids*

COLOR	☐ *Blue*	☐ *Black*	☐ *Red*	☐ *Midnight Purple*	☐ *Silver*
	☐ *Sky White*	☐ *Teal*	☐ *Hot Pink*	☐ *Ultra Yellow*	☐ *Lavender*
	☐ Blue Sapphire	☐ Blk Diamond	☐ Candy Red		

FRAME DIMENSIONS

| Frame Width | ☐ *11"*[*] | ☐ *12"* | ☐ *13"* | ☐ *14"* | ☐ *15"* | (Seat Width 1/2" Narrower) |
| | ☐ *16"* | ☐ *17"* | ☐ *18"* | ☐ *19"* | ☐ *20"* | (*11" Wide by Upholstery) |

| Sling Depth | ☐ 10" | ☐ 11" | ☐ 12" | ☐ 13" | |
| | ☐ 14" | ☐ 15" | ☐ 16" | ☐ 17"[1] | ☐ 18"[1] |

| Cushion | ☐ 2" | ☐ 3" | ☐ 4" | |
| | ☐ Solid Seat[3] | ☐ Omit Cushion | ☐ Omit Seat Sling | |

BACKREST   (Push Handles Std.)   ☐ *Low* (8 1/2"-12")[17]   ☐ *Med* (12"-15 1/2")[17]   ☐ *Tall* (15 1/2"-19")[17]

Backrest Options
☐ 8" Bend (Med & Tall)[17]   ☐ Omit Push Handles[17]   ☐ Depth Adjustable[18, 11]
☐ Omit Depth Adj Solid Back & Hardware   ☐ Omit Depth Adj Solid Back Include Hardware
☐ Swing-Away Adj Stroller Handles (Avail w/ Depth Adj Back Only)   ☐ Solid Back[3, 17]
☐ Backrest Cushion[17]   ☐ Adj Upholstery (Avail w/14"-20" Frame Widths and Med or Tall Back Heights)[17]
☐ Omit Back Upholstery[17]   ☐ Omit Back Post & Upholstery[17]

FRAME SPECIFICATIONS

| Frame Length | ☐ Kids | ☐ *Reg* | ☐ Long | ☐ Hemi[5] | ☐ Long Hemi (17"-18" Deep)[5] |

Hanger Type   ☐ 60°   ☐ 70°   ☐ 90°   ☐ 70° V[19]   ☐ Hemi (60°)   ☐ Omit Hangers
☐ Articulating-Adult (15"-20" Widths)[2]
☐ Articulating-Kids (11"-16" Widths; Std w/2" Footrest Ext Tubes and Adj Flip-Up Footplates)[2]
☐ Impact Guards - Plastic   ☐ Impact Guards - Neoprene

Footplates   ☐ *Composite*[9]   ☐ Plastic Cover   ☐ Reverse   ☐ High Mount[6]
☐ Foam[4]   ☐ Angle Adj[9]   ☐ Angle Adj High Mount[9]   ☐ Omit Footplate
☐ 90° Adj Flip-Up[4, 8]   ☐ 90°/90° Footboard[4, 7]   ☐ Extended[9]
☐ Heel Loops   ☐ Omit Leg Strap

Footrest Ext Tubes[20]   ☐ *Short* (14"-16 1/2"; N/A w/Articulating Legrest)   ☐ *Med* (16 1/2"-19")   ☐ *Long* (19"- 21 1/2")
☐ Omit Ext Tubes

CASTERS   ☐ *8" Pneumatic*   ☐ 8" Polyurethane   ☐ 5" Low-Profile Polyurethane
☐ 6" Pneumatic   ☐ 6" Polyurethane   ☐ Aluminum Caster Rim

Caster Options   ☐ 3/4" Longer Fork Stem Bolt   ☐ 1 1/2" Longer Fork Stem Bolt
☐ Caster Pin Locks   ☐ Omit Caster Wheels   ☐ Quick-Release Caster Stems[21]

ARMRESTS   ☐ *Padded Swing-Away*[17]   ☐ Omit Armrests
☐ Adult - Height Adjustable w/Std Pad (10")   ☐ Adult - Height Adjustable w/Full-Length Pad (14")
☐ Kids - Height Adjustable w/Std Pad (10")   ☐ Kids - Height Adjustable w/Full-Length Pad (14")

Stroller Handles   ☐ Stroller Handles (Reg)[10, 17]   ☐ Stroller Handles (Tall)[10, 17]

AXLE PLATE   ☐ *Std*   ☐ Amputee[11]   ☐ Quad Release Axle Nuts
☐ One-Arm Drive (Attach One-Arm Drive Supplemental Order Form)

REAR WHEELS

| Rim | ☐ Mag[12] | ☐ *Spoke* | ☐ Omit Rear Wheels/Axles |
| Size | ☐ 20" | ☐ 22" | ☐ *24"* | ☐ 26" (3/4" Stem Bolt Std w/26" Wheels) |

Tire   ☐ *Pneumatic*   ☐ Full-Profile Polyurethane[12]   ☐ Airless Insert[12]
☐ Low-Profile Polyurethane[13]   ☐ Kevlar[13]   ☐ High-Pressure Clincher (24", 26" Only)[16]

Handrim   ☐ *Aluminum*   ☐ Plastic Coated   ☐ Long Tabs   ☐ Omit Handrims

Projections   ☐ Vertical[14]   20"/22"   24"/26"
☐ Oblique   ☐ 6   ☐ 8   ☐ 10   ☐ 12

WHEEL LOCKS   ☐ *High-Push*   ☐ Low   ☐ Omit
☐ High-Pull   ☐ Do Not Mount

Wheel Lock Options   ☐ 6" Ext Handles   ☐ 9" Ext Handles
☐ Grade Aids (N/A w/ Polyurethane High-Pressure Clincher Tires or Kids Length Frames.)

ACCESSORIES
☐ Anti-Tip Tubes
☐ Armrest Pouch (Hgt Adj)
☐ Caddy
☐ Crutch Holder
☐ Front-End Stabilizer
☐ Leg Strap
☐ Leg Strap-Double
☐ Spoke Guards
☐ Transfer Board
☐ Tool Kit

Backpack & Seat Pouch
(Specify Color)
☐ Adult _____
☐ Kids _____
☐ Seat Pouch _____

Clothing
(Specify Color and Size)
☐ Long Sleeve Shirt ___
☐ Sweatshirt _____
☐ Golf Shirt _____
☐ T-Shirt _____
☐ Jacket _____
☐ Barrel Bag _____
☐ Hat _____
☐ Eyeglass Holders ___

Lifting Straps
☐ Q2 Low[10, 17]
☐ Q2 Medium[10, 17]
☐ Q2 Tall[10, 17]

Positioning Belts
☐ Long Velcro® Style (67")
☐ Short Velcro® Style (57")
☐ Long Buckle (64")
☐ Short Buckle (54")

Side Guards
☐ Fabric Kids
☐ Fabric Regular
☐ Plastic Kids[15]
☐ Plastic Reg[15]

Touch-Up Paint
☐ Color: _____

Wheelchair Tray Table
☐ Extra Small 10"-12"
☐ Small 13"-14"
☐ Medium 15"-17"
☐ Large 18"-20"

Special Instructions _____
_____
_____
_____
_____
_____

Items in Bold Italic Print are Standard

1. Available only on long frame.
2. N/A w/high-push wheel locks.
3. 8" bend not available; 11"-15" wide, 10"-15" deep only.
4. Not available with heel loops; single leg strap standard.
5. Hemi hangers only.
6. Only available on 60° hangers and hemi hangers.
7. Available only with 11"-16" frame widths.
8. Available only with 11"-16" frame widths and 90° hangers.
9. Available on 14"-20" widths.
10. Omit push handles.
11. Not available with swing-away armrest; height adj. available at swing-away price.
12. Not available on 26" wheels.
13. Only available on 24" wheels.
14. Not available with low-profile polyurethane tires.
15. Not available with height adjustable armrests.
16. Not available with mag wheels.
17. Not available with depth adjustable back.
18. Standard with 20" solid back height and stroller handles.
19. Available with 16"-20" frame widths and composite footplates only.
20. Not available with 90° hangers or articulating legrest-kids.
21. Not available with caster pin locks; not available with 3/4", or 1 1/2" fork stem bolt;

Specifications Subject to Change without Notice

930004 7/93

regarding alternatives which are beyond the scope of this chapter. For older, more intelligent, but more involved individuals with asymmetry or significant tone, a motorized device may be considered. *Three-wheeled scooters* are becoming increasingly popular and are often a wonderful alternative to motorized chairs. The scooters are much less expensive than a standard motorized wheelchair (approximately $2200+ versus $6000 to $7000),[†] they break down to components that are lighter and easier to move from home to car, and they are relatively simple to learn to operate and maintain. Any seating system—from a simple standard molded plastic seat to the most elaborate custom-made system—can be adapted to the scooter. Of concern, however, is that the patient must have bilateral hand use and some degree of reach in order to hold the scooter's handle bars, push the accelerator, and steer. *Traditional motorized wheelchairs* are extremely heavy, do not disassemble easily into component parts, and generally require a van for transport and ramps or a stair-free entrance to the home. Additionally, they are usually quite sophisticated electronically, which may mean frequent fine tuning and adjusting. They usually accommodate environmental control systems, allow for changes in position (e.g., reclining), and can be operated with any number of switches. Traditional motorized wheelchairs require more of a trial-and-error approach to perfect fit and to train the patient, and maintenance may be more involved. The scooter is preferred for a marginal ambulator who requires a device for long distances, whereas the traditional motorized wheelchair is usually reserved for the individual who requires a more extensive mobility system for full-time use. Specialists should be consulted if a traditional motorized wheelchair system is being considered, and one should never be ordered casually by an inexperienced clinician.

Once the chair style has been selected, the size, fit, and options must be determined. The numbered paragraphs that follow correspond to the numbers on the form in Display 13-2.

[†]Prices vary dramatically based on the seating and positioning options required and the need for additional electronic options.

[1] Seat width should allow for growth and should be able to accommodate outerwear for cold winter climates. Most vendors consider 1 inch on each side to be appropriate. Too much room makes it very difficult to propel the wheelchair effectively, especially when arm rests are used. In most pediatric models, chairs can be ordered in 1-inch increments to custom-fit any child. In an x-frame wheelchair, growth for width is achieved by replacing the cross braces and upholstery of the wheelchair. (No growth adjustment is available in a rigid chair.) In the pediatric population, almost all patients are provided with a solid seat, used with a cushion, to avoid the slinging effect of upholstery. Cushions made of 2-inch foam are standard with many wheelchair companies, but many alternatives exist. Cushions can be used not only to protect skin, but to change the patient's placement and alignment within the chair. Increasing the cushion height decreases the back height and armrest height, lowers the foot plates relative to the patient, and changes the patient's effective arm length and access to the wheels. This technique is often used to extend the use of a chair for several months for a patient who is growing tall but who has not outgrown the width of the chair. It is important, when measuring a chair, to remember to account for changes relating to cushion use (Fig. 13-6).

[2] Seat depth should permit comfortable knee flexion without popliteal pressure. In the pediatric population, a solid seat back with hardware placed between the uprights often allows for several inches of growth. The insert is placed forward of the uprights and is moved back as the child grows. However, the most energy-efficient alignment of a patient for propulsion places the greater trochanter over the axis of the back wheel and only 40% of the combined weight of the wheelchair and occupant on the front casters. It is, therefore, unwise to use cushions or allow for excessive seat depth. Axle plate adjustments are available, but the extent of improvement depends on many factors, including the frame size of the chair. The author prefers a sling back for any patient who can tolerate it without being poorly positioned or aligned. This

type of seat back can improve mobility, increase sitting tolerance, and decrease the weight of the wheelchair by eliminating heavy inserts and hardware.

[3] The preferred backrest height is below the scapula, but many patients require additional support. A serious dilemma arises when using a head support for bus transport to school. Automobile safety standards require headrests, and a patient is often safer using a headrest for transportation only (i.e., the patient who has fair head control when in a static position but who experiences fatigue or becomes compromised with excessive movement). It is difficult to mount a headrest on a sling back chair; thus, selection of even a removable headrest often implies changing to a solid back. In certain instances, this combination may be contraindicated for independence and energy-efficient mobility. This problem remains unresolved unless the patient can transfer into a federally approved car seat when in the bus, thus negating the need for a headrest mounted on the wheelchair itself.

[4] Foot plates and leg rests are often dictated by patient size and the wheelchair caster wheel size. Although many therapists believe that 90-degree knee flexion is optimal for weight bearing through a flat foot, this position may not be feasible. Vendors are the best resource for determining which options are available considering the frame size, wheel size, and the patient. More companies are becoming aware of the need for multiple-angle foot plates to allow for the braced and nonbraced foot, but this has proved to be a serious and difficult problem to solve in the past. It is always best to get removable leg rests, and elevating foot gear should only be requested if absolutely necessary, as it is both heavy and difficult to fit properly.

[5] Wheel size is critical in achieving the most energy-efficient propulsion. Ideally, the elbow should be flexed 120 degrees when the handrim is

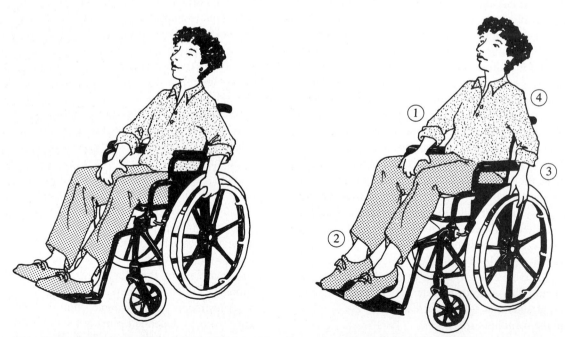

Figure 13-6. A. *Patient is accommodated without cushion.* B. *Use of a cushion will change: (1) Position of arm on armrest; (2) relative leg length; (3) relative arm length in relation to the wheel; and (4) the amount of back support (decreased).*

grasped at the highest point.[8] Pneumatic tires give a smoother ride (adding some shock absorbency) but require maintenance. For small children, the weight of the patient may not justify the need for the extra work; in older, heavier patients, however, the ride on rough terrain is clearly better on pneumatic tires.

[6] Caster size is the ultimate compromise. In the small-framed chair, adjustability of the rear axle is lost if the caster is too big, as the clearance between the two wheels is minimal. Small tires add maneuverability but get stuck in cracks, ditches, and the like. The author recommends the smallest tire that will still allow wheelchair management on the terrain that is navigated most often. The options range from 5- to 8-inch diameter wheels.

[7] Armrest height should be comfortable, should allow the patient to take some weight off the shoulders, and should allow easy access to the wheels. Essentially, the type of armrest should be dictated by ease of management. Many experienced wheelchair users prefer to be without armrests; however, bus drivers, parents, and other caregivers often rely on them for added support when transferring the chair into and out of vehicles.

[8] Brakes should be placed for easiest management and can be operated either by pushing or pulling, depending on the patient's preference. Many companies also offer high- or low-mount options for brakes.

Seat belts and antitippers are a must on children's wheelchairs, especially for new users. Clearly, all the conditions of use and available accessories and options cannot be discussed here, but selection of many of the remaining accessories is based on patient request and may or may not be essential. One should be aware that third-party payers may deny such items as back packs, trays, and utility bags unless they receive specific documentation of necessity.

Once a wheelchair prescription is complete, the therapist should feel satisfied that the decisions made are the best for a given patient. Any misgivings should be discussed with more experienced therapists, another vendor, or a manufacturer's representative. Therapists should always remember that they are ordering expensive equipment and, more importantly, that the equipment selected will affect the quality of the patient's life for the next 3 to 5 years.

Standing

Prone Standers

Prone standers are used frequently for children who require, but cannot achieve, the position of upright standing or its approximation. The child is placed in a prone position on the device. The trunk, buttocks, and lower extremities are all supported. The angle of the board is then increased toward a vertical position, depending on the child's tolerance and the therapist's goals. When the board is at its maximal angle, usually slightly less than 90 degrees, weight bearing is optimal through the lower extremities and feet, although sometimes a kneel-standing position is used. A prone stander is shown in Figure 13-7. The patient benefits from the physiologic changes associated with weight bearing and from the social and perceptual opportunities afforded by an upright position. As the angle of the prone stander decreases to less than upright, the benefits of lower extremity weight bearing will decrease because weight is borne more completely by the trunk.

Several other aspects of the use of the prone stander should be considered. Upper extremity function may range from almost total weight bearing in the child whose prone stander is less than 45 degrees above horizontal to completely free use of the upper extremities in the child who is in an upright position. Extensor muscle function of the neck and back will also vary significantly with various angles. As the patient approaches the upright position, the muscular effort for head righting will decrease. The physical therapist can either facilitate or inhibit muscle activity in various muscle groups by varying the angle of the prone stander.

The therapist must assess the quality of movement shown by the child in the prone stander. The function of the head, neck, scapulae, and upper extremities should be included in this assessment, as

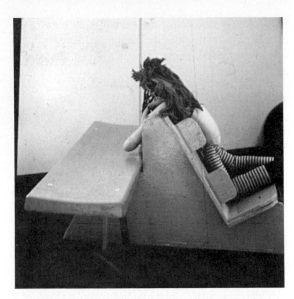

Figure 13-7. *A triwall prone stander covered with enamel paint is used for kneeling.*

should trunk alignment and positioning of the lower extremities. Hyperextension of the neck, exaggerated retraction of the scapulae and holding the upper extremities in the "high-guard" position, and poor symmetry and midline position of the trunk secondary to muscle imbalance are all common postural problems of the child placed in a prone stander. The therapist must consider that proper weight bearing for normal standing requires dynamic pressure through the heels, with the center of gravity passing posterior to the ankle joint; this position is not feasible in a prone stander. Therefore, the use of the prone stander must be evaluated carefully. The prone stander is useful if the physiological benefits of weight bearing are the major goal. If the prone stander is considered for preambulation skills and conditioning, its use may be inappropriate and counterproductive.

When the prone stander is introduced into the patient's program, the entire treatment regimen should be reevaluated. Although the child may appear to adapt well to use of the prone stander for 1 hour each day, longer use or abuse may cause undesirable changes. Increased extensor tone is an example of a change commonly seen with prolonged use of a prone stander. The increased tone may reduce the previously adequate position for sitting and may create difficulties at home and school. This negative effect might require adjustments in the amount of time spent in the prone stander, or it may require a different approach to positioning in the stander.

Supine Standers

A supine stander is an alternative to the prone stander and may better meet the needs of some children whose goal is to achieve an upright position. Similar to a standard tilt table, a supine stander allows weight bearing through the trunk and lower extremities, with the degree of weight-bearing proportional to the angle of the supporting surface. The child is secured around the trunk, hips, and knees with those areas in as close to neutral alignment as is possible. With those criteria achieved, the supine stander is angled toward a 90-degree upright position. Unlike the prone stander, the supine stander does not provide for weight bearing for the upper extremities, and lower extremity weight bearing occurs through the heels rather than the forefeet. The supine stander affords the numerous physiological benefits of upright weight bearing provided by the prone stander, and allows the child to perceive and interact with the environment from an upright posture. Variations of the supine stander are shown in Figures 13-8 and 13-9.

As with all adaptive devices, use of the supine stander must include a careful assessment of the child for compensations, some of which may be pathologic. Commonly noted deviations that occur with a child in a supine stander include thoracic kyphosis with protrusion of the head, hyperextension of the cervical spine, and asymmetry secondary to imbalanced muscle control. If tolerance for an upright position is limited and the child is reclined, increased evidence of asymmetric tonic neck reflex and the Moro reflex may occur. These abnormal reflexes may occur in a supine or semireclined position for any patient with poorly integrated reflex activity. The patient will push into or fix against

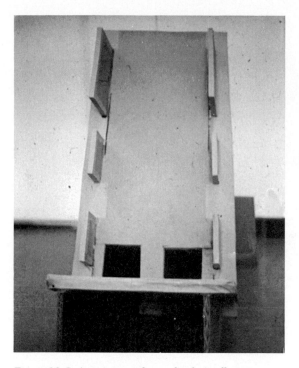

Figure 13-8. *A supine stander made of triwall.*

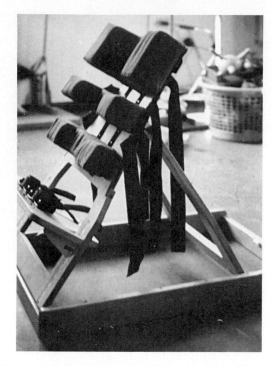

Figure 13-9. *Supine stander made of wood. It is padded for comfort and was designed and built entirely by parents.*

gravity. Because normal development requires the acquisition of antigravity control, the increased reflex activity in a supine position is counterproductive. Upper extremity function for the child in a supine stander usually requires a special table or easel, thus restricting the child's participation in group activities. The supine stander, although used less commonly than the prone stander, has become popular in recent years. As with other pieces of adaptive equipment, periodic evaluation is necessary to determine the long-term benefits and hazards associated with the supine stander.

Side-Lying

Side-Lyers

Side-lyers are particularly useful for young children or large people of low developmental function who may require an alternative to sitting and lying in bed or on the floor. Side-lyers can be elaborately

constructed or be very simple devices with pillows, straps, and other makeshift items. A typical fabricated side-lyer is shown in Figure 13-10. When using a side-lyer, the objective is to place the child in a side-lying position according to the following criteria:

1. The trunk should be as symmetric as possible.
2. The head should be supported in alignment neutral to the trunk.
3. Weight-bearing limbs (upper and lower) should be slightly flexed.
4. Non–weight-bearing limbs should be free to move.

This position encourages play in the midline, dissociation between the limbs, and neutral head and trunk alignment. Straps are commonly used to support the trunk, pelvis, and occasionally, the weight-bearing leg. Pillows usually support the upper leg in a neutral position for abduction or adduction and for internal or external rotation. The device should

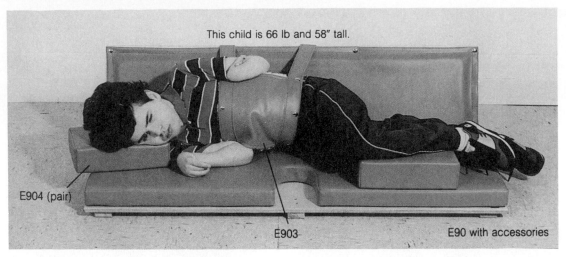

This child is 66 lb and 58″ tall.

E904 (pair)

E903

E90 with accessories

Figure 13-10. *A commercially available side-lyer.*

accommodate the child on either side unless circumstances prevent the child from lying on both sides.

Frequent reassessment is required to ensure that no compensations occur either when using or after being removed from the side-lyer. Areas of potential problems include hyperextension of the neck from pushing against the head support, and flexion and retraction of the shoulder on the non–weight-bearing side. When using a side-lyer, the therapist must be careful when aligning the child with chronic hyperextension of the neck or a tracheostomy. In each of these situations, a rapid attempt to correct the hyperextension may cause an airway obstruction and may compromise the child's ventilation. Although the side-lyer allows for easy manipulation of toys and objects because one hand is fixed in good alignment, the position is not optimal for perceptual development because the child must play with objects in a horizontal plane when the environmental backdrop is vertical (i.e., toys are rotated 90 degrees with respect to the visual field). This ironic occurrence is not a contraindication to using a side-lyer unless the child has obvious or suspected difficulties with perception or cognition. Most children compensate easily for the problem,

especially when sides are alternated, and enjoy these changes of position.

Overall Considerations

Although not a complete list of positioning devices, examples have been provided to illustrate the issues to be considered in choosing and using equipment and the negative consequences that may occur. Negative consequences can be minimized by periodic reassessment of the child and by education of the family and staff. When people who work with the child are aware of the potential negative effects of the equipment, they are more likely to anticipate and recognize early signs of those effects.

Because all physical therapists who work with children and adaptive equipment will be required to suggest the frequency and duration of use, it seems appropriate to discuss the issue of endurance. Unfortunately, a uniform answer rarely exists. Endurance depends on variables that change daily. Rather than suggesting specific times, the therapist may choose to teach parents and staff members about the warning signs of fatigue—difficulty in maintaining the desired posture, increased asymmetry, complaints of discomfort, and verbal requests to be moved. The therapist can then recommend that the device be used until any of those signs are apparent. It may be worthwhile to encourage attempts to increase endurance gradually over the course of several weeks or months, with the realization that minor variations in tolerance will occur daily. Because daily variations in activity level are normal for everyone, we should acknowledge these variations in the handicapped child.

Equipment for Infants and Toddlers

Let us now examine the needs of the infant and toddler and the availability of devices for these younger children. Children in this age group are often undiagnosed, or they may show a developmental delay that may or may not result in a long-term disability. Children who require long periods of hospitalization for cardiac, pulmonary, gastrointestinal, and other disorders are also included in this group, as are children who are normal but whose parents request information about various types of apparatus to aid development.

Hospitalized Children

Normal motor development is an integrated process that requires sensory input and freedom to respond to that input through motor exploration and play. Normal patterns of movement develop when agonist and antagonist muscles learn balanced and synergistic cooperation. Because equipment may disrupt or interfere with this process by limiting or restricting movement, its use in infants and toddlers is almost always discouraged. Movement is often restricted by monitors, telemetry devices, and therapeutic medical equipment when the child is hospitalized. It would be counterproductive to the child's motor development to add to these necessary devices other types of apparatus. The objective for the hospitalized child is often to provide optimal freedom of movement within the limits imposed by medical equipment and practice. Physical therapy for these hospitalized children should encourage increased activity, if safe, and should facilitate movement patterns that, because of the external limita-tions, are difficult for the child to initiate. As the child's medical status improves, or when the child returns home, equipment use should still be limited, except when indicated to promote physical control or safety.

In the United States, car seats for the transport of infants and young children are required in all 50 states. Unfortunately, few guidelines exist for disabled individuals who are unable to use standard car seats or seat belts. This oversight is of serious concern for many parents and professionals working with children.

Strollers and high chairs should be used sparingly, and the child should be in a stable position to allow for optimal oral motor function, head righting and control, and freedom of movement of the upper extremities.

Physical therapy during this period of development should concentrate on encouraging normal, controlled, motor patterns, and devices should not predominate. The therapist working with the young child should make recommendations to the parents about facilitating movement and avoiding static positioning when the child is left alone to play.

As these children grow older, some will outgrow their temporary disability, but others will develop additional symptoms, and a diagnosis may become more evident. Children in the latter group are likely to have continued treatment and equipment needs and should be evaluated as previously outlined.

Ventilator-dependent children represent a small but growing population with major equipment needs. With increasing frequency, the physical therapist will be called upon to assist in the discharge planning and management of ventilator-dependent children. Technologic advances have prolonged life expectancy for many children with chronic illnesses, including those with myelomeningocele and Arnold-Chiari malformation. New, portable ventilators and third-party funding have aided in transforming these once chronically hospitalized children into active members of the community. These children often return home, attend their local school, and participate in recreational and social activities. Such participation requires a transport system for essential life-support equipment, which includes a portable ventilator and battery, electric cascade humidifier (if the patient will be in one setting for many hours), oxygen source, airway suction unit with catheters and hoses, a bag of supplies, and other items. An innovative approach must be taken with this population in order to address their developmental, orthopedic, and respiratory needs. It is essential to find a vendor who is interested in working with the family and who is able to tailor the specific apparatus to the child's unique requirements. A great deal of trial-and-error effort often is expended in an attempt to resolve the problems presented by the weight of the ventilators, unusual balance points, difficult maneuverability, and the child's need to be in close proximity to these devices.

The two systems shown in Figures 13-11 and 13-12 were designed to meet the specific needs of both child and family. Figure 13-11 shows a commercially available double stroller that has been reinforced to house the ventilator in the rear seat with the battery suspended between the seats. The child can recline or sit upright and has use of an age-appropriate and cost-effective device that is both aesthetically pleasing and manageable. Figure 13-12 shows an Alvena frame adapted for a Snug Seat with the battery on the front foot plate and the ventilator positioned behind the seat. The patient is positioned high enough to allow easy access to the equipment stored underneath and to accommodate the comfort of caregivers who may perform suctioning and other procedures. The Snug Seat tilts 45 degrees in space and allows for easy adjust-

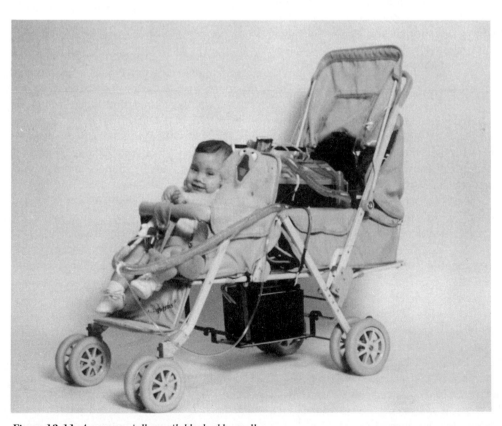

Figure 13-11. *A commercially available double stroller.*

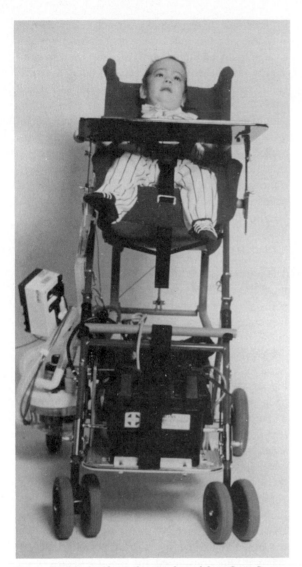

Figure 13-12. *An Alvena frame adapted for a Snug Seat.*

ments for postural changes or growth. As the child grows and independent mobility becomes a concern, manual or motorized wheelchairs can be adapted for the child's use.*

A very special thank you to the DME Shoppe and Joe Thieme, 1572 Shore Road, Naperville, IL 60653, for creating these units and many more similar devices.

Normal Infants and Toddlers

Let us consider the equipment used frequently for normal babies and toddlers, including walkers, swings, and jumpers. It has become common practice for families to purchase these devices for their children, despite little knowledge of their advantages or disadvantages. Swings are probably the most benign device of the three mentioned. There is little evidence to indicate that swings are unsafe for children of this age, particularly if used with supervision by family members. Although swings are pleasant for the child and family, they should be used sparingly because they lack significant stimulation for motor growth and development. Jumpers are devices that are suspended from doorways by large cables, springs, and clamps. The jumper enables the child to bounce up and down by extending the lower extremities and pushing against the floor. Some babies enjoy this device a great deal, whereas others may object to being placed in the device and may become dizzy when they are removed. The child must be supervised constantly to ensure that he or she does not fall, bang against the doorframe, or become entrapped in the cables or springs when reaching out for a toy. Despite these potential hazards, the device can be used for short periods during the day. Like other devices, the jumper impedes development of normal motor skills by eliminating the opportunity to make transitions from one pattern to another and by restricting the learning of new sequences of movement. Even restricted use of the jumper in normal children must be monitored for the development of patterns of exaggerated extensor activity with components of strong internal rotation of the hip. Development of this pattern of movement would be undesirable and would require discontinued use of the jumper. Unlike swings and jumpers, walkers have been implicated in injuries severe enough to be fatal. In 1981, more than 17,000 injuries to children were associated with walkers.[9] Most injuries have been the result of the walker tipping over, falling down stairs, collapsing because of poor structural design, or finger entrapment. Injuries have included abrasions, lacerations, severe head trauma, and death. Many facilities recommend walkers under the mistaken impression that walking skills are helped by these devices. Ridenour studied the effects of frequent and regular use of a walker on bipedal locomotion in human infants. She found that walkers modified the mechanics of infant locomotion in several ways. Infants who used walkers were able to commit numerous mechanical errors while succeeding in bipedal locomotion.[9] The patterns of locomotion with an infant walker are neither normal nor advantageous. Children who use these walkers hold their trunk and lower extremities in flexion. There is also frequent asymmetry as the child leans, and toe-walking is common. These observations, plus the apparent increase in idiopathic toe-walking and scoliosis in young boys, suggest that walkers may have a significant adverse effect on motor development. Although scientific data are needed to confirm this suspicion, most physical therapists discourage the use of walkers by normal infants and strongly discourage their use in infants with documented or suspected neurologic deficits.

Activities of Daily Living

Although not strongly emphasized in this chapter, activities of daily living (ADLs) should be mentioned briefly. ADLs are not major concerns for infants or toddlers with a handicapping condition, but they grow increasingly important as these children grow older and become more capable of caring for themselves. Because families can usually manage the ADL needs of a young child, the issue of ADLs as a therapeutic goal may be overlooked or not considered even though the child becomes more capable as he or she grows older.

Equipment for ADLs, particularly for bathing and toileting, should be assessed according to guidelines similar to those used for other pieces of apparatus described in this chapter. Special toilet seats may improve the function of a child with spasticity who has difficulty voiding because of increased tone. If the child feels secure and confident, he or she will feel relaxed and toileting may proceed more rapidly and easily. When choosing a bathtub seat, both ease of management in the tub and safety of the child are the major objectives. Although many bathtub seats exist, seats that are completely satisfactory for both use and safety are difficult to find for all children, but particularly difficult when the child becomes older and heavier. Vendors should provide sample bathtub seats for both inspection and mock usage trials. The family must decide which tub seat provides the safest and most suitable solution depending on the particular environmental barriers of the home and the physical needs of the child. Occupational therapists should be consulted about recommendations for ADLs.

Conclusions

The purchase, building, and use of adaptive equipment are complex and time-consuming aspects of pediatric physical therapy. These processes are further complicated by the lack of scientific documentation to help with the appropriate and objective choice of equipment. The available options are so numerous that even the most experienced physical therapist is unlikely to feel that all equipment has been considered before making a choice. The safest and most realistic approach to the selection of adaptive devices for children lies in a theoretical construct based on careful evaluation of the child. The goals and status of the child must be known before therapeutic needs can be met with various types of equipment. When this information is known, the therapist can develop a therapeutic program that includes safe and effective use of equipment without unwanted negative effects. When the child's needs and goals are considered, the specific details of the numerous devices available become less intimidating or confusing. Frequent reevaluation by the therapist will ensure that the child receives continuing benefits from adaptive equipment. Input from teachers, aides, and parents will provide invaluable feedback regarding the child's use of the equipment. The scheme suggested in this chapter provides the therapist with the opportunity to document the needs of the child, to select or make the equipment, to evaluate the effects of the equipment, and to reassess the child's status periodically.

References

1. Marks A. On making chairs more comfortable—how to fit the seat to the sitter. *Fine Woodworking.* 1981;31:11.
2. Keegan J. Alterations in the lumbar curve related to posture and sitting. *J Bone Joint Surg.* 1973;35A:7.
3. Akerblom B. *Chairs and Sitting.* Presented at the Symposium on Human Factors in Equipment Design; 1954; Sweden.
4. Knutsson B, Lindh K, Telhag H. Sitting: An electromyographic and mechanical study. *Acta Orthop Scand.* 1966;37:415–426.
5. Keegan J. Evaluation and improvement of seats. *Industr Med Surg.* 1962;31:137–148.
6. Bergan A. *Positioning the Client with Central Nervous System Deficits: The Wheelchair and Other Adapted Equipment.* 2nd ed. New York: Valhalla Press; 1985.
7. Nwaobi O, Brubaker C, Cusick B, et al. Electromyographic investigation of extensor activity in cerebral palsy children in different seating positions. *Dev Med Child Neurol.* 1983;25:175–183.
8. Brubaker C. Ergonomic considerations. *J Rehabil R D* [Clin Suppl]. 1990;27:37–48.
9. Ridenour M. Infant walkers: Developmental tool or inherent danger? *Percept Motor Skills.* 1982;55:1201–1202.

Bibliography

Bull M, Stroup K, Stout J, et al. Establishing special needs care seat loan program. *Pediatrics.* 1990;85:540–547.

Hulme JB, Shaver J, Acher S, et al. Effects of adaptive seating devices on the eating and drinking of children with multiple handicaps. *Am J Occup Ther.* 1987;41:81–89.

Mazur MD, Shurtleff D. Orthopedic management of high-level spina bifida—Early walking compared with early use of a wheelchair. *J Bone Joint Surg.* 1989;71A:56–61.

Stout J, Bull M, Stroup K. Safe transportation for children with disabilities. *Am J Occup Ther.* 1989;43:31–36.

Trefler E, ed. *Seating for Children with Cerebral Palsy—A Resource Manual.* Memphis: University of Tennessee; 1984.

Zacharkow D. *Posture: Sitting, Standing, Chair Design and Exercise.* Springfield, IL: Charles C Thomas; 1988.

Pediatric Physical Therapy,
second edition, edited by Jan
Stephen Tecklin. J. B. Lippincott
Company, Philadelphia © 1994.

14

Susan Kenville Lindeblad

Physical Therapy in Schools

- **Background Information**
- **Legislation**
  Zero Reject
  Nondiscriminatory Evaluation
  Individualized Educational Program
  Parent Participation
  Least Restrictive Environment
  PL 99-457
  Related Services Versus Program
  Transitioning
- **Delivery of Physical Therapy Services in Schools**

Direct Care Services
Indirect Services
Program Development
Treatment
Accountability
- **Roles for Physical Therapy That Extend Beyond Special Education**
  Screening
  Athletics

Background Information

Physical therapy services have been available for many decades in various educational environments within the United States, with physical therapists meeting the needs of children with a variety of disabilities and special needs. Public school therapy, however, has a fairly recent history of availability. Special schools and classes began to appear for crippled children, as they were called, at the turn of the century, and physical therapists began their work in this setting in large cities, such as Boston, Chicago, and Detroit.[1–3] Most of the children served in these early special classes were of normal or near-normal intelligence, and initially, most suffered from poliomyelitis or spastic paralysis.[4,5] Other common diagnoses included cardiac disor-

ders, obstetrical arms or Erb's palsy, bone and joint tuberculosis, club feet, and osteomyelitis.[1,3,5] By the mid-1930s, numerous references in *Physiotherapy Review* related to working with what were then called "crippled and spastic children."[6]

With the discovery of a vaccine for poliomyelitis in the 1950s, there was a remarkable decrease in the population of children with this diagnosis. Their places in the schools, however, were taken by children with various neurologic disorders. The extent and amount of services and therapy available to these children varied from community to community, based upon attitudes of the people, the geographic locations of the schools, and the financial abilities of the families. Children with normal intelligence or mild handicapping conditions continued to have some access to schools; however, children could be denied access to school based upon their ability (or inability) to ambulate in the buildings, their level of toilet training, and their intellectual abilities. Children with mental retardation or severe physical impairments often received no schooling at all, or were sent to day treatment centers or residential facilities.

The 1960s and the Kennedy administration brought a new awareness to the public regarding the handicapped. In 1961, the President's Panel on Mental Retardation outlined the needs of the handicapped and initiated legislative action. Documentaries in the media exposed some of the inhumane care and services for the handicapped. Advocacy became one of the "buzz words" of the time, and advocacy groups became more and more active and powerful.

Legislation

In the legislative arena, a series of landmark court decisions culminated in the enactment of *The Education of All Handicapped Children Act of 1975,* otherwise known as Public Law 94-142 (PL 94-142).

Simply stated, PL 94-142 provides that:

All children regardless of handicapping condition shall receive a free, appropriate, public education. This education is to be provided in the least restricted environment with those related services necessary for the child to function within the educational setting.[7]

The basis of this legislation reverts back to the 8th and 14th Constitutional Amendments and the following Court Decisions:

- In 1954, in the case of *Brown vs. The Board of Education,* the decision made was that separate is not equal, thus the basis for least restricted environment.
- In 1966, PL 89-70 established the Bureau of Education for the Handicapped.
- In 1971 the landmark case of *PARC vs. Commonwealth of Pennsylvania,*[8] the Pennsylvania Association for Retarded Citizens (PARC) filed a class action suit on behalf of 14 specifically named children and all other children who were of similar "class" of trainable mentally retarded people. Prior to this case,

children who were functioning within this level of abilities or lower were excluded in Pennsylvania from public school if a psychologist or mental health professional certified that the child could no longer profit from attendance in school. Any child who had not reached a mental age of 5 years could be denied access to public school. Thus, most children who were mentally retarded were denied public school. The case was resolved in favor of PARC, and all children between 6 and 21 years were to be given a free and appropriate education, regardless of disability. The educational system was ordered to stop applying exclusionary laws; parents were to become involved in planning the program; and re-evaluations were to be made. This court ruling was the basic foundation for PL 94-142.

- In 1972, *Mills vs. District of Columbia Board of Education* expanded the rights of individuals to receive related services, including physical therapy.

This series of major court cases then became instrumental in the development of federal legislation which led to the current status of services. This legislation included the Individuals with Disabilities Education Act (IDEA), PL 94-142 and Part H (PL 99-457).[9]

In 1975, PL 94-142 was enacted into law by the United States Congress.[7] As with all Federal legislation, PL 94-142 was subject to review, renewal, and reappropriation every 10 years. When renewal and reappropriation occurred in 1985/1986, PL 94-142 was renamed the *Individualized Education of Handicapped Act* (IDEA). In addition, Public Law 99-457—The Education of Handicapped Act of 1986, Title I, Part H—was made law via amendment,[9] providing for services to be made available for infants and toddlers, as well as their families.

PL 94-142 had dynamic effects upon the educational system, especially with regard to special needs children. It also had widespread effects upon the delivery of physical therapy in the school setting. PL 94-142 provided for all children to receive a "free, appropriate education, in the least restricted environment, as well as the related services needed to function in the educational setting."[7,10] Each child, regardless of disability, is entitled to a nondiscriminatory evaluation and Individualized Educational Plan (IEP), with zero reject, and IEP planning must provide for parent participation.

Zero Reject

The *zero reject* principle of the right to education provides that any child, regardless of level or type of disability, is entitled to an educational program that is free and appropriate. Programs must meet the needs of the individual children, rather than requiring the child to meet the requirements of the available education.

Nondiscriminatory Evaluation

The evaluation process is an important part of the development of the IEP, and must be done without racial or cultural bias. Generally speaking, evaluation of gross and fine motor development and physical assessment are free of cultural and racial biases. The therapist must be careful, however, not to discriminate. The therapist must also maintain awareness of and adjust for any possible cultural differences that could affect a child's performance in evaluation. For example, a child who is not allowed to play on the floor because of cultural or social constraints may show some delays in gross motor skills.

Individual school districts or states may have developed evaluation tools to assist in the standardization of evaluation as services. Therapists should contact their state's Department of Education for information regarding what tools are available.

Individualized Educational Program

The IEP is a specially designed plan of educational instruction that is developed to meet the special and unique needs of each child. The plan is developed, with participation and input from the educational team, following an evaluation of the child's current needs. The team consists of a representative of the local educational agency (LEA), the teacher, parents, and related services personnel, as appropriate. Children who have the cognitive ability to participate should also be included as members of the team. The format and actual form used to report the IEP varies from school district to school district. The components of the IEP are defined in PL 94-142 and must include the following items:

1. A statement of the present levels of educational performance of the child
2. A statement of annual goals, including short-term instructional objectives
3. A statement of the specific educational services to be provided, and the extent to which the child will be able to participate in regular educational programs
4. The projected date for the initiation of services and the anticipated duration of such services
5. Appropriate objective criteria and evaluation procedures, as well as a determination of schedules, at least annually, to determine if the objectives have been achieved[7]

The role of the physical therapist in the development of the IEP varies within the United States. It is possible that the physical therapist may not be involved in the initial evaluation and IEP. Assessment and treatment by the PT may be suggested at a later time by the parent, the teacher, or other professional once a motor deficit is recognized.

Therapy services may be included in the IEP under a vague objective to facilitate gross motor development, or more specific services may be identified (i.e., to provide instruction in walking within the school). Regardless of how the objective is written, it should always relate to functional skill within the educational setting. Physical therapists are not required to attend or participate in the IEP meetings, but the school or LEA should decide in advance if the therapist needs to attend the meeting or not. When the therapist does not attend the meeting, goals and objectives for physical development and motor domain must be presented, if appropriate for the child. Therefore, the therapist should provide the teacher or parents with adequate information for determining the need for inclusion of these goals in the IEP. When a child is receiving special education services, including physical therapy, the IEP can be used as a realistic framework for planning. The physical therapist should be actively involved in the meeting whenever the child to be discussed has serious motor deficits.

Parent Participation

Parent participation in the educational planning is a central focus of both PL 94-142 and PL 99-457. The parent is a key component in the IEP for both immediate planning and progression and future planning for the child. Initially, some school systems had difficulty in adjusting to parent participation; however, this requirement keeps the primary focus on the individual child and provides for long-term continuity and planning. Parents are, perhaps, the best advocates for their own child, provided they understand their rights and responsibilities. There have been numerous parent training and parent support programs developing across the country to help parents learn about and assume this advocacy role in their child's education. The therapist should be aware of the local availability of parent groups as a resource for information.

Parent participation occurs in a number of ways. The parents must give written permission for the initial evaluation; they may restrict the release of information; they may have access to all educational records relating to their child; their participation is required in the IEP process; they have the right to request a due process hearing; they can serve on local and state advisory panels; and they can participate in public hearings. Many parents exercise these rights and are, therefore, instrumental in obtaining appropriate services for their child. However, some parents are not aware of or do not understand these rights, or may not be as concerned about the education for their child. All of the professionals working in the schools should be well acquainted with both parents' and children's rights to ensure that children receive the appropriate services. Physical therapy is an expensive service that some educators do not believe is educationally necessary. The inclusion of physical therapy in an IEP must often be advocated by the child's parents. If the parents do not ask for their child to receive therapy, frequently, it will not be provided. With this

same thought in mind, if the therapist does not write educationally relevant (as opposed to medically relevant) goals and objectives, therapy may not be justified in the educational setting.

Least Restrictive Environment

Education in the least restrictive environment refers to the concept of mainstreaming, which encourages the integration of children with handicapping conditions with children who are not physically or mentally challenged. Educational agencies must ensure the following:[7]

1. That, to the maximum extent appropriate, handicapped children, including children in public or private institutions or other care facilities, are educated with children who are not handicapped
2. That special classes, separate schooling, or other removal of handicapped children from the regular educational environment occurs only when the nature or severity of the handicap is such that education in regular classes with the use of supplementary aids and services cannot be achieved satisfactorily.

The principle of least restrictive environment supports and provides for children with handicapping conditions to be included in classes with their normal peers, but it also allows for isolated placements when it is considered to be in the best interest of the child. The role of the physical therapist in the least restrictive placement is to work together with the educational system to assist the child to function and succeed in the least restricted environment.

PL 99-457

In 1986, The Education of the Handicapped Act Amendments, PL 99-457, Part H, extended services to infants, toddlers, and preschool children. The Part H amendments provide for a strong commitment to family involvement, multidisciplinary involvement, and coordination of services between public and private agencies.

The rules and regulations promulgated for PL 99-457 are less dogmatic than the earlier version for PL 94-142, and thus extend greater autonomy to the individual states. This makes it difficult to write a single text on the subject, as each state has the ability to develop a plan for the implementation of the act. Therapists, therefore, must request this information about implementation from their own states' Department of Education. There are, however, some common elements to look for, including the definitions for developmental delay, and the team of professionals who may be involved in the care of the infants. There are Child Find services, as well as tracking for services, parent-professional partnerships, lead agency, interagency coordinating councils, and a multidisciplinary team approach. In addition to child evaluation and services, there is also provision for family assessment and services. In place of the IEP, the infant toddler services provide for an Individualized Family Service Plan (IFSP).

Individualized Family Service Plan

An IFSP is required under PL 99-457 for infants and toddlers with special needs. The IFSP is similar to the IEP except that "enhancing the capacity of families to meet the special needs of their infants and toddlers with handicaps" is considered an "urgent and substantial need."[9] The IFSP requires that the infant or toddler and family receive a multidisciplinary assessment and a written plan of intervention.

The family assessment portion of the multidisciplinary team must remain voluntary, and a child may not be excluded from services if the family does not wish to participate in the assessment. The professionals on the team should, however, be able to promote the concept of incorporation of family needs and priorities into the IFSP.

The components of the IFSP, as determined in PL 99-457, must include the following:[9]

1. A statement of the infant's or toddler's present level of physical development, cognitive development, language and speech development, and self-help skills, based on acceptable objective criteria
2. A statement of the family's strengths and needs re-

lating to enhancing the development of the infant or toddler with the handicapping condition
3. A statement of the major outcomes expected to be achieved for the infant/toddler and family, and the criteria, procedures, and schedule used to determine the degree of progress (to be done at least annually)
4. A statement of specific early intervention services necessary to meet the unique needs of the infant/toddler and family, including frequency, intensity, and method of delivering services
5. The projected dates for the initiation of services and anticipated duration of services
6. The name of the case manager from the profession most immediately relevant to the infant's, toddler's, or family's needs who will be responsible for the implementation of the plan and coordination with other agencies and persons
7. The steps to be taken to support the transition of the toddler to services for school-aged children, to the extent that such services are considered appropriate.

As stated, the case manager chosen from the team is the person most relevant to the child's and family's needs. Many states and agencies have difficulty with this concept, and controversy exists over who is most qualified to act as a case manager for the child. The case manager acts as a "gate keeper" for services. This individual specifically coordinates evaluation and treatment, and works to facilitate transition to pre-kindergarten services, and the change from IFSP to an IEP.

Related Services Versus Program

Related services under PL 94-142 include transportation, speech pathology, audiology, psychological services, physical therapy, occupational therapy, recreation, and medical and counseling services, "as may be required to assist a handicapped child to benefit from special education. . . ."[7] This provision is interpreted in a number of different ways. Some people use it to restrict the scope of related services. They have a limited interpretation of the law and require that every objective and activity relate directly to the traditional concepts of education.

Since the 1970s, education in general has become more liberal, and educators are acquiring a more open view of what is educationally relevant. Feeding, dressing, toileting, head control, and mobility are considered to be important components of the educational curriculum for children needing those skills. To meet the overall educational needs of children with handicapping conditions, acceptable objectives in the educational setting may include walking throughout the school to reach classes with nonhandicapped peers, preventing debilitating deformities to allow continued participation in the educational setting, or maintaining a clear airway, thus facilitating the child's concentration in the educational process.

Within PL 99-457, physical therapy is identified not as a related service but as a program. Thus, physical therapy may be the primary need of the child and family, the therapist may be the case manager, and educational goals may be regarded as secondary, at least at an early age. The multidisciplinary team mandated in the federal statute is, in fact, defined in rule as an "interdisciplinary interaction"—"involvement of 2 or more disciplines with provision of integrated and coordinated services including evaluation and assessment."[9]

Transitioning

The enactment of PL 99-457 mandates an additional process—transitioning—in developing the plan for a child. By adding this requirement, there is a built-in need not only to develop a current program for the child, but also to plan for future programming and needs and to assist the family in carryover to the next stages of development and education. Commonly, families have a difficult time making life-style changes, accompanied as they are by new fears and concerns of the unknown. When transition planning and care is included in the IFSP, the family is provided support from the professionals in the programs with whom they are already familiar. Professionals working in early childhood programs, therefore, need to be aware not only of the services they provide but also of the future services available in the pre-kindergarten and educational system. Some states are beginning to take this process one step further and, in junior and senior high school, are beginning to plan for the transition of the child after graduation, or after the child reaches 21 years of age and is no longer eligible for educational services under PL 94-142.

Delivery of Physical Therapy Services in Schools

Delivery models for physical therapy within the school setting are almost as varied as the types of schools and the diagnoses of the children served. The delivery of services also has a number of different parts to be addressed. There has been a great deal written comparing the educational model to the medical model,[11,12] and perhaps this issue has been given too much emphasis in the literature, but therapists and educators may need to keep some basic differences in mind. In the traditional hospital-based medical model, clients are generally dependent upon the staff for all their needs: they are cared for totally. Service can be rather impersonal, staff members wear uniforms that differentiate their duties, and the patients wear embarrassing gowns and wrist bands that differentiate their care. The medical model tends to be restrictive, with many schedules and rules to be followed. The educational model differs from this medical model quite radically. The primary goals in education include the development of independence through learning. The programs are individualized to address each individual child's unique needs, and the schools strive to increase freedom of movement. Pediatric therapists are not likely to wear white uniforms to delineate their medical role or to treat one patient at a time on a sterile plinth. Even though the care delivery models vary in terms of independence, the goals and objectives will maintain a common thread, that of functional skills. Goals and objectives in the medical model are written to address functional outcomes for the patient. When the therapist is addressing the educational needs of the pediatric population, writing goals may be for the functional setting in which the child works, "the school."

Isolation of the physical therapist is one treatment situation that is more prevalent in the educational setting than in other settings. The therapist may be itinerant, traveling to a number of schools in any given day, especially if children are served in their local schools. This isolation may be difficult for the physical therapist, sometimes giving rise to self-doubts about the therapist's abilities. Therapists who work in relative isolation may feel incompetent because no one offers support, or they may be overly confident because no one is there to evaluate their skills. Therapists who work alone should actively seek to join a professional peer group for support, groups such as local pediatric special interest groups or national professional organizations. Planned meetings with other therapists who work in the system are important, and attendance at continuing education programs specially designed to meet the needs of the therapist working with the pediatric population should be mandatory. The therapist may also be encouraged to seek out graduate courses if they are available.

Direct Care Services

Delivery of therapy in a school system should include both indirect and direct services, as both are of equal importance. Direct services by a therapist interested in the care of children should be provided after or at the same time as consultation and management. The therapist should first serve as a consultant—to evaluate the physical environment, safety procedures, and other issues mentioned previously. The therapist then needs to develop management programs for the classroom teacher, physical educator, and parents, as indicated. The therapist should consider providing direct therapy services to the child only *after* these important tasks are completed. This delay of direct services can cause administrative problems and sometimes frustration. Some educators and therapists prefer to de-

fine physical therapy in the narrow spectrum of direct care. Others recognize the broader implications of a total comprehensive management approach in the care of the child and for the carryover of direct care benefits.

Direct services may be provided to a single child for a specified period of time each week, or services may be provided to small groups of two or three children who have similar goals and who may profit from working together with the therapist. This arrangement may be viewed as a least restrictive environment for the delivery of services, as it combines therapy with an opportunity to practice socialization skills.

Indirect Services

Both medical and educational settings employ multidisciplinary approaches to patient care. Educational environments may also use a transdisciplinary approach.[11] The transdisciplinary approach involves role release to the teacher who then serves as the primary direct service provider for all interventions. The therapist provides indirect services to the child by consulting with the teacher. The consultation model reduces the number of individuals who work directly with the child, which provides for greater consistency in care as well as more efficient use of both the child's and the professional's time. This method also offers a greater opportunity to integrate educational and therapeutic interventions. It is also believed to be a more cost-effective system.[11] Some educators believe that this method of consultation and role release reduces the quality of professional services provided to the children and raises serious liability questions.[12] Therefore, it is the responsibility of the professionals involved to develop a strong communication network, working together to exchange information and concerns on a regular basis. Whenever a therapist develops a plan of care to be implemented by another person— whether it be for a therapist assistant, a teacher, or a parent—it is the therapist who is ultimately responsible.

Indirect services may be divided into three basic

categories: management programs, monitoring, and consultation. Indirect services, relating directly to a child or specific small group of children, have been termed *management programs*.[13] According to this service model, the therapist plans, trains, and supervises a program that is administered by another person. A management plan might include positioning that is done by the child's teacher, motor activities and games that are implemented during adaptive physical education sessions, and range of motion exercise or positioning that is done by parents.

Monitoring is also an indirect service whereby the therapist periodically evaluates the children who have been terminated from direct therapy services, or screens those children who are at risk for requiring direct services, but do not yet require that level of care. Monitoring helps to detect deterioration or change in a child's status; to identify the need for modifications in equipment, orthotics, and prosthetics; and to determine whether the management programs are being carried out appropriately by the designated personnel, and if they remain effective.

Consultation as an indirect service can involve recommendations for a specific child, classroom, school, school system, or state agency. Therefore, consultation may address a wide variety of issues, including:

- Recommendations regarding architectural barriers
- Safety programs for schools and buses
- Development of documentation and record-keeping systems
- Development of physical therapy student affiliation programs
- Determinations of space, personnel, and equipment needs
- Inservice education
- Program development, evaluation, and quality assurance

The therapist can also serve as the liaison between the school and the medical community. Moreover, therapists should be very familiar with the State Practice Act so that they can assist in coordinating implementation of school law and the provision of physical therapy.

Program Development

The key to the therapist's intervention is, as always, a comprehensive evaluation to determine the needs of the child and to design an appropriate therapeutic intervention and management plan. After the evaluation is completed, the IEP or IFSP can be developed, and during the team meeting, appropriate behavioral objectives can be written. Behavioral objectives are designed to express the goals for the child in specific, observable, measurable terms. The purpose of behavioral objectives is to provide a focus for physical therapy intervention and a means of communication with teachers, parents, and other professionals. The behavioral objectives help the team target the deficits for programming and enable the team to build upon the strengths of the child.

Behavioral objectives in an educational setting contain the following concepts: conditions, observable behavior, criterion, and relationship to educational need. As an example, the following objective might be written: "Given a simple four-part puzzle, with pieces placed 10 feet from the form board, Lucy will creep reciprocally to retrieve the pieces one at a time to complete the puzzle, in three of five trials with equal weight-bearing on lower extremities." (The educational need here may be the recognition of shapes and sizes in the puzzle.)

The federal mandate is for an IEP/IFSP to be reviewed at least annually. Objectives written for 1 year are referred to as *long-term objectives*. These are usually more general in nature, and are followed by a number of smaller components called *short-term objectives*. The short-term objectives are generally sequential steps leading to the achievement of the long-term objective. Some objectives cannot be divided into smaller components, resulting in a list of unrelated short-term objectives. A number of resources offer assistance in writing behavioral objectives.[10,14–19]

Treatment

The type of physical therapy treatment provided to a school-aged child with a handicapping condition in an educational environment depends upon the specific needs of the child within that particular educational setting. The available resources and philosophy of the school system may also help to define the type of therapy.

The infant and toddler served under PL 99-457 may receive very general developmental, habilitation services. Once the child reaches 5 years of age, or school age, the therapist must keep in mind that the child's primary need is to be involved in education and that therapy is to be designed primarily to help the child achieve educational success. Services may be indirect, direct, or a combination of both. If the appropriate therapy for the child extends beyond the educational needs of the child, it is the therapist's professional obligation to notify the parents and the referring physician so that appropriate therapy can be obtained elsewhere.

Accountability

Physical therapists are accountable for the effectiveness of treatment in all environments. Traditionally, therapists have used anecdotal and narrative record-keeping systems. The behavioral objective, with its specific criterion-based language, lends itself well to a more systematic data collection process. The criteria and conditions given in the behavioral objective determine what items will be measured. When the objectives are written in specific, measurable terminology that can be understood and thus observed by anyone, it becomes possible to collect data on the responses. It is possible to measure the rate or frequency over time; latency, or length of time from stimulus to response; duration, or how long the behavior lasts; topography, or quality of response; force and locus; and whether the child has generalized the behavior to more than one stimulus or situation.

There may be a number of different ways of recording these data, but the therapist should work to develop a system that is efficient and effective as well as easily understood. An additional advantage to this type of outcome assessment is that this approach is frequently used and accepted in the classroom and educational model.

Roles for Physical Therapy That Extend Beyond Special Education

Screening is commonly done in schools to detect various disabilities, such as scoliosis or developmental delays. In addition, physical therapists are increasingly becoming involved in evaluating, preventing, and managing musculoskeletal problems that may affect participation in athletics.[18]

Screening

Several states have adopted laws requiring screening for scoliosis. The physical therapist may be involved in developing a screening program, or may be involved in the primary and secondary screenings. The therapist may provide training for others who will conduct the primary screening, and if a child is identified with a scoliosis for which treatment is indicated, the therapist may be called upon to develop an exercise program and to monitor the condition and program results.

Many school systems evaluate children in preschool or kindergarten for developmental delays. A physical therapist might be involved in setting up and conducting developmental screening tests to detect delays or abnormalities in fine, gross, and perceptual motor development. The therapist may then make recommendations to the classroom teacher and/or parents for activities to assist the child or, if the child is not eligible for services in the school system, may refer the parents to an outside agency.

Athletics

According to Ryan,[20] physical therapists have had little impact on the level of health care for the school athlete because of the salary demands of therapists and because therapists are not qualified to teach academic subjects in high schools. Some physical therapists, however, are becoming involved in school athletics as the injury rate related to participation in school sports increases. Physical therapists who are involved in health care for the school athlete may conduct pre-participation musculoskeletal evaluations, develop age-related and sport-related conditioning programs, and present educational seminars for coaches, parents, and students on the prevention and management of athletic injuries.

Acknowledgment

This chapter is a revision from the first edition, as written by Dr. Susan K. Effgen.

References

1. Batten HE. The industrial school for crippled and deformed children. *Phys Rev.* 1933;13:112–113.
2. Vacha VB. History of the development of special schools and classes for crippled children in Chicago. *Phys Rev.* 1933;13:21–26.
3. Mulcahey AL. Detroit schools for crippled children. *Phys Rev.* 1936;16:63–64.
4. Givins EV. The spastic child in the classroom. *Phys Rev.* 1938;18:136–137.
5. Cable OE, Fowler AF, Foss HS. The crippled children's guide of Buffalo, New York. *Phys Rev.* 1938;16:85–88.
6. Sever JW. Physical therapy in schools for crippled children. *Phys Rev.* 1938;18:298–303.
7. Education for All Handicapped Children Act. Public Law 94-142. U.S. Congress. Senate, 94th Congress, 1975.
8. *Pennsylvania Association for Retarded Children vs. Commonwealth of Pennsylvania.* Civil Action No. 71-42 (3 Judge Court, E.D. Pennsylvania), January 1971.
9. Education of the Handicapped Act Amendments of 1986, Public Law 99-457. U.S. Congress Senate, 99th Congress, 1986.
10. Langdon HJU, Langdon LL. *Initiating Occupational Therapy Programs within the Public School System. A Guide for Occupational Therapists and Public School Administrators.* Thorofare, NJ: Charles B. Slack, 1983.
11. Giangreco MF. Delivery of therapeutic services in special education programs for learners with severe handicaps. *Phys Occup Ther Pediatr.* 1986;6:5–15.
12. Geiger WL, Bradley RH, Rock SL, et al. Commentary. *Phys Occup Ther Pediatr.* 1986;6:16–21.
13. Lindsey D, O'Neal, Haas K, et al. Physical therapy services in North Carolina's schools. *Clin Man Phys Ther.* 1980;4:40–43.
14. Physically and Multiply Handicapped/System Occupational and Physical Therapists: *Resource Manuals for Program for Exceptional Children.* Atlanta, GA: Georgia Department of Education; 1980.
15. Zimmerman J. *Goals and Objectives for Developing Normal Movement Patterns.* Rockville, MD: Aspen Publishers Inc., 1988.
16. Gibson RC. *Special Education Computerized JEP: Physical Therapy and Occupational Therapy.* Johnston, IA: Heartland Education Agency; 1989.
17. *An Introduction to Individualized Education Program Plans in Pennsylvania: Guidelines for School Age IEP Development.* Pennsylvania Department of Education, Bureau of Special and Compensatory Education; 1977.
18. Connolly BH, Montgomery PC. *Therapeutic Exercise in Developmental Disabilities.* Chattanooga, TN: Chattanooga Corporation; 1987.
19. *Physical Therapy Practice in Educational Environments: Policies and Guidelines.* American Physical Therapy Association; 1990.
20. Ryan AJ. An alternative approach to coaching. *Phys Sports Med.* 1981;9:41.

Bibliography

Alberto PA, Troutman AC. *Applied Behavior Analysis for Teachers.* Columbus, OH: Charles E. Merrill; 1982.

Blatt B, Kaplan F. *Christmas in Purgatory: A Photographic Essay on Mental Retardation.* Boston, MA: Allyn & Bacon; 1966.

Campbell PH, Stewart B. Measuring changes in movement skills with infants and young children with handicaps. *J Assoc Persons Severe Handicaps* 1986;11: 153–161.

Evaluation Protocols for Occupational and Physical Therapists in Public School Programs. Florida Department of Education; Tallahassee, FL; 1987.

Ottenbacher KJ. *Evaluating Clinical Change.* Baltimore: Williams & Wilkins; 1986.

PT OT ED: A Quality Assurance Process for PT and OT in the Educational Setting. Pennsylvania Physical Therapy Association; Harrisburg; 1982.

Turnbull HR, Fiedler CR. *Judicial Interpretation of the Education for all Handicapped Children Act.* Reston, VA: ERIC Clearinghouse on Handicapped and Gifted Children; 1985.

Index

Page numbers followed by t, f, and d denote tables, figures, and displays, respectively.

ISBN 0-397-54962-8